CONTEMPORARY NURSING

issues, trends, & management

CONTEMPORARY NURSING
issues, trends, & management

Barbara Cherry, MSN, MBA, RN
Director of Interdisciplinary Programs in Aging
Texas Tech University Health Sciences Center
Lubbock, Texas

Susan R. Jacob, BSN, MSN, PhD, RN
Dean and Professor, School of Nursing
Union University
Jackson, Tennessee

Second Edition

With 70 Illustrations

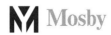

M Mosby

An Affiliate of Elsevier Science

St. Louis London Philadelphia Sydney Toronto

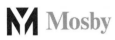

An Affiliate of Elsevier Science

Vice-President, Nursing Editorial Director: Sally Schrefer
Senior Editor: Michael S. Ledbetter
Senior Developmental Editor: Lisa P. Newton
Project Manager: Deborah L. Vogel
Production Editor: Mary E. Drone
Design Manager: Bill Drone
Cover and Interior Design: Renee Duenow

Library of Congress Cataloging-in-Publication Data

Cherry, Barbara, MSN.
    Contemporary nursing : issues, trends & management / Barbara Cherry, Susan R.
Jacob.—2nd ed.
      p. cm.
    Includes bibliograpical references and index.
    ISBN 0-323-01631-6
    1. Nursing. I. Jacob, Susan R. II. Title.
    [DNLM: 1. Nursing—trends. 2. Nursing—organization & administration.]
RT41 .C564 2001
610.73—dc21

SECOND EDITION

NOTICE

Pharmacology is an ever-changing field. Standard safety precautions must be followed, but as new research and clinical experience broaden our knowledge, changes in treatment and drug therapy may become necessary or appropriate. Readers are advised to check the most current product information provided by the manufacturer of each drug to be administered to verify the recommended dose, the method and duration of administration, and contraindications. It is the responsibility of the licensed prescriber, relying on experience and knowledge of the patient, to determine dosages and the best treatment for each individual patient. Neither the Publisher nor the editor assumes any liability for any injury and/or damage to persons or property arising from this publication.

Mosby, Inc.
11830 Westline Industrial Drive
St. Louis, Missouri 63146

Printed in the United States of America

02 03 04 05 TG/FF 9 8 7 6 5 4 3 2

*To all the student nurses whose curiosity and enthusiasm
for nursing created the inspiration to develop this text
and to all practicing nurses who face serious challenges but
reap great rewards for providing high-quality patient care*

Being a Nurse Means . . .

You will never be bored,
You will always be frustrated,
You will be surrounded by challenges,
So much to do and so little time.
You will carry immense responsibility
And very little authority.
You will step into people's lives,
And you will make a difference.

Some will bless you.
Some will curse you.

You will see people at their worst,
And at their best.
You will never cease to be amazed at people's capacity
For love, courage, and endurance.
You will see life begin
and end.

You will experience resounding triumphs
And devastating failures.
You will cry a lot.
You will laugh a lot.
You will know what it is to be human
And to be humane.

Melodie Chenevert, RN

Contributors

Charold L. Baer, PhD, RN, FCCM, CCRN
Professor, Acute Care
Oregon Health and Science University
Portland, Oregon

Toni Bargagliotti, DNSc, RN
Dean and Professor
The University of Memphis
Loewenberg School of Nursing
Memphis, Tennessee

Virginia Trotter Betts, MSN, JD, RN, FAAN
Associate Director for Health Policy Initiatives
Center for Health Services Research
Professor of Nursing
Professor in the College of Graduate Health
    Sciences
University of Tennessee HSC
Memphis, Tennessee

M. Elizabeth Carnegie, DPA, RN, FAAN
Editor Emerita, Nursing Research
Chevy Chase, Maryland

Barbara Cherry, MSN, MBA, RN
Director of Interdisciplinary Programs
    in Aging
Texas Tech University Health Sciences Center
Lubbock, Texas

Laura Day, BSN, MS, RN
Consultant
Federal Dam, Minnesota

Charlotte Eliopoulos, RNC, MPH, PhD
President
Health Education Network
Specialist in Holistic Chronic Care
Glen Arm, Maryland

Alexia Green, PhD, RN
Dean and Professor
School of Nursing
Texas Tech University Health Sciences Center
Lubbock, Texas

Corinne Grimes, MSN, DNSc, RN
Assistant Professor
Texas Women's University
School of Nursing
Dallas, Texas

Susan R. Jacob, BSN, MSN, PhD, RN
Dean and Professor
School of Nursing
Union University
Jackson, Tennessee

Clair B. Jordan, MSN, RN
Executive Director
Texas Nurses Association
Austin, Texas

Marylane Wade Koch, MSN, RN, CNAA, CPHQ
Consultant
Memphis, Tennessee

Robert W. Koch, DNS, RN
Assistant Professor
Loewenberg School of Nursing
The University of Memphis
Memphis, Tennessee

Carrie B. Lenburg, EdD, RN, FAAN
President
Creative Learning and Assessment Systems,
    Inc.
Roane Mountain, Tennessee

Laura R. Mahlmeister, PhD, RN

President, Mahlmeister & Associates
Staff Nurse
San Francisco General Birth Center
San Francisco, California

Leslie H. Nicoll, PhD, MBA, RN

Associate Research Professor
College of Nursing & Health Professions
Senior Research Associate
Edmund S. Muskie School of Public Service
University of Southern Maine
Portland, Maine

Tommie L. Norris, DNS, RN

Assistant Professor
The University of Memphis
Loewenberg School of Nursing
Memphis, Tennessee

Linda C. Pugh, PhD, RNC

Associate Professor
School of Nursing
Johns Hopkins University
Baltimore, Maryland

Anna Sallee, MSN, RN, CCRN

Professor of Nursing
San Jacinto College South
Houston, Texas

Carla D. Sanderson, PhD, RN

Provost and Professor
School of Nursing
Union University
Jackson, Tennessee

Janet C. Scherubel, PhD, RN, CCRN

Adjunct Professor
Loewenberg School of Nursing
The University of Memphis
Memphis, Tennessee

Kathryn S. Skinner, MS, RN, CS

Psychiatric-Mental Health Clinical Nurse
   Specialist
Affiliate Faculty
University of Tennessee College of Nursing
Memphis, Tennessee

Phyllis Skorga, PhD, RN, CCM

Associate Professor
College of Nursing & Health Professions
Arkansas State University
Jonesboro, Arkansas

Margaret Soderstrom, PhD, RN, CS-P, ARNP

Assistant Professor
School of Nursing
Johns Hopkins University
Baltimore, Maryland

Margaret Elizabeth Strong, MSN, RN, CAN

Director Patient Care Services
Methodist Extended Care Hospital
Memphis, Tennessee

Sandra S. Swick, EdD, RN, C

Assistant Professor
Abilene Intercollegiate School of Nursing
Abilene, Texas

Jill J. Webb, PhD, RN, CS

Associate Professor
MSN Program Director
Union University
Jackson, Tennessee

Kathleen M. Werner, MS, BSN, RN

Director Medical/Surgical/Pediatric Nursing
Meriter Hospital
Madison, Wisconsin

Shiphrah A. Alicia Williams-Evans, PhD, RN, CS

Chair and Professor
Department of Nursing
Southwest Tennessee Community College
Memphis, Tennessee

Reviewers

Barbara P. Daniel, RNCS, RCNP, MEd, MS
Cecil Community College
Professor of Nursing
Northeast, Maryland

Debbie Hooser, RN, MSN
Assistant Professor
Baptist College of Health Sciences
Memphis, Tennessee

Johanne A. Quinn, PhD, RN, HNC
King College
Bristol, Tennessee

Yvonne N. Stock, RN, BSN, MS
Professor Nursing
Iowa Western Community College
Co. Bluffs, Iowa

Christine A. Wynd, PhD, RN, CNAA
The University of Akron
College of Nursing
Akron, Ohio

Preface

This second edition of *Contemporary Nursing: Issues, Trends, & Management* comes only 3 years after the first edition was published in 1999. The rapidly changing health care environment requires nurses and other members of the transdisciplinary team to use critical thinking skills to make quick decisions that affect patient outcomes on a daily basis. To do this, nurses must have up-to-date information about current issues and trends that affect professional nursing practice. The content in this book has been updated and expanded to present the most pertinent information regarding contemporary nursing issues and to offer a comprehensive review of the leadership and management knowledge and skills required to practice effectively in the complex and ever-changing health care system.

Among the new topics for this edition are **nursing theory, workplace issues,** and **alternative healing.** More emphasis is placed on **delegation, health policy,** and **evidence-based nursing practice.** Each chapter begins with **real-life vignettes** and **questions to consider while reading the chapter** to stimulate critical thinking. **Integrated learning outcomes** provide students with a clear understanding of behavioral outcomes expected after reading the chapter. **Chapter overviews** introduce the chapters and highlight some of the important points. **Critical thinking activities** that encourage the student to reflect on the content follow each chapter, and **technologic competence** is encouraged by the inclusion of many online critical thinking activities

Unit One: The Development of Nursing

The book opens with a presentation about the exciting evolution of nursing, its very visible public image, and its core foundations, which include nursing theory, nursing education, and licensure and credentialing. These opening chapters provide the reader with a solid background for understanding and studying current and future trends.

Unit Two: Current Issues in Health Care

This unit provides a comprehensive overview of the most current trends and issues occurring today in nursing and health care, including health care financing and economics, the health care delivery system, legal and ethical issues, health policy and politics, cultural and social issues, workplace issues, collective bargaining, nursing informatics and alternative healing. Students, faculty, and veteran nurses will be challenged to critically examine each of these significant issues that are currently shaping the practice of professional nursing and the health care delivery system.

Unit Three: Leadership and Management in Nursing

This unit offers a primer on nursing leadership and management, with a focus on the basic skills that are necessary for nurses to function effectively in the professional nursing role. Chapters examine leadership and management theory and roles, effective communication, delegation and supervision, staffing and nursing care delivery models, quality improvement, and nursing research and evidence-based practice. The updated content in this unit provides the most current information available related to nursing leadership and management and will serve as both a valuable educational tool for students and a very useful resource for practicing nurses.

Unit Four: Career Management

The final unit prepares the student to embark on a career in nursing. Making the transition from student to professional, managing time, understanding career opportunities, finding a good match between the nurse and the employer, and passing the NCLEX examination are all presented with practical, useful advice that will serve as an excellent resource for both students and novice nurses as they build their career in professional nursing.

TEACHING AND LEARNING SUPPORT

Featured in this edition of *Contemporary Nursing* is a dedicated website (http://www.mosby.com/MERLIN/Cherry/) with access to hundreds of active sites keyed specifically to each chapter of the text. These Weblinks are continually updated to provide the most current topics related to the content in the text.

Also new to this edition and available through the Cherry and Jacob website are online resources specifically designed for the instructor. These resources include suggested outlines for lectures, extra credit activities, suggestions for teaching-learning activities, a Test Bank, an Image Collection, and PowerPoint slides. All of these instructor resources are password protected, so please contact your local sales representative for further details.

About the Authors

Barbara Cherry, MSN, MBA, RN

Barbara Cherry received her diploma in nursing from Methodist Hospital School of Nursing in 1973, her BSN from West Texas A&M University in 1980, her MBA from Texas Tech University in 1995, and her MSN from Texas Tech University Health Sciences Center in 1997. Barbara's clinical background is in critical care, medical-surgical, and nephrology nursing. She has over 20 years' clinical and nursing management experience and currently directs the Interdisciplinary Programs in Aging for Texas Tech University Health Sciences Center, Lubbock, Texas. Barbara also is an Assistant Professor for Texas Tech University Health Sciences Center School of Nursing and teaches modules in health policy, quality improvement, budgeting, and health care financing.

Susan R. Jacob, BSN, MSN, PhD, RN

Susan Jacob received her BSN from West Virginia University in 1970, her MSN from San Jose State University in 1975, and her PhD from the University of Tennessee, Memphis in 1993. Her extensive experience as a clinician, educator, and researcher has been focused in the community health arena, specifically home health and hospice. Dr. Jacob's research has addressed the bereavement experience of older adults and enhanced models of home health care delivery. Dr. Jacob is the Dean of the School of Nursing at Union University in Jackson, Tennessee, where she teaches undergraduate and graduate nursing courses such as Professional Nursing Issues, Nursing Research, Nursing Theory, and Intercultural Issues. She is a leader in professional nursing organizations at the state and national level.

Acknowledgments

Our contributors deserve our most sincere thanks for their high-quality, timely work that demonstrates genuine expertise and professionalism. Their contributions have made this book a truly first-rate text that will be invaluable to nursing students and faculty and will serve as an outstanding resource for practicing nursing. We extend a special thanks to our reviewers who gave us helpful suggestions and insights as we developed the second edition.

We would like to express our grateful appreciation to the Mosby staff—Michael Ledbetter, Senior Editor, and Lisa Newton, Senior Developmental Editor—for their very capable and professional support, guidance, and calm reassurance.

Our deepest appreciation goes to the most important people in our lives—our husbands, Mike and Dick, our children, our family, and our friends. Their enduring support and extreme patience have allowed us to accomplish what sometimes seemed to be the impossible.

Contents

4 The Influence of Contemporary Trends and Issues on Nursing Education, 65

Carrie B. Lenburg, EdD, RN, FAAN

5 Nursing Licensure and Certification, 95

Janet C. Scherubel, PhD, RN, CCRN

Unit Two
CURRENT ISSUES IN HEALTH CARE

7 The Health Care Delivery System and Managed Care, 133

Phyllis Skorga, PhD, RN, CCM

8 Legal Issues in Nursing and Health Care, 152

Laura R. Mahlmeister, PhD, RN

9 Ethical and Bioethical Issues in Nursing and Health Care, 198

Carla D. Sanderson, PhD, RN

14 Computers, Informatics, Clinical Information, and the Professional Nurse, 306

Leslie H. Nicoll, PhD, MBA, RN

15 Alternative Healing, 332

Charlotte Eliopoulos, RNC, MPH, PhD

Unit Three
LEADERSHIP AND MANAGEMENT IN NURSING

17 **Effective Communication, 384**
   Anna Sallee, MSN, RN, CCRN

Unit Four
CAREER MANAGEMENT

24 **Contemporary Nursing Roles and Career Opportunities, 541**
Robert W. Koch, DNS, RN

25 **Job Search: Finding Your Match, 562**
Kathryn S. Skinner, MS, RN, CS, and Laura Day, BSN, MS, RN

26 NCLEX-RN Examination, 582

Sandra S. Swick, EdD, RN, C

The Evolution of Professional Nursing

Shiphrah A. Alicia Williams-Evans, PhD, RN, CS,
and M. Elizabeth Carnegie, DPA, RN, FAAN

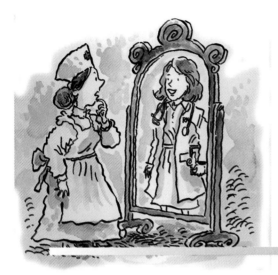

Oh, my, how we've changed.

Vignette

Tabitha Louise Pitts is an 88-year-old nurse who retired from the military 30 years ago. She then began a career as an educator at a state university. She was diagnosed with diabetes mellitus 40 years ago. During the past 3 months she had begun to have difficulty with elevated blood sugar, swelling, and painful urination. Three years ago she had her second below-the-knee amputation. She decided to go to the local health clinic where Dr. Aldora James is an advanced practice nurse. Dr. James is a certified family nurse practitioner with a doctorate in Nursing Science.

After completing the physical examination and analysis of laboratory findings, Dr. James determined that Mrs. Pitts was suffering from end-stage renal disease and brittle uncontrolled diabetes. Dr. James ordered consultations with a nephrologist and endocrinologist to ensure that comprehensive care was provided. Both consulting physicians made a determination that Mrs. Pitts' condition was terminal. Mrs. Pitts was a widow with one son who died 4 years ago in a motor vehicle accident. After reviewing all the possible treatments available, Mrs. Pitts made a decision not to have dialysis.

Dr. James referred Mrs. Pitts to the local hospice. Hospice set up a schedule of twice-a-day home visits to monitor Mrs. Pitts' blood sugar. Juanita Smith was the registered nurse who made these visits. Albee Winthrop, a Psychiatric Mental Health Clinical Specialist, visited with Mrs. Pitts three times each week to

1

provide support and assist her with grief work. Mrs. Winthrop also contacted Mrs. Pitts' minister to ensure that her spiritual needs were met.

Within 3 weeks Mrs. Pitts' condition had worsened. She shared with Mrs. Winthrop that she had feared dying alone ever since her son died. However, because she had hospice care, her line of support expanded to an umbrella of support. Even though the health care that Mrs. Pitts required was affected by capitation, her overall care did not suffer. Parish nurses in her church congregation took turns being with her around the clock. She was never alone, thanks to the services provided by the diversity of nursing care.

Mrs. Pitts reminisced about her experiences in nursing. She recalled that she had seen nursing come full circle. She remembered when it was okay for individuals to die peacefully at home, and she had also seen a time when individuals were rushed to the hospital to die. She marveled at the fact that now an individual could make choices about end-of-life care and "die with dignity, surrounded by caring health professionals."

Questions to consider while reading this chapter
1. What were the challenges faced by nurses in the 1900s?
2. How has managed care affected professional nursing practice?
3. What are the challenges facing nurses in the twenty-first century?

Key Terms

Advanced practice nurse A registered nurse who provides care to clients in the role of certified nurse midwife, clinical nurse specialist, certified nurse anesthetist, or certified nurse practitioner. Formal knowledge and skill are acquired above the basic level of nursing, and since 1994 a master of science degree in nursing is required to obtain certification in these roles (Doheny, Cook, and Stopper, 1997).

Doctor of Nursing Science An advanced terminal degree in nursing that builds on the master's degree to provide scientific ability and knowledge to create, initiate, develop, implement, and evaluate nursing research in all settings. This terminal degree provides the foundation for the nurse scientist to augment clinical, didactic, and research expertise (Doheny, Cook, and Stopper, 1997).

Professional nursing A unique profession that addresses the humanistic and holistic needs and the response patterns of patients, families, and communities to actual and potential health problems. The professional nurse has many roles such as care provider, client advocate, educator, care coordinator, and change agent (Ignatavicius, Workman, and Mishler, 1999).

Florence Nightingale (1820-1910) Considered the founder of organized, professional nursing. She is best known for her contributions to the reforms in the British Army Medical Corps, improved sanitation in India, improved public health in Great Britain, use of statistics, and the development of organized training for nurses.

Learning Outcomes

After studying this chapter, the reader will be able to:
1. Summarize health practices through the course of history.
2. Analyze the impact of historic, political, social, and economic events on the development of nursing.
3. Describe the evolution of professional challenges experienced by nurses of diverse ethnic backgrounds.

CHAPTER OVERVIEW

Throughout the pages of recorded history, nursing has been integrated into every facet of life. A legacy of human caring was initiated when, according to the Book of Exodus, two midwives, Shiphrah and Puah, rescued the baby Moses and hid him to save his life. This legacy of caring has progressed throughout the years, responding to psychologic, social, environmental, and physiologic needs of society. Nurses of the past and present have struggled for recognition as knowledgeable professionals. The evolution of this struggle is reflected in political, cultural, environmental, and economic events that have sculptured our nation and world history (Snodgrass, 1999).

In the beginning men were recognized as health healers. Women challenged the status quo and transformed nursing from the mystical phenomenon to a respected profession (Snodgrass, 1999). The work of Florence Nightingale and Mary Seacole played a major role in bringing about changes in nursing. Using the concept of role modeling, these women demonstrated the value of their worth through their work in fighting for the cause of health and healing. During the twentieth century nurses made tremendous advancements in the areas of education, practice, research, and technology. Nursing as a science progressed through education, clinical practice, development of theory, and rigorous research. Today nurses continue to be challenged to expand their roles and explore new areas of practice and leadership. This chapter will describe the evolution of nursing from prehistoric times through 2000. Box 1-1 summarizes some of the important events in the evolution of nursing.

PREHISTORIC PERIOD

The practice of nursing in the prehistoric period was strongly guided by health beliefs. Nursing and medical practice were delineated by beliefs of magic, religion, and superstition. Individuals who were ill were considered to be cursed by evil spirits and evil gods that entered the human body and caused suffering and death if not cast out. These beliefs dictated the behavior of primitive people who sought to scare away the evil gods and spirits. Members of tribes participated in rituals, wore masks, and engaged in demonstrative dances to rid the sick of demonic possession of one's body. Sacrifices and offerings that sometimes included human sacrifices were made to rid the body of evil gods, demons, and spirits. Many tribes used special herbs, roots, and vegetables to cast out the "curse" of illness.

EARLY CIVILIZATION
Egypt

Ancient Egyptians are noted for their accomplishments at such an early period. They were the first to use the concept of suture in repairing wounds. They also were the first to be recorded as developing community planning that resulted in a decrease in public health problems. One of the main public health problems was the spread of disease through the consumption of water because the water resources were sometimes contaminated. Specific laws on cleanliness, food use and preservation, drinking, exercise, and sexual relations were developed. Health beliefs of Egyptians determined preventive measures taken and personal health behaviors practiced. These health behaviors were usually carried out to accommodate the gods. Some behaviors were also done to expressively appease the spirits of the dead (Ellis and Hartley, 2001). The Egyptians invented the development of the calendar and writing that

BOX 1-1	*Important Events in the Evolution of Nursing*

1751	The Pennsylvania Hospital is the first hospital established in America.
1798	The U.S. Marine Hospital Service comes into being July 16 by an act of Congress. It is renamed the U.S. Public Health Service in 1912.
1840	Two African-American women, Mary Williams and Frances Rose, are listed in the City of Baltimore Directory as nurses.
1851	Florence Nightingale (1820-1910) attends Kaiserswerth to train as a nurse.
1854	During the Crimean War Florence Nightingale transforms the image of nursing; Mary Seacole, a black woman from Jamaica, West Indies, nurses with her.
1861	The outbreak of the Civil War causes African-American women to volunteer as nurses, among whom are Harriet Tubman, Sojourner Truth, and Susie King Taylor.
1863	Harriet Newton Phillips is graduated from the Women's Hospital in Philadelphia.
1872	Another school of nursing opens in the United States: the New England Hospital for Women and Children (in Boston).
1873	Linda Richards is responsible for designing a written patient record and physician's order system—the first in a hospital.
1879	Mary Mahoney, the first trained African-American nurse, is graduated from the New England Hospital for Women and Children, Boston, Massachusetts.
1882	The American Red Cross is established by Clara Barton.
1886	The Visiting Nurses Association (VNA) is started in Philadelphia; Spelman College, Atlanta, Ga., establishes the first diploma nursing program for African-Americans.
1893	Lillian Wald and Mary Brewster establish the Henry Street Visiting Nurse Service in New York; The American Society of Superintendents of Training Schools for Nurses is established (becomes the National League of Nursing Education in 1912 and the National League for Nursing [NLN] in 1952); a nursing program (diploma) is established at Howard University, an African-American school in Washington, DC—the first in a university setting.
1896	The Nurses' Associated Alumnae of the United States and Canada is established (becomes the American Nurses Association [ANA] in 1911)
1898	Namahyoke Curtis, an untrained African-American nurse, is assigned by the War Department as a contract nurse in the Spanish-American War.
1900	The first issue of the *American Journal of Nursing* is published; Jessie Sleet Scales becomes the first African-American public health nurse.
1901	The Army Nurse Corps is established under the Army Reorganization Act.
1902	School nursing is established in New York City, New York, by Linda Rogers.
1903	The first Nursing Practice Acts are passed, and North Carolina is the first state to implement registration of nurses, followed by New Jersey, New York, and Virginia.
1908	The National Association of Colored Graduate Nurses is founded; it is dissolved in 1951.
1909	Ludie Andrews sues the Georgia State Board of Nurse Examiners to secure African-American nurses the right to take the state board examination and become licensed; she wins in 1920.
1912	The U.S. Public Health Service and the National League for Nursing (NLN) are established.
1916	Membership in ANA is derived through the state associations.
1918	Eighteen black nurses are admitted to the Army Nurse Corps after the Armistice is signed ending World War I.
1919	*Public Health Nursing* is written by Mary S. Gardner; a public health nursing program is started at the University of Michigan.
1921	The Sheppard-Towner Act is passed for federal aid for maternal and child health care.
1922	Sigma Theta Tau is founded (becomes the International Honor Society of Nursing in 1985).

BOX 1-1	*Important Events in the Evolution of Nursing—cont'd*

1923	The Goldmark Report criticizes the inadequacies of hospital-based nursing schools and recommends increased educational standards.
1924	The United States Indian Bureau Nursing Service is founded by Eleanor Gregg.
1925	The Frontier Nursing Service is founded by Mary Breckenridge.
1929	The Great Depression begins.
1930	Massive unemployment of nurses occurs.
1931	Estelle Massey Riddle Osborne earns master's degree—the first for an African-American nurse.
1935	The Social Security Act is passed.
1937	Federal appropriations for cancer, venereal diseases, tuberculosis, and mental health are begun.
1939	World War II begins.
1941	The U.S. Army established a quota of 56 black nurses for admission to the Army Nurse Corps; the Nurse Training Act passed.
1943	An amendment to the Nurse Training Bill is passed that bars racial bias.
1945	The U.S. Navy drops the color bar and admits four African-American nurses.
1946	Nurses are classified as professionals by the U.S. Civil Service Commission; the Hospital Survey and Construction Act (Hill-Burton) is passed.
1948	Estelle Osborne is the first African-American nurse elected to Board of the ANA; the ANA votes individual membership to all African-American nurses excluded from any state association.
1949	M. Elizabeth Carnegie is the first African-American nurse to be elected to the Board of a state association—Florida.
1950	The Code for professional nurses is published by the ANA.
1952	National nursing organizations are reorganized from six to two: ANA and NLN.
1954	The Supreme Court Decision, Brown v. Board of Education, asserts that "separate educational facilities were inherently unequal."
1955	Elizabeth Lipford Kent is the first African-American nurse to earn a doctoral degree.
1965	The Social Security Amendment includes Medicare and Medicaid.
1967	Warren Hatcher is the first black male nurse to earn a doctoral degree.
1971	The National Black Nurses Association is organized.
1973	The NLN requires conceptual frameworks in nursing education; the Health Maintenance Organization Act (HMO) is passed.
1974	The ANA receives a grant from the National Institute of Mental Health to initiate a fellowship program to help minorities earn PhDs; the First National Transcultural Conference is held at the University of Utah College of Nursing; the first certification examinations are offered by the ANA.
1975	The American Hospital Association publishes the "Patient's Bill of Rights."
1977	1977 is declared the "Year of the Nurse" by the ANA to help the public better understand nursing.
1978	Barbara Nichols is the first African-American nurse elected president of the ANA; M. Elizabeth Carnegie, an African-American nurse, is elected president of the American Academy of Nursing.
1979	Brigadier General Hazel Johnson Brown is the first African-American Chief of the Army Nurse Corps.
1980	Nita Barrow, Governor General of Barbados, West Indies, is the first African-American nurse knighted as Dame of St. Andrew Order of Her Majesty Queen Elizabeth II; Colorado passes a new nurse practice act that enables nurses to practice independently in private settings; nursing diagnosis evolves as a separate component of the nursing process.
1981	Carolyn Davis becomes the first nurse to head the Centers for Medicare and Medicaid Services (CMS) (formerly the Health Care Financing Administration ([HCFA]); AIDS becomes an increasing epidemic in America.

Continued

BOX 1-1	*Important Events in the Evolution of Nursing—cont'd*

1982	The nurse licensure examination changes to a comprehensive test developed by the National Council of State Boards of Nursing.
1985	Vernice Ferguson, an African-American nurse, is elected president of Sigma Theta Tau International.
1986	The Association of Black Nursing Faculty is founded by Dr. Sally Tucker Allen.
1989	*Promoting Health/Preventing Disease: Year 2000 Objectives* for the Nation is drafted and distributed for public review.
1990	Congress proclaims March 10 as Harriet Tubman Day in the United States, honoring her as the brave African-American freedom fighter and nurse during the Civil War; the Bloodborne Pathogens Standards are established by OSHA—all health care providers are required to use Universal Precautions of Body Substance Isolation when caring for all patients; computers enter most facets of the health care system; the largest number of nurses participate in the war effort: Operation Desert Shield/Desert Storm.
1991	*Healthy People 2000* published.
1992	Eddie Bernice Johnson, an African-American nurse from Texas, is elected to the House of Representatives—the first nurse to be elected to Congress; the ANA Congress of Nursing Practice establishes nursing informatics as a distinct area of nursing practice; hospitals downsize by reducing the number of full-time nurses; home health nursing is rapidly increasing.
1993	The National Center for Nursing Research is upgraded to the National Institute of Nursing Research within the National Institutes of Health.
1994	One hundred and thirty-five million Americans are enrolled in managed care plans (HMOs and PPOs); RN-NCLEX, a computerized nurse-licensing examination, is introduced.
1996	The Commission on Collegiate Nursing Education is established as an agency devoted exclusively to the accreditation of baccalaureate and graduate degree nursing programs.
1997	Rhetaugh Dumas, an African-American nurse, is elected president of the NLN.
1999	The demand for advanced practice nurses is increasing; new drugs are on trial for the treatment of AIDS; nursing assistants or unlicensed assistive personnel (UAPs) are used increasingly as nurse extenders; distance learning is becoming more popular in nursing education; Beverly Malone, the second African-American president of the ANA, is named Deputy Assistant Secretary for Health, Department of Health and Human Services, Office of Public Health and Science; the Institute of Medicine releases its landmark report: *Too Err is Human: Building a Safer Health System.*
2000	M. Elizabeth Carnegie is inducted into the ANA Hall of Fame; the American Nurses Credentialing Center gives its first Psychiatric Mental Health Nurse Practitioner examination; *Healthy People 2010* is published; the National Council of State Boards of Nursing releases new Test Plan, to begin in April 2001.
2001	Beverly Malone is appointed General Secretary, Royal College of Nursing, London. Health Care Financing Administration (HCFA) becomes Centers for Medicare and Medicaid Services (CMS).

Sources: Carnegie ME, 1995; Deloughery GL: *Issues and trends in nursing,* ed. 3, St. Louis, 1998, Mosby; Kalisch P, Kalisch B, 1995; and Donahue MP, 1999.

denoted the initiation of recorded history. The oldest records date back before Christ in sixteenth century BC Egypt. A document containing almost 1000 natural pharmacologic remedies was written to assist in the care and management of disease (Ellis and Hartley, 2001). As in the case of Shiphrah and Puah, the midwives who saved the baby Moses, nurses were used by kings and other aristocrats to deliver babies and care for the young, the elderly, and those who were sick. Other documentation regarding nurses in Egypt is scant.

Palestine

From 1400 to 1200 BC the Hebrews migrated from the Arabian Desert and gradually settled in Palestine, where they became an agricultural society. Under the leadership of Moses, the Hebrews developed the Mosaic Code, which represented one of the first organized methods of disease control and prevention. It contained public health laws that did not allow the eating of a slaughtered animal dead longer than 3 days. Individuals who were thought to have communicable diseases were isolated from the public and could return to their families only after the priest had declared them healed (Ellis and Hartley, 2001). Males who were Hebrew priests and selected women, usually widows and maidens who cared for the sick in their homes, delivered health care. Their efforts were aimed at bringing both physical and spiritual comfort to those in need (Stanhope and Lancaster, 2000).

Greece

From 1500 to 100 BC Greek philosophers sought to understand man and his relationship with the gods, nature, and other men. They believed that the gods and goddesses of Greek mythology controlled health and illness. Temples built to honor Asclepius, the god of medicine, were designated to care for the sick. Asclepius carried a staff that was intertwined with serpents or snakes, representing wisdom and immortality. This staff is believed to be the model of today's medical caduceus. Hippocrates (460-362 BC), considered the "father of medicine," paved the way in establishing scientific knowledge in medicine. Hippocrates was the first to attribute disease to natural causes rather than supernatural causes and curses of the gods. Hippocrates' teachings also encouraged health care providers to look at not just the part of the patient that was sick, but to include the patient's environment (Kalisch and Kalisch, 1995).

In the ancient Greek culture little is documented about nursing. However, attendants who were referred to as "basket healers" assisted the temple priests and physicians. These basket healers often traveled from town to town with physicians to offer their services (Stanhope and Lancaster, 2000).

India

Dating from 2000 to 1200 BC, the earliest cultures of India were Hindu. The sacred books of the Hindu, Vedas, were used to guide health care practices. The Vedas included herbs, spices, displays of magic, and charms. These ingredients were used to rid the body of demons and cure illness. The Indians documented information concerning prenatal care and childhood illnesses. Public hospitals were constructed from 274 to 236 BC and were staffed by male nurses with qualifications and duties similar to those of the twentieth-century practical nurse. The Hindu physicians performed major and minor surgeries, including limb amputations, cesarean deliveries, and wound suturing. Women were primarily responsible for caring for the home and family, and they did not work outside the home. (Ellis and Hartley, 2001; Walton, Barondess, and Locke, 1994).

China

The teachings of Confucius (551-479 BC) had a powerful impact on the customs and practices of the people of ancient China. One tradition that exemplified their belief about health and illness was the yin and yang philosophy. The yin represents the feminine forces, which were negative and passive. The yang represents the masculine forces, which were positive and active.

The Chinese believed that an imbalance between these two forces would result in illness, whereas balance between the yin and yang represented good health (Giger and Davidhizar, 1999). The ancient Chinese used a variety of treatments believed to promote health and harmony, including acupuncture. Acupuncture involves insertion of hot and cold needles into the skin and underlying tissues to manage or cure illnesses such as pain, stroke, or breathing difficulty and ultimately to affect the balance of yin and yang. Hydrotherapy, massage, and exercise were used as preventive health measures (Giger and Davidhizar, 1999). The Chinese also used drug therapy to manage disease conditions and recorded more than 1000 drugs derived from animals, vegetables, and minerals (Walton, Barondess, and Locke, 1994).

Rome

The Roman Empire (27 BC-476 AD), a military dictatorship, adapted medical practices from the countries they conquered and the physicians they enslaved. The first military hospital in Europe was established in Rome. The physicians were enslaved and forced to provide details about their medical practice. Both male and female attendants assisted in the care of the sick. Galen was a famous Greek physician who worked in Rome and made important contributions to the practice of medicine by expanding his knowledge in anatomy, physiology, pathology, and medical therapeutics (Walton, Barondess, and Locke, 1994).

THE MIDDLE AGES

The Middles Ages (476 BC-1450 AD) followed the demise of the Roman Empire (Walton, Barondess, and Locke, 1994). Women used herbs and new methods of healing, whereas men continued to use purging, leeching, and mercury. This period also saw the Roman Catholic Church become a central figure in the organization and management of health care. Most of the changes in health care were based on the Christian concepts of charity and the sanctity of human life. Wives of emperors and other women considered noble became nurses. These women devoted themselves to caring for the sick, often carrying a basket of food and medicine as they journeyed from house to house (Bahr and Johnson, 1995). Widowers and unmarried women became nuns and deaconesses. Two of these deaconesses, Dorcas and Phoebe, are mentioned in the Bible as outstanding for the care they provided to the sick (Freedman, 1995).

During the Middle Ages physicians spent most of their time translating medical essays; they actually provided little medical care. Poorly trained barbers who lacked any formal medical education performed surgery and medical treatments that were considered "bloody" or "messy." Nurses also provided some medical care, although in most hospitals and monasteries female nurses who were not midwives were forbidden to witness childbirth, help with gynecologic examinations, or even diaper male infants (Kalish and Kalish, 1986). In addition, they were not permitted to have contact with male patients, administer enemas, or care for a man with a venereal disease. Nurse midwives provided the bulk of obstetric care within the community (Ellis and Hartley, 2001).

During the Crusades, which lasted for almost 200 years from 1096 to 1291, military nursing orders known as templars and hospitalers were founded. Monks and Christian knights provided nursing care and also defended the hospitals during battle, wearing a suit of armor under their religious habits. The habits were distinguished by the Maltese cross to identify the monks and knights as Christian warriors. The same cross was used years later on a badge designed for the first school of nursing and became a forerunner for the design of nursing pins (Ellis and Hartley, 2001).

THE RENAISSANCE PERIOD

The Renaissance and Reformation periods (1500-1700), also known as the rebirth of Europe, followed the Middle Ages. Major advancements were made in pharmacology, chemistry, and medical knowledge including anatomy, physiology, and surgery.

During this period, as a result of religious dissention between Roman Catholic Christians and the Protestant sects, many monasteries closed, and religious orders were dissolved. Roman Catholics and Protestants dissolved many of their religious facilities known for meeting the health care needs of the people. Contrary to the Catholic teaching, the Protestant church believed that women's duties involved childbearing and caring for the home, not working outside the home. Women of nobility no longer desired to work in hospitals. Individuals who worked as nurses were female prisoners, prostitutes, and those of undesirable character. Nursing was no longer the respected profession it had once been. This period was referred to as the "Dark Ages of Nursing" (Ellis and Hartley, 2001).

During the sixteenth and seventeenth centuries, famine, plague, filth, and horrible crimes ravaged Europe. King Henry VII eliminated the organized monastic relief programs that aided the orphans, poor, and other displaced people. It became common to encounter homeless men, women, and children begging in the streets. Beggars were beaten, branded, and chained to the galleys of boats as punishment for their disgraceful behavior (Ellis and Hartley, 1988).

Out of great concern for social welfare, several nursing groups, such as the Order of the Visitation of St. Mary, St. Vincent de Paul, and the Sisters of Charity, were organized to give time, service, and money to the poor and sick. The Sisters of Charity recruited young women for training in nursing, developed educational programs, and cared for abandoned children. In 1640 St. Vincent de Paul established The Hospital for the Foundling to care for the many orphaned and abandoned children (Ellis and Hartley, 1988).

THE COLONIAL AMERICAN PERIOD

The first hospital and the first medical school were founded in North America. The hospital was the Hospital of the Immaculate built in Mexico City. The first medical school was built at the University of Mexico. In the American colonies, individuals with infectious diseases were isolated in almshouses or pest houses (Kalisch and Kalisch, 1986). Procedures such as purgatives and bleeding were widely used, leading to low life expectancy. Plagues such as yellow fever and smallpox caused thousands of deaths. Benjamin Franklin who was outspoken regarding the care of the sick insisted that a hospital be built to care for the sick. He believed that the community should be responsible for the management and treatment of those who were ill. Through his efforts the first hospital was built in the United States in Philadelphia in 1751. This hospital was called Pennsylvania Hospital (Oermann, 1997). Staff in this and other early hospitals were often untrained, and the public feared that poor patients were used for training purposes. Individuals of wealth did not go to hospitals because they were seen as places to care for the "unfortunate" people (Ellis and Hartley, 1988).

FLORENCE NIGHTINGALE

Florence Nightingale was born in Florence, Italy on May 12, 1820. The Nightingale family was wealthy, well traveled, and well educated. Nightingale was a highly intelligent, talented, and attractive woman. From an early age she demonstrated a deep concern for the poor and suffering. At the age of 25 she became interested in training as a nurse. However, her family, who strongly opposed a nursing career, preferred that she marry and take her place in society (Kelly and Joel, 1996). In 1851 her parents finally permitted her to pursue nurse's training. Nightingale attended a 3-month nursing training program at the Institution of Deaconesses at Kaiserswerth, Germany. In 1854 she began training nurses at the Harley Street Nursing Home and also served as superintendent of nurses at King's College Hospital in London (Kalisch and Kalisch, 1995).

The outbreak of the Crimean War marked a turning point in Nightingale's career. In October 1854 Sidney Herbert, British Secretary of War and an old friend of the Nightingale family, wrote to Nightingale begging her to lead a group of nurses to the Crimea to work at one of the military hospitals under government authority and expense (Dolan, 1978). Nightingale accepted his offer and assembled 38 nurses who were sisters and nuns from different Catholic and Anglican orders (Kelly and Joel, 1996).

Nightingale and her team were assigned to the Barracks Hospital at Scutari. The Barracks Hospital actually was a dilapidated, barnlike building that formerly was used as an artillery barracks. Thousands of cholera victims and hundreds of battle casualties were taken to Scutari. To get to the hospital from the front lines, the wounded and ill soldiers were placed in hospital ships and then had to cross the long and often tortuous Black Sea (Dolan, 1978).

When Nightingale arrived at the Barracks Hospital, she found deplorable conditions. Between 3000 and 4000 sick and wounded men were packed into the hospital that was originally designed to accommodate 1700 patients. There were no beds, blankets, food, or medicine. Many of the wounded soldiers were placed on the floor where lice, maggots, vermin, rodents, and blood covered their bodies. There were no candles or lanterns. All medical care had to be rendered during the light of day (Dolan, 1978).

Despite the distressing conditions at the Barracks Hospital, the army doctors and surgeons at first refused Nightingale's assistance (Kelly and Joel, 1996). However within 1 week, with scurvy, starvation, dysentery, and more fighting erupting, the doctors in desperation called her to help. Nightingale immediately purchased medical supplies, food, linen, and hospital equipment using her own money and that of the Times Relief Fund. Within 10 days she had set up a kitchen for special diets and had rented a house that she converted into a laundry (Kalisch and Kalisch, 1995). The wives of soldiers were hired to manage and operate the laundry service. She assigned soldiers to make repairs and clean up the building. Weeks later she initiated social services, reading classes, and even established coffeehouses for soldiers to enjoy music and recreation (Kelly and Joel, 1996).

Nightingale worked long, hard hours to care for these soldiers. She spent up to 20 hours each day caring for wounds, comforting soldiers, assisting in surgery, directing staff, and keeping records. Nightingale introduced principles of asepsis and infection control, a system for transcribing doctor's orders, and a procedure to maintain patient records. By the end of the Crimean War, Nightingale had trained as many as 125 nurses to care for the wounded and ill soldiers (Dolan, 1978).

Nightingale is credited for using public health principles and statistical methods to advocate improved health conditions for British soldiers. Through carefully kept statistics, Nightingale was able to document that the soldiers' death rate decreased from 42% to 2% as a result of health care reforms that emphasized sanitary conditions. Because of her remarkable work in using statistics to demonstrate cause and effect and improve the health of British soldiers, Nightingale is honored for her contributions to nursing research (Nies and McEwen, 2001).

Nightingale also demonstrated the value of political activism to effect health care reform by writing letters of criticism accompanied by constructive recommendations to British army leaders. Nightingale's ability to overthrow the British army management method that had allowed the deplorable conditions to exist in the army hospitals was considered one of her greatest achievements (Nies and McEwen, 2001).

In 1855, after visiting the frontlines and hospitals in Balaclava, Nightingale contracted "Crimean Fever" and was taken to the Castle Hospital. There she received intensive care from the doctors and nurses she trained. She remained in poor condition for several weeks. Soldiers wept when they heard of her illness and near death. She eventually recovered, but the illness had taken its toll on her overall health.

In 1860 Nightingale established the first nursing school in England. By 1873 graduates of Nightingale's nurse training program in England migrated to the United States, where they became supervisors in the first of the hospital-based (diploma) nursing schools: Massachusetts General Hospital in Boston, Bellevue Hospital in New York, and the New Haven Hospital in Connecticut.

Florence Nightingale's work, from the Crimean War to the establishment of formal nursing education programs, was a catapult for the reorganization and advancement of professional nursing. Until her death in August 1910, Nightingale demonstrated the powerful impact that well-educated, creative, skilled, and competent individuals have in the provision of health care. She is honored as the founder of professional nursing (Kalisch and Kalisch, 1995).

MARY SEACOLE

Mary Seacole was a Jamaican nurse who learned the art of caring and healing from her mother. In her native land of Jamaica, British West Indies, she was nicknamed "Doctress" because of her administration of care to the sick in a lodging house in Kingston (Carnegie, 1995). Seacole learned of the Crimean War and wrote to the British government requesting to join Nightingale's group of nurses. However, she was denied the right to join because she was black. She was concerned about this denial, because many of the British soldiers had lived in Jamaica and she had provided health care to them.

Seacole had served in Cuba and Panama during the yellow fever and cholera epidemics. She had also conducted forensic studies on an infant who died of cholera in Panama. She felt that her experience would be valuable in treating disease in the Crimean War. Therefore she sailed to England at her own expense. She provided a letter of introduction to Nightingale, which was blocked because she was black, even though she was trained by British army doctors (Carnegie, 1995).

After several efforts failed to allow her to join the group, Seacole, who was not a woman of wealth, purchased her own supplies and traveled over 3000 miles to the Crimea. She built and opened a lodging house. On the bottom floor was a restaurant, and on the top floor an area arranged like a hospital to nurse sick soldiers (Carnegie, 1995).

When Seacole finally met Nightingale, the response was still the same: "no vacancies" (Carnegie, 1995). Being denied enlistment did not deter Seacole; she remained faithful and nursed the sick throughout the Crimean War. Her efforts did not go unnoticed by the English people. Long after the war the government finally bestowed a medal on her for her efforts and the services she provided to the sick and injured soldiers.

NURSING IN THE UNITED STATES
The Civil War Period

The Civil War, or the War Between the States (1861 to 1865), was a period of time in which the health care conditions in the United States of America were similar to those of the time of Nightingale and Seacole. There were numerous epidemics such as syphilis, gonorrhea, malaria, smallpox, and typhoid (Oermann, 1997).

The Civil War was initiated by the attack on Fort Sumter, South Carolina, April 17, 1861. During this period of time there were no nurses who were formally trained to care for the sick. However, thousands of men and women from the South and North volunteered to care for the wounded. Hospitals were set up in the field, and there were hospital transports (Carnegie, 1995).

The Secretary of War Simon Cameron appointed a schoolteacher by the name of Dorothea Lynde Dix to organize military hospitals and provide medical supplies to the Union army soldiers. Dix received no official status and no salary for this position.

Nurses served during the Civil War under primitive working conditions. Often maintaining sanitary conditions was not possible. It is recorded that more than six million patients were admitted to hospitals, with approximately one-half million surgical cases. However, approximately 2000 individuals served as nurses (Fitzpatrick, 1997; Kalisch and Kalisch, 1995). This was far less than the number needed to provide adequate care. According to the records that were kept at three hospitals, 181 African-American nurses, both men and women, served between July 16, 1863, and June 14, 1864. Caucasian nurses made $12 per month; African-American nurses made $10 per month (Carnegie, 1995). Three African-American nurses made important contributions to nursing efforts during the Civil War: Harriet Tubman, Sojourner Truth, and Susie King Taylor.

Harriet Tubman served as a nurse in the Sea Islands off the coast of South Carolina. She cared for the sick and was known as the "Conductor of the Underground Railroad." It is also reported that she was the first woman to lead American troops into battle (Carnegie, 1995). Sojourner Truth, known for her abolitionist efforts as well as her nursing efforts, was an advocate of clean and sanitary conditions for patients so they could heal. Susie King Taylor, though hired in the laundry, worked as a nurse due to the growing number of wounded who needed assistance. Having learned to read and write, which was against the law for African-Americans, she also taught many of her comrades in Company E to read and write (Carnegie, 1995).

Many other volunteer nurses made important contributions during the Civil War. Clara Barton served on the front line during the Civil War and operated a war relief program to provide supplies to the battlefields and hospitals. Barton also set up a postwar service to find missing soldiers and is credited with founding the American Red Cross (Oermann, 1997). Louisa May Alcott, who served as a nurse for 6 weeks until stopped by ill health, authored detailed accounts of the experiences encountered by nurses during the war for a newspaper publication entitled *Hospital Sketches* (Kalisch and Kalisch, 1995).

When the Civil War ended, the number of nurse training schools increased. These early nursing programs offered little or no classroom education, and on-the-job training occurred in the hospital wards. The students learned routine patient care duties, worked long hours 6 days per week, and were used as supplemental hospital staff. After graduation most of the

BOX 1-2	*Duties of the Hospital Floor Nurse in 1887*

In addition to caring for your 60 patients, each nurse will follow these regulations:

1. Daily sweep and mop the floors of your ward, dust the patient's furniture and windowsill.
2. Maintain an even temperature on your ward by bringing in a scuttle of coal for the day's business.
3. Light is important to observe the patient's condition, therefore, each day fill kerosene lamps, clean chimneys, and trim wicks. Wash the windows once a week.
4. The nurse's notes are important in aiding the physician's work. Make your pens carefully; you may whittle nibs to your individual taste.
5. Each nurse on day duty will report every day at 7 AM and will leave at 8 PM except on Sabbath, on which day you will be off from 12 noon to 2 PM.
6. Graduate nurses in good standing with the Director of Nurses will be given an evening off each week if you regularly attend church.
7. Each nurse should lay aside from each payday a good sum of her earning for her benefits during her declining years, so that she will not become a burden. For example, if you earn $20 a month, you should set aside $10.
8. Any nurse who smokes, uses liquor in any form, gets her hair done at a beauty shop, or frequents dance halls will have given the Director of Nurses good reason to suspect her worth, intentions, integrity.
9. The nurse who performs her labors, serves her patients and doctors faithfully and without fault for a period of five years will be given an increase by the hospital administration of five cents per day, providing there are no hospital debts that are outstanding.

nurses practiced as private duty nurses or hospital staff (Lindeman and McAthie, 1990). The first nursing textbook, published in 1876, was used by the New York Training School for Nurses at Bellevue Hospital. It was entitled *A Manual of Nursing* (Kalisch and Kalisch, 1995) (Box 1-2).

During the 1890s the nationwide establishment of African-American hospitals and nursing schools gained momentum as African-American musicians, educators, and community leaders became alarmed at the high rates of African-American morbidity and mortality. Because of segregation and discrimination, African-Americans had to establish their own health care institutions to provide African-American patients with access to quality health care and to provide African-American men and women with opportunities to enter the nursing profession. In 1886 John D. Rockefeller funded the establishment of the first school of nursing for African-American women at the Atlanta Baptist Seminary—now known as Spelman College (Salzman, Smith, and West, 1996).

1900 to World War I

In the 1900s states began to require nurses to become registered before entering practice. By 1910 most states had upgraded education requirements to high school, upgraded training, and required registration before practice (Deloughery, 1991; Donahue, 1999).

Lillian Wald, a pioneer in public health nursing, is best known for the development and establishment of a viable practice for public health nurses in the twentieth century. The main location for this practice was the Henry Street Settlement House, located in the Lower East Side of New York City. Its purpose was to provide well-baby care, health education, disease prevention, and treatment of patients with minor illnesses. Nursing practice based at the Henry Street

Settlement House formed the basis of public health nursing for the entire country. Instead of relying on patients visiting the clinic, public health nurses made their way to the various tenements located around Henry Street (Stanhope and Lancaster, 2000; Snodgrass, 1999).

Lillian Wald also developed the first nursing service for occupational health. Ms. Wald believed that prevention of disease among workers would improve productivity. She was able to convince the Metropolitan Life Insurance Company of these ideas. As a result, nursing agencies such as those in place at the Henry Street Settlement House provided skilled nursing services to employees. Another innovation that emerged from this program was the sliding fee scale. Patients were billed according to their income or ability to pay. This innovative nursing service existed for 44 years before it was dissolved by the Metropolitan Life Insurance Company (Stanhope and Lancaster, 2000).

In 1911 Wald chaired a committee formed by members of the Associated Alumnae of Training Schools for Nurses, later to become the American Nurses Association (ANA), and the Society of Superintendents of Training Schools for Nurses, the precursor of the National League for Nursing (NLN). The purpose of the committee was to develop standards for nursing services performed outside of a hospital environment. The committee determined that a new organization was needed to meet the needs of community health nurses. The result of the committee's recommendation was the formation of the National Organization for Public Health Nursing, whose goals were to establish educational and practice standards for community health nursing (Stanhope and Lancaster, 2000).

The ANA and the NLN are still leading nursing organizations today. The ANA has focused primarily on professional aspects of nursing, and the NLN was the only accrediting body for nursing schools until 1996 when the Commission for Collegiate Nursing Education (CCNE), an autonomous arm of the American Association of Colleges of Nursing (AACN) was established as an agency devoted exclusively to the accreditation of baccalaureate and graduate degree nursing programs (Stanhope and Lancaster, 2000).

World War I and the 1920s

During the early 1900s the world was moving rapidly toward global conflict. Germany was arming, and the rest of Europe was trying to ignore the threat. Prosperous was the word used to describe the U.S. economy. Women were granted the right to vote and were moving into the work force on a regular basis.

Advancements in medical care and public health were being made. The primary site for medical care moved from the home to the hospital, and surgical and diagnostic techniques were improved. Pneumonia management was the focus of scientific study. Insulin was discovered in 1922, and in 1928 Alexander Fleming discovered the precursor of penicillin that eventually would be used to successfully treat patients with pneumonia and other infections (Kalisch and Kalisch, 1995).

Environmental conditions improved, and the serious epidemics of the previous century became nonexistent. Lillian Wald, in her book *The House on Henry Street,* linked poor environmental and social conditions to prevalent illnesses and poverty. Wald used this information to lead the fight for better sanitation and housing conditions (Stanhope and Lancaster, 2000).

With the outbreak of World War I (WWI) in 1914, nurses were desperately needed to care for the soldiers who were injured or who suffered from the many illnesses that were a result of trench warfare (Stanhope and Lancaster, 2000). The war offered nurses a chance to advance into new fields of specialization. For example, nurse anesthetists made their first appearance as part of the surgical teams at the front line. More than 20,000 United States–trained nurses served in WWI (Oermann, 1997).

Because many nurses volunteered to provide services during the war, the community health nursing movement in the United States stalled. However, the American Red Cross, founded by Clara Barton in 1882, assisted in efforts to continue public health nursing. The Red Cross nurses originally focused on the rural communities that were not able to access health care services. As the war continued, the Red Cross nurses also moved into urban areas to provide health care services.

During WWI the U.S. Public Health Service, founded in 1798 to provide health care services to merchant seamen, was charged with the responsibility to provide health services at the military posts located within the United States. A nurse, loaned by The National Organization for Public Health Nursing, established nursing services at U.S. military outposts. The responsibilities of the U.S. Public Health Service continued to grow; eventually it was composed of physicians, nurses, and other allied health professionals who provided indigent care and practiced in community health programs (Stanhope and Lancaster, 2000).

Further changes were in store for nursing during WWI. In 1918 the Vassar Camp School for Nurses was established. Its purpose was to provide an intensive, 2-year nurses training program for college graduates. Graduates of the program were given an army reserve commission and would be activated during times of war to meet increased nursing needs. Sponsored by the American Red Cross and the Council of National Defense, the school graduated 435 nurses. The Vassar Camp School for Nurses was a short-lived enterprise. When peace was declared in 1919, the program was permanently disbanded (Stanhope and Lancaster, 2000; Snodgrass, 1999).

In 1921 the federal government recognized the need to improve the health of women and children and passed the Sheppard-Towner Act, one of the first pieces of federal legislation passed to provide funds to assist in the care of special populations (Oermann, 1997). This funding provided public health nurses with resources to promote the health and well-being of women, infants, and children.

Following on these improvements, the Frontier Nursing Service (FNS) was established in 1925 by Mary Breckenridge of Kentucky. Born into a wealthy family, Breckenridge learned the value of providing care to others from her grandmother. Breckenridge began her career in New York's St. Luke's Hospital School of Nursing. After serving as a nurse during WWI, she returned to Columbia University to learn more about community health nursing. Armed with her new knowledge and a passion to assist disadvantaged women and children, Breckenridge returned to Kentucky and the rural Appalachian Mountains (Oermann, 1997; Stanhope and Lancaster, 2000).

Breckenridge believed that the rural mountain area of Kentucky, cut off from many modern conveniences, was an excellent place to prove the value of community health nursing. She established the FNS in a five-room cabin in Hyden, Kentucky. After overcoming serious obstacles such as no water supply or sewage disposal, six other nursing outposts were constructed in the rural mountains from 1927 to 1930. The FNS based its hospital in Hyden and eventually attracted physicians and nurses to provide medical, dental, surgical, nursing, and midwifery services to the rural poor. Financial support for the FNS ranged from fees for labor and supplies to funds raised through annual family dues to donations and fundraising efforts. Nurses working for the FNS traveled a 700-square mile area, many times on horseback, to provide services to approximately 10,000 patients (Oermann, 1997).

Breckenridge established an important health care service for rural Kentucky communities. Equally important was her documentation of the results of community health nursing in rural communities. Breckenridge followed the advice of a consulting physician and collected mortality data on the communities before nursing services actually were started. The results were startling—mortality was significantly reduced—and the need for the nursing services was clearly documented. Breckenridge proved that even in appalling environmental conditions without heat, electricity, or running water, nursing services could make an impact on the health of the community (Stanhope and Lancaster, 2000). The FNS is still in operation today and provides vital service to the rural communities of Kentucky.

The Great Depression (1930 to 1940)

During WWI the United States was prosperous well into the 1920s. However, after the stock market crash in October 1929 the economy quickly dissipated. Millions of men and women became unemployed. Before the depression many people had private duty nurses. However, due to the economy during the depression many nurses found themselves unemployed because numerous families could no longer afford private duty nurses.

Franklin D. Roosevelt, elected President of the United States in 1932, faced a country in shambles. He responded with several innovative and necessary interventions and ushered in the first major social legislation that had been enacted in U.S. history. Entitled the "New Deal," the legislation had several social components that affected the provision of medical care and other services for indigent people across the country (Karger and Stoesz, 1994).

The piece of legislation that had the greatest impact on health care in the United States was the Social Security Act of 1935, which set the precedent for the passage of the Medicare and Medicaid Act that followed in 1965. The main purposes of the 1935 Social Security Act were to provide (1) a national old-age insurance system; (2) federal grants to states for maternal and child welfare services; (3) vocational rehabilitation services for the handicapped; (4) medical care for crippled children and blind people; (5) a plan to strengthen public health services; and (6) a federal-state unemployment system (Karger and Stoesz, 1994).

The passage of the 1935 Social Security Act provided avenues for nursing care, and nursing jobs were created. With funds from the Social Security Act, public health nursing became the major source of health care for dependent mothers and children, the blind, and crippled children. Nurses found employment as public health nurses for county or state health departments (Kovner, 1990). Hospital job opportunities also were created for nurses, and the hospital became the usual employment setting for graduate nurses.

World War II (1940 to 1945)

The United States officially entered World War II (WWII) after the bombing of Pearl Harbor in December 1941. At that time the nursing divisions of all of the military branches had inadequate numbers of nurses. Congress passed legislation to provide needed funds to expand nursing education. A committee of six national nursing organizations, called the National Nursing Council, received one million dollars to accomplish the needed expansion. The U.S. Public Health Service became the administrator of the funds, which further strengthened the tie between the U.S. Public Health Service and nursing (Bullough and Bullough, 1984; Stanhope and Lancaster, 2000).

The war was considered a global conflict, and nursing became an essential part of the military advance. Nurses had to function under combat conditions and to adapt nursing care to meet the challenges of different climates, facilities, and supplies. As a result of their service during WWII, nurses finally were recognized as an integral part of the military and attained the ranks of officers in the army and navy. Colonel Julie O. Flikke was the first army nurse to be promoted to colonel in the U.S. Army and served as superintendent of the Army Nurse Corps from 1937 to 1942 (Deloughery, 1991).

Post World War II Period (1945 to 1950)

The period after WWII was a time of prosperity for the average American. The GI Bill enabled returning veterans to complete their interrupted education. The unemployment rate dropped to an all-time low in the United States. In an effort to provide some type of employment for the returning men, the government mounted a massive campaign to encourage women to return to the more traditional role of mother and wife. Consequently women in all professions, nursing included, chose to return to childbearing and marriage rather than continue employment outside the home.

After WWII, Communism demonstrated its strength more than ever before as the Soviet Union gobbled up the Eastern European countries. North Korea made a grab for South Korea with support from China, resulting in the Korean War. Again, nurses volunteered for the armed services to provide care to patients near the battlefields in Korea, and they worked in the Medical Army Surgical Units, better known as MASH units, where medical and surgical techniques were further refined.

The two decades after WWII saw the emergence of nursing as a true profession. Minimal national standards for nursing education were established by the National Nursing Accrediting service. In 1945 25 State Boards of Nurse Examiners adopted the State Board Test Pool. By 1950 all state boards were participating in the Test Pool and continue to do so today. Nursing continued to improve the quality and quantity of educational programs as the number of nursing baccalaureate programs grew and associate degree programs developed in community or junior colleges (Kalisch and Kalisch, 1995) (Box 1-3).

The end of WWII and the early 1950s marked the beginning of significant federal intervention in health care. The Nurse Training Act of 1943 was the first instance of federal funding being used to support nurse training. The passage of the Hill-Burton Act, or the Hospital Survey and Construction Act of 1946, marked the largest commitment of federal dollars to health care in the country's history. The purpose of the act was to provide funding to construct hospitals and to assist states in planning for other health care facilities based on the

---

BOX 1-3	*Qualities of Good Nurses During Post World War II*

1. Tidy and loyal to the hospital and its personnel
2. Compliant with the orders of the doctors and directives of nursing management
3. Always busy
4. If census was low, fold laundry, clean shelves, prepare supplies to be sterilized
5. Ability to get work done no matter how many patients she had

Source: Martell LK: Maternity care during the post World War II baby boom: the experience of general duty nurses, *West J Nurs Res* 96(3):387-391, 1999.

needs of the communities. Nearly 40% of the hospitals constructed in the late 1940s and the early 1950s were built with Hill-Burton funds. The hospital construction boom created by the Hill-Burton Act led to an increased demand for professional nurses to provide care in hospitals (Williams and Torrens, 1993).

It was also in the early 1950s that the National Association of Colored Graduate Nurses (NACGN) went out of existence. This was the organization that fought for integration of the African-American nurse into the ANA. From 1916 to 1948, African-American nurses in the South were barred from membership in the ANA because of segregation laws in the southern states. With the establishment of individual membership, African-American nurses in the South could bypass their states and become members of the ANA. This type of individual membership continued until all barriers had been dropped in the early 1960s.

In the 1940s the NACGN began to wage an all-out war against discrimination by the southern constituents of the ANA—the route to membership in ANA. This issue was raised by the NACGN on the floor at every national convention of the ANA, and it evoked strong opposition from the southern state constituents. Speaking from the floor of the House of Delegates at the 1946 convention in Atlantic City, a Caucasian nurse from Georgia referred to African-American nurses as "our darkies." Immediately a motion was passed to strike that from the record. However, this comment caused an uproar, and the African-American nurses in the southern states that barred them from membership started the wheels turning to bypass the states and join ANA directly. This arrangement, known as individual membership, was put into effect in 1948.

Nursing in the 1960s

Federal legislation enacted during the 1960s had a major and lasting effect on nursing and health care. The Community Mental Health Centers Act of 1963 provided funds for the construction of community outpatient mental health centers; opportunities for mental health nursing were expanded when funds to staff these centers were appropriated in 1965 with the passage of the Medicare and Medicaid Acts (Karger and Stoesz, 1994). Medicaid, Title XIX of the Social Security Act, was enacted and replaced all programs previously instituted for medical assistance. The purpose of the Medicaid program, which was jointly sponsored and financed with matching funds from federal and state governments, was to serve as medical insurance for those families, primarily women and children, with an income at or below the federal poverty level. Medicaid quickly became "the largest public assistance program in the nation, covering about 9.7% of the population, including more than 15% of all children" (Karger and Stoesz, 1994).

Health departments employed public health nurses to provide the bulk of the care needed by children and pregnant women in the Medicaid population. Services provided by these nurses included family planning, well-child assessments, immunizations, and prenatal care. A physician assigned as the district health officer supervised the nurses. Without the public health nurses and local health departments, many women and children in the inner city areas and rural communities would have been without access to basic health care.

Another important amendment to the Social Security Act was Title XVIII or Medicare, passed in 1965. The Medicare program provides hospital insurance, Part A, and medical insurance, Part B, to all people age 65 and older who are eligible to receive Social Security benefits; people with total, permanent disabilities; and people with end-stage renal disease. As a result of Medicare reimbursement, many hospitals catered to physicians who treated Medicare patients. Medicare patients were attractive to the hospitals because all hospital charges, regardless of amount or appropriateness of services, were reimbursed through the Medicare program (Williams and Torrens, 1993).

As a result of Medicare reimbursement, hospital-bed occupancy increased, which led to increased numbers of nurses needed to staff the hospital. Nursing embraced the hospital setting as the usual practice area and moved away from the community as the preferred practice site. Nursing schools also followed the trend by reducing the number of curriculum hours devoted to community health and concentrated their efforts on hospital-based nursing (Stanhope and Lancaster, 2000).

Another outcome of the Medicare legislation was the home health movement. To receive Medicare reimbursement for home health services, patients had to have (1) home-bound status; (2) a need for part-time or intermittent, skilled nursing care; (3) a medically reasonably and necessary need for treatment; and (4) a plan of care authorized by a physician. Home health agencies were established and began to employ increasing numbers of nurses. The number of home health agencies began to grow in the mid-1960s; and, as a result of Medicare reimbursement and other influences, including a growing elderly population, advances in medical technology, and public demand for increased access to health care, the home health industry has continued unprecedented growth into the 1990s (Rice, 1996). Home health was one of the first employment settings that provided nurses the opportunity to work weekdays only.

Nursing in the 1970s

The women's movement of the 1970s greatly influenced nursing. Nurses not only focused on providing quality care to patients, but they began to focus on the economic benefit of the profession. Nurses demanded fair wages. Hospitals were receiving significant reimbursements for patient care; however, nurses' salaries did not reflect an adequate percentage of that reimbursement. Health care costs soared. This increase in health care costs built the framework for mandated changes in reimbursement. Nursing practice and the educational focus remained in the hospital setting.

During this time nurses played a major role in providing health care to communities and were instrumental in developing hospice programs, birthing centers, and day care centers for the elderly (Stanhope and Lancaster, 2000). Although basic educational programs for nurse practitioners expanded during the 1970s and master's level preparation was developed as the requirement for graduation and practice, certification was also required to practice as a nurse practitioner. Before this time, only certification was required. State Nursing Practice Acts were amended to provide for monitoring and licensing advanced practice nurses.

In 1974 the ANA became concerned about research in the area of ethnic minorities and submitted a proposal to the National Institute of Mental Health for funding a project to permit minority nurses—African-Americans, Hispanics, Asians, and American Indians—to earn PhDs. Of the graduates of the project, the vast majority are on faculties of universities and are conducting research on factors in mental health and illness related to ethnicity and cross-cultural conflict, thereby fulfilling their commitment to advance the cause of quality health care for all people of color.

Despite past laxity, the ANA House of Delegates, at its 1972 convention, did pass an affirmative action resolution calling for a task force to develop and implement a program to correct inequities. The House also provided for the position of an ombudsman to evaluate involvement of minorities in leadership roles within the organization and to treat complaints by applicants for membership or by members of the Association who had been discriminated against because of nationality, race, creed, lifestyle, color, age, or sex. It was also in the seventies that the ANA elected its first African-American president, Barbara Nichols, who served two terms.

Within the structure of many professional organizations is a unit referred to as an academy, which is composed of a cadre of scholars who deal with issues that concern the profession and take positions in the name of the Academy. Nursing, a young profession, has had such an academy, created by the ANA Board, only since 1973. The American Academy of Nursing is composed of clinicians, educators, administrators, and researchers.

At its convention in Atlantic City in 1976, the ANA launched its Hall of Fame to pay tribute to those nurses who not only had paved the way for others to follow, but who also had made outstanding contributions to the profession.

Nursing in the 1980s

The types of patients needing health care changed in the 1980s. Homelessness became a common problem in large cities. Unstable economic developments contributed to an increase in the indigent populations (Karger and Stoesz, 1994). Acquired immune deficiency syndrome (AIDS) emerged as a frightening, fatal disease.

Runaway health care costs became a national issue in the 1980s. Medicare was still reimbursing for any and all hospital services provided to recipients. From 1966 to 1981 the federal contribution to hospital care rose from 13% to 41% (Karger and Stoesz, 1994). In 1983 in an attempt to restrain hospital costs, Congress passed the diagnosis-related group system for reimbursement, better known as the DRG system.

Before 1983 Medicare payments were made to the hospital after the patient received services. Although there were restrictions, the entire bill generally was paid without question. DRGs were implemented to provide prospective payment for hospital services based on the patient's admitting diagnosis and thereby to reduce the overall cost. Hospitals now were to be reimbursed one amount based on the patient's diagnosis, not on hospital charges. The system was developed by physicians at the Yale-New Haven Hospital and addressed approximately 468 diagnoses classified according to length of stay and cost of procedures associated with the diagnosis (Nies and McEwen, 2001).

As a result of the DRG reimbursement system, hospitals were forced to increase efficiency and more closely manage hospital services, including the patient's length of stay, laboratory and radiographic testing, and diagnostic procedures. Case management and critical pathways were developed to more efficiently manage patient care, and case management became a new area of specialization for the professional nurse.

Despite the high cost of health care, medicine prospered. Medical care advanced in areas such as organ transplantation, resuscitation and support of premature infants, and critical care techniques. Physician specialization and advances in medical technology flourished. Medical specialties such as nephrology, cardiology, endocrinology, orthopedics, neurosurgery, cardiovascular surgery, and advanced practices for obstetrics all led to improved health care services—and costs—in the hospital setting. The advanced technology also led to the development of outpatient surgery units.

Outpatient surgery services blossomed and provided a quick and efficient site for surgery that did not require extended hospital stays. Costs were greatly reduced because of fewer staff members needed for coverage, fewer supplies, and reduced facility costs. Nurses were interested in employment opportunities in outpatient facilities because they afforded a chance to work only during the day with no weekend assignments.

As the concern over increasing health care costs heightened, use of ambulatory services increased, and enrollment in health maintenance organizations grew. Advanced nurse practitioners increased in popularity as cost-effective providers of primary and preventive health care. A growing number of nurses moved from the hospital setting into the community to practice in programs such as hospice and home health. Consumers began to demand bans on unhealthy activities such as smoking in public. Health education became more important as consumers were encouraged to take responsibility for their own care (Stanhope and Lancaster, 2000). Even the terminology changed; the individual once known as the patient became known as the client or consumer and was afforded respect as a person who purchases a service.

Public health programs struggled to survive as counties and states cut health department budgets. A landmark study conducted by the Institute of Medicine (1988) entitled *The Future of Public Health* indicated a dismal picture for public health. The study determined that public health had moved away from its traditional role and core functions, and no strategy was in place to bring public health back to its original purpose (Stanhope and Lancaster, 2000). Inadequate funding for public health continues to be a problem, and hopefully in the near future public health will be restored to its original function and purpose.

Toward the end of the 1980s the American Medical Association announced its answer to the nursing shortage. It proposed to establish a 9-month program to prepare Registered Care Technologists. This proposal incensed unified nurses who fought it. As a result, the proposal came to naught (Schorr and Kennedy, 1999).

Also in the late eighties several nursing scholars suggested that nursing research needed to be firmly focused on the substantive information required to guide practice, rather than on philosophic and methodologic dilemmas of scientific inquiry. The creation of the National Center for Nursing Research in 1985 at the National Institutes of Health brought with it an increase in federal resources for nursing research and research training (Hinshaw, 1999).

Nursing in the 1990s

The 1990s began with alarm over the state of the U.S. economy. Government statisticians reported an alarming increase in the national debt complicated by slow economic growth. In the early 1990s average household incomes were stagnating. More women with families entered the workforce to afford the increasing cost of living. More nurses selected jobs in which they could work more hours in fewer days for more money, sometimes sacrificing the fringe benefits, which would allow them to work a second job or earn higher pay through shift differential for working evening and night shifts. Creative shifts such as the 10-hour day, 4-day work week or the 12-hour day, 3-day work week became commonplace in health care facilities. Just as in the 1980s, the cost of health care continued to increase with the technologic advancements in medical care.

There also were growing concerns in the 90s about the health of the nation, which prompted the Healthy People 2000 initiative. Many diseases associated with preventable causes characterized mortality in the United States. In 1990 more than two million U.S. residents died from diseases such as heart disease, cancer, cerebral vascular disease, accidents, chronic obstructive pulmonary disease, liver cirrhosis, tuberculosis, and human immunodeficiency virus infection. Factors contributing to these common disease states relate to lifestyle patterns, behaviors, and habits. More youth were at risk because of behavior such as smoking cigarettes, using abusive drug substances, eating poorly balanced diets, failing to exercise, having sex with multiple partners, and being subjected to acts of violence. *Healthy People 2000: National Health Promotion and Disease Prevention Objectives* was published in 1991 by the U.S. Department of Health and Human Services as a nationwide effort to help states, cities, and communities identify health promotion and disease prevention strategies to address these health risk problems.

The AIDS epidemic radically changed the process for infection control among health care workers in health care institutions across the nation. Recapping needles, wearing latex gloves, and using isolation precautions were issues that triggered much dialog and debate among health care workers. Health care workers were mandated to use preventive measures in the form of Universal Precautions; all contact with blood and body fluids from all patients was considered potentially infectious.

Exposure to hazardous materials also became a major issue of concern, not just for health care workers but also for the general public. Chemical and radioactive substances that created dangerous exposure and health risks were increasingly used in the workplace. Employers were held legally accountable for informing their employees of the actual or potential hazards and for reducing their exposure risk through training and the use of protective equipment. The hazardous materials issue was especially important in nursing and medicine, particularly with regard to exposure to carcinogenic chemicals used in drug therapy and in environmental infection control.

In 1990 the increasing costs of Medicaid and Medicare triggered political action for health care reform. Findings of a federal commission appointed to evaluate the American health care system include (Kalisch and Kalisch, 1995):

- Fifteen percent of the gross national product was related to health care expenditures (this amounts to approximately one trillion dollars annually).
- The United States spent more than twice as much as any industrialized nation for health care services.
- Americans were living longer, which indicated a growing demand for home health and nursing home care, as well as increased Medicare expenditures.

It became apparent that, if health care spending continued to increase, the U.S. economy would be in danger of collapse. Thus the health care system moved toward managed care in an attempt to control health care expenditures. The managed care movement has had a tremendous impact on nursing. To control costs, more health care is being provided in managed care environments.

The focus of managed care was on providing more preventive and primary care, using outpatient and home settings when possible, and limiting expensive hospitalizations. Massive downsizing of hospital nursing staff occurred, with an increasing use of unlicensed assistive personnel to provide care in hospitals. There was an increasing demand for community health nurses and advanced practice nurses to provide primary care services. The nurse of the 1990s had to be focused on delivering health care services that (1) encompassed health risk assessment based on family and environmental factors, (2) supported health promotion and disease prevention, and (3) advanced counseling and health education (Oermann, 1997).

In June 1993 the National Center for Nursing Research was redesignated the National Institute of Nursing Research. Moving nursing research into the National Institutes of Health enhanced the interdisciplinary possibilities for collaborative investigation. There was a rapid growth of nursing research during the 1990s. Multiple research programs focused on important health issues such as health promotion across the life span. Nursing research is also beginning to inform health care policy through federal commissions and agency programs (Hinshaw, 1999).

In the 1990s a partnership was forged between mandatory state licensure authorities, which set practice standards at the level of entering associate degree graduates, and national, nongovernmental bodies that certify graduate-prepared specialists. These national certifying agencies were intensely engaged in improving methods for determining the continuous competence of certified nurse practitioners within the swift current of health care change. The consumer's voice in the partnership was heard via collaboration with advocacy organizations and the appointment of more public members to licensing, certifying, and accreditation boards. Voluntary credentialing bodies recognized that, if they were to serve effectively, they had to engage in active public information campaigns to inform consumers about their health care choices (Styles, 1999).

Nursing in the Twenty-First Century

Professional nurses in the twenty-first century are faced with many challenges within the dynamic state of health care. Changing duties, responsibilities, and conflicts amidst nursing shortages and public concern over patient safety and quality of care characterize present-day practice. These changes require professional nurses to have core competency in critical thinking, communication, assessment, leadership, and technical skills, as well as knowledge of health promotion/disease prevention, information technology, health systems, and public policy. In addition to the issues of access, cost, quality, and accountability in health care, nurses today are challenged by an aging population, consumer health values, and an increasingly intercultural society. Evidence-based practice is more prevalent than ever and continues to improve health outcomes for individuals, groups, communities, and the nation. The nursing profession with over 2.6 million members has a tremendous opportunity to unite efforts to shape health care and the profession.

SUMMARY

Nursing is a dynamic profession that has evolved into a theory and research-based practice. From its unorganized and poorly defined beginnings, a profession based on the framework of competence, autonomy, determination, and human caring evolved. The challenges and struggles have paralleled the path of world history and have brought about significant changes in the profession. From the men who led the path, to the women who brought dignity and respect to their philosophy of caring, to the pioneers who brought about unity in the profession plagued by a history of racism, sexism, and sometimes disgrace, nursing has become recognized as a profession critical to the health of the nation. Despite a myriad of challenges, the practice of nursing has been distinguished and qualified by the intellect, skill, commitment, and contribution of countless sisters, deaconesses, and individuals such as Seacole, Dix, Barton, Wald, Breckenridge, and Nightingale.

Through periods of war, socioeconomic change, and health care reform, nurses have played a vital role in initiating change to improve the health care arena. Nurses have provided the integrity to maintain the quality of care in all health care settings. The evolution of the practice from the treatment of disease to health promotion and disease prevention has led the way in determining the type of providers needed to care for patients in the future. This

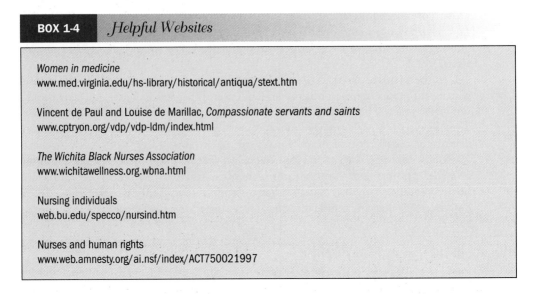

evolution will continue to provide the foundation for the scope of practice, educational curricula, scholarship, and research necessary for nurses to lead and manage the health care environment of the future. Nurses will continue to increase knowledge, manage technology, and maintain ethical standards to provide high quality care to individuals, families, and communities throughout the world (Box 1-4).

Critical Thinking Activities

1. How have the historical aspects of nursing affected nursing as we know it today?
2. Compare and contrast various contributions made by nurse pioneers, and describe how this affects your philosophy of nursing.
3. What was the historical significance of racial segregation and the impact of racial integration on professional nursing? Explain why this is important.
4. What is your vision for the profession of nursing in the future?
5. What are some of the challenges facing the nursing profession that you see in the future?

REFERENCES

Bahr L, Johnson B: *Collier's Encyclopedia,* vol 18, New York, 1995, Collier's.

Bullough VL, Bullough B: *History, trends, and politics of nursing,* Norwalk, Conn, 1984, Appleton-Century-Crofts.

Carnegie ME: *The path we tread: blacks in nursing: 1854-1994,* ed 3, New York, 1995, National League for Nursing.

Doheny MD, Cook CB, Stopper MC: *The discipline of nursing: an introduction,* ed 4, Stamford, Conn, 1997, Appleton Lange.

Delougherty GL: *Issues and trends in nursing,* St Louis, 1991, Mosby.

Dolan J: *Nursing in society: a historical perspective,* Philadelphia, 1978, WB Saunders.

Ellis JR, Hartley CL: *Nursing in today's world: challenges, issues and trends,* Philadelphia, 1988, JB Lippincott.

Ellis JR, Hartley CL: *Nursing in today's world: challenges, issues and trends,* Philadelphia, 2001, JB Lippincott.

Fitzpatrick MF: The mercy brigade, *Civil War Times* 36(3):34-40, 1997.

Freedman D: *The anchor bible dictionary,* New York, 1995, Doubleday.

Giger J, Davidhizar R: *Transcultural nursing: assessment and intervention,* ed 2, St Louis, 1999, Mosby.

Hinshaw AS: Nursing research and the explosion of knowledge. In Schorr TM, Kennedy MS, editors: *One hundred years of American nursing,* New York, 1999, JB Lippincott.

Ignatavicius M, Workman L, Mishler MA: *Medical surgical nursing: a nursing process approach,* ed 3, Philadelphia, 1999, WB Saunders.

Kalisch P, Kalisch B: *The advance of American nursing,* ed 2, Philadelphia, 1986, JB Lippincott.

Kalisch P, Kalisch B: *The advance of American nursing,* ed 3, Philadelphia, 1995, JB Lippincott.

Karger HJ, Stoesz D: *American social welfare policy: a pluralist approach,* New York, 1994, Longman.

Kelly L, Joel L: *The nursing experience: trends, challenges and transition,* ed 3, New York, 1996, McGraw-Hill.

Kovner AR: *Health care delivery in the United States,* ed 4, New York, 1990, Springer Publishing Company.

Lindeman C, McAthie, M: *Nursing trends and issues,* Springhouse, Pa, 1990, Springhouse Corporation.

Nies MA, McEwen M: *Community health nursing: promoting the health of populations,* ed 3, Philadelphia, 2001, WB Saunders.

Oermann MH: *Professional nursing practice,* Stamford, Conn, 1997, Appleton and Lange.

Rice R: *Home health nursing practice: concepts and application,* ed 2, St Louis, 1996, Mosby.

Salzman J, Smith D, West C, editors: *Encyclopedia of African-American culture and history,* vol 3, New York, 1996, Macmillan Library Reference USA; Simon and Schuster Macmillan.

Schorr TM, Kennedy MS: *One hundred years of American nursing,* New York, 1999, JB Lippincott.

Snodgrass, M.E: *Historical encyclopedia of nursing,* Santa Barbara, 1999, ABC-CLIO.

Stanhope M, Lancaster J: *Community and public health nursing,* St Louis, 2000, Mosby.

Styles MS: *The new wave of credentialing.* In Schorr TS, Kennedy MS, editors: *One hundred years of American nursing,* New York, 1999, JB Lippincott.

Walton J, Barondess J, Locke S: *The Oxford medical companion,* New York, 1994, Oxford University Press.

Williams SJ, Torrens PR: *Introduction to health services,* ed 4, Albany, NY, 1993, Delmar Publishing.

US Department of Health and Human Services, Public Health Service. *Healthy people 2020: national health promotion and disease prevention objectives,* Washington, DC, 1991, USDHHS.

SUGGESTED READINGS

Anteau CM, Williams LA: What we learned from the Oklahoma City bombing, *Nursing* 36(5):52-55, 1998.

Aronitz F: Competition for the education of nurses, *Community College Week* 13(6):2-4, 2000.

Bezyack ME: Advanced practice: is it right for you? *Am J Nurs* 96(1):15-25, 1996.

Carnegie ME: Black nurses at the front, *Am J Nurs* 84(10):1250-1252,1984.

Carnegie ME: *The path we tread: blacks in nursing: 1854-1984,* Philadelphia, 1986, JB Lippincott.

Collins H: Mission for the millennium: choke out remains of polio, *Charlotte Observer,* March 14, 1999, pp 1A, 10A.

Donahue MP: Nursing: the finest art—an illustrated history, St Louis, 1999, Mosby.

Donaldson MS, Vanselow NA: The nature of primary care, *J Fam Pract* 42(2):397-421, 1996.

Shelton K: A brief history of black women in the military, *Precinct Reporter* 3(9):2-4, 1996.

2

The Contemporary Image of Professional Nursing

Toni Bargagliotti, DNSc, RN

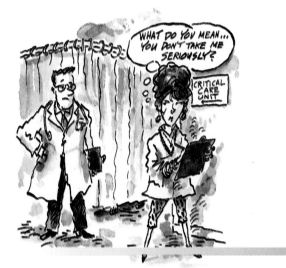

Each nurse forms the image of nursing
every day.

People are always blaming their circumstances for what they are. I don't believe in circumstances. The people who get on in this world are the people who get up and look for the circumstances they want, and if they can't find them, make them.

GEORGE BERNARD SHAW

Vignette

Mary is a senior nursing student who asks a faculty member, "Why can't we wear different scrubs and jewelry to clinical? Have you seen what nurses wear? I don't know what difference it makes anyway. Patients don't care what we're wearing. They care that we know how to take care of them. You know, 2 months after we graduate, we'll be wearing what everyone else does. Yes, I know we look better than everyone else does. But why?"

Questions to consider while reading this chapter
1. How does the image of a nurse differ from that of a physician?
2. Why shouldn't nurses wear jewelry?
3. How does the nurse's appearance affect the patient's opinion of the quality of care the nurse provides?

Learning Outcomes

After studying this chapter, the reader will be able to:

1. Explain the contributing factors to the nursing shortage.
2. Describe the image of nursing in art, media, literature, and architecture over time.
3. Identify nursing actions that convey a negative image of nursing.
4. Suggest strategies that would enhance the image of nursing.
5. Create an individualized plan to promote a positive image of nursing in practice.

Key Terms

Architecture The art of building.

Art Any branch of creative work, especially painting and drawing, that displays form, beauty, and any unusual perception.

Literature All writings in prose or verse.

Media All the means of communication such as newspapers, radio, and television.

Stereotype A fixed or conventional conception of a person or group held by a number of people that allows for no individuality.

CHAPTER OVERVIEW

This chapter describes how the image of nursing has been shaped and suggests strategies that nurses can use to forge a positive public and professional image of their practice. Because nurses have been the subjects of artists, sculptors, and writers for thousands of years, an historic perspective is used to illustrate the contextual background for the evolving image of this profession. Examples from nursing practice are used to illustrate how different approaches to the same situation continually shape the image of nursing.

IMAGES OF NURSING

When you imagine a nurse, what mental picture comes to mind? Do you think of *Life* Magazine's (1942) nurse in a starched white uniform with a cap; NBC's Emmy award–winning character, Carol Hathaway, RN, Head Nurse in *ER;* Universal Studio's Greg Focker, RN, in *Meet the Parents* (2000); or your colleagues with whom you practiced yesterday? The contemporary image of professional nursing in the United States is an ever-changing kaleidoscope created by the 2.2 million men and women of all ages, races, and religious beliefs who are registered nurses. Adding to this multifaceted collage are the numerous snapshots of nurses and nursing as portrayed in television commercials, bumper stickers, art, poetry, architecture, postage stamps, television dramas, television serials, movies, newspaper comic strips, stained glass windows, and statues. Second in size to the profession of teaching, nurses have been alternatively described as either saints or sinners, powerless or powerful, admired or ignored. Their practice has captured the attention of historians, economists, and sociologists who have studied this unusual group of people. Although nursing is the profession for which sentimental women need not apply, historians have described nurses as those who were ordered to care.

From these many perspectives of nursing, how and why has nursing been portrayed in art, literature, film, and the media? What does the public believe about nursing? How can professional nurses create a positive image?

Since Florence Nightingale reduced mortality rates from 42% to 2% in a Crimean hospital constructed over an open sewer, nurses have been reformers who are expected to use limited resources to address unlimited "wants" for health care. The request for Nightingale's nursing services in the Crimean was born out of newspaper reports about the devastating health care conditions in the Crimean War. Today the latest congressional report, ABC's *20/20* episode entitled Disappearing Nurses, and Gallup poll results indicate the value that the public places on nursing practice.

Although over the years at various times nurses have become concerned with their public image and media portrayal, the extensive work of Kalisch and Kalisch (1995) outlining the image of nursing in film and media over time permanently etched the image issue into the professional radar screen. Although image concerns may appear to be self-serving, the deepening national concern about the emerging nursing shortage of unprecedented magnitude is focusing considerable attention on the way that nursing is publicly imaged. Whether nursing shortages emerge from the public image of nursing or images of nursing emerge from nursing shortages, the two are inextricably related. Understanding the current shortage provides the fundamental basis for a discussion of the image of nurses.

THE NURSING SHORTAGE

This emerging nursing shortage that has already arrived in many areas of the United States has steep supply and demand side features. For example, the Georgia Hospital Association has reported a 13% statewide vacancy rate, increasing to 19% in metropolitan Atlanta (Crawshaw, 2000). How did this happen?

Consider the following data: the average age of a new nursing graduate is 33, and from a community college the average age of a registered nurse (RN) is 44, and the average age of nursing faculty is 50 (Buerhaus, Staiger, and Auerbach, 2000). By 2015 more than half of U.S. RNs are predicted to retire. The graying of American nurses is occurring because of two factors outside of nursing: (1) the declining birth rate of potential nurses every year following the boomer generation (1946-1960), and (2) the women's movement in the 1970s that opened new career opportunities for women (Buerhaus, Staiger, and Auerbach, 2000). However, the most serious concern is that since 1995, the overall number of students entering nursing has declined each successive year (AACN, 2000). The intertwining of the image of nursing and the nursing shortage is found in one succinct conclusion: nursing would be able to attract more young people if media images of nurses included more than "being on strike or laid off or involved in a mercy killing" (Jaklevic and Lovern, 2000).

An aging baby boomer generation and the increasing complexity of health care fuel the demand side of the shortage. By 2006 the U.S. Bureau of Labor Statistics predicts that job opportunities for RNs will have increased by 21% in comparison to a 14% job growth in all other occupations (AACN, 1998). By 2020 the need for hospital RNs alone will have increased by 36% (AACN, 1998), whereas the supply of full-time equivalent nurses will remain at year 2000 levels (Buerhaus, Staiger, and Auerbach, 2000). As noted by a public finance analyst with Moody's Investor's Service, since "hospitals are competing with medical groups, insurers, and dot-coms for a shrinking pool of qualified nurses" (Jaklevic and Lovern, 2000), the need to increase RNs by 36% is a conservative estimate addressing the needs of only one practice site.

NURSING IN ART, LITERATURE, AND ARCHITECTURE

Although the way that nursing has been portrayed in art, literature, and architecture over time may seem to be unrelated to the contemporary image of nursing, the mental image of contemporary nursing is enmeshed with these earliest images.

Art and literature have been the way in which people describe the human condition and cultural values of their time. Throughout history, new social and political institutions and rulers have made social and political statements of arrival through architecture, which "symbolizes the activity of the institution and tells us something about its importance within a culture" (Kingsley, 1988, p. 63); nursing has made similar statements. It has been suggested that it was through the architecture of hospital-based schools of nursing that nursing established both its self-image and public image as a profession in the United States (Kingsley, 1988).

In these earliest descriptions of nurses and nursing are found the enduring fundamental and essential tensions that exist within the profession today. Also within the art, literature, and architecture of nursing is found the eternal question asked by those who know they will one day require nursing care: "Can I trust and entrust my life to this nurse?" Although people hope that nursing is a vocation, a "calling" that requires education, commitment, and dedication, they fear that it is only a job requiring minimal training that one endures for the lack of other opportunities or until something "better" is available.

Antiquity Image of Nursing

The earliest literary reference to nursing chronicles the actions of two nurse midwives in approximately 1900 BC in Exodus 1 of the Old Testament, which indicates that the practice of two midwives became the vehicle through which the Israelites, the Jewish race, and the resultant Judeo-Christian heritage survived.

Nurse midwives and baby nurses, who were untrained servants, have been portrayed in art since the sixth century BC (Kampen, 1988). Found in eleventh century AD art are the first male images of nurses. Notably the nursing order of the Knights Hospitallers of St. John of Jerusalem in their black robes with a white Maltese cross were artistically portrayed as soldiers, rather than providers of nursing care (Kalisch and Kalisch, 1995). The next artistic renderings of nursing care, provided by other than servants or family members, would occur as the result of the twelfth century AD Christian writings on the Seven Corporal Works of Mercy that were performed to achieve salvation in the next life (Kampen, 1988). In these paintings the nurse would be portrayed as a woman in a religious order or as a person of wealth performing nursing as an act of Christian mercy.

These meager artistic renderings of nurses convey four images that continue to be familiar to contemporary nurses. Nurses were advocates and protectors, untrained servants, soldiers, or well-respected caregivers. For more than 600 years nursing appeared infrequently in art or literature.

Victorian Image of Nursing

In 1844, when Nightingale was "called" to become a nurse, Charles Dickens immortalized a different kind of nurse through Sairy Gamp, the nurse for whom nursing was endured because of the lack of other opportunities. For Sairy Gamp, a drunken, physically unkempt, uncaring nurse in *Martin Chuzzlewit,* nursing provided a way to profit from the sick and dying.

Reflecting the concern of Victorian England for untrained caregivers, Dickens advised Sairy of the advantages of "... a little less liquor, and a little more humanity, and a little less regard for herself, and a little more regard for her patients, and perhaps a trifle of additional honesty" p. 894).

Fortunately Sairy's literary arrival was followed by Longfellow's portrayal of the heroic Nightingale in "Santa Filomena" (1857). As important as Nightingale was to the improved health care of British soldiers and to the development of modern nursing, the ever increasingly positive images of Nightingale occurred solely because she was able to succinctly demonstrate the aggregate outcomes of nursing practice. To do so, she became one of the earliest users of the emerging body of knowledge called statistics and developed the pie chart that continues to remain in common use. Notably, nursing emerged at a time of turbulent social change and reform in Great Britain. At that time women did not have the basic rights of citizenship.

Early Twentieth-Century Nursing

Toward the end of the Nightingale period at the turn of the century, nurses in war settings vividly capture the attention of artists. The most compelling image is Bellows' 1918 canvas, *Edith Cavell Directing the Escape of Soldiers from Prison Camp* (Donahue, 1985). World War I (WWI) Germany shocked the world with its 1915 firing squad execution of Edith Cavell, founder of the first nursing school in Belgium, who aided soldiers escaping prison camps. The art of heroic nursing expressed in several famous paintings reflected the reality of WWI nurses who were also the recipients of 3 Distinguished Service Crosses, 23 Distinguished Service Medals, 28 French Croix de Guerre's, 69 British Military Medals, and 4 U.S. Navy Crosses (Donahue, 1985). Notably American nurses who served in World War I were not commissioned in the military services.

The arrival of nursing as a profession and a "calling" and the central importance of nurses to hospitals was clearly evidenced in the architecture of grand and imposing nursing schools that were attached to hospitals. They were deliberately designed with impressive entrances and private rooms, as well as lobby and recreational areas of gymnasiums, swimming pools, and tennis courts to attract women who were, in the words of the Board of Governors of the New York Hospital Training School, "women of refinement" (Kingsley, 1988, p. 69). Hutchinson, who donated funding for the Charity Hospital School of Nursing in 1901, indicated that the care provided to nurses would be directly proportional to the quantity and quality of care provided to patients (Kingsley, 1988). The size of these residences is grandly reflected in the Cook County Hospital School of Nursing completed in 1935 that was 17 stories tall and occupied a complete city block (Kingsley, 1988).

The 1930s—Nursing As Angel of Mercy

The popular 1937 CBS radio series and later RKO movie serial, *Dr. Christian,* portrayed the all wise country doctor whose loyal nurse was a dedicated, intelligent, and caring professional in a traditional white uniform (Kalisch and Kalisch, 1995).

On a grander scale, Warner Brother's *The White Angel* (1936), chronicled the professional life of Florence Nightingale. Endorsed by the American Nurses' Association (ANA), *The White Angel* clearly portrayed Nightingale's persistence and head-to-head confrontation with medicine. Anticipating that the medical staff would deny her nurses rations, she brought provisions for them. When the medical staff locked her out of the hospital to which she had been sent, Nightingale sat outside in the snow until patients and soldiers required physicians to admit these nurses. As Jones (1988) noted, *The White Angel* clearly conveyed to the public that nursing is a holy vocation, that nurses have professional credentials, but that the career choice is opposed because women belong at home. A subtle inference of the film is that Nightingale was smart enough to overcome the obstacles of medicine.

In 1938 Rich's tall and imposing white limestone statue, the *Spirit of Nursing*, was placed in Arlington National Cemetery to "honor the compassion and bravery of military nurses" (Donahue, 1985, p. 433). Similarly, Germany's 1936 stamp commemorated nursing as a symbol of community service with a larger-than-life nurse compassionately overlooking people (Donahue, 1985).

The 1940s—Nurse As Heroine

Considered to be the most positive movie about nursing, *So Proudly We Hail* is the 1942 story of nurses in Bataan and Corrigedor. The film, starring Claudette Colbert, portrayed a small group of nurses rerouted to the Philippines after the attack on Pearl Harbor. Soon cut off from supplies and replacements as the Japanese took over the Philippines, these nurses provided care with few supplies and no staff to the thousands of soldiers in the Philippines. Norman's *We band of angels: The story of American nurses trapped on Bataan by the Japanese* (1999) tells via their diaries and interviews the gritty, difficult, and heroic story of these nurses who served on Bataan.

Nursing was depicted on a 1940 Australian stamp as a larger-than-life figure looking over a soldier, a sailor, and an aviator; in Costa Rica's 1945 stamp of Florence Nightingale and Edith Cavell; and in the 1945 commissioning of the *USS Higbee*, a U.S. Navy destroyer named in honor of a Navy nurse (Donahue, 1985).

After nursing's glorious contributions to WWII, nurses returned home to find low salaries, long hours, too few staff, and too many patients. However, nursing continued to be glamorized through the *Cherry Ames* series, the *Sue Barton* series, and other romance novels.

Nursing in the Anti-Establishment Era of the 1960s

In the 1960s the modern-day version of Sairy Gamp would be drawn by Ken Kesey (1962) through the character of Nurse Ratched in *One Flew Over the Cuckoo's Nest*. This best-selling novel later became a play and motion picture (1975) that won six Oscars, including Best Picture of the Year. Nurse Ratched or "Big Nurse" represented the "establishment" that insisted on conformity and stifled creativity. Entrusted with the care of the mentally ill, Nurse Ratched, a military nurse in a starched white uniform, was the ultimate power figure who cruelly punished patients to cure their psychosis through conformity to a "system" (Fiedler, 1988). As Dickens had done with Sairy Gamp, Kesey described Nurse Ratched from the perspective of a patient.

In this case, the fun-loving, mentally healthy McMurphy was a patient who went to a mental hospital as a way to shed other responsibilities. He challenged the routine of the ward. When Nurse Ratched's attempts to control the mentally healthy McMurphy via tranquilizers and shock treatments failed, she caused him to be lobotomized. Although Kesey's scathing portrayal of "Big Nurse" provided a somber reminder to the profession of patient rights, *One Flew Over the Cuckoo's Nest* also made a significant social statement about mental health care and the growing revolution of the 1960s. Notably, President Kennedy's movement of the mentally ill from institutionalization in large state hospitals to community-based mental health care found widespread public acceptance.

The reality of the turbulent period of the 1960s is that nurses were prominently in the forefront of public health initiatives that were President Johnson's first salvo in the War on Poverty. Nurses were also dramatically shaping the future course of health care through the development of coronary care units, intensive care units, hemodialysis, and Silver and Ford's first nurse practitioner program in Colorado. Advances in nursing knowledge in these areas were also fueled by two unrelated events: (1) the nation's experience with massive trauma in Vietnam, and (2) the monitoring techniques developed for the space program. A U.S. Bureau of Labor study indicated that salaries of nurses were woefully inadequate in comparison to other, far less trained American workers (Kalisch and Kalisch, 1995).

Nursing in the Sexual Revolution of the 1970s

Media images of the nurse in the 1970s were formed amidst a sexual revolution and a growing anti-military American culture. War would again provide the media backdrop. The 1976 stamp, *Clara Maas, She Gave Her Life,* commemorated the 100th birthday of Maas, a 25-year-old nurse who died after deliberately obtaining two carrier mosquito bites so that she could continue providing care to soldiers with yellow fever in the Spanish-American War (Donahue, 1985). Her modern day counterparts would be nurses in *M*A*S*H.*

The nursing profession viewed *M*A*S*H* (1972-1983) as professionally destructive through the negative portrayal of Hot Lips Hoolihan and the nurses of the 4077th Army MASH unit in Korea. The sexual exploits of nurses and physicians and the uncaring Margaret provided few positive images. However, for the American public who were receiving a daily dose of *M*A*S*H* in the news footage of Vietnam on nightly news, *M*A*S*H* presented a glimmer of reality. Continuous front-line exposure to the massive trauma of young men did not immunize these nurses from caring or from the horrors of what they were seeing. They coped with its horrors with a sense of humor and irreverence toward "the system." Nurses serving in Vietnam would later be imaged in the television series, *China Beach.*

Similarly, the less popular *M*A*S*H* spin-off series, *Trapper John, MD,* depicted a negative image of nursing while providing at least one strategically important image for the profession: the portrayal of the wise African-American nurse whose "take" on the situation was always accurate. At the time of the series, the profession had fewer than 5% African-American nurses. To place this in history, it was not until 1964 that the Louisiana State Nurses' Association became the last state to fully admit African-American nurses for membership from all districts of the state (Carnegie, 1995).

Nursing in the 1980s to 1990s

Portraying an actual event, the complexities of nursing are realistically described by the character of Nurse Rivers in *Miss Evers' Boys.* Through the character of Miss Evers, the play tells the true story of Nurse Rivers who was hired to recruit young African-American men into the infamous Tuskegee experiment designed to describe the long-term effects of syphilis. When her patients asked her to obtain the new treatment of penicillin for them and she sought to do so, the physician investigators required her to discourage them from treatment. Their reasoning, designed to exploit and manipulate her, presents her with several moral dilemmas that she had not been educated to manage. As the narrator of the story, Nurse Rivers introduces non-nurses to the dilemmas of nursing practice and the consequences of misplaced faith and trust in physicians.

In 1997 three films used war and nursing as a backdrop: *The English Patient, Love and War,* and *Paradise Road.* In *The English Patient,* the 1997 Best Picture of the Year, it is the RN who recognizes that the severely burned, dying patient in WWII, known as the English Patient, cannot continue to be transported to a safer area. She volunteers to stay behind in an abandoned building to care for him until he dies. As she creates an environment to care for him, his story is told. The nurse is a nonjudgmental caregiver whose care brings him peace before he dies.

In *Love and War,* the story of the young Hemingway in WWI and the nurse he loved is told. The nurse saved young Hemingway's leg from certain amputation by irrigating and debriding the wound with the newly discovered Dakin's solution. In this story the nurse, who is far more knowledgeable than the physician about how to save this leg, does so despite orders not to do so.

Paradise Road tells the true story of women in a Japanese prisoner-of-war camp. Although the nurse is not the central figure, it is she who leaves the camp to obtain quinine to treat an older woman who, in her last days, learns a human value system. For her efforts the nurse is physically tortured.

In contrast to these heroic media portrayals of nursing was the Nicole Miller advertisement in *Golf* (June, 1997) designed to sell golf clothes to men. Four practicing New York physicians were pictured on a golf green with the caption "Playing doctor." Draped around the physicians were young female models in white bikini bathing suits with nursing caps and tennis shoes. As a result of rapid written response from nurses and the American Organization of Nurse Executives (AONE), the company withdrew the advertisement and apologized to Nicole Miller customers and readers of *Golf* magazine (Wood, 1997).

Artistic views of nursing during this period focused on caring. In the Vietnam War Women's Memorial, the central figure is the nurse in battle fatigues cradling the head of a soldier for whom she is providing care. Evident in the bronze statue is the fatigue of the nurse and her care for this dying soldier.

Architecturally nursing in the 1980s continued to "arrive" through its buildings. The award-winning University of Oregon Center for the Health Sciences School of Nursing in Portland provides an excellent contemporary example of the current emphasis in American nursing education. Oriented with commanding views of the mountains, this building of glass and wood reflects the timber-based industry of Oregon and the inextricable linkage between nursing and its community. The nursing research level, with its many nursing research laboratories, reflects the primary mission of the school, which is to generate nursing knowledge. It also reflects the breadth of nursing research that is conducted. The importance of personal interaction in an Internet world is found throughout the building in conversational areas and in the widened hallways that encourage people to personally engage with one another.

The Image of Men

Notably absent in these media portrayals of nurses are the men who are entering nursing in increasing numbers. Perhaps one of the most positive film portrayals of men who are nurses occurs in *Meet the Parents,* a comedy released in December 2000. In this film the aspiring son-in-law is Greg Focker, RN, a wonderful character who humorously addresses and rises above the worst of all stereotypes that are endured by men in this profession. Men who are nurses are also interspersed throughout the fictional television series *ER* and the documentary series *Trauma: Life in the ER.*

IMAGEMAKERS OF NURSES

As noted in Box 2-1, during the 1980s and 1990s nurses moved into highly public national roles.

Nurses of America Campaign

In 1990 the Tri-Council of Nursing with funding from the Pew Foundation implemented the Nurses of America (NOA) media campaign. NOA was designed to convey to the public that nurses are expert clinicians who are able to interpret technical data in usable ways, as well as coordinate and negotiate health care. In collaboration with the American Advertising Council, several television and print advertisements of nursing, such as "Anyone can care, but not everyone can be a nurse," or "By 10:00 AM, Susan Smith, RN had saved a life," began to appear. As a part of the NOA campaign, Suzanne Gordon, a journalist with the *Boston Globe,* and Bernice Buresch, a journalist with *U.S. News and World Report,* "media" trained many nursing leaders across the United States.

A strategically important part of the NOA campaign was raising the consciousness among nurses of the invisibility of nursing in the news media. For example, a story that captured the news media of that time was that of a New York jogger who had sustained life-threatening head injuries as a result of being severely beaten while jogging in Central Park. Although her recovery was predominantly the result of the excellent intensive care nursing that she received, nursing was never mentioned in the news coverage. Similarly, a study of sources quoted by journalists in health coverage in *The New York Times, LA Times,* and the *Boston Globe* indicated

---

| **BOX 2-1** | *Imagemakers of Nursing* |

Dr. Carolyne K. Davis, RN
Director of Health Care Finance Administration (HCFA) during the Reagan Administration. Implemented the Medicare capitated reimbursement system based on diagnosis-related groups (DRGs)

Sheila Burke, MPH, RN
Chief of Staff, Senate Majority Leader, Bob Dole. Senior political advisor during Dole presidential campaign

Dr. Shirley Chater, RN
Director of the Social Security Administration during the first Clinton Administration

Dr. Ada Sue Hinshaw, RN
Director of the first National Center of Nursing Research, now the National Institute of Nursing Research (NINR), National Institute of Health

Dr. Beverly Malone, RN, ANA president (1996-2000)
Deputy Assistant Secretary for Health, United States Department of Health and Human Services (DHHS); member of the US delegation to the World Health Assembly

Dr. Beverly Malone, RN (2001-present)
General Secretary, Royal College of Nursing, London

that nurses accounted for 10 of more than 900 citations (Buresch, Gordon, and Bell, 1991). In fact, nurses ranked last after patients. Sigma Theta Tau International's Woodhull study of 20,000 articles published in 16 newspapers, magazines, and other health care publications (1998) indicated that nurses were cited only 4% of the time in the more than 2000 articles about health care.

THE ENDURING PUBLIC CONCERN WITH NURSING

The effects of the emerging nursing shortage were chronicled in the *20/20* episode, "Disappearing Nurses," which aired on ABC on November 26, 1999. This episode accurately described that staffing shortages can mean too few RNs, inadequately trained RNs, or the inappropriate use of unlicensed personnel.

Against this backdrop of nursing images that extend from antiquity to the latest CNN broadcast is the question of the image that will be created by nurses today. Although attention and concern about the professional image of nursing might superficially seem to be a self-serving exercise, the many historical images of nursing indicate otherwise.

The literary and media images of nursing from saint to sinner are not conflicting views. They represent the eternal question asked by people since the beginning of time, "Can I trust and entrust my life to this nurse?" The first lessons learned in life are that pain hurts. People have quickly understood that health is essential to the enjoyment of life. Illness is to be avoided. Illness and death are certainties of life that require care. As a consequence of living, people know their own contemporary version of the Biblical story of Job. Serious and debilitating illnesses more often lead to a loss of social support from friends than a rallying of support.

People want to believe that, when they need health care, their nurse will be a knowledgeable, caring, committed, and dedicated person. They want to believe that the nurse will, as Virginia Henderson indicated, perform nursing care that does for them what they would otherwise do if they had the necessary strength, ability, and knowledge. Perhaps as fearful as entrusting their lives to someone else is the fear of entrusting knowledge of their most intimate selves to someone who may not treat them kindly. To be sick is to entrust the most intimate physical functions, fears, and concerns to a nurse (Fagin and Diers, 1983). People know that whatever public facades about their real relationships to "kith and kin" they can maintain when healthy will be immediately stripped bare during illness. They also know that a stranger, the nurse, will soon know their most intimate secrets of "personhood at its worst" when they are ill . They hope for a Nightingale who will overcome all obstacles to reduce their mortality from 42% to 2%, but they fear a Sairy Gamp or a Nurse Ratched who will neglect or control them in harmful ways. Because they have chosen not to be a nurse, they wonder how anyone else can.

From a sociologic perspective the conflicting metaphors of nurse as ministering angel, battle-ax, physician's handmaiden, and naughty nurse have not served the profession well (Kitson, 1997; Cunningham, 1999). As Cunningham (1999) and others have noted, the angel image also carries with it the belief that pay is not relevant compared with the privilege of doing good. Moreover, any suffering that can be experienced by nurses will only add to their virtue. Cunningham (1999) and others have further suggested that in a patriarchal society men who are ill ridicule nurses as battleaxes or sexually provocative people as a way to reverse the power relationship they felt when under the care of nurses. None of these stereotypes have served the profession well.

What the Public Believes About Nursing

Two recent Gallup polls illustrate what the public believes about nursing. For the second consecutive year nurses were ranked highest among all professions for having the highest professional standards of honesty and ethics, with more than 79% of the American public indicating that nurses have very high or high standards. In this poll pharmacists rated second at 67%, and physicians were at 63% (The Gallup Organization, 2000a). In a second Gallup poll (The Gallup Organization, 2000b) concerning health care, 86% were generally satisfied with the nurses and doctors with whom they had contact, and 85% would be pleased if their son or daughter became an RN (Woody, 2000).

From a somewhat different perspective, Floyd (2000) reported that a Harris poll conducted for Sigma Theta Tau found that the public sought nursing advice in four areas: (1) self-care or immediate postoperative care of someone else, (2) over-the-counter health care products, (3) administration and side effects of prescription medications, and (4) interpreting physician-provided information.

Recognizing the influence that high school guidance counselors and nonnursing university professors have on nursing and prenursing students, Lippman and Ponton (1989; 1993) tested the opinions that these two important groups held about nursing. Their randomly selected samples of nonnursing university professors (n = 539 across 19 campuses) and high school guidance counselors (n = 313) characterized nurses as knowledgeable, essential health care providers who were not perceived to be physician handmaidens. (Lippman and Ponton, 1989, 1993). Interestingly, both groups strongly favored university nursing education over hospital-based and associate degree programs and strongly indicated their belief that baccalaureate preparation of nurses was essential to quality health care. They both strongly disagreed with or left blank items related to nursing as a sex object or to statements that "Nurses do 'it' better." A professor summarized the beliefs of many with the comment that the sexually related questions were "dumb questions."

A high school guidance counselor provided a revealing comment that "There seems to be a problem with large numbers of disgruntled nurses in the population—usually nonpracticing—who have been very influential with my students. They tend to be mothers, aunts, sisters, and friends" (Lippman and Ponton, 1993, p. 133). When nurses wonder why they are not more highly regarded by young people, they may want to consider how they are portraying their profession in casual conversation with others.

Five years later Huffstutler and colleagues' secondary analysis of responses from nonnursing university professors, students, and others (1998) indicated that these respondents most closely associated nursing with caring, although they differed in the ways that they described caring. This finding reflects the nursing-sponsored image-building campaigns of the early 1990s that imaged nurses as caring.

All of these findings indicate that nurses are well regarded and trusted by the public. Perhaps, more important, they pose the interesting question for nurses about why they deride their profession to others and wear tee shirts and other apparel with derisive comments about nursing, such as "Nurses do IT better," "Nurses get to the POINT," and "run a Code naked?"

What Nurses Believe About Nursing

A most telling study about the public image of nursing compared the beliefs of nurses (n = 173) with other health professionals (n = 520) (physicians, administrators, and others in a Veterans Administration hospital). In this study nurses were rated most highly as careerists who do what needs to be done and are self-sacrificing, moral, and noble. However, nurses significantly differed from their counterparts by rating themselves higher on doing what needs to be done and higher as a sex object (Schweitzer et al., 1994).

THE REALITY OF THE CONTEMPORARY STAFF NURSE

> The reason for the existence of the modern health care institution—the hospital, the nursing home, the mental hospital, the home care agency—is to deliver nursing. If surgery could be done safely and economically on the kitchen table, and if people could survive it, it would be. If diagnosis and management of serious medical illness could be done in office practices in 8.5-minute visits, it would be. If the chronically mentally ill could be taken care of at home, and protected from the world and from themselves, they would be. If the demented, the frail, the paralyzed, the very old could be cared for at home, they would be and it would be a whole lot cheaper because public policy would not contemplate channeling the money to family caregivers: they're supposed to want to do it anyway (Diers, 1988, pp. VIII-2 and VIII-3).

Logically it could be inferred that nurses would be highly valued since their practice settings exist to deliver their services and new practice settings are emerging daily. The public highly values their profession. Nursing's heroic and noble public image has been etched in stone and in stained-glass windows in larger-than-life proportions. However, Shindul-Rothchild, Berry, and Long-Middleton's survey (1996) indicated that almost one in four nurses planned to leave the profession. Forty percent of nurses would not recommend their practice setting for the care of a family member. Why?

Clash Between Beliefs and Reality

Mills and Blaesing (2000) found that nurses who were more likely to be satisfied with their career over time held three values: (1) the sense of professional status, (2) the belief that they made a difference (patient care rewards), and (3) pride in their profession. Those belief systems soon clashed with the health care reform that occurred during the 1990s.

Health care changes in the 1990s shifted practice boundaries with the widespread marginalization of professional nursing care. Multiskilled unidentifiable workers replaced 20% to 50% of RNs in downsizing and rightsizing efforts that left nurses doing more and supervising the unskilled with 20% fewer staff than other industrialized nations (Brannon, 1996; Gordon, 1997; Kitson, 1997). Although these changes were attributed to managed care and the Budget Reconciliation Act of 1997, Grando's historical research (1998) indicates that these same events occurred in the 20-year post WWII period. During this nursing shortage administrators tested the elasticity of nursing with unlicensed persons as a deliberate strategy to avoid increasing salaries.

The mega corporate environments that emerged in the 1990s diminished nursing staffs to increase the margin, while increasing administrative staffs to consume 25% of the hospital dollar. Far outstripping physician income, Gordon (1997) cites a 1995 survey that indicated the average compensation for chief executive officers of small hospitals to be $188,500; in larger hospitals, $280,900; and in the nation's seven largest for-profit health maintenance organizations (HMOs), $7 million.

Although they experienced significant downsizing, nurses and their employers conveyed and continue to convey to patients that hospitals and other health care settings provide caring, individualized, holistic care. Home health care agencies marketed nursing as "a part of your family," although Coffman's study (1997) indicated that families perceive the home health nurse to be a "stranger in the family."

Ironically, although nursing beliefs about the care they would provide were highly congruent with the marketing claims of the nurse's employer, these claims placed the nurse in direct conflict with a system internally determined to provide essential rather than "nice to have" care. Nurses, expecting to have adequate, competent staff and to be rewarded for providing caring, individualized, holistic care, instead faced a quite different reality. The employer asked only one question: How much was provided for how little to ensure that customers were delighted rather than satisfied, healthy, or healthier?

When patients realize that their expectations are not being met, they are rightfully angry. Even when it may be possible for them to understand that the system will only provide minimal care, there remains one additional thorny problem. If the nurse were their advocate, as nursing has so claimed, why didn't the nurse or nursing *fix* the system to provide all that was promised (Kelly, 1989)? Patients who believed that their care would be caring, sensitive, and individualized are stunned by what occurs and angry when they are discharged home requiring skilled nursing care that they must now provide for themselves (Barnum, 1991; Kelly, 1989).

Second, in terms of nursing practice, there was a significant mismatch about the claims of managed care and what actually occurred. Productivity and work redesign literature centered on accountability and identification of core processes. Achieving cost savings through the elimination of nonvalue-adding activities such as supervision of recurring tasks underscores a principle that has been advanced by nurses during most of the twentieth century. Since managed care focused on outcomes, the nursing care that prevents hypostatic pneumonia, decubitus ulcers, fractured hips from falls, overmedication of the elderly, and undermedication of pain would be recognized. The nursing care that promotes wound healing, early treatment of dysrhythmias, immediate treatment of chemotherapy reactions, and faster recovery through critical pathways would at last be recognized and rewarded. Since patients would be discharged earlier, patient and family teaching would become central rather than peripheral to nursing practice. However, the outcomes of health care changes that occurred during the 1990s are well documented in the Institute of Medicine study on the costs and extent of health care errors.

That nurses would be dissatisfied with their practice arena is not surprising. The changing health care system has dramatically increased their workload, devalued their practice, dramatically reduced the margins of error, and resulted in harm to the patient.

WHY IS THIS HAPPENING?

Kersbergen (2000) has conceptually characterized these changes as the shift of health care from an altruistic to a business model. The enduring mismatch between the way in which nursing care is marketed and the way in which it is provided makes it centrally important for nurses to understand how reimbursement shifts changed historical relationships. This reimbursement climate inverts the physical/financial proximity relationship between nurses and patients (Patterson, 1992). As indicated in Fig. 2-1, nurses who are in closest proximity to patients are the most distant provider from the actual purchaser of care who determines what the care will be.

Although patients may want nursing care, the amount and type of care they will receive is negotiated through multiple parties (hospital financial officers, insurers, and employers) whose concerns are solely economic. At the same time, nurses and patients believe that nurses buffer patients from these same parties. Notably, the least knowledgeable persons, the purchasers of care (employer, insurance company) who will never be affected by the care, are the persons who determine care.

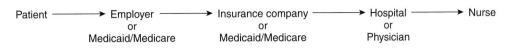

FIG. 2-1 Purchasing relationship between patient and nurse.

Second, in a competitive marketplace, two fundamental economic assumptions are operative: (1) scarce resources and (2) unlimited wants. Since buyers will always seek alternative ways to purchase goods or services at a lower cost, substitutes are used. Predictably, downward substitution rapidly occurred in health care (Patterson, 1992). These two economic principles predict that the extent of downward substitution will always be directly related to how knowledgeable the buyer (hospital, insurer, employer) is about nursing care.

Numbers—the Only Language in a Business Model

Nightingale was influential because she reduced mortality rates by 40%. She counted and made the data known. When numbers talk, nursing is reduced to a whisper when there are no data (Hadley, 1996). Historically nursing has justified patient care on a case-by-case basis rather than on aggregate data about populations of patients. Regrettably this language does not provide the cost-benefit data that are now required to justify cost. What is the medication error rate by nursing unit, by nurse, by type of nurse, or by skill mix? How many infection-free catheter days are normative for Foley catheters inserted by RNs vs. unlicensed persons? What is the fall rate for high-risk patients? What is the postoperative infection rate by procedure by unit? What happens to any of the above when the skill mix is changed?

Quantifying problems is not only essential for purchasers of care, who are nonproviders, but is equally essential and effective within hospitals. For example, take the common problem of a varying census on different nursing units that is experienced by all hospitals. In one hospital with this long-standing problem, a new nursing service administrator decided to define the problem, not in terms of percentages of occupancy as it is traditionally defined, but in terms of outcomes. Using an average month, the number of personnel moves to staff 100 beds was actually counted and found to be 400. When the hospital administrator was asked if he knew that it took 400 personnel moves to staff 100 beds in an average month, the problem became quickly definable in one sound byte. A consultant was immediately engaged for assistance.

Managed care manages health care services from a cost/benefit rather than altruistic perspective. Effectively providing care in this climate requires demonstrating the economic value of services. Clearly, the profession was not well positioned to thrive in this climate. However, historically the profession has not always considered the downstream effect of its actions.

Nursing's Contribution

Nursing literature indicates that the profession has been plagued by a number of problems. It is female dominated by people who are socialized to be anti-intellectuals as evidenced by the marginal percentage of nurses with advanced degrees. Further, the way in which nursing students are taught implies that for nurses knowledge is burdensome. Nursing professors admonish students to learn so that patients will be not be harmed or killed, while their medical counterparts teach their students that knowledge enables them to do something and subsequently, that knowledge is power (Christman, 1991; Barnum, 1991). Multiple education entry points blur the substantive difference in roles, creating confusion not only with the public, but also within the profession (Christman, 1991; Christman, 1998).

From a different perspective, Aaronson (1989) has contended that nursing fails to understand the basic premise of social exchange theory: societal rewards are in direct relationship to the scarcity of the service provided. By contrast, medicine understands it well. Following the release of the Flexner report (1910), which recommended the closure of 400 medical schools and the retention of only 35 high-quality university-based schools, medicine immediately closed these schools. Within 15 years of making that decision, medicine became the most highly valued occupation in the United States (Christman, 1998). Since that time, medicine has controlled the numbers of physicians and secured a legal monopoly as the sole gatekeeper to health care.

The response to the Flexner report is instructive because in 1910 medicine had a questionable knowledge base at best. On the other hand, in 1910 nursing was the one service that substantially reduced hospital mortality rates. Although nursing was far more powerful because of its demonstrated results, it was unwilling to use this influence. Nursing did not respond to similar reports and recommendations. Medicine is only one example; teachers are another. As Christman (1998) noted, nurses have been "studied more and have responded less" than other professional groups (p. 211).

Ninety-one years later nursing continues to exert no control over enrollments or length of the educational experience. Indeed, nurses continue to allow nonnurses to practice nursing. Although Bowman (1993) has rightfully indicated that individual nurses are not to "blame" for all of the image issues confronting the profession, individual nurses have made and continue to make contributions to the negative image of nursing.

Changing Physicians' Image of Nursing

An enduring mystery and common experience for nurses is how to address a medical problem with the primary customer of the hospital, the physician. Unlike the nurse who is an employee, the physician is an independent contractor who brings revenue in the form of patients to the employer of the nurse. Although physicians are revenue generators for health care agencies, in exchange for hospital privileges physicians agree to be self-governing and to abide by a set of medical staff bylaws. All medical staff bylaws include a disciplinary process that begins with the section chief who is required to address documented patient care problems.

Consider the following actual clinical situation.

A nephrologist complains in a meeting with a nursing service administrator, the Chief of Medical Staff, and the physician liaison that he is not being notified by nursing about his patients and that nurses do not know how to take care of his dialysis patients.

RESPONSE 1	ANALYSIS
Nurse 1 tells the nephrologist how well prepared the nursing staff are; this is the first complaint of this type that has been received.	Denies the problem
However, nursing is short-staffed, and there are a lot of agency nurses.	Excuses 1 and 2
She will investigate.	First positive response
However, without a specific incident and patient, she may not be	Excuse 3, which clearly conveys that nursing is not accountable and that the problem will continue able to directly address the problem.

RESPONSE 2	ANALYSIS
Nurse 2 carefully takes notes and limits her comments to clarifying comments while the physician becomes increasingly more derogatory. She concludes with the need to investigate and indicates that a written report will be sent to all parties. The physician is thanked for bringing this to her attention.	Positive action
The investigation indicates that multiple nurses over time and in different units have all phoned the nephrologist, who loudly announces that they have awakened his baby and abruptly hangs up the phone. Second, this is a difficult physician who never has time to discuss his patients when making rounds. Specific examples of unanswered questions are obtained.	
The written findings are prepared, and nurse 2 poses only one question, "Since the physician is not able to 'take calls' after 5:30 PM, the patient care issue that concerns nursing is the question of who will be covering his patients."	
Outcome: Within 2 weeks his hospital privileges were quietly rescinded.	

All too often, when nurses practice with a physician whose practice is substandard or who is highly volatile, they believe that this behavior is a nursing problem. Rather it is a medical problem that must be addressed by medicine via their staff bylaws. Only when nurses disengage, factually document the problem in patient care terms rather than in personality issues, and forward this in writing to a nurse manager *and* the appropriate section chief, can the problem be resolved.

Just as nursing's involvement with medical problems is confined to appropriate notification, so should medicine's involvement with nursing be. When a physician notifies and informs a nurse about a nursing problem, a more positive answer is, "Thank you. Let me investigate the problem and get back to you." Lengthy detailed discussions are seldom useful. When the nurse makes an error, a simple apology and sincere statement of corrective action is sufficient.

Second, ongoing problems between nurses and physicians are communication and time. Consider how often a physician is paged for a problem and phones the unit but no one knows the problem or who paged the physician. There may be a need for a change in orders, but the nurse who requested the order is away from the unit or engaged with another patient when the physician makes rounds. A simple note, such as a post-it note, works.

Effect of Communication Patterns on Image

In observing nurses, Buresch and Gordon (1996) have noted the ongoing subtle self-sabotage of nurses in multiple ways. Nurses refer to nurses by first name, whereas physicians are Dr. Last Name. During teaching rounds in hospitals noted for high nurse-physician collaboration, nurses frequently position themselves behind residents and interns, contributing little. Similarly, nurses and physicians differ in the way they approach each other. For example, when a nurse sought a physician to inquire about a patient issue and found her in discussion with another physician, the nurse left. However, minutes later, the same physician interrupted the nurse who was in conference with other nurses, who all allowed the interruption.

The Look of Nursing

In the 1970s nurses successfully shed the uniform of "authority in gleaming white" nursing cap, uniform, sensible shoes, and white hose that, according to Curtin (1994a), required pupil accommodation to adjust from the glare. Today nursing expresses its professional autonomy by dressing for success in the corporate boardrooms with business attire (Andrica, 1995).

Meanwhile, as one Emergency Department staff nurse wrote, staff nurses are in "T-shirts with Mickey Mouse logos, 'Run a Code Naked' and the name of a local bar; college sweatshirts, stretch pants, mismatched jogging suits . . . stained and wrinkled clothes (Zimmerman, 1996, p. 267), and tennis shoes. Although Zimmerman humorously notes that these nurses appeared to be dressed for a "come as you are party," they were in fact practicing in an Emergency Department. The clear message nurses are conveying is that the nurse should not be taken seriously and has little regard for the seriousness of the situations to be encountered.

And the Public Says . . .

Multiple studies indicate that consumers prefer the traditional white nursing uniform (Mangum et al., 1991; Kucera and Nieswiadomy, 1991). However, younger students and faculty are less conservative in their thinking than older students and faculty who prefer white uniforms (Newton and Chaney, 1996). Lehna and colleagues' study of nursing attire as an indicator of professionalism (1999) indicated that the 12 RNs and a layperson could not answer whether the changing dress of nurses projected a negative image nor could they describe professional dress other than as a total package that "they knew when they saw it." Nonetheless, few professionals wear pink, purple, and blue flowered shirts outside of a clinical area. Few adults wear wrinkled, faded, pajama-styled, drawstring clothing outside of their homes. In an Emergency Department where the normative attire of "scrubs" resulted in increasingly "sloppy," mismatched scrubs, a patient told a 28-year-old nurse dressed in a T-shirt and jogging pants that "you're just a kid out of high school telling me what to do" (Zimmerman, 1996).

Molloy (1996) indicated that airlines changed the attire for flight attendants when it was noticed that persons dressed in "cute" designer uniforms could not command the attention of passengers in an emergency. When attire was changed to a more business-like suit, flight attendants were better able to direct passengers and command attention in emergency situations. The current array of nursing attire projects an image statement that could not be occurring at a less opportune time. Although it is unlikely that nurses would return to gleaming "whites," conservatively colored "scrubs" with a white laboratory coat monogrammed with John Smith, RN, present a far more professional appearance than is currently found in many clinical settings. Notably, when professional nursing is being marginalized, the loss of a uniform appearance has resulted in the inability of patients and families to distinguish between the nurse and the housekeeper (Carpenito, 1995).

BELIEVE IN NURSING

Creating a different image and a different reality requires one simple action. Nurses have to believe in nursing, in who nurses are, and in what nurses do. This requires valuing nursing; valuing the name of nursing; and reclaiming the name, the birthright, and the practice.

Valuing Nursing

Everyone employed in a nursing department is not a nurse. Although this may seem to be an obvious observation, nurses *behave* as if it were true. Consider how often nursing staff meetings include all staff nurses, assistants, ward clerks, and so on. Nurses need to be the first people to ask why. Discussions of unit problems or directions for the future need to be held first and separately with professional nurses. The dialog would be considerably different and far more useful. Including everyone in a staff meeting indicates to assistive staff that they are expected to offer opinions about professional nursing practice.

Although the initial response to separate staff meetings may be that it would be too time-consuming, the alternative is far more likely. The time would be spent far more productively for nurses and other staff. Although nurse managers periodically meet with other hospital managers, they more frequently have nurse manager meetings to discuss care issues that involve nursing.

The devaluing of nursing occurs daily in discussions with patients, families, and physicians. Ninety-nine percent of the time when an intervention occurs with a patient in a hospital or home health care agency, it is the nurse who recognized the problem (Reichstein, 1991; Gordon, 1997).

Reclaiming the Name of Nurse

As the International Congress of Nursing (ICN) determined in 1985, the term "nurse" is reserved for an RN (Holleran, 1991). Referring to anyone else or allowing anyone else to use this title undermines the profession. Nurses should not introduce an aide, a multiskilled worker, or a licensed practical/vocational nurse (LPN or LVN) to a patient, family, physician, or anyone else, as Mr. Smith's nurse. The only person with the legal scope of practice in all 50 states to be anyone's NURSE is an RN. The LPN is a valuable assistant created to do the "practical" tasks, hence the name. However, all nursing practice acts require nursing care to be planned and directed by an RN. Introducing anyone else in the role of THE NURSE is misleading. A patient care assistant is identified to others as the nurses' assistant. Similarly, health teaching, advice, direction, and progress reports to patients, physicians, or others comes only from THE NURSE. When nurses meet patients, they advise them that their questions should be directed to THE NURSE, not the assistant.

In more and more settings nurses are encountering employers who refer to all employees, including professional nursing staff, as associates. In some settings nurses are being prohibited from including the designation *RN* on their nametags. Monogrammed scrubs and laboratory coats with first initial, last name, RN, avoids this discussion.

On a daily basis news stories identify many people as nurses who are not RNs. When this occurs, the public believes that a nurse did whatever is being reported. The image of nursing will improve when all nurses correct inaccurate labeling of nurses and false assumptions.

Reclaiming Personal Identity

Gordon (1994), a journalist intrigued by the image of nursing, made two significant observations about the way in which nurses refer to themselves and to other nurses. The first is the increasingly common use of first names, which is deadly for the profession since "nonpersons have only first names." However, nurses often introduce themselves as "Hi, I'm Susie and I'm your nurse." As Curtin (1994b) humorously noted, "The mind boggles at the thought of a physician introducing himself in like manner: 'Hi! I'm Dick, I'm your doctor,' or a lawyer greeting a client with 'Hi! I'm Larry the lawyer' " (p. 10). Second, the method used to dehumanize people to encourage their conformity is to remove their name. For this reason, prisoners are not referred to by their name. The use of first names, no names, and referral to everyone as the nurse has led to professional concerns that patients have no idea who the nurse is (Letters, 1996). More important, the information they may receive from the nursing assistant may well be believed to be from the RN.

Although some nurses have claimed that the use of a last name may place them in danger, this is a difficult claim to support. However, prominently wearing a hospital identification badge with full name, social security number, and other identifiers may. Nurses who are proud of their profession and take pride in their accountability are proud to use their last name in a professional setting.

In a Southern California Kaiser hospital, RNs began using business cards when a nurse manager noticed that, after an Emergency Department nurse instructed a patient to phone if there were any problems, the patient asked for her name and number, which the nurse had to sheepishly write on a scrap piece of paper (Bream and Poblador, 1995). To implement this change, nurses first had to become comfortable giving patients, families, or unfamiliar physicians their business card.

Initially nursing resistance occurred because they did not believe "it" was important. "It" was their personal identification as a nurse. Second, some were concerned that if they had no credentials after their name other than RN, they would appear less knowledgeable. Third and most important, some preferred anonymity because they were concerned about being too identifiable and therefore accountable. Ironically, after a year of use, business cards made it possible for patients to proclaim to others the excellence of the nurse's practice.

Reclaiming the Birthright

Before anyone else believed that a nurse extender could replace nurses, nurses gave away their role to others through patient assignments. Curtin (1994a) astutely indicated that the place of the nursing assistant, LPN/LVN, multiskilled worker, or whoever else may be invented is *not* at the bedside. His or her place is at the side of nurses. These roles were designed to extend, not replace.

Changing the Song

As Mattera (1999) notes, turning to Landers, a syndicated columnist, is probably not the best approach to solving the problem. In her January 27, 1999 syndicated column, Ann Landers wrote: "I've had a ton of letters with a litany of complaints (from nurses). The profession is clearly in a state of jeopardy. And now I would like some suggestions on how to fix it." Mattera's frustrated response indicated that "two million creative problem solvers ought to be able to fix the things that are bothering nurses without jeopardizing the hospital bottom line. Because if you can't accept the reality that hospitals need to exist at a certain profit level, and figure that into your problem-solving, then you'll have designed a perfect nursing environment that no one will put into practice" (p. 7).

On a More Positive Note

Notice how often nurses, who are widely accepting of patients from different backgrounds, different cultures, and different perspectives, are unable to think positively about others in health care. For nursing to be valued, medical care cannot be valued. For health promotion to be valued, illness care cannot be valued. Valuing critical care practice requires devaluing wellness care. For associate degree education to be valued, baccalaureate education is not. For baccalaureate education to be valued, graduate education is not. For graduate education to be positive, doctoral education is not. For female nurses to be valued, male nurses are not. For day nurses to be good at what they do, night nurses are not. For collective bargaining to be useful, those who do not bargain collectively do not care. For staff nurses to be positive, nurse managers must be negative. For nurse managers to be positive, nursing administrators must be negative. In short, for any nurse who perceives any other nurse to be different in any way requires that one or the other must be negatively viewed.

The context for nursing has not changed since Nightingale sat in the snow waiting to be allowed to enter the hospital at Scutari. Instead of collectively going head to head with those who oppose nursing practice, contemporary nurses have gone head to head with each other as they epitomized the sociologic concept of "like against like," termed *horizontal violence,* that is highly indicative of oppressed group behavior (Roberts, 2000).

For far too long, many nurses consider any professional issue in terms of a personal involvement. If it does not affect me, it is somebody else's problem. Nurses who disagree with some minor component disagree with the entirety in public and in private. Imagine the difference if nurses told everyone what nurses do well and confined the disagreements in-house. What if nurses thought carefully before disagreeing with each other about minor issues to thoughtfully conserve energy for important issues? What if nurses looked to each other rather than everyone else for consultation and assistance.

Valuing the Future of the Profession

In 1875 Dr. Howard, a Montreal medical professor, suggested that the new nursing profession should require the same preliminary education as the medical profession requires, with the exceptions that natural science should have a higher place than the classics and professional education should extend over 3 years. Howard was quickly drowned out by numerous medical papers in the late 1800s and early 1900s that argued to "attempt to give nurses instruction as to the reason why . . . would be, in the majority of instances, to inflict a heavy task upon them and to lift them more or less out of their proper sphere . . . to give them more than an insight into it is to demand for them complete education as medical practitioners. . . ." Similarly, Aaronson (1989) cites the president of the Pennsylvania State Board of Medical Examiners who said in 1909 that "The instruction commonly prevalent in hospital training schools is not only absurdly too comprehensive, but dangerous. It is sufficient to almost entirely result in nurses assuming the right to usurp the functions of physicians."

As health care becomes increasingly more complex, nursing remains the only health profession that vehemently claims to require less education. Christman (1998) rightfully notes that "knowledge not possessed" cannot be used by even the most highly motivated of nurses. With the expansion of science doubling exponentially every 2 years, the nursing educational issue becomes less understandable (Christman, 1998).

While nurses were debating the "issue" for 30 years, physical therapy moved from baccalaureate to graduate education, and pharmacists moved from a baccalaureate to a doctoral program while obtaining excellent physical assessment skills and the right to administer medications. The interesting question posed by Christman (1991) is how nursing could justify the "ethics of deliberately and willfully withholding the benefits of science from patients by preserving mediocre preparation" (p. 212).

The irony is the 1965 entry into practice issue would have benefited all nurses since all RNs would retain their licenses. Notably, changing the educational requirements for nursing education has never required "opening" any nursing practice act for legislative approval.

Changing the rules and regulations for education is within the purview of the state Boards of Nursing comprised of nurses. Entry into practice is an issue that affects the future, not the present. Imagine how different history would be today if a different path had been chosen. Notably, in Australia diploma nurses were the strongest supporters of baccalaureate entry into practice. Following minimal discussion, baccalaureate education is their national requirement.

CREATING A NEW IMAGE

Envision a new world where nurses value nursing, and image it daily. Nurses take themselves seriously and dress the part. Nurses are highly visible to patients, families, and physicians because they have reclaimed their birthright and their practice. Since nurses are clear about the role boundaries between themselves and those who extend their practice, others are also. Nurses are "stuck like glue" together. Negative comments about a colleague are made to the colleague and to no one else. Professional nurses recognize that their greatest benefit—and one of the most efficient and powerful uses for their money—is the less than 1% of their salary that they spend for membership in the American Nurses Association, the National League for Nursing, Sigma Theta Tau International, and their specialty organization. They look forward to annual meetings because they provide an excellent opportunity to meet colleagues and discuss issues and practice innovations.

Since all nursing is valued, nurses recognize the value of caring, health promotion, and health teaching, as well as the value of illness care. They celebrate that nurses save lives everyday. In the modern medical climate, nurses supervise assistive personnel and use their authority to ensure that patient care delivery is excellent. Nurses value nursing's metaphor as mothering, class struggle, equality, and conscience for medicine (Fagin and Diers, 1983) because it is worn with style. To this legacy they add astute businessperson, researcher, caregiver for the family, and entrepreneur.

In this new world nurses believe in nursing, in self, and in their colleagues. It is significant to the future of nursing that nurses safeguard nursing's public image in local newspapers, television and media dramas, and daily practice (Box 2-2). However, nurses must realize that they themselves play a part in forming the image of nursing on a daily basis.

BOX 2-2 *Helpful Websites*

American Nurses' Association Press Releases
www.nursingworld.org/pressrel/2001/index.htm

American Association of Colleges of Nursing Press Releases
www.aacn.nche.edu/Media/NewsReleases/newslist.htm

National League for Nursing Press Releases
www.nln.org/pressreleases/index.htm

Sigma Theta Tau International Nursing Honor Society-Media
www.nursingsociety.org/

Critical Thinking Activities

1. The earliest Western image of nursing is that of patient advocate in 1900 BC. Four thousand years later, what is nursing's highest priority advocacy role in contemporary society?
2. Recent studies have indicated that nurses are the most highly trusted health professional group. What component of nursing's contemporary image places nurses in this position of trust? What threatens this position?
3. You are a trauma nurse who takes care of a U.S. Senator following a life-threatening car accident. He credits you with saving his life. When he becomes president, he invites you to the White House and asks you to tell him the most important thing he can do to reform the health care system. In one sentence, what would you say?
4. In an ideal health care setting, what would be the most important image of nursing?
5. If you wanted to artistically portray a twenty-first century nurse, what would the nurse be wearing?

REFERENCES

Aaronson LS: A challenge for nursing: re-viewing a historic competition, *Nurs Outlook* 37(6):274-279, 1989.

Aides relieve nursing shortage, *Life* 12(1):32-34, 36, 1942.

American Association of Colleges of Nursing: With demand for RNs climbing, and shortening supply, forecasters say what's ahead isn't typical shortage cycle, *AACN Iss Bull,* February, 1998.

American Association of Colleges of Nursing: *Nursing school enrollments decline as demand for RNs continues to climb,* Washington, DC, February 17, 2000, AACN.

Andrica DC: Professional image: What counts? *Nurs Econ* 13(6):375, 1995.

Barnum B: Nursing's image and the future, *Nurs Health Care* 12(1):19-21, 1991.

Bowman AM: Victim blaming in nursing, *Nurs Outlook* 41(6):268-273, 1993.

Brannon RL: Restructuring hospital services: reversing the trend toward a professional work force, *Int J Health Serv* 26(4):642-654, 1996.

Bream TL, Poblador A: Business cards at the bedside, *Am J Nurs* 95 (2), 71-72, 1995.

Buerhaus PI, Staiger DO, Auerbach DI: Why are shortages of hospital RNs concentrated in specialty care units, *Nurs Econ* 18 (3):111-116, 2000.

Buresch B, Gordon S: Subtle self-sabotage, *Am J Nurs* 96(4):22-24, 1996.

Buresch B, Gordon S, Bell N: Who counts in news coverage of health care? *Nurs Outlook* 39(5):204-208, 1991.

Carnegie ME: *Paths we tread: blacks in nursing worldwide, 1854-1994,* ed 3, New York, 1995, National League for Nursing Press Pub. No. 14-2678.

Carpenito LJ: Bring back the nurse's cap (editorial), *Nurs Forum* 30 (4):3-4, 1995.

Christman L: Perspectives on role socialization of nurses, *Nurs Outlook* 39(5):209-212, 1991.

Christman L: Who is a nurse? *Image: J Nurs Scholarship* 30 (3):211-215, 1998.

Coffman S: Home-care nurses as strangers in the family, *West J Nurs Res* 19(1):82-96, 1997.

Crawshaw J: Critical care nursing shortage is nationwide, *Crit Care Alert* 8 (9):105, 2000.

Cunningham, A: Nursing stereotypes. Nursing Standard, 13(45) 46-47, 1999.

Curtin L:. The heart of patient care (editorial opinion), *Nurs Manage* 25(5):7-8, 1994a.

Curtin L: 25 years: a slightly irreverent retrospective, *Nurs Manage* 25(6):9-32, 1994b.

Dickens C: *Martin Chuzzlewit,* New York, 1910, Macmillan Co.

Diers D: The mystery of nursing: Secretary's Commission on Nursing: support studies and background information, vol II, Rockville, Md, 1988, Department of Health and Human Services, pp VIII-1-VIII-10.

Diers D: On waves . . . , *Image: J Nurs Scholarship* 24(1):2, 1992.

Donahue MP: *Nursing: the finest art: an illustrated history,* St Louis, 1985, Mosby.

Fagin C, Diers D: Nursing as metaphor, *N Engl J Med* (2):116-117, 1983.

Fiedler LA: Images of the nurse in fiction and popular culture. In Jones AH, editor: *Images of nurses: perspectives from history, art, and literature,* Philadelphia, 1988, University of Pennsylvania Press.

Flexner A: *Medical education in the United States and Canada,* New York, 1910, Carnegie Foundation.

Floyd A: The public's use of nurses for health care advice, *J Nurs Scholarship* 32(3):220, 2000.

The Gallup Organization, Healthcare (September 11-13, 2000). Retrieved January 26, 2000(a) from the World Wide Web: www.gallup.com/poll/indicators/indhealth2.asp

The Gallup Organization. Honesty/ethics in the professions (November, 2000). Retrieved January 26, 2000(b) from the World Wide Web: www.gallup.com/poll/indicators/indhnsty_ethcs2.asp

Gordon S: Guest editorial. What's in a name? *J Emerg Nurs* 20(3):170, 1994.

Gordon S: What nurses stand for, *Atlantic Monthly* 279(2):81-88, 1997.

Grando V: Making do with fewer nurses in the United States, 1945-1965, *Image: J Nurs Scholarship* 30 (2):147-149, 1998.

Hadley EH: Nursing in the political and economic marketplace: challenges for the 21st century, *Nurs Outlook* 44(1):6-10, 1996.

Holleran C: Inside view. Was it a nurse? Why the confusion? *Int Nurs Rev* 38(3):62, 1991.

Huffstutler SY et al: The public's image of nursing as described to baccalaureate prenursing students, *J Professional Nurs* 14(1):7-13, 1998.

Jaklevic MC, Lovern E: A nursing code blue: few easy solutions seen for a national RN shortage that's different from prior undersupplies, *Mod Healthcare* 30(12):42-44, 2000.

Jones AH, editor: Images of Nurses: *Perspectives from history, art, and literature,* Philadelphia, 1988, University of Pennsylvania Press.

Kalisch PA, Kalisch BJ: *The advance of American nursing,* ed 3, Philadelphia, 1995, JB Lippincott.

Kampen MB: Before Florence Nightingale: a prehistory of nursing in painting and sculpture. In Jones AH, editor: *Images of nurses: perspectives from history, art, and literature,* Philadelphia, 1988, University of Pennsylvania Press.

Kelly LS: Editorial. Image, niceness and the illusion of quality, *Nurs Outlook* 37(6):5, 1989.

Kersbergen AL: Managed care shifts health care from an altruistic model to a business framework, *Nurs Health Care Perspect* 21(2):81-86, 2000.

Kesey K: *One flew over the cuckoo's nest,* New York, 1962, New American Library/Signet.

Kingsley K: The architecture of nursing. In Jones AH, editor: *Images of nurses: perspectives from history, art, and literature,* Philadelphia, 1988, University of Pennsylvania Press.

Kitson AL: John Hopkins address: does nursing have a future? *Image: J Nurs Scholarship* 29(2):111-115, 1997.

Kucera KA, Nieswiadomy RM: Nursing attire: the public's preference, *Nursing Manage* 22(10):68-70, 1991.

Lehna C et al: Nursing attire: indicators of professionalism, *J Professional Nurs* 15(3):192-199, 1999.

Letters to Debates and disputes, *Nursing '96* 16 (2):6, 1996.

Lippman DT, Ponton KS: Nursing's image on the university campus, *Nurs Outlook* 37(1):24-27, 1989.

Lippman DT, Ponton KS: The image of nursing among high school guidance counselors, *Nurs Outlook* 41:129-134, 1993.

Longfellow HW: Santa Filomena, *Atlantic Monthly* 1 (11):22-23, 1857.

Lusk B: Professional classifications of American nurses, 1910-1935, *West J Nurs Res* 19(2):227-242, 1997.

Mangum S et al: Perceptions of nurses' uniforms, *Image: J Nurs Scholarship* 32(2):127-130, 1991.

Mattera MD: Ann Landers, again! *RN* 62(3):7, 1999.

McConnell EA: Making the invisible visible, *Nursing '95,* 24(4):53-54, 1995.

Mills A, Blaesing SL: A lesson from the last nursing shortage: the influence of work values on career satisfaction with nursing, *J Nurs Admin* 30(6):309-315, 2000.

Molloy J: *The new woman's dress for success,* New York, 1996, Warner Books.

Morrow H: Nurses, nursing, and women, *Int Nurs Rev* 35(1):22-25, 27, 1988.

Muff J: Of images and ideals: a look at socialization and sexism in nursing. In Jones AH, editor: *Images of nurses: perspectives from history, art, and literature,* Philadelphia, 1988, University of Pennsylvania Press.

Newton M, Chaney J: Professional image: enhanced or inhibited by attire? *J Professional Nurs* 12 (4):240-244, 1996.

Norman EM: *We band of angels: the untold story of American nurses trapped on Bataan by the Japanese,* New York, 1999, Random House.

Patterson C: The economic value of nursing, *Nurs Econ* 10(3):192-203, 1992.

Pritchett P: *New work habits for a radically changing world,* Dallas, 1996, Pritchett and Associates.

Q and A: *J Emerg Nurs* 21(12):165-166, 1995.

Richardson J: Let our voices build, not destroy, *J Nurs Admin* 23(6):5, 1993.

Reichstein J: Let's make nursing the visible profession, *Nursing '91* 11:148-149, 1991.

Roberts SJ: Development of a positive professional identity: liberating oneself from the oppressor within, *Adv Nurs Sci* 224:71-82, 2000.

Shindul-Rothchild J, Berry D, Long-Middleton E: Where have all the nurses gone? Final results of our patient care survey, *Am J Nurs* 96(11):24-39, 1996.

Schweitzer SF et al: The image of the staff nurse, *Nurs Manage* 25(6):88-89, 1994.

Sigma Theta Tau International: *The Woodhull study on nursing and the media: health care's invisible partner,* Indianapolis, 1998, Sigma Theta Tau Center Nursing Press.

Tomey AM et al: Students' perceptions of ideal and nursing career choices, *Nurs Outlook* 44:27-30, 1996.

Vonnegut K Jr: *Welcome to the monkey house,* London, 1968, Jonathan Cape.

White KR, Begun KW: Profession building in the new health care system, Nurs Admin Q 20(3):79-85, 1996.

Wood W: Demeaning portrayal of RNs angers AONE, *Nurseweek* 10(12):3, 1997.

Woody M: Future practice, *Reflect Nursing Leadership,* First Quarter, 2000, p 34.

Zimmerman PG: Guest Editorial. Dressing the part, *J Emerg Nurs* 22(8):267-268, 1996.

SUGGESTED READINGS

American Nurses Association: *Nursing's agenda for health care reform,* Washington, DC, 1992, American Nurses Publishing.

Anderson CA: From the editor: Are nurses becoming invisible? *Nurs Outlook* 43(3):103-104, 1995.

Kaler SR, Levy DA, Schall M: Stereotypes of professional roles, *Image: J Nurs Scholarship* 21(2):85-89, 1989.

Theories of Nursing Practice

3

Margaret Soderstrom, PhD, RN, CS-P, ARNP, and Linda C. Pugh, PhD, RNC

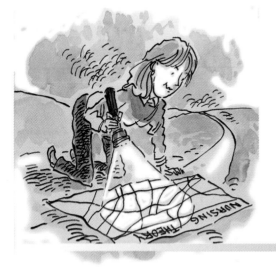

Nursing theory provides the direction
for research practice.

*Science is built up with facts, as a house is with stones. But a collection of facts is no more
a science than a heap of stones a house . . .*

JULES HENRI POINCARE, 1909, FRENCH SCIENTIST AND MATHEMATICIAN

Vignette

The little boy kicked the stone, using first one shoed foot, then the other. He did not pay much attention until he saw the shiny marks showing through the stone's surface. Only then did he stop and pick it up. Something about its composition fascinated him. It was at that moment that he heard his mother call and ran off in the direction of her voice. The stone sat for weeks as layers of dirt gathered on it. Another stone, swept against it by the wind, comfortably nestled close. Over time the two stones gathered substance as they continued to attract other stones of various sizes and shapes. The pile of stones became larger in height and width. Adjoining stones varied in form and content. Eventually, as one might imagine, quite a mass developed. Years later, a man who was a scientist noticed a large hill composed of stones. Out of the corner of his eye, he observed a shiny surface on one of the stones located near the bottom. It was somehow familiar. Curious, he carefully studied the hill before him. Slowly, he began separating the many stones into piles, organizing and defining what initially appeared to be scattered meaningless entities. Eventually he used scientific equipment to assist in this endeavor. There were occasional setbacks, each assisting in providing feedback and refining the process. Once sorted, the purpose of every item became evident. Each one was carefully laid. He could finally accept the premise. It was the beginning, a scientific foundation for future ideas and the generation of new directions. It remained consistently sturdy, resilient, and withstood the test of time.

MARGARET SODERSTROM, 2001

Questions to consider while reading this chapter
1.   What is nursing theory?
2.   How is nursing theory different from the theory of other disciplines?
3.   How does theory relate to nursing practice?

Key Terms

Nursing science The collection and organization of data related to nursing and its associated components. The purpose of this data collection is to provide a body of scientific knowledge, which provides the basis for nursing practice.

Nursing theory The compilation of data that defines, describes, and logically relates information that will explain past nursing phenomena and predict future trends. Theories provide a foundation for developing models or frameworks for nursing practice development.

Concept An idea or a general impression. Concepts are the basic ingredients of theory; examples of nursing concepts include health, stress, and adaptation.

Conceptual model Deals with concepts that are associated because of their relevance to a common theme.

Construct Labels given to ideas, objects, or events.

Proposition Statement that proposes the relationship between and among concepts.

Schematic model A diagram or visual representation of concepts, conceptual models, *or* theory.

Learning Outcomes

After studying this chapter, the reader will be able to:
1.   Differentiate between a science and a theory.
2.   Identify the criteria necessary for science.
3.   Identify the criteria necessary for theory.
4.   Explain a nursing theory and a nursing model.
5.   Discuss two early and two contemporary nursing theorists and their theories.
6.   Explain the impact of nursing theory on the profession of nursing.

CHAPTER OVERVIEW

Nursing theory is to nursing as world history is to the world. Without an idea of where one has been, how can one know how, why, when, or where to go? Nursing theory provides nurses with a focus for research and practice. One may consider using a theory as one considers using a map or a flashlight that guides direction while making available a variety of ways to get where one is going. Yet it has been a curiosity to note that the worth of studying nursing theorists and their theories and the role of responsibility these theories contribute toward the evolution of nursing science has been under appreciated. Odd though it may sound, some of the naysayers tend to be nursing students. Nursing theory is not usually the favorite subject of undergraduates who would much rather practice technical "hands-on" skills. Whether this is a maturation issue or an issue of knowledge and experience remains undetermined by nursing faculty and the profession itself. The philosopher Eden Phillpots said, "The universe is full of things patiently waiting for our wits to get sharper" (Bronowski, 1972). Let us hope they will.

This chapter in no way reflects the breadth and depth of nursing theorists and their theories. There are many scholarly works devoted to this topic. Instead, it is a survey, a general overview, a smattering of nursing theories, with chosen segments that are intended to assist in providing the idea, the notion, and indeed, the semblance of what a theory is and how it is critical to the profession of nursing. Readers interested in perusing the theoretic basis for nursing practice will find resources for further exploration at the end of the chapter.

SCIENCE AND THEORY

Science is a method of bringing together facts and giving them coherence and integrity. Science assists one in understanding how the unique yet related parts of a structure fit and become more than the individual parts summed. In the above metaphor the stones represent the facts, the process of laying the stones represents the science, and the future ideas and new directions represent the theory.

Science is both dynamic and static: dynamic in figuring out how a phenomenon happens, static in describing what happens. The criteria for a scientific inquiry involve five aspects: hypothesis, method, data collection, results, and evaluation. These five aspects are described in Box 3-1.

A theory is defined as a group of related concepts that explain existing phenomena and predict future events (Barnum, 2000). Theory development functions in a parallel manner to

---

BOX 3-1	*The Five Aspects of Scientific Inquiry*

Hypothesis
Ask the question that is to be the main focus. It usually includes independent and dependent variables.

Method
Decide what data will be collected to answer the question. Decide on and identify the step-by-step procedure that will be used to collect these data. Make sure this process can be easily replicated.

Data collection
Implement the step-by-step procedure that has been determined to answer the question.

Results
On the conclusion of the data collection, statistically identify the outcomes. Establish parameters (e.g., level of significance) that will determine whether or not the data are relevant.

Evaluation
Examine the results to determine the relevance of outcome data in answering the hypothesis. Determine the significance and identify the potential for future research.

scientific process. It is a microanalytic part of the whole macroanalytic scientific process. Even though Freud and Jung each had their individual theories about the psychology of man, their theories were focused on specific ideas taken from the entire knowledge base surrounding psychology and psychotherapy and its scientific premise. Similarly, Albert Einstein's theory of relativity was but a fraction of the existing scientific knowledge base of mathematics at the time. Yet it is an undisputed fact that these theorists changed the thinking of the time and were responsible for the evolution of their philosophic and scientific interests (Anastasi, 1958). The criterion for theory acceptance involves six factors: inclusiveness, consistency, accuracy, relevance, fruitfulness, and simplicity. See Box 3-2 for an explanation of these six factors.

The importance of theories in the evolution of science is unquestioned. Nursing has evolved as a profession and as a science in a similar manner. Nursing theories have explained, explored, defined, and delineated specific areas. Beginning with the work of Florence Nightingale in 1860, nursing theorists have taken the vast pool of scientific information available and focused on precise target areas of interest. In so doing, theoretic models have been conceptualized to guide nursing actions, interventions, and implementation.

Nursing Science

As might be expected, there are several definitions of nursing science (Abdellah, 1969; Jacox, 1974). Although these definitions differ, they generally support the premise that, simply put, nursing science is a collection of data related to nursing that may be applied to the practice of nursing. These data encompass a vast array of knowledge that spans all of nursing and its

---

BOX 3-2	*Criterion for Theory Acceptance*

Inclusiveness
Does the theory include all concepts related to the area of interest?

Consistency
Can the theory address new entities without having its founding assumptions changed?

Accuracy
Does the theory explain retrospective occurrences? Does the theory maintain its capacity to predict future outcomes?

Relevance
Does the theory relate to the scientific foundation from which it is derived? Is it reflective of the scientific base?

Fruitfulness
Does the theory generate new directions for future research?

Simplicity
Does the theory provide a road map for replication? Is it simple to follow? **DOES IT MAKE SENSE?**

diversity. This knowledge guides the practice of nursing to better serve clients through prevention, education, and health maintenance.

Theories, Models, and Frameworks

"Theories and conceptual models are the primary mechanisms by which researchers organize findings into a broader conceptual context" (Polit, Beck, and Hungler, 2001, p.144). Different terms are used in relation to conceptual contexts for research. These terms include theories, models, frameworks, schemes, and maps. Terms are often used differently by different writers resulting in a blurring of terms (Polit, Beck, and Hungler, 2001).

Theory. Theory is generally considered an abstract generalization that presents a systematic explanation about how phenomena are interrelated. Therefore traditionally a theory must have at least two concepts that are related in a way that the theory explains (Polit, Beck, and Hungler, 2001).

Conceptual Model. A conceptual model deals with concepts that are assembled because of their relevance to a common theme. The term conceptual framework is used interchangeably with conceptual model. Conceptual models, or frameworks, also provide a conceptual perspective regarding interrelated phenomena, but they are more loosely structured than theories. There are many conceptual models of nursing that offer broad explanations of the nursing process. Four concepts basic to nursing that are included in these models are: (1) nursing, (2) person, (3) health, and (4) environment. The various nursing models define these concepts differently, link the concepts in various ways, and emphasize differently the relationships among the concepts. For example, Roy's Adaptation Model emphasizes the patient's adaptation as a central phenomenon, whereas Martha Rogers emphasizes centrality of the individual as a unified whole. Theses models are used by nurse researchers to formulate research questions and hypotheses.

The terms conceptual model or framework and nursing theory are often used interchangeably. In this chapter the nursing theories described may also be referred to as conceptual models. The term model is also used in reference to a diagram depicting the theory. In this chapter the term model will refer to a schematic model, which is a diagram or visual representation of the conceptual model or theory.

Nursing Theory

Theory and theoretic thinking guide research and practice. The basic ingredients of theory are concepts. Examples of nursing concepts include health, stress, and adaptation. Propositions are statements that propose the relationship between and among concepts (Polit, Beck and Hungler, 2001). Theories provide us with a frame of reference, the ability to choose concepts to study, or ideas that are within one's practice. A theory helps guide research, and research helps validate theory.

In the research model the researcher decides what to study and how and why the area of interest is important to the practice of nursing. In the practice model the clinician decides what areas to directly assess, when to assess, and which intervention to implement. These decisions may or may not be knowingly based on a model or theory. Regardless, often the outcome supports the notion that behavior replicates a theoretic model, even though the clinician may be unaware that he or she is using a theoretic model in the practice process.

TABLE 3-1	*The Language of Nursing Theory*	
LANGUAGE OF NURSING THEORY	**DEFINITION**	**EXAMPLES**
Concept	Labels given to ideas, objects, events; a summary of thoughts or a way to categorize thoughts or ideas	Comfort, fatigue, pain, depression, environment
Construct	A group of concepts; they are deliberately invented	Intelligence, motivation, learned helplessness, obesity
Conceptual Model	A structure to organize concepts (ideas)	Roy's *Adaptation Model*
Philosophy	Values and beliefs of the discipline	Watson's *Philosophy and Science of Caring*
Theory	The organization of concepts or constructs that shows the relationship of the ideas with the intention of describing, explaining, or predicting; the purpose is to make scientific findings meaningful and generalizable; our goal in science has been to explain, predict, and **CONTROL!**	Self-care, adaptation, caring, behavioral system, unitary man, hierarchy of needs, interpersonal relationship, humanistic, nurse-client transactions

Just as in any other area-specific unit, nursing theory has its own unique language. The words of this language identify linkages between the database of scientific nursing knowledge and the extracted information taken from this source for nursing theory. The interpretation of these words translates uniquely to the theory investigated. This application, or language of nursing theory, is the structure, or framework, from which one understands the theory. Table 3-1 presents the language of nursing theory, along with definitions and examples.

Schematic Models

A schematic model is something that demonstrates concepts, usually with a picture. It is a visual representation of ideas. The model depicts concepts and shows how the concepts are related with the use of images such as arrows and dotted lines (Polit, Beck, and Hungler, 2001). For example, a blueprint is a pictorial demonstration of a particular type of house one might build. A model airplane is a detailed miniature replication of the original full sized version. Diagramming a sentence outlines the specific parts (adverb, adjective, verb, subject, object, phrases) that make that particular sentence complete. Similarly, a nursing model gives a visual diagram or picture of concepts. Whether that is a critical pathway, decision tree, medication protocol, or other nursing related practice, the model allows one to view the interrelated parts of the whole in picture form. A model of a nursing theory does the same thing. From the earliest model, offered by Florence Nightingale, nursing theory has been described and explained using this medium. Schematic models are used for clarifying complex concepts. The language of theory is translated into picture form, offering a comprehensive view, or model, of the theory. The schematic model shows how the concepts are related. A model, like a blueprint of a building, allows one to see the layout, including outlines of all features specific to the theory. Although it is not the same as understanding every minute detail about the structure, its intent is to provide an overview, which at a glance is informative and descriptive.

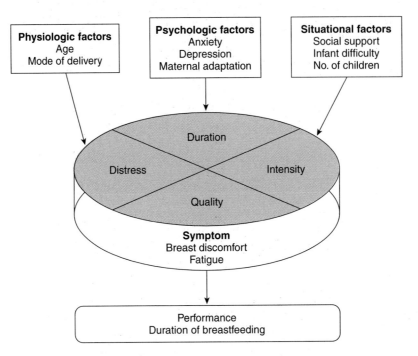

FIG. 3-1 The theory of unpleasant symptoms.

Levels of Theory

Many persons refer to the level of a nursing theory, which can range from broad in scope to a smaller, more specific scope. For example, Grand Theory is often broad in scope and may describe and explain large segments of human experience. Rogers' Theory of Unitary Man describes the entire nursing process. Other levels include Middle Range Theory and Practice Theory, which are smaller in scope and may refer to a specific population such as Jacob's Grief of Older Women (Jacob, 1996) or to a specific situation such as Good and Moore's balance between analgesia and side effects (Good and Moore, 1998). Today nurses often use these middle range theories that are smaller in scope and simpler to understand to guide their daily practice.

An example of a theory that is smaller in scope is the Theory of Unpleasant Symptoms (Lenz et al., 1997), which examines symptoms that are influenced by physiologic, psychologic, and situational factors as they relate to performance. The model of this theory is presented in Fig. 3-1.

FLORENCE NIGHTINGALE: THE FIRST NURSING THEORIST

If theory means to put concepts in a form in which relationships are described and predictions are made, then Florence Nightingale was the first nursing theorist. Nightingale did not deliberately set out to develop theory; rather her goal was to ease the suffering of soldiers and citizens of England. However, many important influences in her life directed her toward theory development:

- A classic education (philosophy [science], French, Italian, Greek, Latin, the arts, and history)

BOX 3-3	*Nightingale's Definitions of Nursing*

Nursing is an art, and an art requiring an organized practical and scientific training.
Nursing is putting us in the best possible conditions for nature to preserve health—to prevent or restore or to cure disease or injury.
Nursing is therefore to help the patient live.

- Upper class life, great wealth, and a prominent social life (operas, parties, balls)
- Religion and spirituality (she spent much time daydreaming about how she could serve God and experienced four visions from God)
- Era of reform throughout England (Industrial Revolution and dichotomy among the classes)

Despite her wealth and upper class existence, Miss Nightingale was very dissatisfied with life. In 1852 she wrote a monograph, *Cassandra,* and pointed out the hopelessness inherent in being a woman in this day. "The family? It is too narrow a field for the development of an immortal spirit . . . . The system dooms some minds to incurable infancy, others to silent misery. Marriage is the only chance (and it is but a chance) offered to women for escape from this death; and how eagerly and how ignorantly it is embraced" (Nightingale, 1992, pp. 37-38). Her diary writings have been interpreted at times to be suicidal. Often depressed, Nightingale resorted to dreams as an escape from her unhappiness and discontent. Her personality and her own individual lifestyle (dogmatic, practical, a critical observer who was fascinated by numbers and recorded everything she saw and experienced) set her apart. She was self-willed, unhappy, and dissatisfied at times in spite of having beauty, a brilliant social career, and an education of which few men of her day could boast. She had enjoyed the best of music and art and the companionship of charming and important people. However, in refusing marriage and the round of social gaiety, she was revolting against the restrictions placed on women of her day, and she struggled to be allowed to work in a serious way.

Thus Florence Nightingale eventually convinced her family to allow her to attend nurses training and so began her distinguished career in developing professional nursing. Nightingale is well remembered for her significant contributions to professional nursing in the areas of theory of practice, nursing education, scholarship, and statistics. See Box 3-3 for Nightingale's definition of professional nursing.

Nightingale's Theory of Practice

Nightingale's theory of practice was documented for nurses and laypersons alike and served as the foundation for the promotion of health. This theory was referred to by Nightingale as the "Canons of Nursing" and guided the practice of professional nursing. A description of these canons, or standards, follows.

Ventilation and Warming. In the concept of ventilation and warming, Nightingale is very precise to "keep the air he breathes as pure as the external air without chilling him" (Nightingale, 1859, p. 8). Plenty of ventilation is necessary to carry off the noxious elements from a sick person's lungs and skin.

Noise. "Unnecessary noise, or noise that creates an expectation in the mind is that which hurts a patient" (Nightingale, 1859, p. 25). The nurse should guard against sudden noise, thoughtless chatter, and whispering in a patient's room. The effect of music may be beneficial.

Variety. Variety is another concept that helps alleviate suffering. Beautiful objects, brilliant colors, cut flowers, perhaps different things to do (e.g., handwork), and even pets would alleviate the boredom felt by those suffering.

Diet. The fourth concept is diet. "Sick cookery should half do the work of your poor patient's weak digestion" (Nightingale, 1859, p. 38). Nightingale reviews some of the common substances (gruel, arrowroot puddings, and egg flip) given to the sick.

Light. "It is the unqualified result of all my experience with the sick that second only to their need of fresh air is their need of light" (Nightingale, 1859, p. 47). Take the patient outside for direct sunlight. Keep rooms well lighted with no bed curtains or dark windows.

Chattering Hopes and Advices. Chattering hopes and advices is an attempt to cheer the patient by attendants and friends. Nightingale warns against this because she determines this to be false hope and hollow advice. She clearly appeals: "Leave off this practice of attempting to cheer the sick by making light of their danger and by exaggerating their probabilities of recovery" (Nightingale, 1859, p. 54).

Cleanliness (Health of Houses). Nightingale's attention to cleanliness takes up a large portion of her book. She writes that health depends on this. Describing the care of bed and bedding and of rooms and walls, she states the exact steps needed to clean each. In addition, she details how to clean the sick person so as to prevent poisoning by the skin. She describes the patient's feeling of well-being after washing and drying. The nurse needs to wash her own hands with friction as well. Some believe that Nightingale's success was based on cleaning up the hospitals.

Because of these significant contributions to nursing and to improving the health of both soldiers and citizens alike, Nightingale was highly recognized. Her honors, decorations, medals, and citations may be seen in the United Services Museum in Whitehall, London. She was the first woman to ever receive the British Order of Merit by King Edward VII. One of her biographers (Cook, 1942) said: "She was not only 'The Lady with a Lamp' throwing light into dark places but also a kind of galvanic battery stirring and sometimes shocking the dull and sluggish public to life and action."

SURVEY OF SELECTED NURSING THEORIES

A brief discussion of selected nursing theories follows. The date identified indicates the year in which the theory was first presented as a theory. However, most theories have continued to be refined and modified. A summary of the major nursing theorists with a brief description of their theory or conceptual model is presented in Table 3-2. This summary table provides the reader with information to guide further exploration of nursing theory. Box 3-4 provides online resources to begin further exploration of nursing theories.

TABLE 3-2	*Summary of Major Nursing Theorists and Theory Description*
DATE AND THEORIST	**THEORY DESCRIPTION**
1860: Florence Nightingale	Investigated the impact of the environment on healing
1952: Hildegard E. Peplau	Explored the interpersonal relationship of the nurse and the client and identified the client's *feelings* as a predictor of positive outcomes related to health and wellness
1960: Faye Abdellah	Client-centered interventions
1961: Ida Jean Orlando	Nurse-client relationship; deliberate nursing approach using *nursing process,* which stressed the action of the individual client in determining the action of the nurse; focus is on the present or short-term outcome
1966: Virginia Henderson	Nursing assists patients with fourteen essential functions toward independence
1967: Myra Estrin Levine	Four conservation principles of inpatient client resources (energy, structural integrity, personal integrity, and social integrity)
1970: Martha E. Rogers	Science of unitary man: energy fields, openness, pattern, and organization; nurse promotes synchronicity between human beings and their universe/environment
1971: Dorethea Orem	Nursing facilitates client self-care by measuring the client's deficit relative to self-care needs; the nurse implements appropriate measures to assist the client in meeting these needs by matching them with an appropriate supportive intervention
1971: Imogene King	Goal attainment using nurse-client transactions; addresses client systems and includes society, groups, and the individual
1974: Sister Callista Roy	Client's adaptation to condition using environmental stimuli to adjust perception
1977: Madeline Leininger	Transcultural nursing and caring nursing; concepts are aimed toward caring and the components of a culture care theory; diversity, universality, worldview, and ethnohistory are essential to the four concepts (care, caring, health, and nursing)
1979: Margaret Newman	Central components of this model are health and consciousness followed by concepts of movement, time, and space, all components are summative units, described in relationship to health as well as to each other
1979: Jean Watson	Philosophy and science of caring and humanistic nursing; there are 10 "carative" factors, which are core to nursing; this holistic outlook addresses the impact and importance of altruism, sensitivity, trust, and interpersonal skills
1980: Dorothy E. Johnson	Behavioral system model for nursing; separates the psychologic and the physiologic aspects of illness; role of the nurse is to provide support and comfort to attain regulation of the client's behavior
1981: Rosemarie Rizzo Parse	Man-living-health: man, by existing, actively participates in creating health according to environmental influences; individual is regarded as an open system wherein health is a process
1989: Patricia Benner and Judith Wrubel	Primacy of caring; the practice of nurses depends on the experience absorbed by engaging in five practice areas (novice, advanced beginner, competent, proficient, and expert) in the seven domains of nursing practice (helping, teaching-coaching, diagnostic and patient monitoring, effective management of rapid change, administration and monitoring of therapeutic interventions and regimens, monitoring and ensuring the quality of health care practices, and organizational work-role competencies)
1995: Betty Neuman	Systems model: wellness-Illness continuum; promotes the nurse as the agent in assisting the client in adapting to and therefore reducing stressors; supports the notion of prevention through appropriate intervention

Dorothea Orem (1971): Self-Care Deficit Model: Self-Care, Self-Care Deficits, and Nursing Systems

When the client incurs an insult that renders him or her incapable of fully functioning, there is a self-care deficit, which makes nursing intervention necessary. The object of Orem's theory is to restore the client's self-care capability to enable him or her to sustain structural reliability, performance, and growth through purposeful nursing intervention. The aim of such intervention is to help the client cope with unmet care needs by acquiring the maximum level of function. This would be to either regain previous function or maximize available function present after the insult, hence restoring a sense of well-being.

Hildegard E. Peplau (1972): Interpersonal Relations As a Nursing Process: Man As an Organism That Exists in an Unstable Equilibrium

When the client incurs an insult that renders her or him incapable of moving forward because of existing stressful environmental conditions, anxiety increases. This condition creates a situation wherein the option is to either move in a backward direction or to plateau. Nursing intervention in Peplau's model focuses on reducing the related incapacitating stressors through therapeutic interpersonal interaction. Intervention involves the nurse assisting the client with mutual goal setting. These goals may address exploration of the identified problem, identification of viable options, and implementation of available resources for resolution. Nursing interpersonal process is present and interactive, using associated and appropriate nursing intervention skills, which incorporate the roles of the nurse as resource person, educator, mentor, transfer agent, and counselor. Peplau's model requires that the nurse have a self-awareness and insight regarding her or his own behaviors. This awareness may be applied in identifying and working through those behaviors unique to the client's schema. Fig. 3-2 presents Peplau's Psychodynamic Nursing Model.

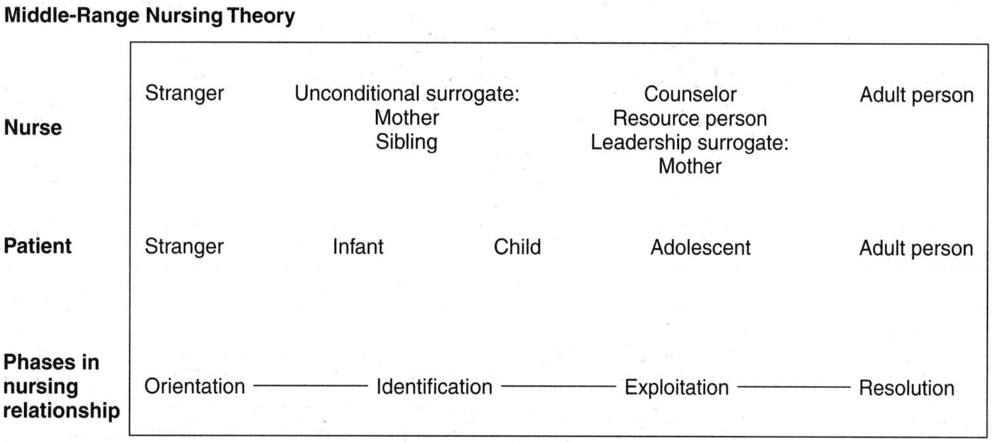

Middle-Range Nursing Theory

Nurse	Stranger	Unconditional surrogate: Mother Sibling	Counselor Resource person Leadership surrogate: Mother	Adult person
Patient	Stranger	Infant Child	Adolescent	Adult person
Phases in nursing relationship	Orientation ———— Identification ———— Exploitation ———— Resolution			

FIG. 3-2 Hildegard E. Peplau's Psychodynamic Nursing Model. Phases and changing roles in nurse-patient relationships. (From Peplau HE: *Interpersonal relations in nursing,* New York, 1952, GP Putnam and Sons, p. 54.)

Martha E. Rogers (1970): Science of Unitary Human Beings: Humans As Energy Fields That Interact Constantly With the Environment

When the client/human unit incurs an insult that renders him or her out of balance with the universe, nursing interventions must be geared toward helping the client/human unit attain an increasing complex balance and synchronicity with the universe. Essential to Rogers' theory is the belief that each being is unique and consists of more than the collective sum of parts and that each being is continuously evolving in a forward momentum as it interacts continuously with the surrounding environmental field. Using the right side of the brain to recognize every human unit's capacity for imagery, sensation, and emotion and the left side of the brain for language, abstraction, and thought is a brain integration that is necessary to support the notion of human-environmental synergy.

Sister Calista Roy (1974) Adaptation Model: Assistance With the Adaptation to Stressors To Facilitate the Integration Process of the Client

When the client incurs an insult that renders him or her in need of environmental modification, the nurse will be the change agent in assisting the individual with this adaptation. By helping the "biopsychosocial" client modify external stimuli, adaptation will occur. In the case of illness, the outcome will be a diminished or absent integration of the constantly changing setting known as the illness environment, with the constantly changing human who is interacting with the existing outside surroundings. To attain wellness, adaptation must occur through this integration. The nurse's role is to promote this adaptation by modifying and regulating peripheral stimuli to enable the client's adaptation and integration with a supportive healing environment. In so doing, the nurse will be instrumental in assisting the client with the areas of health and well-being, life worth and value, and self-respect and dignity. Sister Calista Roy's Adaptation Model is depicted in Fig. 3-3.

Grand Nursing Theory

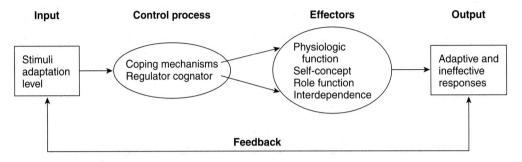

FIG. 3-3 Sister Calista Roy's Adaptation Model. Person as an adaptive system. (From Roy C: *Introduction to nursing: an adaptation model,* ed. 2, Englewood Cliffs, NJ, 1984, Prentice Hall, p. 30.)

Jean Watson (1978): Model of Human Caring: Transpersonal Caring As the Fulcrum: Philosophy and Science As the Core of Nursing

When the client incurs an insult that renders him or her in need, the transpersonal process between the client and the nurse is considered a healing nursing intervention. An assumption of Watson's theory is that all persons require human caring to quell need. Hence the transpersonal process of "caring," or the caring between nurse, environment, and client, is essential to healing. Caring promotes the notion that every human being strives for interconnectedness with other humans and with nature. The nurse who implements these carative factors is the facilitator in the goal of restoring congruence between client's perceived self and the existent self through the promotion of health and equilibrium. The expectation is that the client will experience balance and harmony in mind-body-soul. Harmony, or wellness will prevail, whereas disharmony, or illness, will be altered, eliminated, or circumvented.

FUTURE OF NURSING THEORIES AND THEORISTS

At no time in history have so many health care concerns been the primary focus of federal and state legislative agendas. Questions are being asked in the twenty-first century about how health care is being conducted and managed. It is imperative that nurses be on the front lines to provide testimony in response to these queries.

The nursing shortage, scarce resources, health maintenance organizations, managed care, Medicare, welfare to work plans, confidentiality issues, parity of reimbursement, advanced practice nurses and their scope of practice, mandatory overtime, whistle-blower protection, prescriptive authority, licensure, multistate compacts, telemedicine, and many other policy issues that directly affect nursing practice are coming before the U.S. Congress and individual state legislative bodies for practice-related decisions. The direct impact on nursing cannot be overemphasized.

As nursing continues to operate in an environment of continuing change, outcome data will be analyzed in an effort to provide quality care and access to that care for all clients in need of health care services. Therefore one may predict that established nursing theories will be reevaluated and modified accordingly. New theories will be created and developed that may help answer the health care questions of the twenty-first century. Simply put, nursing theories in the twenty-first century will embrace complex environmental changes that incorporate new technologies such as genetics, computers, noninvasive surgery, robotics, decreasing energy sources, increasing pollutants under a thinning ozone layer, environmental hazards, new diseases, and antibiotic resistant illness that affect the clients of today differently from those clients as recent as 5 years ago.

SUMMARY

Let the reader beware. As stated at the beginning of this chapter, the information provided is in no manner a substitute for a comprehensive analysis of existing nursing theories and theorists. More exist than are presented here, and, in fact, several comprehensive texts may be accessed that cover these theories in depth. However, this chapter offers an overview of theory in the attempt to familiarize readers with the idea of theory. Selected theories are described to that end. One should identify nursing theories as ideas that have shaped and continue to shape the nursing profession in practice and research. It is our intention to assist students with understanding that practice and research are interdependent entities. In other words, practice and research cannot efficiently or efficaciously exist one without the other. Like the metaphor at the beginning of this chapter, without the existence of the stones (scientific data), the separation into specific concentrated yet related areas (theory) could not have happened.

Critical Thinking Activities

1. Read an article in a recent issue of *Nursing Research;* identify the conceptual or theoretic framework and examine how the major variables in the study reflect concepts described in the conceptual or theoretic framework.
2. Select a nursing theory that you find most interesting and then: (a) explain the reason for choosing that particular theory, and (b) discuss how the theory could guide nursing practice using relevant examples from your clinical experiences.
3. Interview a master's- and/or a doctoral-prepared nurse and ask the nurse to discuss how a specific theory has influenced her or his nursing practice and has guided her or his nursing research.

REFERENCES

Abdellah FG: The nature of nursing science, *Nurs Res* 18(5):393, 1969.

Anastasi T: Heredity, environment, and the question "how"? *Psychol Rev* 65:197-208, 1958.

Barnum BS: *Nursing theory: analysis, application, evaluation,* Philadelphia, 2000, JB Lippincott.

Bronowski J: *The origins of knowledge and imagination,* New Haven, Conn, 1972, Yale University Press.

Cook E: *The life of Florence Nightingale,* New York, 1942, MacMillan.

Good M, Moore SM: Clinical practice guidelines as a source of middle range theory: focus on acute pain, *Nurs Outlook* 44:74-79, 1998.

Jacob S: The grief process of older women whose husbands received hospice care, *J Adv Nurs* 24:280-286, 1996.

Jacox AK: Theory construction in nursing: an overview, *Nurs Res* 23(1):4, 1974.

Lenz ER et al: The middle-range theory of unpleasant symptoms: an update, *Adv Nurs Sci* 19(3):14-27, 1997.

Nightingale F: *Notes on nursing: what it is, and what it is not (commemorative edition),* Philadelphia, 1992, JB Lippincott.

Nightingale F: *Notes on nursing: what it is, and what it is not,* London, 1859, Harrison and Sons.

Polit D, Beck C, Hungler B: *Essentials of nursing research,* New York, 2001, JB Lippincott.

SUGGESTED READINGS

Benner P: *From novice to expert: excellence in power in clinical nursing practice,* Menlo Park, Calif, 1984, Addison Wesley.

Chinn P, Kramer M: *Theory and nursing: integrated knowledge development,* St Louis, 1999, Mosby.

Johnson BM, Webber PB: *An introduction to theory and reasoning in nursing,* Philadelphia, 2001, JB Lippincott.

King I: *Toward a theory for nursing: general concepts of human behavior,* New York, 1971, John Wiley & Sons.

Leddy S, Pepper J: *Conceptual bases in professional nursing,* Philadelphia, 1998, JB Lippincott.

Leininger MM: *Transcultural nursing: concepts, theories and practices,* New York, 1978, John Wiley & Sons.

Levine M: The four conservation principles of nursing, *Nurs Forum* 6:93, 1967.

Newman MA: *Health as expanding consciousness,* St Louis, 1986, Mosby.

Nicoll L: *Perspectives on nursing theory,* Philadelphia, 1997, JB Lippincott.

Orem DE: *Nursing concepts of practice,* ed 6, New York, 1971, McGraw-Hill.

Parse RR: *Man-living-health: a theory of nursing,* New York, 1981, John Wiley & Sons.

Peplau HE: *International relations in nursing,* New York, 1952, GP Putnam.

Tomey AM, Alligood MR: *Nursing theorists and their work,* ed 4, St Louis, 1998, Mosby.

4

The Influence of Contemporary Trends and Issues on Nursing Education

Carrie B. Lenburg, EdD, RN, FAAN

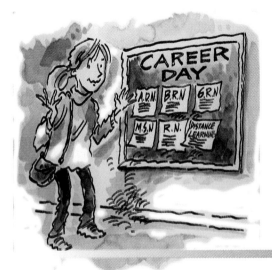

Educational diversity promotes access and career development.

Vignette

Carolee was young and eager and wanted to be a nurse; so she enrolled in the local diploma school, which was the only option. Completing the program made her feel more confident, and she now wanted a BSN so she could teach nursing. However, her family had few resources and could not pay for her schooling. Thus Carolee moved to another city, where she worked part-time and went to school full-time for one semester and then reversed the process for the next semester until she finished the 3-year RN to BSN program. It was hard work and tiring, but she felt great when she finally graduated with her BSN. But trends were changing and by the time she finished that program, a master's degree in nursing was required to teach. And so, to reach her goal, she had to complete yet another degree. She worked and saved but didn't have nearly enough to start. Then she learned that the federal government offered "traineeships" that paid all tuition and fees to MSN students because of the nursing shortage. Fortunately, Carolee's application was approved and she earned her MSN as a full-time student in 1 year. After working several years as a nurse educator, she began studying for a doctoral degree in education, which she completed in 3 years, again with funding from a government fellowship. Carolee's education story took place several years ago. At every step trends and expectations for practice changed, but her ambition and confidence also changed. As it was then, so it is today. Those who want to be competent nurses and leaders must change with the times, search for opportunities, and be persistent. The need for change never ends.

Questions to consider while reading this chapter
1. What is the minimal education requirement for a nurse?
2. How have current trends in society, health care, and nursing influenced nursing education?
3. What feasible opportunities exist for you to advance your education beyond the current degree you are seeking?
4. What local, state, and national resources are available to learn more about nursing education?
5. What is your commitment to ongoing professional development?

Key Terms

Community-oriented curriculum Emphasizes health promotion, disease prevention, and health restoration in the context of extended family, community, and populations as clients, throughout the educational program.

Competency outcomes The results, or end-products, of planned study and experience that are focused on designated abilities required for practice.

COPA model Competency Outcomes and Performance Assessment model developed by C. B. Lenburg as a framework to promote initial and continuing competence in education and practice for students, faculty, nurses, and others.

Contemporary issues The problems, questions, and concerns that are current for the present time, whenever that may be. Contemporary is always the present time.

Continuing competence The ongoing development and improvement of those abilities and skills required for a given practice or role.

Core practice competencies The constellation of eight skill categories developed by Lenburg as essential for contemporary nursing practice: assessment and intervention, communication, critical thinking, human caring relationships, teaching, management, leadership, and knowledge integration.

Educational mobility The progressive movement from one type or level of education to another. Examples are progression from technical or diploma education to academic degree programs such as LPN to RN, RN to BSN or MSN, or nonnursing to a nursing degree. Programs usually include various flexible advanced placement options.

Initial competence Designated or required knowledge and abilities learned and validated during the basic education program for a particular level.

Performance-based assessment Evaluation of abilities based on objective demonstration of the competencies required rather than on evaluation of knowledge about those abilities. This may include performance in actual or simulation situations and in physical hands-on activities or the observable evidence of such skills as planning, writing, speaking, or problem solving.

Learning Outcomes

After studying this chapter, the reader will be able to:
1. Integrate knowledge of current trends and issues in society into a more holistic perception of their influence on nursing, nursing education, students, and faculty.
2. Integrate knowledge of current trends and issues into a personal contemporary philosophy of ongoing professional development and practice.

3. Differentiate among various types of conventional and mobility nursing education programs and the issues associated with them.
4. Access pertinent information resources related to evolving trends and issues as a component of ongoing professional development.

CHAPTER OVERVIEW

Nursing education (and practice) is influenced by a number of emerging trends in society, some of which are described in this chapter; others also are important and are discussed elsewhere in this book. The selected trends are presented with related issues for students and faculty to provide a broader view of education. The American society is increasingly diverse; thus each trend precipitates different issues and problems. Trends result from issues in the past, just as these issues will lead to other trends in the future; this is the never-ending process of change. These trends are complex and overlapping but are presented here as separate categories to emphasize their importance; all of them influence nursing education. The chapter is brief and should be considered as a guide to more in-depth resources, including the print and Internet website references listed at the end of the chapter; explore them as much as possible.

The most influential trend is the rapid development of knowledge and information fueled by expanding communication technology and the Internet. This in turn precipitates expectations for nearly instant access and response to almost everything and results in multiple problems for students and faculty. A related trend is the increasing urgency for competence, focused on specified outcomes and validated through objective performance assessment methods. Competency outcomes and performance-based evaluation now are required and are more stringent to safeguard consumers, nurses, and employers; therefore they are essential in nursing education. Other trends focus on ethics and bioethical developments and personal choice. Expanding scientific research and innovations have led to amazing new treatment modalities, but also to a multitude of issues. Expectations of personal freedom of choice raise ethical issues related to abortion, the right to die, and lifestyle preferences. Several highly interrelated trends include the changing characteristics of the population and the political and economic influences on health and health care. Collectively they have influenced the trends of community- and consumer-oriented health care, interdisciplinary health care, use of alternative health practices, and increased collaboration among various agencies and institutions. Two other trends that affect nursing education are the increasing shortage of qualified nurses, faculty, and students and the increasing stress related to personal and professional responsibilities.

These trends influence the number and types of nursing programs for basic and experienced students. Students and the effective contemporary practitioner need to understand these trends and issues to cope with them and help change them into more positive trends (ANA, 1999). At the end of the chapter, interactive learning activities are suggested under each learning outcome.

TRENDS AND ISSUES IN CONTEMPORARY NURSING EDUCATION

In many ways nursing education is the same as it always has been: concerned with preparing nurses with enough knowledge and skills to meet the health care needs of the community with compassion. How it does this is shaped by a number of trends and issues in society, which change continually and with increasing complexity. This chapter presents a concise review of selected trends and related issues that influence the content, expected outcomes, learning processes, and assessment methods of nursing education today. Heller, Oros, and Durney-Crowley (2000) summarize similar trends that influence nursing. Baer (2000) and Kalisch and Kalisch (1995) are basic resources for detailed content; also review AACN (1999b), ANA (1976, 1991), and Schorr and Zimmerman (1990).

Table 4-1 lists ten trends and summarizes issues related to students and faculty. These trends and issues illustrate nursing's complex environment and help to explain how and why nursing education needs to change and function in contemporary society. The final trend focuses on nursing education itself and on its continuing and emerging issues. Although listed separately, the trends actually should be viewed as a constellation of factors that simultaneously influence nursing education and practice. Box 4-1 lists major organizations concerned with nursing education; they provide relevant current data.

BOX 4-1	*Selected Organizations Relevant to Nursing Education: General Description and Purpose*

American Academy of Nursing—The organization of top leaders in all facets of nursing: practice, education, administration, research, organizations, and government; the think tank of the profession; promotes advancement of all aspects of nursing; publishes position papers, conference proceedings, and documents to advance nursing.

American Association of Colleges of Nursing—The organization of deans and directors of baccalaureate and higher degree nursing programs; establishes standards for programs, concerned with legislative issues that pertain to professional nursing education; publishes the *Journal of Professional Nursing, The Essentials of Baccalaureate Degree Programs* (1997), and other related documents pertaining to the BSN and higher degree education.

American Nurses Association—The major national nursing organization concerned with broad scope of practice issues; standards of practice, scope of practice, ethics, legal, employment; a federation of state nurses associations; publications related to array of practice issues and standards.

American Nurses Credentialing Center—National credentialing center offering certification examination in 28 areas; sets standards and protocols for certification; promotes certification for relevant specialty areas in nursing practice; publishes materials related to certification.

Commission on Collegiate Nursing Education (CCNE)—A subsidiary of AACN with responsibility for establishing and implementing standards for the accreditation of baccalaureate and graduate degree programs in nursing.

National Council of State Boards of Nursing—Organization of all state boards; coordinates licensure activities on national level; conducts studies as basis for creating licensure examination; developed computerized licensure examinations; works with other organizations to promote nursing standards and regulation.

National League for Nursing (NLN)—The national organization of nurse educators, with councils for four types of programs (LPN, diploma, ADN, and BSN); only nursing organization that includes lay citizens concerned with nursing and health care. NLN also has councils for nursing informatics, research in nursing education, wellness centers, and other focused concerns; accredits home health care agencies (CHAPS); multiple types of print and visual publications.

NLN Accreditation Commission—Formed in 1997 as a subsidiary of NLN with responsibility for establishing and implementing standards for the accreditation of all types of schools of nursing; follows guidelines from the U.S. Department of Education.

National Student Nurses Association—Organization of statewide student nurse associations; concerned with education and career issues; provides student perspectives to other national nursing organizations.

Internet address to locate many other organizations: www.lib.umich.edu/hw/nursing/organ.html.

TABLE 4-1	*Summary of Trends and Issues That Influence Nursing Education*	
MAJOR CONTEMPORARY TRENDS	**RELATED ISSUES FOR STUDENTS**	**RELATED ISSUES FOR FACULTY AND THE PROFESSION**
1. Knowledge expansion, use of technology and Internet	■ Information overload; virtually unlimited global content via technology, Internet; discern current and accurate information; outdated textbooks ■ High faculty expectations; limited time ■ Achieve core practice competencies	■ Constant change of content and curriculum ■ Limited time to learn, integrate, help students ■ Changing technology, health care; expanding web of contacts; expected rapid response ■ Limited time for reflection and creativity
2. Practice-based competency outcomes and evidence-based content	■ Learning experiences focused on core practice competency outcomes, professional skills beyond technical psychomotor skills ■ Integration of "best practices," evidence-based standards, research findings into practice	■ Curriculum and faculty development time, work; focus outcomes and core competencies ■ Different conceptual model, more practice specific; evidence-based standards of care ■ Initial and continuing competence; linked to licensure, multistate regulations; accreditation
3. Performance-based competency learning and assessment methods	■ Multiple teaching-learning methods: interactive group work, collaboration, in and out of class, projects, problem-based learning, self responsibility, accountability for competence; interdisciplinary learning; use computers to access resources ■ Competency assessment based on performance examinations; licensure requirements	■ Major changes for teachers and students re roles, methods, content; less lecture; learner responsibility, interactive learning strategies ■ Different kind of preparation, focus on specific outcomes; core competencies ■ Assessment of competence using specific performance examinations, increase objectivity, consistency; multistate regulations
4. Sociodemographic, cultural diversity, economic and political changes	■ Increased aging, ethnic diversity; requires respect for differences, preferences, customs ■ Violence in society, workplace; safety concerns ■ Different content, client care, clinical sites ■ Economic and political change influences health care delivery and access to clinical experiences	■ Changes in student and consumer populations require respect for diversity, changes in content and clinical experiences; emphasis on geriatrics, cultural diversity; health promotion; violence in society ■ Changes in time, effort, expertise to prepare ■ Political, economic influence on care delivery

Continued

TABLE 4-1   *Summary of Trends and Issues That Influence Nursing Education—cont'd*

MAJOR CONTEMPORARY TRENDS	RELATED ISSUES FOR STUDENTS	RELATED ISSUES FOR FACULTY AND THE PROFESSION
5. Community-focused, collaborative, interdisciplinary, alternative approaches	■ Broad scope of nursing; clinical experiences throughout community; continuum from acute care to health promotion, hospitals to home, rural to global settings ■ Requires more planning, travel time, expenses, arrangements; different skills, communication ■ Multiple teachers, preceptors, varying abilities ■ Interdisciplinary collaborative learning ■ Community, congregation groups, service-learning projects; global community ■ Alternative health practices; diversity	■ Community concepts integrated throughout program; work with multiple agencies, community groups, congregations to promote health; service-learning; rural to global issues ■ Need more time and planning to learn, implement different focus, content, methods, settings; interdisciplinary collaboration ■ Students in multiple locations simultaneously; concern re instruction, assessment by preceptors; varied expectations, goals ■ Alternative health practices; diversity
6. Consumer-oriented society	■ All expect value, quality, individual consideration, attention ■ Increased litigation, medical/nursing errors; focus on safe, competent care ■ Increased individual responsibility, accountability for learning and health ■ Consumer initiatives for involvement and protection; balance standards and preferences	■ Changing relationships among teachers, students, nurses, clients; impact on program ■ More concern re individual consumer's needs; shared authority, responsibility for health ■ Litigation; errors in medical, nursing practice; expectation for safe competent care ■ Balance standards and preferences of students and faculty
7. Ethics and bioethical concerns	■ Integrate into professional practice acceptance of the individual's right of choice regarding life and death issues, health care methods ■ Alternative solutions to ethical dilemmas; issues re diverse beliefs, gray zones instead of black and white absolutes; separate personal opinions and professional practice	■ Teach ethics, bioethical concepts, changes; diverse interpretations and actions ■ Teach alternative solutions to ethical dilemmas; focus on competencies of assessment, reflective judgment, communication, caring ■ Accountability for ethical competence; separate personal and professional practice

8. Increasing shortage of nurses, students, faculty, and support personnel	■ Shortage of staff results in limitations in clinical learning; heavy workload, fewer preceptors with less time to help students ■ Fewer qualified faculty results in higher ratios ■ Students need more, not less, clinical learning; have more responsibility with less individual help; consequences for competence	■ Too few qualified teachers and preceptors ■ Fewer and less academically able students with economic problems need more help ■ Decreasing enrollments, graduations, and aging of nurses results in issues for future of profession ■ Issues re recruitment, teaching, counseling
9. Increasing professional and personal responsibilities	■ High stress re competing demands of school, home, work; interferes with meeting competency outcomes and completing programs; own health ■ Required to validate initial and continuing competence, lifelong learning, preparation to meet professional expectations	■ High stress re changes in curriculum, teaching methods, technology, rapid change in clinical settings and regulations; fewer resources ■ Changes in student body; need more help ■ Required clinical practice, research, publications, service; increasing demands on professional and personal life increase stress
10. Diversity, flexibility, mobility, and delivery of education programs	■ Increased adult responsibilities influence learning and completion; need multiple-entry, multiple-exit mobility or other flexible options ■ Expenses and time re education, care of dependents; conflict of work and study ■ Pros and cons of mediated, Internet courses, programs; self-directed learning	■ Issues re philosophy, curriculum development and implementation for diverse students; entry into practice debates, conflicts ■ Diverse mobility options take more time, energy, resources; students at a distance ■ Problems developing using Internet, other mediated courses; issues of instruction and assessment, quality and accountability for education, practice; legal, ethical concerns

Knowledge Expansion and Use of Technology and the Internet

With the ever-expanding developments in computer technology, the volume of knowledge is expanding exponentially. From e-mails to complex research documents and video images, nurses and students, like everyone else, are communicating more frequently, with more contacts and with the speed of light. This ability to access and disseminate unlimited information almost instantly has enormous benefits but also presents major issues. Computer-accessible knowledge has become the potential content for nursing and other courses and the standards for practice. Textbooks and journal articles are considered nearly obsolete by the time they are published, and an expanding array of websites has become a major learning resource. Websites generally are more interactive than texts and link to multitudes of other helpful resources (Nicoll, 2000; Skiba, 1997). Even though updated frequently, they also become outdated quickly. Students easily can become lost in the interesting web of links while they search for assignments and communicate with others in class or around the world. Thus it actually may take more time to find and learn content, although it provides broader, more specific, and more accurate information.

Herein lies the conflict and the issues: almost unlimited information is available, but it requires more time and skill to navigate the web and learn, even though most students seem to have less time for study (Focus, 1999; Mallow and Gilje, 1999). Learning from the Internet requires disciplined focus and clear guidelines and expected outcomes related to assignments. It also develops skills in analytic thinking, decision making, and reflective judgment, all of which are essential competencies for nursing practice but are not easily learned. Other issues relate to time management, the integration of all the information available, keeping up with changes in technology, and meeting the expectations for immediate responses to an ever-widening web of contacts.

Like students, faculty also have similar issues related to knowledge and technology expansion, the scope of information, and the time to use it. They have to make rational decisions about what and how much students need to learn at a given level, and they, too, can become entranced by and lost in the learning opportunities available on the Internet. Teachers also have to learn and keep updated with content and technology to be able to effectively help students stay ahead of the curve. Unlike students, faculty also are constantly in the process of making curriculum and course revisions and modifying teaching and evaluation methods—all of which are time-consuming and greatly influenced by the knowledge and technology explosion.

Practice-Based Competency Outcomes

Trends in business and commerce often find their way into higher education and nursing education. The current emphasis on using competency outcomes to set directions and goals related to real-world practice is one of them. To focus on outcomes is to focus on results. In business the outcome of spending time and resources based on actual needs is what counts in determining financial success. The same is true for nursing practice and nursing education. What really matters is that students (nurses) achieve the competency outcomes that specify the skills actually needed in practice. They are the measurable results of time and efforts spent in learning. Competence in realistic practice-based outcomes is the target, the goal to be reached.

However, this outcomes approach is very different for most teachers and students from the past ways of thinking, teaching methods, and evaluation. It is not just changing words. For teachers it requires considerable rethinking and time to revise course syllabi, reassess and specify the competencies nurses actually need for practice in the changing and complex contemporary health care environments, and design ways to help students learn them. For students it means a change from memorizing class notes and readings to learning to integrate knowledge, make decisions, and be competent and confident in the abilities contained in course outcomes. Practice-based competency outcomes specify the destination students need to reach, the interactive learning strategies are the directions and guidelines for getting there, and performance-based assessment confirms they have arrived at the right place. The process is important, but achieving final competency outcomes is the bottom line. These changes in the entire education process pose threats and concerns to all the stakeholders that need to be resolved (Bargagliotti, Luttrell, and Lenburg, 1999).

Redefining practice-based competencies is a complex issue, and, although many educators and organizations are engaged in this process, no single method has emerged as predominant. Lenburg (1999a, b) created the Competency Outcomes and Performance Assessment (COPA) Model (see Fig. 4-1, p. 78) as a way to change and reorganize the curriculum to emphasize competence and assessment. Using this framework, she developed a master list of eight core practice competency categories under which all of the skills nurses use in practice can be listed. They include assessment and intervention, communication, critical thinking, caring relationships, teaching, management, leadership, and knowledge integration (Box 4-2).

Competency outcomes incorporate these practice-based skills, as well as the course content. Learning strategies and performance examination are based on outcomes and content. Several articles describe the model, process, and related issues as used by others (Luttrell et al., 1999; Redman, Lenburg, and Walker, 1999). Critical thinking is perhaps the most pivotal competence, as seen in many resources (Critical thinking, 2000; Rubenfeld and Scheffer, 1995).

Others have suggested different models, competencies, and expected outcomes for students and practitioners (Curley, 1998; Eichelberger and Hewlett, 1999). Nursing organizations continue to revise standards to focus on competencies. Explore the websites in Table 4-2 for the most current information for groups such as the American Association of Colleges of Nursing (AACN), the American Nurses Association (ANA), the Joint Commission on Accreditation of Healthcare Organizations (JCAHO), the National Federation of Specialty Nursing Organizations (NFSNO), the National League for Nursing Accreditation Commission (NLNAC), and the Pew Commission (Bellack and O'Neil, 2000). These emerging trends and issues related to competency outcomes have a direct impact on nursing education and practice.

BOX 4-2	*Lenburg's Eight Core Practice Competencies*

- Assessment and Interventions
- Critical Thinking
- Communication
- Teaching
- Human Caring Relationships
- Management
- Leadership
- Knowledge Integration

TABLE 4-2	*Helpful Websites**

NAME OF SOURCE	ADDRESS	COMMENTS
Nursing organizations and associations directly or indirectly concerned with nursing education		
American Association of Colleges of Nursing	aacn.nche.edu	BSN and Higher degree schools
American Association for History of Nursing	aahn.org	Membership, contacts, publication
American Holistic Nurses Association	ahna.org	Publications, certificate program and CE course listings
American Nurses Association	nursingworld.org	Links to organizations,, publications, *Am Nurse*, career, lists
American Nurses Credentialing Center	nursingworld.org/ancc/	Information re certification programs, requirements
American Organization of Nurse Executives	aone.org (ahaonlinestore.com)	Information; publications re nursing leadership, administration
Commission on Collegiate Nursing Education	aacn.nche.edu/accreditation/index.htm	Accreditation of BSN and higher degrees
International Council of Nurses	icn.ch	ICN resources and links
International Parish Nursing Resource Center	advocatehealth.com/about/faith/pnursctr.html	Information and links to resources
More about Parish nursing	csbsju.edu/library/Internet/parish.html	Links to resources
National Council of State Boards of Nursing	ncsbn.org	Info re NCLEX and regulations
National Federation of Specialty Nurs Orgzs	nfsno.org	Resource re specialty nursing organizations; conferences
National League for Nursing (NLN)	nln.org	Info re schools, testing
NLN Accrediting Commission	nlnac.org	Info re accreditation of all types of nursing schools
National Student Nurses Association	nsna.org	Info for students; see: www.toledolink.com/~ornrsg/
Sigma Theta Tau International	nursingsociety.org	Honor society information; research directory; case studies
Southern Nursing Research Society	snrs.org	Example: regional organization; research; new online journal
Midwest Nursing Research Society	mnrs.org	Example: regional organization; links to resources
Examples of online journals		
Online Journal of Issues in Nursing	nursingworld.org/ojin/	Hosted by American Nurses Assoc, at Kent State University
Southern Online Journal of Nursing Research	www.snrs.org	S. Nursing Research Society (began 2000)

Websites of resources concerned with health, nursing, and/or education (each address begins with www. unless otherwise noted)

Resource	Address	Description
Agency for Health Care Quality and Research	ahcpr.org	US Dept of HHS; proceedings: working conditions, safety, etc.
Alternative health care	wholenurse.com	Resource links, information re alternative health practices
American Hospital Association	ahapolicyforum.org/policyresources	Nursing shortage and workforce issues
College Guide (was Peterson's)	ecollege.com	Links to colleges by type, state; other useful resources
Distance learning channel	ed-x.com	Listing of about 3000 courses
Fuld Institute of Technology in Nursing	fitne.net (or: ev.net/fitne)	For educators; publications, links; Nightingale Tracker system
Health and Environment resource	noharm.org	Patient safety, products; coalition of 250 nursing and others
Health: multiple links to resources	healthweb.org/index.cfm	Links to multiple health resources
Healthy People 2010	health.gov/healthypeople	Publication; other links; also via www.firstgov.gov
Institute of Medicine	iom.edu	Publications, other links, via National Academy of Sciences
Lippincott publisher: multiple links	nursingcenter.com	Links to journals, schools, organizations, publications; computers in nursing, nursing research, CE, virtual university, etc.
Martindale's Health Science Guide	sci.lib.uci.edu/HSG/Nursing.html	To: HSG/Nursing.html. Martindale Virtual Nurse Ctr; links
National Library of Medicine	locatorplus.gov/	National Library locator, databases; information retrieval
Nightingale Institute for Hlth and Environment	nihe.org	Resource to promote healthy environment
Nursing Ethics Network	bc.edu/nursing/ethics	New resource, Boston College; RN ethics survey; helpful links
Nursing: multiple links to resources	nursingnet.org	Links to resources; allied health, continuing education, etc.
Nursing: multiple links; alpha listings	inurse.com	Links to institutions; organizations; continuing education, etc.
Nursing: multiple web resources	http://ublib.buffalo.edu/libraries/units/hsl/internet/nsgsites.html (note specific address)	
Nursing: Univ. of MI: multiple resources	healthweb.org/	Organizations; practice, education
Pew Health Professions Commission	futurehealth.ucsf.edu/	Publications re health care changes; service learning projects; abstracts for computers in nursing, nursing research, others
Robert Wood Johnson Foundation	rwjf.org	Colleagues in Caring project; multiple others; grants
Slack publisher: multiple links	slackinc.com/allied/	Excellent resource: links to journals, schools, organizations, etc.
Southern Regional Electronic Campus	electroniccampus.org	Links to online resources, courses, college programs in south
U.S. Government resources (extensive)	firstgov.gov	Excellent links to official resources, social security, documents

Continued

*This list represents *examples* of Internet resources as beginning points. It is not a complete or "best" list; it is a suggested sampling. At the time of this writing, addresses are operational; but be aware that they may change, become obsolete, or be discontinued; others are added frequently. Most addresses listed below begin with "http://www." unless otherwise indicated. Note that some have hyphens or other symbols, and some are case sensitive in which the capital letters MUST be used exactly as specified. Some search engines to use to find sites on the Internet include Altavista, Excite, and Yahoo. Use Metacrawler to search search engines.

TABLE 4-2 *Sample of Online References Related to Nursing Education and Related Resources—cont'd*

NAME OF SOURCE	ADDRESS	COMMENTS
Websites of resources concerned with health, nursing, and/or education (each address begins with www. unless otherwise noted)—cont'd		
U.S. Government: major links to resources	medlineplus.gov	Links re disease, health, NLM, NIH, DHHS, clinical trials, etc.
U.S. Government: consumer gateway links	healthfinder.gov (healthfinderkids.gov)	Links to health, consumer-focused, support groups; one for kids
U.S. Government: Div of Nursing	bhpr.hrsa.gov/	Nurse survey; databases available, by state; available 2/01
Virtual Nurse	virtualnurse.com	Links to career, education, resources; excellent resource and links
Wall Street Journal	wsj.com	Current news re health (Health Journal), education, technology
Yahoo nursing and health site	dir.yahoo.com/health/nursing/	Excellent resource links; journals, lists
College and university websites†		
California State Univ., Dominguez Hills	csudh.edu	State-wide mobility program; distance learning
Case-Western Reserve Univ.	cwru.edu	Multi-option; international; research; nursing informatics
Excelsior College (Regents College)	excelsior.edu	External degrees: AND, BSN, masters programs
George Mason Univ.	gmu.edu	Campus and Mobility programs; WANRR (research resource)
Indiana Univ/Purdue Univ.	iupui.edu	Multiple programs and sites; nursing informatics
Minnesota Virtual Univ.	mnvu.extension.umn.edu/	Virtual university offerings, distance learning
Univ. of Alabama, Birmingham	uab.edu	Campus and distance programs
Univ. of Colorado Health Sci Center	uchs.edu	Undergraduate and graduate Internet courses, programs
Univ. of Kansas	kumc.edu	Campus and distance programs
Univ. of Maryland	umd.edu	Multiple programs; mobility; nursing informatics
Univ. of Phoenix Online	phoenix.edu	Multiple online Internet programs; courses
Univ. of Texas, Austin	utexas.edu	Campus; multiple options; nursing informatics
Univ. of Washington	son.washington.edu	Campus; research focus; multiple programs

†Most colleges and universities offer some form of distance learning, and/or online courses; some offer entire degrees. Some are cited that offer a major, or courses in nursing informatics. Some examples of different types of educational institutions located throughout the country are cited with web addresses; use these as a format guide to locate others of interest. Please note: Specific addresses, names, and/or offerings may change subsequent to this publication. (In most instances the address follows " http://www.".)

Performance-Based Learning and Assessment Methods

A change in methods used to promote learning and evaluate competence is another trend closely linked to competency outcomes. In the era of cost containment, finding the most effective and efficient ways for students to become competent is paramount. Related issues include:

- Changes in roles of teachers and learners
- Refocusing responsibility and accountability
- Shifting the perception of students from passive receivers of information to active learners responsible for being competent in the array of specific practice-based skills

In actual clinical practice, nurses must be competent in creative and effective problem solving, communication, teaching, caring, and management. Rather than lectures and multiple-choice tests, these skills are learned more effectively through activities such as problem-based learning, case studies, and diverse projects in many community agencies. In addition to hospitals and extended care agencies, settings include congregational health, parish nursing, hospice care, homeless clinics, rural migrant workers, schools, and prisons (Brendtro and Leuning, 2000; Mathews-Smith et al., 2001; Mundt, 1997; Palmer, 2001; Solari-Twadell and McDermott, 1999).

The concept of evaluation also is changing to focus on documenting actual competence in the most realistic circumstances. This requires performance examinations that specify the critical elements, or behaviors, that must be met according to the standard for practice (Lenburg, 1999b; Luttrell et al., 1999; Scanlon, Care, and Gessler, 2001; Tracy et al., 2000). Developing a structured portfolio is another method used to document competence (Serembus, 2000; Trossman, 1999). The rapid expansion of knowledge and technology and related changes in competency outcomes in education and practice require major changes in teaching-learning methods and evaluation of performance.

These trends precipitate issues for students and teachers. Both need to change ideas about learning. Sometimes students think it is easier just to figure out "what the teacher wants" and "study for the test" rather than engage in interactive group projects in and out of class that require more decision making, group process, and time. It is easier to take written tests than to demonstrate actual competence through performance examinations that require 100% accuracy of specified critical elements. Yet demonstration of competence is what employers expect, consumers need, and practitioners must do. Memorization is not adequate; abilities to assess, solve problems, and communicate effectively in diverse circumstances require far more skill. The increase in reported medical-related errors also vividly emphasizes the need for more effective performance validation (IOM, 1999; NCSBN, 1997-2001)

Issues for faculty also include creating interactive learning strategies and making arrangements for them. This means contracts with many agencies, working with preceptors and community leaders, and having students in multiple settings simultaneously. Again, the issues are time, creativity, and a very different way of thinking about learning. It also means creating more complex performance examinations both in class and in clinical settings to help students gain confidence and demonstrate achievement of essential competencies (Fig. 4-1). No easy task, but one required in contemporary education and practice.

Sociodemographic, Cultural Diversity, and Economic and Political Changes

From rural to metropolitan areas throughout the United States the population is undergoing significant transformation (Baer et al., 2000; Nursing, 1994). Many articles and websites

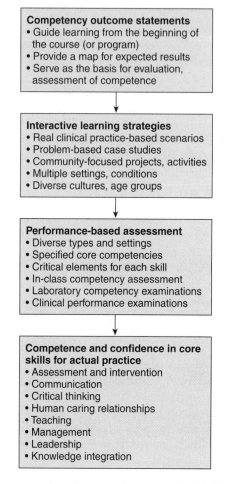

FIG. 4-1 Competency Outcomes and Performance Assessment (COPA) Model: from initial outcome expectations to competence in practice.

provide details about the aging of the population (i.e., the rapidly growing percentage of those over 65 and even 85 years of age). Others describe the number of ethnic minority groups and the increasing number of those in poverty, homeless, or under-insured. Other changes of note include differences in lifestyle choices and arrangements. For example, the definition of "family" is radically different as evident in the number of single individuals living with other singles, single-parent households (many by design) and same-sex couples (with and without children). Other changes pertain to economic and political trends related to population and to health care delivery. These changes present many issues for nursing and education; students are urged to explore the following references: Hurst and Osban, 2000; Lutz, Herrick, and Lehman, 2001; and Lenburg et al., 1995. Increasing violence in society and the workplace is another concern among health care providers and educators (Melamed, 2000; ANA, 1999).

Some of the issues for students are the distinct differences among patients in their responses to illness, treatments, and caregivers, which are based on differences in age, culture, religion, and life experiences in family and community (Ryan et al., 2000). Additional factors pertain to the heritage of their geographic location. For example, issues related to nursing care may differ considerably among those in areas that are rural or urban, mountains or plains, north, south, east, or west. Ways of healing and caring may include many alternative, non-medical, natural remedies and embrace the benefits of religion, rituals, and traditions (LaSala et al., 1997; Moylan, 2000). How the nurse responds to these modalities may make all the difference in the therapeutic relationship and outcome of care.

Effective and thoughtful nursing care is individualized according to client characteristics and circumstances, which is why students need to learn as much as possible from sociology, cultural diversity, psychology, religion, economics, history, and literature, as well as basic sciences. Moreover, learning the stories of diverse peoples, their customs, life experiences, and expectations is interesting and expands human understanding and creativity for personal and professional life.

Issues for faculty include the need to modify curriculum and learning experiences to help students prepare for increasing diversity in the population and healing modalities, in health care costs, and in the consequences of inadequate insurance or resources to support health. Teachers need time to learn about and establish trusting and caring relationships among leaders in various communities and to create new learning opportunities. Case studies (i.e., projects related to community health and ethnic and lifestyle diversity) are essential.

Community-Focused Interdisciplinary Approaches

These societal trends described in the preceding paragraphs helped create the current focus on community-focused health with an interdisciplinary emphasis. The large-scale economic and political influences to reduce health care costs also played a part. For example, the extraordinary expansion of knowledge and creative treatment technologies made it common practice for complex surgery to be performed in ambulatory settings on an outpatient basis or for drugs to be used instead of surgery. In addition, diverse health-conscious groups slowly made progress to change the national orientation from "illness care" to promoting health more efficiently and effectively. Another contributing factor is the increasing emphasis on health of the family as a whole and on entire communities and populations (Kiehl and Wink, 2000; Lutz, Herrick, and Lehman, 2001). The concept of community now is perceived as groups of individuals who share particular characteristics that shape their collective relationships, regardless of where they are located. Some examples are religious communities, ethnic communities, and homeless communities. The concept of community agencies also is redefined; acute hospitals are viewed as one of many community resources rather than in a totally different category. These changes require a radically different philosophy of care, one that creates a culture of interdisciplinary collaboration. This health care culture incorporates concepts of shared responsibility for health promotion among individuals, family, community, and multiple care providers. More than ever, family and neighbors need to become competent caregivers and members of the health care team.

The issues for teachers and students flow from these changes in philosophy, from "nursing as illness care in hospitals" to "nursing as health promotion and care management for individuals in the context of family, and family within the community." This requires a different perception and integration of core practice competencies (see Box 4-2); care delivery is more complex since general hospitals have become large critical care units, and less acute patients receive care in ambulatory settings or at home. Thus many acutely ill and post surgical patients now need illness nursing care, as well as health promotion, in their homes or other settings (Mathews-Smith et al., 2001; Mitty and Mezey, 1998; Ryan et al., 2000). Patients in hospital, at home, or in extended care settings are sicker and need interdisciplinary care that often is coordinated and managed by nurses.

This new reality poses a bipolar dilemma: how to prepare nurses who will be competent to manage illness and health care to diverse clients dispersed throughout the community and at the same time able to provide critical care to patients in hospitals who are sicker and stay for shorter periods of time. These changes require reorganization of the curriculum so that multiple aspects of community health and illness care are emphasized in courses throughout the program rather than in one course in community public health. Students need very different clinical experiences dispersed throughout the community and under the supervision of preceptors and nursing staff (Kiehl and Wink, 2000; Bringing healthcare, 1996). Like a row of dominoes falling, these changes pose yet more issues.

Some issues for students include changing their image of where they will work, the kinds of patients they will care for, and the skills they will use. Although many will work in acute care hospitals, others will provide care in diverse community settings to those who are culturally diverse or elderly and have multiple chronic and/or acute conditions that require long-term nursing management. This requires skill in all core practice competencies, especially creative problem solving, interdisciplinary collaboration, and ability to use computers and communication technology effectively and independently (Engelke and Britton, 2000). The Nightingale Tracker system is an example of such technology currently being tested by the Fuld Institute for Technology in Nursing Education (FITNE); access its website and reports through www.fitne.net.

Other issues include working with preceptors and staff in multiple locations with less one-on-one instructor interaction. This requires planning, time, and resources for travel to diverse clinical locations and out-of-class peer group work and projects. But it provides opportunities for students to learn collaboration and diverse approaches to care in multiple settings and to develop confidence and competence. Useful experiences may include projects in congregational health, parish nursing, rural health care, and alternative health practices (Brendtro and Leuning, 2000; Palmer, 2001). Service-learning projects also are relevant parts of community health (Green and Adderley-Kelly, 1999; White and Henry, 1999). Explore websites in Table 4-2.

Consumer-Oriented Society

As consumers have become more knowledgeable about illness care, health promotion, and the consequences of errors in care, they also have become more assertive about their rights to competent and prudent care. The economics and politics of health care and access to comprehensive information via the Internet have promoted more consumer involvement in setting health care standards and policies (Lewis, 2000; see Table 4-2 for multiple websites). Consumers are more active on health-related boards and committees and consumer advocacy groups. Their involvement has helped bring attention to needed revisions and also has precipitated some issues that influence nursing education.

For example, nurses need to change their approach from "giving care" to the patient, to "working with" the patient as a member of the health care team. This involves a different emphasis on interpersonal communication and making decisions for outcomes. A more informed and engaged patient is better able to make effective decisions, and thus patient teaching is a core practice competence. Interactive learning and service-learning projects are valuable ways for students to learn to work with consumers in planning projects to promote safety and health and community responsibility for health (Hurst and Osban, 2000; White and Henry, 1999).

Other issues pertain to the increasing number and consequences of serious medical errors made by health care professionals. These errors have led to an increased number of lawsuits with high associated costs, which further increase the cost of health care and tarnish the belief in the quality of health care in this country. The Institute of Medicine (IOM, 1999) conducted a major study, which was widely reported in professional journals and national newspapers; nursing organizations also responded (ANA, AACN). A large percent of errors are attributed to nurses, and therefore nursing faculty and administrators are increasingly concerned with ensuring the competence of students and nurses. These issues have in large part supported the need to insist on competency-based performance examinations in schools of nursing and as part of employer annual evaluations, and accreditation (JCAHO, 2000)

Ethics and Bioethical Concerns

Another trend closely connected to those in the preceding paragraphs is patients who have different ways of responding to illness, care providers, and therapies, which raises ethical issues of who is right and who has the right to prevail. This is particularly relevant regarding end-of-life issues (Rushton and Sabatier, 2001).

Issues for students include the separation of professional practice behaviors from personal beliefs and preferences and acceptance of the concept of "a gray continuum" instead of simplistic black-and-white interpretations. Diversity of backgrounds also conveys diversity in interpretation of behaviors, events, and language. Some of the most controversial issues include the right of individual choice regarding abortion, organ transplant, preference in sexual partners, and euthanasia or right to die a dignified death. Other issues may include the use of alternative remedies that may not be in the mainstream, even among those who engage in complementary health practices.

Teachers have similar issues related to which content to include in courses and clinical experiences and how to help students become more respectful of diversity in life practices. One part of the solution is to teach ethical concepts and to use case studies, guided learning experiences, and focused discussions to explore ways of interacting with patients/clients who present behaviors or responses that are very different from the expected norm. The need to explore these ethical issues will become even more essential as the characteristics of the population change further (Riley and Fry, 2000).

Increasing Shortage of Nurses, Students, and Faculty

A recurring trend over many decades is the shortage of qualified staff nurses, teachers, and students. In addition to Chapter 12 in this book, several references provide historical and current details regarding the numbers and causes (e.g., Baer, 2000; Heller, Oros, and Durney-Crowley, 2000; and Nursing shortage, 2001). Most current information and discussion of the consequences also are provided on the website for AACN (2000b), ANA (1999), NFSNO, and other specialty organizations (see Table 4-2). One of the most dire consequences is the increasing number of errors in patient care as reported by the Pew Commission (Bellack and O'Neil, 2000). Two primary aspects of the trend include the predicted short- and long-term shortage and the increased aging of the profession. The current nursing workforce of nurses, teachers, and students is older than ever, and fewer personnel are available. The average age of nurses is in the mid-40s; and, as fewer younger students enter nursing, the average age will continue to rise (Buerhaus, 2001; Buerhaus, Staiger, and Auerbach, 2000).

The shortage and aging of nurses have serious consequences and issues for students, teachers, and the profession. Inadequate clinical staff results in lower quality of care and fewer preceptors with enough time to work with students. More nurses work part time and for agencies, which means that some students may be in clinical settings without adequate supervision or may have fewer opportunities for specific learning experiences. They also may be exposed to nurses with inadequate educational background to help them integrate content and practice and thus precipitate undesirable practices. Therefore students must take more individual responsibility for competence.

Similarly, staff shortage has consequences for teachers as they arrange for supervised learning experiences for students in multiple and diverse clinical settings throughout the community. These conditions may lead to frustration and disappointments, as well as limited competence in the very abilities required for contemporary professional practice. These circumstances present special concerns for students in distance learning and Internet-based programs who are more dependent on qualified nurses to be preceptors.

The number of qualified student applicants is declining, and many of those who enroll are older and/or have prior education in nursing or in other fields (Frik, Speed, and Pollock, 1996). They often seek kinds of learning experiences that are different from those of young students, and they may find course offerings and experiences frustrating. Nursing programs also are faced with shortage of qualified teachers because of the declining number of master of science in nursing and doctoral graduates prepared in education, which in turn, may lead to higher student-teacher ratios at a time when the complexity of clinical learning requires even more one-on-one supervision. These issues require multilateral planning by teachers, students, the profession, and the broader community.

Increasing Professional and Personal Responsibilities

In the context of all these trends, another one with multiple related issues has become increasingly evident. Students, teachers, and nurses confront increasing life responsibilities and associated stressful demands on time and resources. In summary, they simultaneously must cope with the explosion of new information and technology; changing health care systems; more precise expectations for learning outcomes; more interactive and out-of-class methods of learning; different expectations for competent performance; shortage of nurse preceptors and teachers; and multiple cultural, ethical, and legal aspects of an ever-changing society. In addition, most also have the responsibility of caring for dependent children, as well as aging parents.

At the same time, the profession requires its members to keep current and pursue planned professional development. Complexities in practice increase the need for nurses, teachers, and administrators to document continuing competence for relicensure and recertification. Changes in multistate regulations also draw attention to the need for initial and continuing competence (Gaffney, 1999). In many states continuing education is mandatory, and state boards of nursing have changed or are in the process of changing requirements to validate continuing competence (see websites for NCSBN and specific states, such as California, Kentucky, Tennessee). The American Nurses Association has cited the continuing competence of nurses as one of its focus issues of concern (ANA 1999; ANA, 2000; multiple issues of *The American Nurse,* 2001).

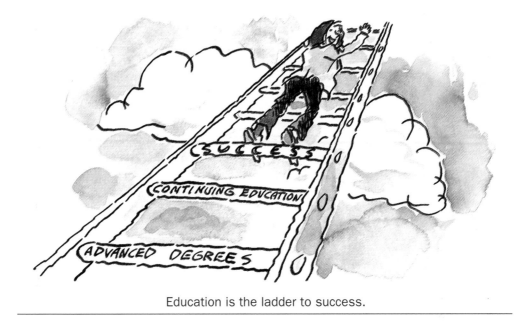

Education is the ladder to success.

The related issues are almost universal, and solutions are difficult and multifaceted. The high stress levels associated with both professional and personal demands have consequences for one's own health and that of those around them. These issues illustrate how important it is for all of those involved in the educational process to be more caring, understanding, respectful, and helpful to each other. Teachers, students, administrators, staff nurses, employers, family, and friends need to learn anew the meaning of "caring community" in the context of rapid change.

DIVERSITY, FLEXIBILITY, MOBILITY, AND DELIVERY OF EDUCATION PROGRAMS

A brief review of the major types of education programs that prepare nurses for licensure is presented here to set the stage for summarizing some contemporary issues related to diversity, flexibility, mobility, and distance delivery of programs. Details about numbers of programs and students are provided by the National League for Nursing (NLN) (1997); also see the AACN website for a 2001 report. The continued development of these programs illustrates issues in nursing during the past 100 years. Table 4-3 provides a concise overview of program types; several references are cited for more detail, including some very interesting ones that focus on the historic context for today's issues (Baer et al., 2000; Kalisch and Kalisch, 1995) (see also Chapter 1). Moreover, an increasing number of nursing schools are developing partnerships with communities and changing the curriculum to promote more competent and effective health care (Kiehl and Wink, 2000; Lutz, Herrick, and Lehman, 2001).

Licensed Practical Nurse Programs

Practical nurse programs provide the shortest but most restricted option for individuals seeking a nursing license. Typically licensed practical nurse (LPN) programs are 9 to 12 months in

TABLE 4-3	*Types of Nursing Education Programs*

TYPE OF PROGRAM AND CREDENTIAL	TYPE OF INSTITUTION	LENGTH OF PROGRAM	PURPOSE AND SCOPE
Practical/vocational nurse program; prepares for LPN/LVN license	High schools, hospitals, vocational-technical schools	9-12 mo	Basic technical bedside care; hospitals, nursing homes, home care; offices in LPN positions
Diploma; prepares for RN license	Hospitals, some in conjunction with colleges	2-3 y	Basic RN positions; hospitals and agency care
Associate Degree Nursing; prepares for RN license	Community and junior colleges	2 y	Basic technical care in RN positions, primarily in institutions
Baccalaureate Degree Nursing; BSN, prepares for RN license	Colleges and universities	2-4 y (depends on type option)	Basic professional practice as RN; management, community and public health settings; prepares for graduate school and certification; basic programs are 4 y and mobility options may be only 2 y
Master's Degree Nursing; MSN	Universities	1-2 y beyond BSN degree	Advanced clinical practice, management, education, leadership positions
Doctoral programs; PhD, EdD, DSN, DNSc, ND degrees	Universities	Varies	Advanced practice in clinical, educational, administrative settings; leadership position

length and may be offered by high schools, adult education and vocational technical schools, or hospitals. In California and Texas the term *vocational nurse* is used, and graduates who are licensed are called LVNs. Each state board of nursing sets responsibilities and scope of practice. The LPN/LVN usually is required to work under the supervision of a registered nurse (RN) or other licensed person, and scope of practice focuses on technical nursing procedures and treatments. Variations in which some of the more technical aspects of care they can administer are determined by each state board. LPNs/LVNs are employed in many different types of settings, including hospitals, nursing homes, offices, and other structured settings. In 1995 more than 1100 LPN/LVN programs produced approximately 44,000 graduates, although the number was 2% less than the previous reporting period (NLN, 1997).

For many reasons some individuals want or need to begin a career in nursing in LPN/LVN programs. Once licensed, they can obtain employment, and subsequently many continue on to various programs that prepare for registration as a professional nurse (RN). Some of these opportunities are presented in the section for mobility programs. Although helpful in many settings, LPN preparation is considered by many to be inadequate for the complexities of contemporary nursing care.

Hospital Diploma Programs

The oldest and most traditional of nursing education programs that prepare for professional licensure are hospital-based diploma programs. These programs were initially developed in the United States in the late 1800s in general hospitals in cities such as Boston, New York, Hartford, and Philadelphia and subsequently spread across the country. They began as training programs by physicians and lasted a few weeks. Soon the nurse graduates began developing courses and teaching them from the nursing perspective, and programs were extended from 1 to 2 years in length. In later years all diploma programs were 3 years in length and had fairly uniform courses of study and clinical hours. Linda Richard and other early graduates wrote initial nursing textbooks and began offering specialty training to staff hospitals and clinics (Kalisch and Kalisch, 1995). This was a major turning point in nursing.

As the number of hospitals expanded, the need for nurses likewise increased, and essentially every hospital developed its own training program. At their peak in the 1950s and 1960s, approximately 1300 diploma programs were in operation. Many changes in society related to education and health care also influenced nursing education, and by 2000 the NLN reported only 86 diploma schools still operating. These remaining programs now are more like the newer associate degree programs than the earlier diploma programs and typically are 2 years in length and follow an academic calendar, even though they include considerably more hands-on clinical experience. In fact, many of them have arrangements with colleges to offer arts and sciences and in some cases dual credentials, an associate degree, and a hospital diploma.

Associate Degree Programs

In the late 1950s a different trend in nursing education began to emerge in response to social, political, and educational changes in society and to a growing shortage of RNs. During World War II (WWII) the need for RNs who could be prepared in a much shorter time was critical. The Cadet Nurse Corp, a shortened version of the diploma program, was developed and proved to be very successful. From this necessity, nurse leaders learned that nurses could be prepared in less time and still meet RN licensure and practice requirements. This shortened program, offered in colleges, was in the context of the newly developing community college movement that offered 2-year associate degree programs in many technical fields. These associate degree programs reinforced the ideas of shorter college study, the integration of content into more comprehensive courses, and the differentiation of technical education in a college setting from the more conventional 4-year degree program that prepared students for graduate study.

After WWII communities all over the country rapidly applied new federal funding to develop community colleges and public and private junior colleges. They prepared many more citizens for newly created and more technical jobs required for the era of expansion and industrialization. This also was an era in which the idea of a college education for the ordinary person was not just a remote dream. With military benefits for education tuition and funds for institutions, the 2-year college degree allowed thousands of men and women to rise above their heritage to earn a college degree that was within their means and to fill jobs needed by new business and industry.

At the same time, the increasing complexity and expansion of medical care required more and better prepared RNs. A few educators began to create a new 2-year nursing program for the community college, which required courses in arts and sciences and a more integrated approach to nursing content and clinical learning (Kalisch and Kalisch, 1995; Montag, 1959). These pioneers reasoned that nursing belonged in college settings along with other disciplines to provide a better education for nurses and women and to establish more respect and recognition for nursing's contribution to the community's health. As the number of community colleges grew and the need for nurses increased, community college nursing programs became a logical proposal for development and expansion. Baer and colleagues (2000) and Kalisch and Kalisch (1995) provide details; Dillon (1997) and Simmons (1993) provide brief and interesting summaries of associate degree in nursing (ADN) education.

This is a vivid example of how changes in society influence the evolution of nursing education; it was another significant "first" in nursing and an important part of the evolving professionalization of nursing as a discipline. For the first time it was possible for all nurse education programs to be offered in college settings and for all graduates to earn a college degree. The original concept was that technical RNs (associate degree nurses) would work with professional RNs (nurses with a bachelor of science in nursing [BSN]), as a team. ADN programs were so successful that they became the new career pathway for thousands of students; today the majority of RNs are ADN graduates. By 2000 approximately 885 ADN programs were listed by the NLNAC. During the same time the number of 4-year BSN programs slowly but steadily increased. Thus the combination of 2-year ADN and 4-year BSN programs became the undergraduate backbone of the profession and a progressive model for students, educators, and employers (see Table 4-2 for websites).

Baccalaureate Degree Nursing Programs

In 1909 the efforts of progressive physicians and nurses resulted in a nursing program offered by the University of Minnesota; however, it was a diploma model and did not offer a college degree. During the next decade more than 15 similar programs were developed by other universities. It was not until 1924 that Yale University offered the first separate department of nursing whose graduates earned the baccalaureate degree. The 28-month program required scientific studies and clinical work and had the prestige and authority of other departments, with its own dean and budget (Kalisch and Kalisch, 1995). This was another first in the history of nursing education.

It took years of effort and many progressive nursing leaders to convince college administrators, physicians, and other nurses that nursing care could be improved and the profession advanced through collegiate education. They envisioned nursing as a professional discipline exceeding far more than the technical hands-on care provided by less educated nurses. They believed that nurses could provide more comprehensive and compassionate care and be more effective if they had a solid foundation in the arts and sciences before or during the 4-year nursing program offered by colleges and universities. To a large extent this debate continues to this day. The number of colleges and universities offering the BSN degree slowly continued to increase, and by 2001 the AACN reported 570 basic BSN programs; 609 offer RN-BSN options.

BSN degree programs typically require 2 years of arts and sciences as the foundation for 2 years of nursing courses, most requiring 120 to 130 semester credits for the degree. Nursing courses include typical content related to the care of patients with medical, surgical, pediatric, obstetric, and psychiatric conditions, although course titles differ considerably. They also include courses in community and public health, beginning research, management, and leadership. The broader scope of professional practice also emphasizes the need for courses such as epidemiology, statistics, and pathophysiology. Other differences are the expanded focus that includes the family and community and the emphasis on health promotion and illness prevention, with an increasing part of clinical experiences in diverse community settings. Graduates of BSN programs take the same NCLEX-RN licensure examination as diploma and ADN graduates. An increasing number of specialty areas require the BSN degree as part of the certification process, and admission into master's programs usually requires the BSN degree.

Master's Degree Nursing Programs

In the 1960s and 1970s the increasing complexity of health care; the need for qualified nurse educators, administrators, and clinicians; and the increasing number of BSN graduates stimulated the federal government to provide support for the development of a master of science in nursing (MSN) degree and other types of programs. In 1977 most nurse administrators were diploma graduates (46%); only 28% had MSN or doctoral degrees (Kalisch and Kalisch, 1995). Efforts of lobbyist and nurse leaders resulted in federal funding for nursing programs, student tuition, and building construction. Traineeship and fellowship grants enabled thousands of RNs to return to school to earn BSN and advanced degrees to prepare for positions in education, administration, practice, and research. Until the late 1970s MSN programs primarily focused on preparing educators and administrators, but in the next decade the curriculum trend shifted to an overwhelming emphasis on clinical practice, with little attention to these functional areas. By the 1990s, both the negative and the positive consequences of these decisions became apparent.

Currently most MSN programs are designed to prepare advanced nurse practitioners and clinical specialists in a wide array of specialty areas. The extraordinary and rapid changes in health care during the 1990s highlighted the cost-effective and quality care benefits of using advanced practice nurses to provide primary health care previously unavailable or provided by physicians. In the past two decades nurses have waged intensive and persistent legal battles to change state laws to permit nurse practitioners to write prescriptions, receive reimbursement for care, and operate independent nurse practices and health centers. The resulting recognition and expanded scope of practice changed the definition and roles of advanced practice nurses and increased the number of MSN students. Most nurse educators and managers and administrators in nursing care facilities now are required to have a master's degree. These factors have had a marked influence on the MSN curriculum and the number of programs available. In 2001 the AACN listed 382 master's degree nursing programs.

Different MSN education options are available, the most common of which is for graduates of BSN programs; other options are designed for graduates of nonnursing degree programs and for nurse doctorate (ND) programs and are especially attractive during periods of nursing shortages. A growing number of universities offer multiple options and clinical specialty majors in response to changes in health care needs. Financial constraints, changes in education philosophy, and computer technology have provided incentives for universities to develop more programs that offer flexible distance learning and mobility options, especially for part-time students. The current trend is MSN programs that can be completed almost entirely through Internet courses. Some programs use computerized online courses and other mediated arrangements such as audio and/or video teleconferencing, closed statewide computer and/or video networking, correspondence courses, and various types of cognitive and performance examinations (Skiba, 1997; Wambach et al, 1999). Some require short periods of intensive on-campus classes or assigned clinical experiences with designated preceptors. Technology has made it possible for nurses to meet requirements for higher degrees and still meet other obligations and constraints. Explore websites in Table 4-2.

Doctoral Programs

Nurse pioneers developed the first doctoral programs for nurses at the turn of the last century at Teachers College, Columbia University. The first nurse graduated in 1932 with an EdD degree in nursing education; later New York University offered a PhD program in 1934. More than 30 years elapsed before doctoral programs in nursing were offered: the doctor of nursing science degree (DNS, DNSc). In 2001 the AACN survey reported 77 nursing doctoral programs.

Currently four types of doctoral degrees are used by nursing students: (1) the Doctor of Education (EdD) for those interested in education; (2) the Doctor of Philosophy (PhD) for those interested in research; (3) the Doctor of Nursing Science (DNS or DNSc) for those interested in advanced clinical nursing practice; and (4) the Doctor of Nursing (ND) for those with BS degrees in other fields who want to pursue doctoral preparation for entry into nursing practice. The ND degree, which prepares nurses for basic licensure (NCLEX-RN), was first offered at Case Western Reserve University in 1979. Shortly after, Rush University and the University of Colorado Health Science Center offered programs, and others followed thereafter. Some schools offer options combined with another major such as business, law, or informatics. Henry (1997) reviewed various aspects of trends in doctoral education; see Newman (1997) and Classic Image (1997) for interesting articles.

APPROVAL AND ACCREDITATION OF NURSING PROGRAMS

All nursing programs must meet the rules and regulations of the State Board of Nursing for the particular state involved. A program must go through a rigorous approval process before it is officially approved to enroll students; thereafter it is reviewed periodically to ensure that it continues to meet the specified criteria.

All colleges and universities must meet additional regulations and standards established by regional accrediting bodies, which function under federal authority to ensure that the academic institutions actually offer the programs they proclaim. Accreditation by regional bodies (such as the Southern Association of Colleges and Schools) requires years of planned activities and report writing followed by site visits by evaluators, with final decisions ultimately made by a review board.

In addition, professional schools usually seek an additional voluntary accreditation by a professional association that is approved to accredit by the U.S. Department of Education. The NLN accredits all types of basic nursing programs. The AACN accredits baccalaureate and graduate degree nursing programs through its subsidiary organization the Commission on Collegiate Nursing Education.

Students must know the accreditation status of the schools they attend or plan to attend. Accreditation means that the school has established academic and professional standards. Graduate schools often require that prospective students have attended an accredited program. Some financial grants for additional study also include this requirement.

FLEXIBLE EDUCATION, MOBILITY, AND DISTANCE LEARNING PROGRAMS

Nursing literature over the past 30 years substantiates the need for the effectiveness of various mobility and distance delivery programs. During the early 1970s NLN conducted an extensive Open Curriculum study involving some 200 programs, some of which were summarized by

TABLE 4-4	*Basic Entry and Mobility Options and Patterns*
PROGRAM ENTRY OPTIONS	**MOBILITY OPTIONS: CONTINUE TO:***
Licensed practical nurse program	Associate degree
	Baccalaureate degree
Hospital diploma program	Baccalaureate degree
	Master's degree
	Nurse doctorate
Associate degree program	Baccalaureate degree
	Master's degree
	Nurse doctorate
Baccalaureate degree program	Master's degree
	Nurse doctorate
	DNS, DSc, others
Master's degree program	Philosophy doctorate
	Education doctorate
	Nurse doctorate
	DNS, DSc, others
Nurse doctorate	Master's degree
	Philosophy doctorate
	Education doctorate
	DNS, DSc, others
Nonnursing degree	Baccalaureate degree
	Master's degree
	Nurse doctorate
	Doctoral degrees

*Options vary considerably among and even within colleges and universities; prerequisites and requirements differ considerably. New combinations with Internet-based and other distance learning options are being developed or revised.

Most common types of education mobility approaches:

1. Advanced placement: use examinations, bridge courses, combination to award credit
2. Articulation: agreement among institutions, even statewide, to arrange curriculum on continuum for ease in transition to next degree; career ladder, 2-plus-2, etc., concepts
3. Escrow/bypass: award credit for prior learning based on success in current courses
4. External learning converted via examinations and special assessment; transfer credits
5. Blanket credit: advanced placement based on record of prior school and licensure

Combination of approaches: two or more methods used with same students; different methods used for different students, depending on degree options

Lenburg and Johnson (1974). Explore more current discussions (AACN, 1998; Baer et al., 2000; Kalisch and Kalisch, 1995; AACN, 2000a; ANA, 1991; Lenburg, 1975.

During the 1990s mobility and distance learning programs became more acceptable and have proliferated. Organizations such as the AACN, the NLN, the National Council of State Boards of Nursing, and others have published position statements related to mobility options, even though they were initially resistant to them (AACN 1998; NLN, 1993). Also refer to organization websites and historical references. By the year 2000 most BSN programs had flexible options for RN students, and many ADN programs had options for LPNs (Frik, Speed, and Pollock, 1996; Redmond, 1997). Table 4-4 summarizes the multiple points of entry into licensed nursing and some of the options for continued educational mobility.

The oldest and most controversial distance mobility program in nursing is the New York Regents College external degree, renamed Excelsior College in 2001. Its ADN program was initiated in 1972 and the BSN in 1976, both of which were fully accredited shortly thereafter, albeit with considerable controversy (Lenburg, 1975). Nearly all of its students are LPNs or RNs, although a prior license is not required; many students with health-related certificates or degrees have completed the programs. A master's degree program in nursing informatics was added in 2000. These options offer the most extensive national and international mobility program, as they are based entirely on assessment of knowledge through standardized written examinations, clinical competence through extensive nursing performance examinations, and the evaluation of arts and sciences either through prior college credit or college proficiency examinations. Literally thousands of nurses have completed degrees this way and have continued through graduate school and into leadership positions in nursing, substantiating their success (Lenburg, 1990). Other nursing programs have adopted these ideas and, with the expansion of computer and communications technology, have expanded opportunities further. Explore websites for Excelsior College, University of Phoenix Online, and others in Table 4-2.

Career ladder programs designed as 1-plus-1 or 2-plus-2 options have been offered for many years by some schools and currently by several states. Examples of statewide programs are those offered by Georgia (Kish et al., 1997); Iowa (McClelland et al., 1997), and Maryland (Rapson, 2000); also see websites for Colorado and Kentucky. A different model is illustrated by the consortium of 25 nursing programs in northeast Ohio. Cooperating leaders from these schools named the project the Nursing Education Mobility Action Group (NEMAG) and successfully developed the ACCESS model in the early 1990s. It continues to assist LPNs and RNs in that region to earn ADN and BSN degrees using options such as the transition course or the escrow/bypass methods. The 5-year evaluation of the project supported its effectiveness and efficiency (Nichols, Lenburg, Soehnlen, 2000; Rolince et al., 2001). Project LINC is another innovative mobility program for working adults; it was initiated in New York City and was so successful that it subsequently has been implemented in several other states (Westmoreland et al., 1998). Benjamin-Coleman and colleagues (2001) provide a review of a decade of distance learning program.

Changes in the social, political, financial, and philosophical climates; the knowledge and technology explosion; research from past experiences; and the continuing shortage of nurses have combined to make education mobility and distance learning opportunities a necessity and a reality throughout the country. The long-standing debate over "entry into practice" continues as nursing pursues its professionalization destiny (AACN, 1999a; AACN, 1999b, 2000a; NLN, 1993). Many nurse leaders have long considered mobility programs a method to achieve this goal. A review of websites for universities and colleges illustrates how widespread distance learning options have become, including some schools that offer entire degree programs or a number of courses via the Internet. For example, see websites for the offerings in California, central Florida, Colorado, Kansas, and Maryland.

Trends and issues that influence nursing education make it even more important to comply with quality standards and accreditation and to emphasize competency outcomes for students and graduates. Changes in number and qualifications of students and shortage of faculty and finances make it necessary to develop effective learning strategies for students. This includes advisement, tutoring, peer mentoring, and mediated learning programs to promote competence especially among older, rural, or minority students (Griffiths and Tagliareni, 1999; Ramsey et al., 2000). Although distance programs and Internet courses are often more convenient, they also present challenges for students. Some factors relate to access to current hardware and software technology and the time, ability, and money to use it. Students also need discipline and determination to pursue courses and clinical learning when a teacher is not present and learning is the responsibility of the learner, who also may be working full time and managing a household with multiple other responsibilities. Multiple entry–multiple exit programs also require planning and budgeting of time and resources for self and family, including consideration for the unexpected.

SUMMARY

This chapter has presented 10 major trends and related issues for students and faculty in education programs. To a large extent these issues influence the content, learning process, and evaluation methods used in all types of programs. They also influence the persistence of multiple types and levels of programs for entry into practice and the acceptance of diverse mobility and distance learning programs, all of which are increasingly using the Internet and electronic databases and resources in learning and practice. As students integrate current trends and attempt to resolve issues, they are learning to create the trends for the next generation; they are participating in nursing history in the making. As active learners, they integrate the words of Oliver Windell Holmes, who said: "The mind once stretched with a new idea never regains its original dimensions."

Critical Thinking Activities for Each Outcome (Use combinations of learning activities)

1. Integrate knowledge of current trends and issues in society into a more holistic perception of their influence on nursing, nursing education, students and faculty.
   Learning Exercises:
   a. List the major trends and associated issues in rank order of importance (relevance) to you from most important (1) to least important (10) and write a rationale for the top three.
   b. Create a chart that reflects your sense of the importance of these trends in nursing before and after studying this chapter. List the trends on the left; then use one column for before and another one for after the study of trends. Use a rating scale of 1 to 5, with 5 indicating most important, to reflect your perceptions of each trend on nursing.
   c. Analyze reflectively at least three issues you have experienced in nursing education and how they relate to the broader trends described in the chapter.
   d. Write a one-page reflective summary of your perception of the nursing profession and nursing education that incorporates four to five of the trends described in the chapter.
2. Integrate knowledge of current trends and issues into a personal contemporary philosophy of ongoing professional development and practice.
   Learning Exercises:
   a. In a small work group discuss changes in philosophy of nursing among group members related to the major trends and issues presented in the chapter.
   b. Summarize key points that support the need for ongoing professional development by group members.
   c. Write a personal philosophy of nursing (one to two paragraphs) that integrates elements of four or five trends presented.
   d. Outline a plan for continuing professional development that incorporates elements of at least 5 trends presented.

3. Differentiate among diverse conventional and flexible mobility nursing education programs and the issues related to them.
   Learning Exercises:
   a. Create a defining features matrix that identifies the major characteristics and differences among programs that prepare individuals for registered nurse licensure.
   b. Create a pro and con grid to summarize issues related to various flexible and educational mobility options.
   c. List at least three issues presented by major nursing organizations with their positive or negative positions related to diverse entry points into the profession.
   d. Critique the major issues related to Internet-based nursing degree programs (or clinical courses) and the corresponding justification for having them.

4. Access pertinent information resources related to evolving trends and issues as a component of ongoing professional development.
   Learning Exercises:
   a. In a small group, analyze several issues that are particularly relevant to members of the group and classify them under one or more of the trend headings.
   b. Submit a list of questions that could be used as guidelines to analyze issues and their merit within the context of broader trends and the goals of nursing education. (Include questions re what, who, why, when, where, and how.)
   c. Access three additional websites not listed in the chapter and describe their usefulness for ongoing professional development in the context of trends and issues.

REFERENCES

American Association of Colleges of Nursing: *Position statement: education mobility,* Washington, DC, 1998, AACN, www.aacn.nch.edu.

American Association of Colleges of Nursing: *White paper: distance technology in nursing education,* Washington, DC, 1999a, AACN, www.aacn.nche.edu.

American Association of Colleges of Nursing: *Position statement: nursing education's agenda for the 21st century,* Washington, DC, 1999b, AACN, www.aacn.nche.edu.

American Association of Colleges of Nursing: *Position statement: baccalaureate degree in nursing as minimal preparation for professional practice,* Washington, DC, 2000a, AACN, www.aacn.nche.edu.

American Association of Colleges of Nursing: *Nursing school enrollments decline as demand continues to climb,* Washington, DC, 2000b, AACN.

American Nurses Association: *One strong voice,* Kansas City, Mo, 1976, ANA.

American Nurses Association: *Nursing's agenda for healthcare reform,* Kansas City, Mo, 1991, ANA.

American Nurses Association: ANA to focus on core issues, *American Nurse,* Nov/Dec 1999, pp 17, 19. (See www.nursingworld.org/tan for multiple other articles re profession issues: adequate staffing, continuing competence, patient safety, advocacy, and workplace health and safety; also re organization unity.)

Baer ED et al: *Enduring issues in American nursing,* New York, 2000, Springer.

Bargagliotti T, Luttrell M, Lenburg CB: Reducing threats to the implementation of a competency-based performance assessment system, Online *J Iss Nurs,* Sept 1999, www.nursingworld.org/ojin.

Bellack JP, O'Neil EH: Recreating nursing practice for a new century: recommendations and implications of the Pew Health Professions Commission's final report, *Nurs Health Care Perspect* 21:14-21, 2000.

Benjamin-Coleman R et al: Distance education: a decade of distance education: RN to BSN, *Nurs Educator* 26:9-12, 2001.

Brendtro MJ, Leuning C: Nurses in churches: a population-focused clinical option, *J Nurs Educ* 39:285-288, 2000.

Bringing healthcare to the streets (Special issue), *Nurs Health Care* 17:entire issue, 1996.

Buerhaus PI: Aging nurses in an aging society: long-term implications, *Reflections Nurs Leadership* 27(1): 35-36, 2001, www.nursingsociety.org.

Buerhaus PI, Staiger DO, Auerbach DI: Implications of an aging registered nurse workforce, *JAMA* 283 (22):2948-2954, 2000.

Classic Image: Perspectives from Image past (Special issue), *Image J Nurs Scholarship* 29:123-131, 1997.

Critical thinking and evidence-based practice (Special issue), *J Nurs Educ* 39(8):entire issue, 2000.

Curley MAQ: Patient-nurse synergy: optimizing patients' outcomes, *Am J Crit Care* 7(1):64-72, 1998.

Dillon P: Changing directions: the future of associate degree nursing, *Nurs Health Care Perspect* 18:20-24, 1997.

Eichelberger LW, Hewlett PO: Competency Model 101: the process of developing core competencies, *Nurs Health Care Perspect* 20:204-208, 1999.

Engelke MK, Britton BP: From black bags to interactive workstations, *Reflections Nurs Leadership* 26(4):30-32, 2000.

Focus on technology (Special issue), *J Nurs Educ* 38:entire issue, September 1999.

Frik SM, Speed DJ, Pollock SE: A special pathway for registered nurses with baccalaureate degrees in fields other than nursing, *J Nurs Educ* 35:152-156, 1996.

Gaffney T: The regulatory dilemma surrounding interstate practice, Online *J Iss Nurs,* May 1999, www.nursingworld.org/ojin. See other articles, same focused issue.

Green PM, Adderley-Kelly B: Partnership for health promotion in an urban community, *Nurs Health Care Perspect* 20:76-81, 1999.

Griffiths MJ, Tagliareni E: Challenging traditional assumptions about minority students in nursing education: outcomes from Project IMPART, *Nurs Health Care Perspect* 20:290-295, 1999.

Heller BR, Oros MT, Durney-Crowley J: The future of nursing education: 10 trends to watch, *Nurs Health Care Perspect* 21:9-13, 2000.

Henry B: Editorial: professional doctorates for professional practice, *Image J Nurs Scholarship* 29:102, 1997.

Hurst CP, Osban LB: Service learning on wheels: the Nightingale mobile clinic, *Nurs Health Care Perspect* 21:184-187, 2000.

Institute of Medicine (IOM): To err is human: building a safer health system, National Academy of Science Press, 1999, www.iom.edu/. See nursing response: www.aacn.nche.edu and www.nursingworld.org.

Joint Commission on Accreditation of Healthcare Organizations: criteria, journals, news, 2000, www.jcaho.org.

Kalisch PA, Kalisch BJ: *The advance of American nursing,* ed 3, 1995, Philadelphia, 1995, JB Lippincott.

Kiehl EM, Wink DM: Nursing students as change agents in the community: community-based nursing education in practice, *Nurs Health Care Perspect* 21:293-297, 2000.

Kish C et al: Georgia's RN-BSN articulation model, *Nurs Health Care Perspect* 18:26-30, 1997.

LaSala KB et al: Rural health care and interdisciplinary education, *Nurs Health Care Perspect* 18:292-298, 1997.

Lenburg CB: *Open learning and career mobility in nursing,* St Louis, 1975, Mosby.

Lenburg CB: Do external degree programs really work? *Nurs Outlook* 36:234-238, 1990.

Lenburg CB: Redesigning expectations for initial and continuing competence for contemporary nursing practice, Online *J Iss Nurs,* September 1999a, www.nursingworld.org/ojin.

Lenburg CB: The framework, concepts and methods of the competency outcomes and performance assessment (COPA) Model, Online *J Issu Nurs,* September 1999b, www.nursingworld.org/ojin.

Lenburg CB, Johnson W: Career mobility through nursing education, *Nurs Outlook* 32:250-254, 1974.

Lenburg CB et al: *Promoting cultural competence in nursing education,* Washington, DC, 1995, American Academy of Nursing.

Lewis D: Direct to consumer, *Reflections Nurs Leadership* 26(4):24-26, 2000.

Luttrell MF et al: Redesigning a BSN curriculum: competency outcomes for learning and performance assessment, *Nurs Health Care Perspect* 20:134-141, 1999.

Lutz J, Herrick CA, Lehman BB: Community partnership: a school of nursing creates nursing centers for older adults, *Nurs Health Care Perspect* 22:26-29, 2001.

Mallow GE, Gilje F: Technology-based nursing education: overview and call for further dialogue, *J Nurs Educ* 38:248-251, 1999.

Mathews-Smith G et al: A new module in caring for older adults: problem-based learning and practice portfolios, *J Nurs Educ* 40:73-78, 2001.

McClelland E et al: The Iowa articulation story: collaboration works, *Nurse Educ* 22(2):19-24, 1997.

Melamed A: Nurses attack hidden dangers of health care, *American Nurse,* November/December 2000, p 17, www.nursingworld.org/tan/.

Mitty E, Mezey M: Integrating advanced practice nurses in home care: recommendations for a teaching home care program, *Nurs Health Care Perspect* 19:264-270, 1998.

Montag ML: *Community college education for nursing,* New York, 1959, McGraw-Hill.

Moylan LB: Alternative treatment modalities: the need for a rational response by the nursing profession, *Nurs Outlook* 48:259-261, 2000.

Mundt MH: A model for clinical learning experiences in integrated healthcare networks, *J Nurs Educ* 36:309-316, 1997.

National Council of State Boards of Nursing (NCSBN): National council studies continued competence: committee develops personal accountability profile, *Issues* 18(2):1, 1997. (Also see www.ncsbn.org/ through 2001.)

National League for Nursing: A vision for nursing education, New York, 1993, Author, www.nln.org.

National League for Nursing: *Nursing datasource 1997.* Volume 1, *Trends in contemporary nursing education,* New York, 1997, Author.

Newman MA: The professional doctorate in nursing: a position paper, *Image J Nurs Scholarship* 29:361-362, 1997 (reprint of 1975 article in *Nurs Outlook* 23:704-706).

Nichols EF, Lenburg CB, Soehnlen JJ: Evaluation of a collaborative articulation mobility project using escrow and transition course methods, *Nurs Health Care Perspect* 21:188-195, 2000.

Nicoll LH: *Nurses' guide to the Internet,* ed 3, Philadelphia, 2000, JB Lippincott, www.lww.com.

Nursing bridging worlds (Special issue on cultural diversity and health issues), *Nurs Health Care* 15:227-261, 1994.

Nursing shortage: Feature issue, Online *J Iss Nurs,* Feb 2001, entire issue, www.nursingworld.org/ojin/topic/14.

Palmer J: Parish nursing connecting faith and health, *Reflections Nurs Leadership* 27(1):17-18, 2001.

Ramsey P et al: The NURSE center: a peer mentor-tutor project for disadvantaged nursing students in Appalachia, *Nurse Educ* 25:277-281, 2000.

Rapson MF: Statewide nursing articulation model design: politics or academics? *J Nurs Educ* 39:294-301, 2000.

Redman R, Lenburg CB, Walker, P: Competency assessment: methods for development and implementation in nursing education and practice, Online *J Iss Nurs,* September 1999, American Nurses Association.

Redmond GM: LPN-BSN: education for a reformed healthcare system, *J Nurs Educ* 36:121-127, 1997.

Riley JM, Fry ST: Nurses report widespread ethical conflicts, *Reflections Nurs Leadership* 26(2):35-36, 2000 (also see: www.bc.edu/nursing/ethics).

Rolince P et al: A regional collaboration for educational and career mobility: the nursing education mobility action group, *Nurs Health Care Perspect* 22:75-80, 2001.

Rubenfeld MG, Scheffer BK: *Critical thinking in nursing: an interactive approach,* Philadelphia, 1995, Lippincott.

Rushton CH, Sabatier KH: The nursing leadership consortium on end-of-life care: the response of the nursing profession to the need for improvement in palliative care, *Nurs Outlook* 49:58-60, 2001.

Ryan M et al: Learning to care for clients in their world, not mine, *J Nurs Educ* 39:401-408, 2000.

Scanlon JM, Care WD, Gessler S: Dealing with the unsafe student in clinical practice, *Nurs Educ* 26:23-27, 2001.

Schorr T, Zimmerman A: *Making choices, taking chances: nursing leaders tell their stories,* St Louis, 1990, Mosby.

Serembus JF: Teaching the process of developing a professional portfolio, *Nurse Educ* 25:282-287, 2000 (see references cited in this article).

Simmons J, editor: *Perspectives—celebrating 40 years of associate degree nursing education,* New York, 1993, National League for Nursing.

Skiba DJ: Transforming nursing education to celebrate learning, *Nurs Health Care Perspect* 18:124-129ff, 1997.

Solari-Twadell PA, McDermott MA, editors: *Parish nursing—promoting whole person health within faith communities,* Thousand Oaks, Calif, 1999, Sage.

Tracy SM et al: The clinical achievement portfolio: an outcomes-based assessment project in nursing education, *Nurs Educ* 25:241-246, 2000.

Trossman S: The professional portfolio: documenting who you are, what you do, *Am Nurse,* March/April 1999, www.nursingworld.org/tan/.

Wambach K et al: Beyond correspondence, video conferencing, and voice mail: Internet based master's degree courses in nursing, *J Nurs Educ* 38:267-271, 1999.

Westmoreland D et al: Replicating Project LINC in two midwestern states: implications for policy development, *Nurs Health Care Perspect* 19:166-174, 1998.

White SG, Henry JK: Incorporation of service-learning into a baccalaureate nursing education curriculum, *Nurs Outlook* 47:257-261, 1999.

Nursing Licensure and Certification 5

Janet C. Scherubel, PhD, RN, CCRN

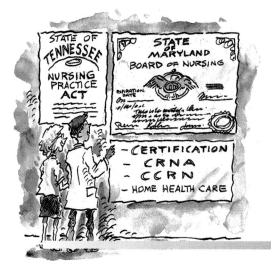

Professional and legal regulations
ensure safe, competent nursing care.

Vignette

Three nurses are discussing their nursing practice licenses. Joe Branch, a senior nursing student, is preparing for initial licensure. Mary Stone's license is due for renewal. Carmella Larkin has just moved into the state. As the three are talking about these changes in their practice, Georgio Gonzales, a nurse practitioner, joins the group. Georgio recently completed a certification examination and is interested in becoming certified for advanced practice. All the nurses have a general knowledge of the requirements for licensure and certification but lack the specific information needed to legally practice within the state. Mary suggests contacting the State Board of Nursing. The nurses agree that this is a sensible idea, and Mary leaves to phone the Board of Nursing. On returning Mary informs the group that the answers to all their questions may be found in the state's Nursing Practice Act and accompanying Rules and Regulations. Further the State Board of Nursing office will send free copies of both documents to each nurse.

The situation described here is not uncommon. Nurses need specific, current information on licensure and renewal of licensure. The most comprehensive sources for this information are the state Nursing Practice Act and the State Board of Nursing. These resources provide accurate advice on the relevant provisions for practicing nursing within each state and the United States territories. All nurses and nursing students should obtain copies of their state's practice act and become familiar with its contents.

Questions to consider while reading this chapter
1. Who establishes the "rules" for nursing practice—the state or the employer?
2. Do graduates from different types of nursing education programs require different types of licenses?

95

3. If a nurse graduate passes the NCLEX-RN, does that person still need a license?
4. What happens if a nurse's license expires? Can the nurse still practice?
5. Must a nurse complete graduate school and take an examination to be an advanced practice nurse?
6. Are the regulations governing advanced practice the same in all states?

Key Terms

Accreditation Process by which schools of nursing are approved to conduct nursing education programs.

Advanced practice nurse Legal title for nurses prepared by education and competence to perform independent practice.

American Nurses Association Professional organization that represents all registered nurses.

American Nurses Credentialing Center Independent agency of the American Nurses Association that conducts certification examinations and certifies advanced practice nurses.

Certification Process by which nurses are recognized for advanced education and competence.

Compact state A term of law. In the context of the Mutual Recognition Model, a state that has established an agreement with other states allowing nurses to practice within the state without an additional license. The interstate compacts have been enacted by the state legislatures.

Commission on Collegiate Nursing Education (CCNE) A subsidiary of colleges of nursing with responsibility for accrediting baccalaureate and higher-degree nursing programs.

Continued competency Program initiatives to ensure nurses knowledge, skills, and expertise beyond initial licensure.

Grandfathered Statutory process by which previously licensed persons are incorporated into revisions or additions in nursing practice acts.

International Council of Nursing Professional organization that represents nurses in 119 countries around the world.

Licensure by endorsement Process by which nurses licensed in one state may seek licensure in another without repeat examinations. The requirements are included in state nursing practice acts or accompanying rules and regulations.

Mandatory continuing education State-level educational requirements for renewal of license.

Mutual recognition of nursing Program developed by the State Boards of Nursing, Inc. The model proposes interstate compacts so that nurses licensed in one jurisdiction may practice in other compact states without duplicate licensure.

National Council of State Boards of Nursing, Inc. Organization whose membership consists of the board of nursing of each state or territory.

National League for Nursing Professional organization whose members represent multiple disciplines. The National League for Nursing conducts many types of programs, including accrediting nursing education programs.

Nursing practice act Statute in each state and territory that regulates the practice of nursing.

State Board of Nursing Appointed board within each state charged with responsibility to administer the nursing practice act of that state.

Sunset legislation Statutes that provide for revocation of laws if not reviewed and renewed within a specified time period.

Learning Outcomes

After studying this chapter, the reader will be able to

1. Explain the development of licensure requirements in the United States.
2. Summarize current licensure requirements in the context of historical developments.
3. Analyze the various components of a nursing practice act.
4. Discuss mutual recognition of nursing practice and identify compact states.
5. Differentiate among requirements for certification for advanced practice in different specialties.
6. Use appropriate resources to obtain current information on licensure and certification.
7. Describe the development of certification requirements for advanced practice in the United States.

CHAPTER OVERVIEW

To be a registered nurse! That is the goal of every student nurse. A worthy goal reached through study, clinical practice, and successful completion of the NCLEX-RN, the National Council Licensure Examination–Registered Nurse. In this chapter the reader will learn how and why nursing licensure developed, steps necessary to becoming licensed, licensure regulations, and the responsibilities of a registered nurse (RN).

After licensure as an RN, nurses still must maintain and increase their knowledge and skills. Some may wish to specialize in a particular area of nursing or expand their practice. Nurses with these goals may seek certification in a specialty field. This chapter describes certification, the means to achieve certification, and the organizations that administer certifying examinations. Whether it is licensure or certification, the nursing profession is continually progressing. Legal requirements to practice are continually revised to ensure the protection of the public. Just as in the past, nurses face issues and challenges as they seek to increase their competence and the nursing services they provide to patients and clients. Today it is no different. In this chapter issues related to licensure and certification are explored. Finally, future challenges emerging on the horizon are identified.

THE HISTORY OF NURSING LICENSURE
Recognition: Pins and Registries

The aim of caregivers since early times has been to be identified and recognized for one's skills and achievements. At first caregivers, particularly in the monasteries and convents of the medieval period, were identified by the habits they wore. Frequently special insignia designated health personnel. During the Crusades, a large Maltese cross adorned the black habits of the Knights Hospitalers of St. John of Jerusalem on the battlefield (Kalisch and Kalisch, 1995). These forms of identification allowed others to recognize their particular skills in caregiving and healing. More recently, nurses wore a readily identifiable symbol of their school of nursing, the nursing cap.

Today, as in the past, the school of nursing pin identifies graduates from a particular school of nursing. Early in each school's history, the students and faculty crafted the pin. The pin's emblems and text symbolize the philosophy, beliefs, and aspirations of the nursing program. Students receive it at graduation in a pinning ceremony. Nurses wear their pins proudly as evidence of their achievement, learning, and skill. It is one way in which they distinguish themselves as distinct health care providers with a special body of knowledge and clinical skills.

Nursing programs also maintain a record of all graduates. Florence Nightingale started this practice by creating a list of graduates in 1860 at the St. Thomas' School of Nursing in

England. This list became known as the "registry" of graduate nurses. The registry of nurses initiated by Nightingale provided institutions and clients with the means to identify graduates of nursing programs and ascertain the skills and knowledge of graduates. Today nursing programs around the world continue the tradition started by Nightingale and maintain a registry or listing of all graduates of the nursing program.

Purpose of Licensure

As nursing programs proliferated, variations developed among the programs. Entry criteria differed, and educational programs were structured to meet specific employer needs. A simple registry of graduates was not sufficient to ensure minimal levels of competency in all graduates, regardless of the training program. Another process was necessary to distinguish those sufficiently trained to provide nursing care from untrained or lesser-trained individuals. Graduate nurses, physicians, and hospitals joined to resolve the issue. The outcome was the development of criteria for licensure of nurses. Then as now, the primary purpose of licensure is the protection of the public.

Early Licensure Activities

As early as 1867, Dr. Henry Wentworth Acland suggested licensure of English nurses. However, it was not until 1896 that licensing nurses was first attempted in the United States. Nursing programs in the United States developed in much the same manner as was the pattern in England. Before the late 1800s many hospitals began training programs to prepare nursing staff for their own institutions. The programs varied based on the needs of the hospital, the availability of physicians and nurses for training students, and resources devoted to the training. To develop a standard for nurses and to improve the mobility of nurses between institutions, the Nurses Associated Alumnae of the United States and Canada, the organization that later became the American Nurses Association (ANA) in 1911, advocated licensure of nursing program graduates. But the group met with much resistance from hospitals, physicians, and nurses. These first attempts at licensure failed for lack of support (Kelly and Joel, 1996).

Nurses worldwide mounted an extensive educational campaign explaining the purposes and safeguards inherent in licensure, and in 1901 the International Council of Nurses passed a resolution that each nation and state examine and license its nurses. In 1903 North Carolina, New Jersey, New York, and Virginia were the first states to institute permissive licensure. The licensure rules were voluntary. These permissive licenses permitted but did not require nurses to become registered.

Under permissive licensure, educational standards were set at a minimum of 2 years of training for nurses. State boards of nursing were established with rules for examinations and revocation of the license. Nurses not passing the examination could not use the title of RN. Therefore, in addition to protecting the public from unskilled practitioners, these rules were an early move to protect the title of RN. The New York State Board of Regents began a registry of nurses successfully completing all requirements. In 20 years, by 1923, all states had instituted examinations for permissive licensure. Each state's licensure examinations varied in content, length, and format and included written, oral, and practice components. The early work in examinations for licensure was the forerunner of today's licensure and certification requirements (Kalisch and Kalisch, 1995).

The early state efforts in licensing nurses were commendable. Nonetheless, there was considerable variability between states in nursing education requirements, the licensure examinations, and the nursing practice acts themselves. The widespread variability in nursing practice acts prompted the ANA and later the National Council of State Boards of Nursing to design model nursing practice acts. The model acts provided a template for states to follow. The first was published in 1915. These model practice acts have been revised and updated as nursing practice advanced (Kelly and Joel, 1996). The latest revision of the model nursing practice act occurred in 1994 (National Council of State Boards of Nursing, 1994). The model nursing practice act proposes a definition of nursing, the scope of practice for the RN, descriptions of advanced practice nursing, requirements for prescriptive authority of nurses, and guidelines for disciplinary actions against nurses who violate sections of the act. Separate sections of the model act provide guidelines for State Boards of Nursing and the necessary requirements for entry into practice. From these model acts, each state or jurisdiction developed a unique practice act. Although the individual act addresses the needs of that jurisdiction, each includes the sections described in the model act. The nursing practice act for any state may be obtained by contacting that state or territorial board of nursing. A listing of state boards of nursing addresses and Internet addresses is provided (Appendix B).

Mandatory Licensure

Once each state had established permissive licensure, the next movement was toward a requirement that all nurses must be licensed. This practice is termed mandatory licensure. Likewise, efforts were promulgated to standardize nursing testing procedures. In the mid 1930s New York was the first state to require mandatory licensure, although this requirement was not effective until 1947. After World War II the ANA formed the National Council of State Boards of Nursing. The council was comprised of a representative of each state and jurisdiction in the United States. As part of its original activities, the Council advocated a standardized examination for licensure. This sponsorship led to the National League for Nursing administering the first State Board Test Pool Examination in 1950. The written examination included separate sections on medical-surgical nursing, maternity nursing, nursing of children, and psychiatric nursing. This format for examination continued for over 30 years, and many of today's nurses took these examinations.

The next major event in licensure efforts occurred in 1982 with the development of the first NCLEX examination. The test was revised to include all nursing content within one section of the examination. In addition the format was changed to present questions in a nursing process format. Just as with previous versions of licensing examinations, the NCLEX has evolved over time. Paper and pencil testing was replaced with computerized adaptive testing in 1994. Extensive information on the NCLEX may be found in Chapter 26 of this text.

COMPONENTS OF NURSING PRACTICE ACTS

As discussed previously, each state develops rules and regulations to govern the practice of nursing within that state. These rules are in the nursing practice acts or rules and regulations to administer the act. Many nursing practice acts are patterned after the ANA or the National Council of State Boards of Nursing, Inc. model practice acts, and all contain comparable information.

Purpose of Act

Each act begins with a purpose. All nursing practice acts include two essential purposes. First, each includes statements that refer to protecting the health and safety of the citizens of the jurisdiction. The act describes the qualifications and responsibilities of those individuals covered by the regulations. Likewise the act delineates those excluded from the practice of nursing. These provisions ensure the protection of the public. The second purpose is to protect the title of RN. The legal title, RN, is reserved for those meeting the requirements to practice nursing. Only those licensed may use the designation of RN. Thus unlicensed personnel are prevented from using the title of Registered Nurse.

Definition of Nursing

In each state or jurisdictional nursing practice act the practice of professional nursing is defined. The definition of nursing is of utmost importance because it delineates the scope of practice for nurses within the state. That is, each act outlines the activities nurses may legally perform within the jurisdiction. Many states follow the guidelines incorporated in the model practice act, although each is specific and delineates practice within that state or jurisdiction. For example, some states describe nursing as a process that includes nursing diagnosis, whereas other states list broad areas of nursing activities. To prevent the acts from becoming outdated, there are no lists of skills or procedures in the acts. As nursing knowledge and practices advance, new techniques are frequently allowable because of the generalized nature of the definition of nursing.

Many jurisdictions incorporate definitions of advanced practice nursing within one definition of nursing. In other states the definitions of advanced nursing practice and the scope of practice for advanced practice nurses are separately defined. The format of the act will be readily apparent with review of the nurse practice act.

Each state or jurisdiction establishes laws regulating practice within its borders. Therefore it is imperative for the nurse to know and understand the definition of nursing in the states in which he or she practices. Further, jurisdictions retain the rights to govern practice within the jurisdiction, even in the presence of a mutual recognition agreement with other compact states. This retention of states rights is an essential component in the Mutual Recognition Model.

Licensure Requirements

A section of each nursing practice act describes the requirements and procedures necessary for initial entry into nursing practice, or nursing licensure. An initial requirement in all jurisdictions is graduation from high school and an accredited nursing program. Candidates for licensure must submit evidence of graduation as defined by each state.

At present North Dakota is the only state requiring a baccalaureate degree for licensure as a professional nurse. This requirement was initiated in 1987. In North Dakota the nurse graduating from an associate degree program may be licensed as a technical nurse. In all other states, graduates of diploma, associate degree, or baccalaureate nursing programs may be licensed as RNs.

Additional requirements for licensure may include the mental and physical health status of the applicant. In addition, jurisdictions may conduct a review of prior legal convictions. This is especially important in reference to felony convictions. Some states have appended provisions related to recreational drug abuse. Finally, most states require statements from the school of nursing attesting the eligibility of the candidate for licensure. Frequently a transcript of coursework, a diploma, or a letter from the dean of the program attesting to the graduation of the applicant is necessary. Once again, as the laws are continually being revised to reflect the current practice of nursing, it is incumbent on the individual to be cognizant of the current licensure requirements in all states in which he or she intends to practice.

Regardless of individual state requirements, all nursing practice acts require candidates for practice to successfully complete the NCLEX-RN licensure examination. In some states it is possible to obtain a temporary permit to practice, pending receipt of success on the licensure examination. This practice was especially prevalent in past years, as in some states it took several months for results of the licensure examinations to be reported. Now, however, with the prompt response from the testing services, the need for temporary permits to practice is becoming less frequent.

A temporary permit is still available for nurses moving from one state to another. To obtain a license to practice in another state, the nurse applies for licensure by endorsement. Nurses licensed in one jurisdiction may apply for licensure in a second jurisdiction by submitting a letter to the second State Board of Nursing. Typically evidence for the new license is similar to that for initial licensure. In addition, proof of the nurse's current license to practice, as well as any restrictions imposed on the license by the first state, is required. These procedures will continue for all states not participating in the Mutual Recognition Model. For those states designated as compact states, the nurse should contact the State Board of Nursing to determine the appropriate procedures for nursing practice. Regardless of the type of nursing practice act, the nurse is still responsible for ascertaining the requirements to practice within each jurisdiction.

Renewal of Licensure

In addition to outlining requirements for initial licensure, each nursing practice act includes the requirements and information necessary to renew one's nursing license. These regulations define the length of time a license is valid, generally from 2 to 3 years. In addition, any specific requirements for renewal of licensure are stated.

Mandatory Continuing Education

The nurse will find information on mandatory continuing education for renewal of licensure in the section on license renewal. All nurses are expected to remain competent to practice through various means of continuing education. In 1976 California was the first state to institute mandatory continuing education for renewal of licensure. Since that time a number of states have instituted requirements of continuing education for renewal of licensure. The number of hours necessary varies, depending on the jurisdiction, ranging from 20 to 40 hours over a 2- to 3-year period. An additional obligation has been instituted in some jurisdictions. These jurisdictions require specific continuing education content such as health care ethics or the state nursing practice act. Clinical course content may be designated for specific health problems such as sexually transmitted infections, human immunodeficiency virus–acquired immune deficiency syndrome, and family violence. In other states the Board of Nursing allows the nurse wide latitude in meeting the requirements for renewal of licensure.

ROLE OF REGULATORY BOARDS TO ENSURE SAFE PRACTICE
Membership of the Board of Nursing

An important section of every nursing practice act is the designation of a regulatory board of nurses and consumers to administer the nursing practice act. Frequently this responsibility is assigned to a State Board of Nursing. The practice act outlines guidelines for membership on the board. In addition, procedures by which members are appointed to the Board of Nursing are designated. In most cases, the members are appointed by the Governor's office. Interested individuals or organizations, such as the state nurses association may submit names to the Governor for consideration.

Duties of the Board of Nursing

The responsibilities and duties of the Board of Nursing are delineated in detail. Specific duties of the board may be outlined in the act itself or in the enabling laws. These enabling administrative statutes are frequently designated as Rules and Regulations for the Practice of Nursing. It is through the work of the Board of Nursing that nursing licenses are granted and renewed and disciplinary action taken when provisions of the act are violated. Just as all nurses need to be cognizant of their nursing practice acts, nurses should also become familiar with the role of the State Board of Nursing.

A major responsibility of the Board of Nursing is responding to concerns about a nurse's practice. The review of a nurse's potential malfeasance, violation of the act, or other state and federal laws are within the responsibilities of the Board of Nursing. The nursing practice act describes the due process and procedures for this review. The Board of Nursing will then assign appropriate disciplinary action. These activities are a key responsibility of the Board of Nursing. Actions may include restrictions on the license or suspension or revocation of a nurse's license when provisions of the act are violated. Just as all nurses need to be cognizant of their nursing practice acts, nurses should become familiar with the role of the State Board of Nursing.

SPECIAL CASES OF LICENSURE
Military and Government Nurses

There are many nurses whose practice takes them throughout the country on a regular basis. For example, many nurses are members of the military or join the military nursing services after graduation. The Veterans Administration or Public Health Service employs thousands of nurses. These nurses serve in many jurisdictions, as well as outside the United States boundaries. It is not necessary for these nursing personnel to obtain a nursing license in each jurisdiction in which they practice. The graduate takes the NCLEX-RN examination in one state. On successful completion, as an employee of the United States government, he or she may practice in other jurisdictions without additional licensure requirements.

Foreign Nurse Graduates

A growing number of nurses practicing in the United States completed their nursing education in another country. The nurses met the requirements for practice in those jurisdictions. When these nurses move to the United States, they take a special examination administered by the Commission on Graduates of Foreign Nursing Schools. The examination is given in English and tests the knowledge required to practice in this country. On successful completion, the foreign nurse graduate may apply for a license to practice in this country.

International Practice

In a similar manner nurses licensed in the United States may want to practice in other countries. Nurses interested in these opportunities may contact either the International Council of Nurses or the nursing regulatory board of the country in which they wish to practice.

REVISION OF NURSING PRACTICE ACTS

Nursing practice acts, just as other sections of states codes, are written and passed by legislators. Just as in any legislative endeavor, many governmental agencies, administrators, consumers and special interest groups seek to influence the legislation. These groups become actively involved in developing the accompanying rules and regulations. For example, physicians, dentists, pharmacists, licensed practical nurses, certified nursing assistants, emergency personnel, and physician's assistants are just a few of the health care providers who are directly affected by the scope and definition of nursing practice. Likewise, organizations such as schools, hospitals, home health agencies, and extended care facilities are vitally concerned with the role of nurses today. Because of these multiple interest groups, the nursing practice act as finally passed or amended by the state legislature represents the aims and concerns of many, not only nurses. Review of a state's practice act reveals the influential parties involved in creating the act. Each group participates in defining the scope and practice of nursing and regulations affecting nursing practice within the jurisdiction. Because of these varied interests, it is essential for nurses to understand the practice act and the additional legislation that influences and controls their practice. Further, as proposals to amend the nursing practice act are promulgated at the state level, it is imperative for all nurses to be involved in this process. The resulting laws affect your profession, your practice, and your livelihood.

Sunset Legislation

One example of legislative activity affecting nursing practice acts is sunset legislation. Sunset laws are found in many states. These laws are intended to ensure that legislation is current and reflects the needs of the public. When sunset provisions are included in nursing practice acts, the act must be reviewed by a specific date. If the act is not renewed, it is automatically rescinded. This review process allows for revisions to update practice acts to be consistent with current nursing practice. Many nursing practice acts contain provisions of sunset legislation. It is through these activities that the scope of nursing practice is updated and the diagnosis of nursing problems has been incorporated into many definitions of nursing. Other changes include requirements for mandatory continuing education for renewal of licensure. Equally important, sunset laws have provided the means to define advanced practice nursing and incorporate prescriptive authority for advanced practice nurses.

DELEGATION OF AUTHORITY TO OTHERS

The rapid expansion of health care providers, changes in health care delivery systems, and efforts to control health care costs have led to participation of many types of unlicensed personnel in the provision of health care. These personnel present a challenge to RNs working with them. Questions arise as to who can delegate what activities to which unlicensed provider groups. Guidelines for delegation have been developed by many nursing organizations, including the ANA and the National Council of State Boards of Nursing. However, the most current regulations may be found in the nursing practice acts of individual states. Because regulations differ among states, each nurse must identify and understand the regulations for the state in which he or she practices. Chapter 18 presents a detailed discussion of delegation and supervision.

CURRENT LICENSURE ACTIVITIES
Mutual Recognition Model

Efforts to provide common definitions of nursing practice, standards of education, and testing for entry into practice across state boundaries have been very successful. Nonetheless, most nurses are still required to apply for licensure in each state in which they practice. With the increased mobility of nurses, the telecommunications movement, and the necessity of caring for clients across long distances, state boards of nursing have recognized the need to provide practicing nurses with more than procedures of endorsement of their initial license. This need has led to further changes in nursing licensure. In 1997 the Delegate Assembly of the National

TABLE 5-1	*Compact States Are Those That Have Enacted Legislation Supporting Mutual Recognition Among States*

STATE	DATE ENACTED	DATE EFFECTIVE
Utah	March, 1998	January, 2000
Arkansas	February, 1999	July, 2000
Maryland	April, 1999	July, 1999
Texas	June, 1999	January, 2000
Wisconsin	December, 1999	January, 2000
North Carolina	July, 1999	July, 2000
Nebraska	February, 2000	January, 2001
South Dakota	February, 2000	January, 2001
Iowa	March, 2000	July, 2000
Mississippi	April, 2000	July, 2001
Delaware	June, 2000	July, 2000
Maine	August, 2000	July 2001
Idaho	March 2001	July 2001

From National Council of State Boards of Nursing, Inc., February 2001, www.ncsbn.org.

Council of State Boards of Nursing moved to a new level of nursing regulation. The assembly approved a resolution endorsing a mutual recognition model of nursing regulation. Through this model individual state boards will develop an interstate compact allowing nurses licensed in one state to practice in all other states and territories. Nurses will be responsible for following the laws and regulations of those states, although they will not be required to apply for individual state licensure (National Council of State Boards of Nursing, 2001).

A number of issues associated with mutual recognition concern nurses. On the other hand, mutual recognition would greatly facilitate interstate practice and movement of nurses to areas of shortage. A national database would provide information on individual nurses' practice and tracking mechanisms. On the other hand, concerns relate to monitoring nurses who practice in multiple jurisdictions, nurse privacy, and due process rights. Differences in practice requirements in different states may cause nurses confusion as to their rights and responsibilities. As may be seen in Table 5-1 and Fig. 5-1, currently thirteen states have enacted legislation to allow mutual recognition compacts. Many of these began in 2000, with the remainder in 2001.

The results of mutual recognition compacts will affect all nurses. Nursing students and graduates must remain apprised of changing conditions. The most comprehensive and current sources of information are the Internet sites for the American Journal of Nurses and the National Council of State Boards of Nursing. In addition, the Online Journal of Nursing at the American Journal of Nursing website and the individual state boards of nursing can provide current information to interested nurses.

Continued Competency

As discussed in preceding paragraphs, the primary purpose of nurse licensure is protection of the public. Thus mandatory continuing education was instituted as a strategy to ensure

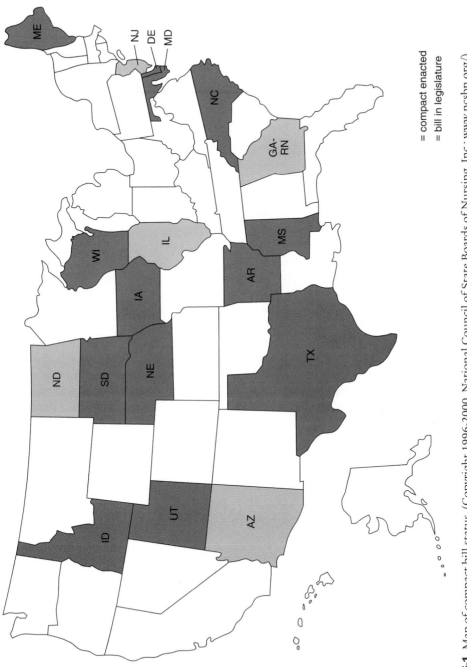
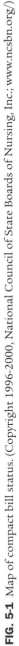

= compact enacted
= bill in legislature

FIG. 5-1 Map of compact bill status. (Copyright 1996-2000, National Council of State Boards of Nursing, Inc.; www.ncsbn.org/)

that nurses were competent to remain in practice. These programs have continued for a number of years. However, a growing number of nurses believe that more is required than just attending seminars to demonstrate the degree of competence. Consortiums of nurses in a number of states are examining other alternatives for renewal of licensure. These requirements may include clinical practice hours, portfolios, and other exemplars of practice.

There is increasing concern for patient safety and treatment in today's health care system. Models of continued competency are but one attempt by professional nurses to ensure that patients and clients receive safe, effective nursing care. Another strategy in this quest is establishing programs of certification of advanced practice nurses.

CERTIFICATION
Purpose of Certification

There are distinct differences between licensure and certification. At the most basic level, licensure establishes minimal levels of practice, whereas certification recognizes excellence in practice. Because of this difference, the background, requirements, and practice opportunities for licensure and certification differ markedly.

Just as with the development of nursing licensure, at its inception certification was not legally required; rather it was voluntary. In an effort to recognize nurses who had completed additional education and demonstrated competency in clinical practice, a number of nursing graduate schools and nursing specialty organizations offered certification programs. In the 1970s and later, advanced clinical courses were designed for nurses as a certificate program. The programs varied in length and content and did not offer a full master's course of study in nursing.

A second distinct difference in licensure and certification pertains to the organizations that grant certification. Whereas licensure is granted and governed by legislation and administered through the State Boards of Nursing, certification is awarded by nongovernmental agencies. Typically these agencies are professional nursing specialty organizations. These organizations have created certification boards that are separate from the parent organization to conform to Department of Education requirements. See Appendix A for a list of specialty organizations.

The first field of nursing practice to certify practitioners was nurse anesthesia in 1946. Since that time the National Association of Nurse Anesthetists has maintained strict standards for education, certification, and practice of practicing nurse anesthetists. The policies and procedures established by nurse anesthetists provided a model for subsequently certifying advanced practitioners in nursing. Similarly in 1961 the American College of Nurse Midwives, founded in 1955, began certifying nurse midwives.

As certificate programs developed, it became apparent that standardization in programs was a necessity. In 1975 the ANA convened a national study group at the University of Wisconsin–Milwaukee to explore the issue. Seventy-five nursing specialty organizations attended. The report of the group recommended the formation of a central organization for certification of nurses. This report, in conjunction with efforts of many nurses, resulted in the formation of the American Nurses Credentialing Center. At present the American Nurses Credentialing Center (2001) has certified more than 200,000 nurses in 25 areas of specialty practice (Box 5-1).

Subsequently in 1991 the American Board of Nursing Specialties organized with eight members: the ANA and the certifying boards of occupational health nurses, neuroscience nurses, rehabilitation nurses, nurse anesthetists, nutritional support nurses, nephrology

| BOX 5-1 | *American Nurses Credentialing Center Areas of Certification* |

Specialist certification
Cardiac rehabilitation nurse
College health nurse
Community health nurse
General nursing practice
Gerontologic nurse
Home health nurse
Medical-surgical nurse
Nursing administration
Nursing continuing education/staff development
Pediatric nurse
Perinatal nurse
Psychiatric and mental health nurse
School nurse

Clinical specialist programs
Adult psychiatric mental health nursing
Child and adolescent psychiatric and mental
     health nursing

Community health nursing
Gerontologic nursing
Home health nursing
Medical-surgical nursing

Nursing administration certification
Nursing administration advanced

Modular certification
Ambulatory care nursing
Nursing case management

Nurse practitioner programs
Acute care nurse practitioner
Adult nurse practitioner
Family nurse practitioner
Gerontological nurse practitioner
Pediatric nurse practitioner
School nurse practitioner

nurses, and orthopedic nurses. This specialty board represents the majority of nursing organizations that certify nurses. Their mission is to ensure high standards and quality in education, evaluation, and practice of certified nurses. These efforts are further indication of nurses' commitment to protection of the public and the patients that nurses serve.

Certification began as a voluntary effort controlled by nursing organizations. State agencies were not involved in the credentialing process. This is still the case, although state nursing practice acts now include requirements for nurses to practice in these advanced roles. Thus state practice acts first contained provisions requiring certification for nurse anesthetists and nurse midwives. With the development of additional advanced practice roles, all states have included requirements of certification in their regulations for advanced practice nurses (National Council of State Boards of Nursing, 2001). These definitions frequently are included in the nursing practice act. A number of states differentiate the advanced practice of nursing by including separate titles for nurse practitioners and clinical nurse specialists. Although many states require a master's degree in the specialty area for practice, this is not the case in all jurisdictions (Hawkins and Holcombe, 1995). In addition, all states incorporate specific provisions for prescribing medications (McDermott, 1995).

Steps to Certification

The best strategy for nurses wishing to practice in an expanded role is to become informed of specific requirements in their chosen field. First the nurse should contact both the American Nursing Credentialing Center and the specialty organization in his or her area of practice to determine the education, experience, and examination requirements necessary to become certified. Concurrently every nurse should contact the state boards of nursing in the state(s) in

BOX 5-2	*Helpful Websites*

ANA www.nursingworld.org	ANCC www.nursingworld.org/ancc
ICN www.nursingworld.org/icn	National Council of State Boards of Nursing www.ncsbn.org
NLN www.nln.org	

which he or she wishes to practice and obtain information on legal requirements to practice in those jurisdictions. After gathering the requirements to practice, the nurse should develop a plan of action to complete the necessary advanced course work, clinical practice requirements, and examinations. By completing the requirements of these agencies, the advanced practice nurse may practice in an expanded role. In addition to the certifying agencies, the nurse may wish to contact other advanced practice nurses. These nurses will serve as valuable colleagues to the new advanced practice nurse.

SUMMARY

Nursing practice acts provide protection of the public and protection of the title of RN. This is accomplished through the development of specific regulations regarding education and examination of competence to practice. Each act contains guidelines for disciplinary action to protect both the public and professional nursing. The nursing practice act of each jurisdiction addresses the needs of the state and the responsibilities of nurses practicing within that state. It is important for all nurses and students of nursing to become familiar with the regulations guiding their own practice. Box 5-2 contains Internet addresses for nursing organizations with which RNs should become familiar.

As health care delivery evolves and nursing practice advances, it is necessary to make changes in the nursing practice act so that it remains responsive to the needs of all. Nurses must be part of this process. Collaboration with professional nursing organizations, the State Board of Nursing, and individual nurses will enable nursing to continually meet the needs of patients.

Critical Thinking Activities

1. Obtain a picture and description of your school/college of nursing pin. Examine each component of the pin and learn the meaning ascribed to it. Reflect on how the nursing program exemplifies the symbolism of its pin. Think about your own nursing practice and in what ways it represents the meaning of your nursing school pin.

2. Contact the board of nursing in your home state/jurisdiction and obtain a copy of your nursing practice act with the accompanying rules and regulations. Read the act carefully and identify the definition of nursing and the scope of nursing practice. Compare your current nursing practice with

the legal definition of nursing. List the requirements for initial licensure and subsequent renewal of a license. Identify the behaviors or practices that lead the Board of Nursing to discipline nurses and the resultant consequences.

3. Compare your nursing practice act with those of adjoining states. How are the definitions of nursing practice and scope of practice similar and different? How can you obtain a license to practice in another state?

4. With the growth of telehealth and telenursing, nurses are practicing across state lines without ever leaving home. What are the implications of practicing in another state? How do the states adjoining your state regulate telehealth?

5. Use the list of compact states in Table 5-1 to identify their geographic proximity to your home state. What effect will mutual recognition have on your nursing practice?

6. Use texts, journals, or the Internet to identify current issues related to nursing licensure. Determine how these issues will affect the nursing practice act and nursing practice within your state or jurisdiction. Select and investigate one issue and formulate a position statement on the issue. Identify key organizations (e.g., the state nursing association and a nursing specialty organization). Contact the organizations and determine their position on the issue. In collaboration with other students, faculty, and nursing organizations, develop strategies to become involved in and influence the outcome of nursing practice issues.

7. Select a clinical area that interests you. Contact the American Nurse Credentialing Center and the clinical specialty nursing organization to determine if the specialty offers certification at an advanced practice level. Obtain information and requirements for certification in your chosen field. Identify strategies to prepare for certification.

8. Use the nursing practice act of your state to identify the scope of practice, regulations, and requirements for certified advanced practice nursing.

9. Seek out nurses certified in advanced practice. Learn from them about their role and the issues facing them in their practice. Select and investigate one issue and determine strategies to influence the outcome of this issue.

Online Activities

1. Use the Internet addresses provided and contact the Board of Nursing in your home state/jurisdiction. Download a copy of your state's nursing practice act and the accompanying rules and regulations. Read the act carefully and identify the definition of nursing and scope of nursing practice. Compare your current nursing practice with the legal definition of nursing. List the requirements for initial licensure and subsequent renewal of a license. Identify three behaviors or practices that lead to disciplinary action of nurses by the Board of Nursing and the consequences of those actions.

2. Select a state/jurisdiction that is contiguous to your home jurisdiction. Use the Internet address for the board of nursing in that state. Compare your nursing practice act with those of adjoining states. How do the definitions of nursing practice and scope of practice differ? How can you obtain a license to practice in another state? How do the states adjoining your state regulate telehealth?

3. Contact the National Council of State Boards of Nursing, Inc. at www.ncsbn.org. Explore the website. Find the map of compact states and identify their geographic proximity to your home state. What effect will mutual recognition have on your practice in your home state?

4. Contact the National Council of State Boards of Nursing, Inc. at www.ncsbn.org. Explore the website. Learn more about the NCLEX examination.

5. Contact the ANA at www.nursingworld.org. Explore this site. Read the ANA information on nurse licensure and the mutual recognition model.

6. From the ANA Internet site, link to your home jurisdiction's nursing association. Bookmark this Internet site for future use. Explore the site. Identify two issues affecting nursing in your state and what nurses in your state are doing about the issues. Determine the date of the next state nursing association meeting.

7. Select a clinical area that interests you. Contact the American Nurse Credentialing Center at www.nursingworld.org/ancc/. Determine if the clinical specialty area offers certification at an advanced practice level. Obtain information and requirements for certification in your chosen field.

8. Use a search engine to locate a nursing specialty organization for your favorite clinical specialty. Go to the nursing organization site and explore the site. Determine what avenues are available for advanced practice nurses. Does the specialty organization offer a certification examination?

REFERENCES

American Nurses Credentialing Center: ANCC Board Certification, 2001, www.nursingworld.org/ancc/certify/cert/catalogs.

Hawkins JW, Holcombe JK: Titling for advanced practice nurses, *Oncol Nurs Forum* 22(suppl):5-9, 1995.

Kalisch PA, Kalisch BJ: *The advance of American nursing,* ed 3, Philadelphia, 1995, JB Lippincott.

Kelly LY, Joel LA: *The nursing experience: trends, challenges, and transitions,* ed 3, New York, 1996, McGraw-Hill.

McDermott KC: Prescriptive authority for advanced practice nurses: current and future perspectives, *Oncol Nurs Forum* 22:25-30, 1995.

National Council of State Boards of Nursing: *Model nurse practice act,* Chicago, 1994, National Council.

National Council of State Boards of Nursing: *Mutual recognition,* 2001, www.ncsbn.org.

Financing Health Care and Economic Issues

Marylane Wade Koch, MSN, RN, CNAA, CPHQ

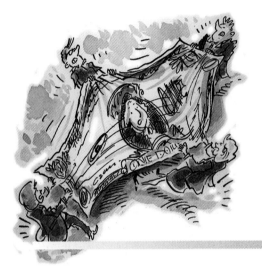

There is a tug-of-war for the shrinking health care dollar.

Vignette

As a home care nurse for many years, my patients primarily have been older adults. Knowing Medicare coverage guidelines for service was critical to the financial success of the home care agency. Today in the home care agency, I am caring for patients of all ages with varying reimbursement guidelines for services. These guidelines differ among managed care organizations (MCOs) and insurance companies. When I first took this job, understanding Medicare coverage guidelines was a new challenge. Now even more is required. Nurses now need extensive knowledge of managed care and the economic influences on professional practice to provide patient care.

Questions to consider while reading this chapter

1. Often the role of the professional nurse is influenced by the employer's ability to pay for the costs associated with staffing and providing quality health care services. Is this a passing trend or is this just doing business today in the evolving health care environment?
2. What does health care economics have to do with me as I provide patient care?
3. Why do I need to understand health care economics and its implications for my practice? Isn't that the role of the finance department or business office at my workplace?

4.   With so many variations in health care insurance, I have a hard time understanding my own policy coverage. What role do I have in assisting my patients/clients in understanding their insurance or coverage options? Can being a more informed consumer add value to my practice?

Key Terms

Capitation   A method of reimbursing providers (usually physicians) with a fixed payment typically expressed as a per-member-per-month payment that is paid in advance for future anticipated contracted health services.

Centers for Medicare and Medicaid Services (CMS) (formerly the Health Care Financing Administration [HCFA])   The federal government agency that administers Medicare and Medicaid.

DRGs (diagnosis-related groups)   Refers to reimbursement based on a predetermined fixed price per case or diagnosis for clients in 468 categories.

GDP (gross domestic product)   The total output of all goods and services in the country.

Health Care Financing Administration (HCFA)   The federal government agency that administered Medicare and Medicaid until 2001.

Marginal   An economic term that refers to the change in some variable (e.g., the number of tests performed).

Medicaid   A jointly sponsored state and federal program that pays medical services for the aged, poor, blind, disabled, and families with dependent children.

Medicare   A federally funded health insurance program for persons age 65 years and older who qualify for Social Security benefits, the disabled, and persons with end-stage renal disease.

Third party   An organization other than the patient and the supplier (hospital or physician), such as an insurance company, that assumes responsibility for payment of health care charges.

Learning Outcomes

After studying this chapter, the reader will be able to:

1.   Analyze major factors that have influenced health care access and financing since the middle of the twentieth century.
2.   Analyze the relationship between market issues and health care resource allocation.
3.   Integrate knowledge of health care resources, access, and financing into managing professional nursing care.
4.   Critique the relationship between contemporary economic issues and trends and professional nursing practice.

CHAPTER OVERVIEW

In the past two decades the costs of health care have continued to increase, with economic issues taking a more central role in health care decision-making. Hospital managers know that for many patients the hospital will receive a predetermined payment, regardless of length of stay and specific treatments. Physicians recognize that the prescribed course of treatment for their patients may be analyzed by a peer review committee. The costs that their patients incur may be compared with those of other physicians or against cost benchmarks. Businesses require employees to cover larger amounts of their health insurance premiums or pay larger deductibles and copayments. Health insurance companies "manage" care, sometimes placing limits on medical care coverage or on the site of care delivery. These dramatic and relatively new developments are all driven by the new economics of health care.

The objective of this chapter is to describe and explain the major economic issues and trends driving the critical changes in health care delivery and financing. The chapter has five sections. The first section reviews trends and major changes in health care financing. The second area of discussion is an analysis of the allocation of medical care resources, with emphasis on the dominant issues of access and cost containment. The third section is a discussion of the general approaches available for making health care allocation and delivery decisions. The fourth section explores the mix of health financing methods, distinguishing the varied roles of government and private funding. The final section discusses the major issues of the new health care world of managed care and its impact on nursing.

HISTORY OF HEALTH CARE FINANCING

Several underlying themes have driven health care financing in the United States. Among these are the role of physicians in health care decision making, the broad objective of providing the "best" possible care to everyone, the rapidly increasing sophistication and cost of medical technology, economic incentives, and the fee-for-service payment mode. For many years two of these factors, physician domination in decision making and the fee-for-service payment mode, were intertwined. This fed into the lack of cost consciousness in health care.

The simultaneous occurrence of the physician's decision-making role and fee-for-service payments was combined with the driving motivation in the health care system to provide the best possible care for all patients, regardless of cost. Costs were rarely discussed between provider and patient, so the cost of care almost appeared to be an afterthought for bill-paying time. Medical tests or procedures were provided if the physician determined that additional care might offer any marginal aid or provide any marginal diagnostic information.

Especially beginning in the 1960s, the approach of "if it helps at all, do it" was furthered by the rapid pace of technologic change. New and sophisticated technologies significantly enhanced physicians' ability to provide treatment. The more tests or procedures performed, the greater the earnings because physician income was tied to procedures. Instead of attempting to allocate medical resources to the highest medical need, there was an economic incentive to provide as much care as possible and the highest available quality of care in all cases. However, as the quality of care, available technologies, and medical revenues increased, this situation caused overuse of health services and rapid cost inflation.

Although health care was overused in many cases and costs were increasing, patients as consumers of medical care remained largely insulated from the effects of cost inflation. Most patients were covered by some form of insurance or "third-party payment" mechanism. They were not paying the "full cost" for their care or even for their health insurance premiums. These costs generally were subsidized by their employers or by taxpayers through such programs as Medicare and Medicaid. Insurance provided payments for the additional costs generated by any extra services provided. Because patients were not aware of the costs of their health care, providers had little incentive to be concerned about costs. The lack of cost consciousness in the demand for medical care generated "perverse economic incentives." Providers received more income for using more services and had no financial risk for their use of additional resources. Practitioners were often motivated to provide additional services, because they earned more income from each procedure they performed. This practice of overuse occurred, regardless of the cost of procedures or the total cost of treatment.

Medicare was implemented in 1965 to provide health insurance coverage for those age 65 and older who are eligible for social security benefits, those with end-stage renal disease, and the eligible disabled population. By the early 1980s increased medical usage (increased intensity of care) and high inflation, as well as a growing elderly population and high overall inflation, generated large increases in the total Medicare bill. The rapid growth of Medicare expenditures became a major factor in the federal budget deficit, which caused the Centers for Medicare and Medicaid Services (CMS) (formerly the Health Care Financing Administration [HCFA]) to rethink the entire Medicare payment system. This led to a revolution in health insurance reimbursement.

Health Care Financing Revolution

Table 6-1 shows the dramatic increases in national health expenditures between 1965 and 1998; National Health Expenditures as a percent of gross domestic product rose from 6% to 14.5% (National Health Statistics, 1999). The significance of this growth is that, for every dollar spent for goods and services in the United States, 14.5¢ goes to pay for health care. The health care financing revolution was initiated in 1983, when Medicare moved from a retrospective or cost-based reimbursement approach to a new prospective payment system (PPS) based on diagnosis-related groups (DRGs). This shift was critical for hospitals because Medicare is the largest single payer of hospital charges. Medicare provided one third of hospital revenue or a total of 87 billion dollars in 1997 (Komisar et al., 1997).

Under DRGs each Medicare patient is assigned to one of the nearly 500 diagnosis groupings based on his or her primary diagnosis when admitted to the hospital. For that patient's care, Medicare limits its total payment to the hospital to the amount preestablished for that DRG. For example, for the diagnosis of congestive heart failure, Medicare pays the hospital a set amount to cover the average length of stay for this diagnosis. This contrasts sharply with the previous approach under which hospital patients incurred costs for all prescribed therapies and Medicare subsequently reimbursed these charges according to its fairly generous payment schedules.

TABLE 6-1	*National Health Expenditures: Selected Years 1965–1998*			
NATIONAL HEALTH EXPENDITURES	**1965**	**1980**	**1990**	**1998**
Amount in billions of dollars	41.1	247.3	699.4	1149.1
Percent of gross domestic product	5.7	8.9	12.1	13.5
Amount per capita (dollars)	202	1052	2689	4094
	Percent of total expenditures			
Hospital care	34	42	37	33
Physician services	20	18	21	20
Dentist services	7	5	5	5
Nursing home care	4	7	7	8
Home health care	0.2	1.0	1.9	2.5
Drugs and other medical nondurables	14	9	9	11

Source: National Health Statistics Group, Office of Actuary, National Health Expenditures, 1998, Health Care Financing Review, vol. 24, no. 2, HCFA pub.no. 03420, Health Care Financing Administration, Washington: U.S. Government Printing Office, Winter, 1999.

Since 1983 if hospital costs are greater than the DRG payment for a patient, the hospital incurs a loss, but if costs are less than the DRG amount, the hospital makes a profit. Hospitals face a real economic incentive to reduce length of stay and minimize procedures performed. Reimbursement amounts for the same DRG classification may vary somewhat between hospitals. Variations are based on whether it is a teaching hospital, which receives an additional payment to support medical education, and whether it is an urban facility, which receives higher reimbursement than a rural hospital. Although DRGs originally applied only to hospital payments for Medicare patients, once the reimbursement revolution began, similar or comparable reimbursement arrangements were initiated by private insurance companies.

DRGs also had an immediate and profound effect on hospital administration and cost accounting. Implementation of the DRG system substantially expanded the role of hospital management, including nurse administrators. First, it was apparent that gains were made primarily from the careful diagnosis of patients according to their highest potential DRG classification. This initiated new roles for hospital-based nurses in utilization management to assist in determining the appropriate DRG for patients. Utilization nurses play a pivotal role in determining the appropriate DRG, with its resulting length of stay for patients. Second, hospital record keeping and accounting methodologies also were revolutionized. It became necessary for hospitals to adapt new and highly specific Medicare cost accounting procedures. These procedures mandate that all internal hospital costs be carefully allocated to each of the DRG categories. Experienced nurses with business knowledge bring needed technical background and skills to these new accounting and utilization management tasks, thereby expanding opportunities for nurse managers or administrators.

By the early 1990s, based on the success of DRGs in reducing the rate of growth of Medicare payments (although not the total amount), the financing revolution was extended with a new approach to physician reimbursement. The Medicare fee schedule for physician payments was revised completely. The old fee scheme was replaced with a new one determined by an innovative Resource-Based Relative Value Scale (RBRVS). The objective was to bring the payments for different types of medical services more in line with the physician skills required and the actual time spent on specific procedures. For example, when Medicare initially covered cataract surgery, it was a relatively rare and lengthy procedure. However, over time cataract correction has become one of the most frequently performed Medicare surgical procedures. The procedure became so rapid and relatively easy to perform that it was viewed by CMS as overpaid. The RBRVS system sought to correct the disparity between Medicare's high payments for this type of procedure and relatively low payments for more hands-on primary care. Payments to primary care and internal medicine physicians were increased, and many fees to specialists were reduced. For example, fees to general practitioners and internists for lengthy initial examinations were increased, whereas fees for many surgical procedures were decreased.

Managed Care

As the shift to prospective payment occurred under Medicare, private insurance companies also developed alternate health care financing modes, which generally are termed managed care. Managed care organizations (MCOs) encompass several different approaches, such as health maintenance organizations (HMOs) and preferred provider organizations (PPOs). A commonality of these forms of payment is a method for review and oversight of the medical goods and services used. Under managed care the insurance company, a peer review organization, or another review mechanism is used to bring cost consciousness to bear on medical decision making. In this process a reviewer evaluates the patient's medical options, keeping the concept of cost effectiveness in mind. Coverage may be denied for procedures that are considered unnecessary, excessive, or experimental, which is in strong contrast to the previously pervasive "if it helps, do it" approach.

In developing managed care, private insurance goals are the same as those sought by Medicare DRGs. The goal is to overcome some of the problems of retrospective payment of charges such as inefficiency, overuse, and excess charges. Because more than 70% of all private insurance is provided by employers for their workers, insurance companies also were pushed by their largest business customers to decrease the rapid rate of growth of insurance premiums and health care costs. Business health insurance costs were increasing 20% a year by the late 1980s. More and more firms began to "self-insure" their workers. This is a process by which the company establishes reserves and manages its own health benefits program rather than paying premiums to an external insurance company. Firms learned that this could result in substantial savings as they managed their own health plans

As businesses saw increased health care costs reduce their profits, they became concerned about the effects of health costs on their international competitiveness. For example, during the 1980s at least $800 of the price paid for a new car in the United States went to pay for health care for the workers who manufactured the car. In contrast, health care coverage for the workers producing a car in Japan during that same time only cost the manufacturing company about $150.

The widespread and rapid expansion of managed care in the 1990s was a response to numerous factors, including cost inflation, overuse, an increasing number of persons who are uninsured ("uncompensated" care), and the effects of health costs on business profits and international competitiveness. Therefore employer health insurance markets have moved rapidly from conventional insurance plans to MCOs. In only 2 years, from 1993 to 1995, coverage of employees by conventional insurance declined from 49% to 27%, whereas managed care coverage increased from 51% to 73% (Managed Care, 1997). This trend is expected to continue and is having a major impact on inflation of health costs.

The Employer Health Benefits 2000 Annual Survey conducted by the Kaiser Family Foundation and the Health Research and Educational Trust demonstrates a move by businesses to limit the availability of plan types offered to workers. About 65% of workers are still given a choice of more than one plan. However, survey results showed significant change in the availability of different types of plans. An example is the percentage of workers offered a PPO option increased from 45% in 1996 to 66% in 2000 (News Briefs, 2001). Fewer workers were offered conventional and HMO plans. With an increase in managed care, the private insurance market is accomplishing one of the goals sought by national health insurance proposals—slowing the rate of growth of health care costs.

Inflation and Cost Containment

Cost containment was "the health issue" from the mid-1970s through the 1980s because health care costs increased much more rapidly than prices of most other goods and services. Health care inflation is measured by the medical care component of the overall Consumer Price Index (CPI), which is the primary measure of U.S. price changes. In the early 1990s medical care inflation slowed considerably, decreasing from 8% in 1990 to 4% in 1999. (U.S. Dept. of Labor, 2000) Several factors influenced this positive trend of slower health care inflation. Inflation in general declined. General inflation affects health care because hospitals, clinics, and other providers have to hire workers and purchase supplies, energy, and all other inputs at higher prices or wages.

The largest share of health expenditure is for hospital-based care, which has achieved reduced inflation. DRGs led to decreases in hospital admission rates and patients' average length of stay. Patients are being discharged from hospitals "quicker and sicker." Therefore outpatient procedures and the use of home health and primary care clinics have increased. These changes have helped reduce inflation. Hospitals also are using cost-cutting techniques such as decreasing inventories, joining purchasing groups, and using physician review. Drug companies have been forced to limit price hikes, and generic products are often prescribed for patients. In addition, new cost containment and utilization control strategies under managed care, as well as increased cost sharing by patients, have helped slow inflation. Thus the measures that have been taken in recent years by insurers, other payers, providers, and consumers have reduced inflation in health care to more manageable levels, leaving access as the dominant health issue to be solved.

Access Issues

Because health care cost inflation has significantly slowed in the 1990s, the dominant health issue is access, particularly for the uninsured or underinsured. Lack of access to health care today primarily reflects a lack of insurance coverage, so access is an issue of financial access. Before the passage of Medicare and Medicaid legislation in 1965, few Americans had health insurance, but since then the percentage of persons having health care coverage has increased. The 17.5% uninsured under age 65 represent about 41 million people with no health insurance (U.S. Department of Health and Human Services, 2000). They include the working poor who are employed by small firms without insurance coverage and part-time workers, as well as indigents, some acquired immune deficiency syndrome patients (who have lost coverage), and other groups.

Medicaid is intended to improve access to health care for the poor. However, even though Medicaid recipients have improved access when compared with the uninsured, Medicaid recipients are only about half as likely to obtain needed health services (Berk and Schur, 1998). The poor are more likely to lack a usual source of care, less likely to use preventive services, and more likely to be hospitalized for avoidable conditions than those who are not poor (U.S. Department of Health and Human Services, 2000).

Although the lack of insurance often is a serious problem for households, it also presents problems for providers and for all insurers. The uninsured and underinsured populations generate uncompensated or indigent care costs and bad debt for health care providers. These unpaid costs then must be covered by those who do pay so that the hospital can continue operating, a process known as "cost-shifting." Thus providers increase their charges against households and public and private insurers, who pay for their own care and some contribution for the care of the uninsured population. This in turn increases insurance premiums, which makes it even more difficult for many households and businesses to afford coverage. However, in the new era of managed care and with the growth of HMOs and PPOs, the ability of providers to shift costs has decreased dramatically. The problem of uncompensated care and cost-shifting is a major reason that many people advocate some form of national health insurance coverage.

In addition to the problem of the uninsured population, there are several other barriers to health care access. For those living in rural or inner-city areas, there may be location or geographic problems of access. These may be straightforward transportation issues or may involve the lack of specialists, new technology, or specialized facilities in many regions of the country and in some inner cities. Access to health care may be hampered by long waiting periods that require patients or their families to miss extended periods of work, with lost wages representing a financial opportunity cost of obtaining care. One unique access problem is related to the nature of transplantation technology. In this case, the access issue is how to allocate the limited number of organs available.

The next sections look closer at the issues of financing and access to examine what generates health care costs. Questions regarding the allocation of resources to health care and the production of medical goods and services are examined.

ALLOCATION OF HEALTH CARE RESOURCES
Health Resources

The health care system of any society consists of its entire package of health care delivery and financing mechanisms, combined with its health and medical institutions and any additional institutional framework that affects health. Although the health care systems of different countries may appear to be different, there actually are only a limited number of ways in which health care resources can be allocated for the production and distribution of medical care.

Health care resources include all the inputs devoted to producing medical care and health care: (1) "labor" such as nurses, physicians, technicians, pharmacists, and administrators, including their education, skills, and training; (2) "capital," including all the medical facilities and equipment available; (3) "land," the actual land area for hospitals and other facilities; and (4) "entrepreneurship," which encompasses the skills and risk taking that business persons bring to health businesses, especially to starting new ventures. Because all these resources are "scarce" or limited in the amounts available at any given time, decisions have to be made that involve choices about how to best use them. Basic decisions (choices) must be made in the production and provision of health care (i.e., in the allocation of scarce resources to health and medical care).

Resource Allocation Questions

Each society has to answer several basic underlying questions to decide how to allocate its resources to health care. First, what combination of medical goods and all other goods do we want to produce in the economy using our scarce resources? This means how much or what share of the total production of all goods and services should be health care. In 1998 14% of the Gross Domestic Product (GDP) was allocated to health care, with a value of more than $1 trillion. CMS projects that national health expenditures will double to reach $2.6 trillion by 2010, representing 15.9% of the GDP, having declined to 13% in 1999 (Health Care Financing Administration, 2000). If the share of total expenditures devoted to health increases, then some nonhealth goods and services will need to be eliminated, transferring the resources or inputs from the things given up to medical care.

The second resource question to be answered is: what combination of specific medical goods and services do we want to produce in the health care sector of the economy? Or what types of health and medical care do we choose to produce? Do we prefer a high-tech, institution-based mix of health services emphasizing therapeutic (crisis-oriented) medical care, or do we choose a prevention-oriented health system emphasizing primary care and wellness? Such choices are made either explicitly or implicitly. For example, if it is decided to allocate more scarce health resources to hip replacements for elderly osteoporosis patients, then there are fewer medical resources to allocate to maternal and child health. Thus the maternal and child care eliminated to obtain additional hip surgeries is the real cost of performing more of the hip procedures, another example of "opportunity cost."

The third question is: who should receive the medical goods and services? This actually is a distribution question, and the answer may depend largely on who has the health insurance coverage to finance the purchase of health care. If the society has some form of national health insurance, this indicates that it has decided that all of its citizens should have financial access to medical care. In contrast, in the United States we only provide federal or state funding for defined groups that have eligibility for specific programs such as Medicare and Medicaid. Some defined groups have established (or legislated) "rights" to medical care, but the entire population does not.

The way a society answers these basic questions defines that society's type of health care system. Although there are many variations, there are a fairly limited number of approaches to economic decision making and allocating resources in health care. The major systems for allocating resources include (1) a competitive market system, (2) a market system, but with government regulation of the markets, (3) centralized government planning and/or a single-payer financing system, or (4) some combination of the first three options.

MARKET ALLOCATION ISSUES

There is no advanced industrial country with a purely competitive market system for the allocation of health care resources. The United States and South Africa are the only industrialized Western countries that do not have a national health insurance system covering of all their citizens. Most of the European countries have a substantial amount of central government planning in their health systems, with Great Britain being a primary example of a fully centralized or nationalized system. Almost all of the health care resources in the British National Health Service (e.g., hospitals, clinics, nursing homes) are owned and run by the government.

Regulated Market System

In contrast to other countries, the health care system in the United States predominantly relies on decision making through the market system of the U.S. economy, although most U.S. health care markets are regulated by federal or state legislation. To describe our health care system, first consider exactly what is meant by a market. A market is simply a means by which a buyer and a seller come together. It may be a place such as a pharmacy or a clinic, but market transactions also can be accomplished by telephone (a prescription can be called in, charged, and delivered) or even by computer (prescription can be emailed with the payment information). Then, do health services received from a Veterans Administration (VA) hospital involve a market transaction if there are no charges? The answer to this question would be *no,* because this transaction implies a transfer of in-kind services from taxpayers to the VA patient and is a nonmarket transaction or an entitlement given to veterans.

In a regulated market system examples of regulation include requirements of minimum nurse staffing in long-term care facilities, laws regarding the disposal of medical waste products, and regulations affecting the conduct of medical laboratories. In addition, all licensure and certification laws or qualifying examinations represent regulation of medical professionals. Thus we have a market system for most health care goods and services, but virtually no area escapes regulation.

Competition

A market system implies private ownership of resources and private decision making by consumers about their purchases and by businesses about producing and selling. These decisions are made largely on the basis of the prices of goods and services. For a market system to function effectively and efficiently, it needs to be competitive. Competition implies that (1) there are numerous buyers and sellers in the market, so no single seller or group of sellers can manipulate the price; (2) the products of all suppliers in the market are exactly the same; (3) consumers and sellers are well informed about market conditions and prices; and (4) new resources are free to enter or leave this market.

Although we have a regulated market system for producing health care, there are numerous reasons why these markets are not really competitive. Consumers cannot be well informed about what health care to purchase without a doctor's diagnosis. Also it may be difficult for consumers to get information about the prices of services until after the services are provided. Once the patient visits the physician, the physician is likely to be in charge of numerous subsequent decisions, so the doctor in effect becomes an "agent" for the patient. Further, the physician's income may be affected by what is ordered for the patient. In other words, the physician's reimbursement incentives may encourage overuse or underuse. However, a competitive market system assumes that buyers are capable of making independent decisions.

Another issue in assuming that health care markets can be competitive is "third-party payments" or insurance payments for medical care. A competitive market system assumes that people make their decisions to purchase something on the basis of its price, but health care consumers often pay less than the "full price" because their insurance pays some or all of the cost. If an employer bought "shoe insurance" for employees so they only had to pay a coinsurance payment of perhaps $10 (or possibly only 20% of the full price) for shoes, how many pairs would an employee buy? And would the employee buy more expensive or cheaper shoes? This is exactly the issue that insurance coverage or third-party payment brings to confound medical care markets. The effect of health insurance on health care markets is to create a two-tier price system—the provider charges the gross price, but insured consumers face another price, the lower net price or out-of-pocket price at the time of use. The result is that the consumer perceives health care as cheaper than it is and is motivated to purchase more and possibly to overconsume. This situation has become an important determinant of the increase in managed care.

Production Functions

One further question needs to be addressed in describing resource allocation in our health care market system: What specific health resources (inputs) do we want to use to produce final medical goods and services (outputs)? There also are choices in answering this question because many health services can be produced in more than one way. A useful approach for analyzing this type of production decision is to develop alternative "production functions" that state how much output (Q) can be produced by combining different sets of inputs. For example, inpatient days of care, a typical measure of hospital output, could be produced by hospitals hiring different combinations of staff and personnel, including physicians (Dr), registered nurses (RN), licensed practical nurses (LPN), nurse aides (NA), laboratory technicians (LT), pharmacists (Ph), support staff such as janitorial and kitchen workers (W), and administrators (A). To provide days of service, all hospitals also must have other inputs, such as rooms/beds (R) representing the hospital facility, technology (T) representing all the equipment, energy (E) representing what is needed to keep the hospital open (including practice insurance), and laboratories (L) indicating all laboratory facilities. Compare the following three production functions that describe alternative input combinations for producing inpatient hospital days:

1. Q15f (Dr, R, T, E, L)
2. Q25f (Dr, RN, R, T, E, L)
3. Q35f (Dr, RN, LPN, NA, LT, Ph, W, A, R, T, E, L)

Each of these three production functions states that the quantity of inpatient days is a function of (depends on) some combination of inputs or resources, including labor resources. The first indicates that physicians are the only hospital workers and provide all the care given (e.g., run all tests, deliver meal trays, send bills). The second indicates that the hospital personnel includes physicians and nurses providing all the care and other services and management. Alternately, care could be provided by combining many types of hospital personnel, as seen in the third production function. Each of these alternative production functions also shows the nonlabor inputs necessary to keep the hospital running.

Cost Functions

If the market prices (P) of each of the inputs are added to a production function, it can be transformed into a cost (C) function. The prices of labor inputs (personnel) would be their competitive market salaries or wages, or what the hospital actually has to pay to hire and retain staff. Using cost functions for the three production functions presented previously, the total cost of a hospital day could be derived by substituting numbers of employees, quantities of inputs, and actual prices into the alternative cost functions shown in Box 6-1.

Comparing the total costs derived for these three cost functions allows the hospital administration to make decisions about how to produce days of hospital care efficiently and effectively. Economic efficiency implies minimizing the cost of production or that the most output is being achieved for the value of the inputs. This concept indicates that the hospital is unlikely to operate under either of the first two cost function options described in Box 6-1. The salaries of physicians and RNs are higher relative to assistive staff who might perform the less complex medical services (perhaps taking blood pressure), and they are certainly higher than wages of other staff who can perform nonmedical tasks. This explains why hospitals have been motivated to hire more assistive personnel, such as LPNs and nursing assistants, to the extent permitted by staffing regulations.

BOX 6-1 *Alternative Hospital Cost Functions*

(1) $C(Q_1) = f(Dr \cdot P_{Dr} + R \cdot P_R + T \cdot P_T + E \cdot P_E + L \cdot P_L)$

(2) $C(Q_2) = f(Dr \cdot P_{Dr} + R_N \cdot P_{RN} + R \cdot P_R + T \cdot P_T + E \cdot P_E + L \cdot P_L)$

(3) $C(Q_3) = f(Dr \cdot P_{Dr} + R_N \cdot P_{RN} + LVN \cdot P_{LVN} + NA \cdot P_{NA} + LT \cdot P_{LT} + PH \cdot P_{Ph} + W \cdot P_W + A \cdot P_A + R \cdot P_R + T \cdot P_T + E \cdot P_E + L \cdot P_L)$

Job Growth and the Health Care Industry

An additional resource issue relates to health care as a driving force of new job growth throughout the economy. Between 1988 and 1992 the health services industry created 1.4 million jobs or half of all the new jobs produced in the United States. Since the long economic expansion of the 1990s began in March 1991, two thirds of all the new jobs created were in health care. This job growth is predicted to continue, but at a slower rate, declining from 4% to 5% to 3% to 4%. The surge of job creation in the health industry is likely to decline as the restructuring of health care delivery continues.

SOURCES OF HEALTH CARE FINANCING

The more than $1 trillion (more than $4000 per capita) spent on health care in the United States in 1998 was financed by combinations of private and public sources. The payment mode affects the delivery of medical goods and services through close interactions between the health delivery markets and the payment mechanisms. Paying for health services and supplies for individuals, which constitutes almost 60% of total health care expenditures, is a major concern in health care financing. Other health expenditures are for areas such as health research, health professional education, and capital investment in medical facilities construction.

Most health care for individuals is paid either by households through direct out-of-pocket payments or by third-party public or private insurers. Third-party payers include private insurance companies, independent health plans, government health programs, and claims payment agents (U.S. Census Bureau, 1998). Seventy percent of people in the United States have a private insurance plan, usually through employment or a union; the government provides health coverage insurance for 24.3% of the people. In addition, some health care is paid by charitable organizations, foundations, or other sources.

Household Out-of-Pocket Payments

In 1994 private sources (i.e., nongovernment) accounted for 55% of total national health expenditures; this share is projected to decline slightly by 2005. Households pay approximately one third of these private expenditures for health services and supplies from their own personal resources (out-of-pocket); the remaining two thirds is covered mostly by private insurance payments. Elderly households (with people age 65 years or older) spend a much larger share of their income on out-of-pocket health expenditures than do nonelderly households. Despite their universal Medicare coverage, the elderly spend 21% of their income on health care, compared with only 8% of the nonelderly's income (Komisar et al., 1997).

Medical savings accounts (MSAs) represent a new and somewhat controversial form of health insurance introduced on a trial basis in 1996. The project, originally scheduled to end December 31, 2000, has received a 2-year extension. An MSA is an innovative type of insurance plan that combines a personal savings account with a high deductible health insurance policy. In general, MSA plans allow the individual to deposit pretax income into a savings account to be used for qualified (allowable) medical expenses, including routine health care costs up to the insurance policy deductible. The plan can also allow flexibility for the type of medical services the employee needs, such as extra dental care or maternity coverage. As insurance premium costs rise, employers may find this option appealing, as a transition to a defined contribution plan rather than a defined benefit plan (Perrin, 2001).

Private Insurance

Private insurance accounts for most of the remaining two thirds of privately financed health care. It is important to remember that the cost of providing health insurance to employees is passed on by the employer to the consumer in the pricing of goods and services. Thus all people pay a part of health care costs in every purchase they make. In the 1990s private insurance has increasingly followed the lead of Medicare in implementing the medical reimbursement revolution. Payment mechanisms have shifted to capitated payments or prospective reimbursement under an array of PPOs and point-of-service (POS) arrangements. HMOs represent a form of managed care that may have capitation payments or fee-for-service payments to providers. An HMO is a way of organizing and delivering health care that combines delivery with the payment mechanism (insurance), usually by prepayment or capitation. HMOs reduce costs by constraining use, particularly by reducing inpatient hospital use. A PPO is based on contractual arrangements between the insurer and provider, under which the provider gives lower prices and the insurer agrees to motivate its entire group of insured members to use that particular facility or physician group. PPOs reduce barriers to price shopping—they provide a list of providers to consumers and give patients a financial incentive to use these providers. POS arrangements give consumer patients somewhat more flexibility in selection of providers but also involve contracts between medical providers and insurers. Thus it is no longer possible to separate payment and delivery modes because major payment mechanisms combine the two.

Tax Subsidies of Private Payments

Private sources of health expenditures are subsidized by the government if they represent tax deductions or nontaxable income. The income tax code allows households to deduct health expenditures that total more than a certain percentage of their income and also contributions to health philanthropy. Further, private insurance premiums paid by employers also are subsidized as a fringe benefit that is not a taxable income. The deductibility of these health expenditures represents tax revenue losses to the federal government. In addition, cities subsidize health care real estate through property tax exemptions for nonprofit and public hospitals.

Public Insurance

Government is the biggest influence in the health insurance market, generating half of hospital revenues and more than one fourth of physician incomes. The largest health insurance program is Medicare, covering approximately 13% of the U.S population (U.S. Census Bureau, 1998). Since enactment of the program in 1965, the population covered by Medicare has doubled, and it is projected to increase to 55 million within 20 years. Medicare is an entitlement program based on age or disability criteria rather than on need. Medicare Part A covers inpatient hospital services, skilled nursing facilities (SNFs), and home health benefits. Hospital coverage has deductible and coinsurance requirements and some coverage limitations. Payments to home health and SNFs are 15% of Medicare spending and are increasing rapidly. Managed care coverage of Medicare beneficiaries also is growing and is expected to double in the next 10 years (Kaiser Family Foundation, 1997). As noted previously, the introduction of DRGs in Medicare hospital reimbursement initiated the health financing revolution that is still ongoing.

In contrast to Medicare, which is a federal program with national eligibility criteria, Medicaid is a joint federal-state program for which states establish some of the eligibility criteria based on their Aid to Families with Dependent Children (AFDC) income eligibility levels. The federal government established minimum coverage that states may supplement. Medicaid covers 10.3% of the population, primarily disabled persons, AFDC households, and those in nursing homes who qualify based on their low income level (U.S. Census Bureau,1998). Thus a program designed to provide health care access to impoverished families, particularly children, has become the primary payer of long-term care nationwide, covering almost half of all nursing home costs. In addition Medicaid is required to cover the deductibles and co-payments for Medicare beneficiaries who are impoverished and termed dual eligible. More than 30% of Medicaid payments covered services for the elderly in 1994, when total Medicaid payments exceeded $118 billion. For most states Medicaid represents the fastest growing component in the state budget.

Impacts of Payment Modes

The shift to increased managed care has resulted in many changes. There have been clear increases in efficiency in the delivery of care, such as more efficient use of medical services and some decreased prices of services. The hospital share of health care expenditures is decreasing, and there is evidence of decrease in the number of hospitals, especially in rural areas. Other attempts to increase efficiency include the growth of free-standing clinics, more outpatient use, cuts in programs and eligibility, and new options for patients. Nonetheless, after all the efficiency changes, health costs remain the fastest increasing element in federal and state budgets.

The type of reimbursement also influences provider behavior, emphasizing the importance of the underlying economic incentives that providers face. Because patients are being discharged earlier and sometimes in less stable condition, patient care is shifting from acute care to more community-based sites such as community mental health centers, home health agencies, and multiple other community sites.

The economic incentives in medical settings have shifted toward more cost-effective care. Managed care and utilization reviews are shifting the health care system toward increased preventive care and away from its long-standing emphasis on acute care.

IMPLICATIONS FOR NURSING: MANAGING CARE

Nurses represent a major professional force in the delivery of health care services in the United States today. Never has there been greater opportunity to advance the practice of professional nursing. Innovation and excellence in all nursing practice is needed to contain costs while attaining positive, measurable outcomes.

All professional nurses have a role in managing care in the setting where they work. Practitioners are needed to provide cost-effective care for wellness, acute care, and chronic illness. Educators are necessary to inform the public of ways to improve health and practice prevention and how to manage chronic disease. Administrators are necessary to organize health care services for optimal resource management with high-quality outcomes at reasonable costs. Professional nursing practice spans a variety of settings from acute, institutional, or hospital care to outpatient care to community-based clinics, physician offices, and home care agencies. Each setting holds practice challenges in providing and managing care that is efficient, affordable, and of high quality. These trends mandate that nurses have a clear understanding of the economic and financing issues underlying the continuously developing roles of nurses.

Many opportunities for nurses in today's health care environment are economically and politically driven. Changes in the financing of health care services directly affect professional nursing practice. Markus (1990) outlined several reasons why payment reform is important to nursing:

1. The rules of payment are important as a reflection of the value and worth society places on health care services for the public.
2. Government policy influences the public's openness to secure services from various professionals such as nurse practitioners.
3. Financing impacts salaried employees because health care providers build job opportunities based on payment sources. For instance, if a professional service is covered under reimbursed allowances, jobs in that service will be offered by the provider.
4. Payment modes will determine if a particular nursing role will be reimbursed, affecting specialties and professional autonomy.

As national health care concerns change, the financing rules will reflect the concerns and attitudes of policy makers and hopefully the public at large. In particular, Medicare payment changes will increasingly impact nursing practice as the elderly population dependent on this health insurance increases.

In Nursing's Agenda for Health Care Reform (1991) the American Nurses Association emphasizes the need for more primary care management. Under this proposal consumers would be allowed to choose the least costly access to health care through community-based programs. Wellness and preventive care would be a major thrust, with regulatory and payment barriers removed. This process has allowed for direct reimbursement of services and care management provided by nurse practitioners, clinical specialists, and nurse midwives under certain guidelines, allowing nurses to demonstrate economic value with positive care outcomes. Because there are political obstacles to these cost-efficient solutions, nurses must be politically active in influencing necessary legislative changes.

The goal of the Pew Commission report, *Healthy America: Practitioners for 2005* (1991), was to assist schools in preparing health care professionals to meet future demands. Thomas W. Langfitt, MD, president of the Pew Charitable Trust, delineates two possible paths for health care reform: (1) reorganization of the health care system, and (2) refinancing the present system to allow access and contain costs (Pew Health Professions Commission, 1991).

These paths for reform are grounded in five major trends delineated as affecting the future of health care practitioners:

1. Efficiency and effectiveness through coordinated care
2. Diversity and aging in the population
3. Tensions in expansion of science and technology
4. Consumer empowerment
5. Values that shape health care

Each of these trends is significant to a better understanding of the role nursing can play in health care. Nurses must learn how to proactively position themselves educationally and professionally to work with the new economic challenges of health care. These trends are examined in the following discussion and are applied to professional practice to demonstrate care management in an ever-changing economic environment.

Efficiency and Effectiveness of Care

Health care financing has progressed from physician-dominated decision making in a fee-for-service mode with third-party and retrospective payment to prospective and capitated payment. Nurses provide services as a resource or input into the health care delivery system to produce patient care and care management. Nurses can affect care management in many ways, including nursing process, case management, utilization management, and education. Because resources are limited and decisions are based on service costs, administrators may combine nonnursing resources with limited nursing resources to decrease the total costs of production of services. Professional nurses are pressured to demonstrate excellent clinical resource management and to design care delivery that provides a less costly service that satisfies the customer requirements.

Coordinated Care. Integrated or coordinated care is one way to decrease duplication of services and reduce wasted health care resources. This type of care has brought about the use of more case management and integration of services for cost-efficient care. More care is being delivered in the community through home care, outpatient clinics, and ambulatory care centers at less costly rates as inpatient hospital-based care decreases. These changes in the health care environment require professional nurses to understand basic principles of financial and resource management.

Case Management. Case management is a role in which nurses can demonstrate cost effectiveness in managed care. Opportunities exist for nurses who understand the overall structure and processes of the health care industry and who bring skills of critical thinking, as well as patient advocacy. Understanding current health care economics is critical to this role. The American Association of Managed Care Nurses has as its mission: (1) to be recognized as the "expert" in managed care nursing, (2) to establish standards for managed care practice, (3) to positively impact public policy regarding managed health care delivery, and (4) to assist in educating the public on managed care. To learn more about the American Association of Managed Care Nurses, Inc., visit their website at www.aamcn.org or call 1-804-747-9698.

Disease Management. Disease management programs provide another opportunity for professional nurses to impact effectiveness and efficiency of health care services. Although there is controversy over whether or not these programs consistently deliver improved care in a cost effective way, reports continue to be positive. For example, a coronary artery disease (CAD) management program, targets the treatment of heart disease, a cost that consumes the largest percentage of U.S. health expenditures. The related cost estimates for health expenditures and productivity losses were $326.6 billion in 2000. At Universal Healthcare in Buffalo, New York, results were measured after just 1 year of implementation of a CAD management program, increasing the rate of annual lipid profile testing from 76% to 81%. In the years 1996 to 1999 the rate of Medicare patients on beta blockers following a myocardial infarction increased from 54% to 98%. (Shaw, 2001). Cedar-Sinai Medical Center in Los Angeles is addressing uncontrolled hypertension through a disease management program. This disease management program has resulted in statistically significant lower blood pressures and reduced provider visits and provider costs (Hatcher, 2001).

Outcome Measures. Nurses will be most successful when they can demonstrate efficiency of care with measurable, effective outcomes. Nurses must know how much their services cost and at what price services can be offered. They must be innovative in minimizing resource use, demonstrating the resulting decrease in costs and responding to the economic incentives of prospective payment and capitation. Rewards will come to those health care professionals who can manage the costs of disease and teach the value of good health. Practitioner value and accountability will be found in clinical and financial management.

Population Diversity and Aging

In the United States today more than 13% of Americans are age 65 years or older. The average life expectancy is 77 years, with women living on the average beyond 80 years. The fastest growing segment of the U.S. population is persons age 85 years and older. This trend translates to an increase of health care expenditures consumed by older adults. Management of health expenditures for the elderly will be paramount for a successful financial model for health care services in the United States.

The aging population means a renewed emphasis on care for chronic disease. Nurses can add value to their practice with an ability to delay the onset of chronic illness through education and prevention. Nurses have opportunities to develop and implement disease management programs and measure their effectiveness. The increasing number of elderly in the United States brings many economic and professional challenges as nurses bring value to their care through special education in geriatrics and care of the older adult. Opportunities will be available for nurses to participate in care management in various long-term care settings.

The U.S. population also is becoming more ethnically and racially diverse, with the number of minorities growing at a rate double that of whites (Nies and McEwen, 2001). Diversity brings new cultural practices and disease patterns with economic and care implications, and the increase in minority populations brings a new labor source to health care. Increased diversity in professional and nonprofessional health care workers could change the current availability and cost for the services of professional nurses.

Expansion of Technology

Improved technology for diagnostic and therapeutic practice is under examination for cost efficiency vs. outcome delivery. The U.S. health care delivery system must balance the health contributions of the improved technology with the accompanying costs. Other issues that the United States must face are those of quality of life, access to care, risk–benefit analysis, and individual consumer choice.

U.S. consumers have long lived with access to high levels of technology with little concern for costs. Nurses will be key players in educating patients and families about the cost-to-benefit ratio of certain technologies and will assist in selecting alternatives. One example is found in the increased use of pharmaceuticals; more advanced drugs are marketed with varying degrees of actual documented benefit over existing ones. Many patients are afraid to trust generic drugs, although they are less expensive. The nurse can be a link to educating the public regarding the potential gain in use of a more expensive drug vs. a less costly alternative. This is most important to older adults and others on fixed incomes who may already be spending a large portion of their income on health care.

The technology of the Internet offers promise for innovative programs (Box 6-2). The e-Case Management program at Wilson Medical Center, an integrated delivery system in North Carolina, uses a web-based approach to case management and claims dramatic improvement in quality of care and decreased costs. Information can be accessed from any site through the Internet at any location, which promotes continuity of care. Technology offers tools that can enhance care management (Durrer and Wright, 2001).

BOX 6-2	*Online Health Care Financing Resources*

American Association of Managed Care Nurses
www.aamcn.org

American Case Managers Association
www.acmaweb.org

Centers for Disease Control and Prevention
www.fedstats.gov

Health Care Financing Administration
www.hcfa.gov

Joint Interim Committee on Managed Care
www.senate.state.mo.us/mancare/mc-main.htm

Managed Care: Challenges and Opportunities for Nursing
www.ana.org/readroom/fsmgdcar.htm

Managed Care Magazine online
www.managedcaremag.com

Medicare www.medicare.gov
Medicare managed care www.hcfa.gov/medicare/mgdcar.htm

U.S. Census Bureau
www.census.gov

Information technology is of utmost importance to the professional nurse. The ability to gather and analyze health-related information and data for improved care is critical. Information technology is expensive but offers many opportunities in managing health care costs. Combining clinical skills with information technology skills can provide significant advantage to the success of professional nurses and new avenues for professional nurses to demonstrate their ability to provide cost-effective outcomes measurement.

Consumer Empowerment

Consumers or patients are health care customers demanding quality health care services at affordable rates. To be selected for services and products, providers are challenged to assess and meet customer requirements. The health care marketplace generates choices among services and products and alternative prices. Nurses must respond to marketplace opportunities and provide customer-focused care, which means putting the customer or patient first—a philosophy that nurses can totally support.

Economic forces are motivating the shift toward a model of health promotion and preventive care to achieve cost-effectiveness. This brings a new relationship with the consumer, emphasizing cost-sharing through individual choices in health practices. For instance, the insurance rate may be higher, or benefits may vary, based on unhealthy individual practices such as smoking, drinking, or taking drugs. Again, customer choice has economic implications in the health care marketplace of the future.

As managed care grows, recent legislation is in place to protect Americans enrolled in managed care plans. The new rule protects individuals with special health care needs to ensure continued access to care as they transition from fee-for-service to a managed care plan and assess quality and appropriateness of care. Information for beneficiaries about the managed care plan must be comprehensive and easy to understand. Another important aspect is the requirement for state rate-setting to ensure that capitation rates are actuarially sound. Other aspects of the legislation include access to services, patient-provider communication, network adequacy, marketing activities, and a grievance system. These changes encourage empowerment and protection of the health care consumer (New Patient Protections, 2001).

Nurses have many opportunities in a consumer-empowered marketplace. Nurse practitioners can demonstrate their ability and skills to deliver customer-focused primary care at reasonable costs as a cost-effective alternative to physician services. Opportunities for advanced practice nurses include primary care, case management, utilization management, quality improvement, patient advocacy, triage, education, and resource management. Nurses can take the lead in demonstrating the value of wellness and teaching health consciousness. Written materials for all levels of education will be needed, providing yet another opportunity for nurses who publish.

SUMMARY

Changes in the focus of the U.S. health care delivery system have brought new challenges for professional nurses. Box 6-3 outlines many of the trends occurring in health care. Health care has moved from emphasis on illness to emphasis on wellness and prevention, including the shift from acute care services to preventive and community-based services such as ambulatory care and home care. This shift mirrors the change in focus from hospital or institutional-based services to noninstitutional services such as home care.

Financing of health care services has gone from fee-for-service, or cost-based, to prospective payment and managed care. In the past, health care services were primarily directed by the physician, whereas today there are more diverse decision makers through managed care. The concept of "if it helps at all, do it" regardless of cost has yielded to practice based on outcomes measurement and cost-effectiveness.

In the past, "state-of-the-art" technology was introduced and used regardless of price. Today technology is used and respected as important to health care delivery but only with demonstrated outcomes, for the appropriate service, and at the right price. Information technology is critical to move to data-driven decision making. The current paper patient records are being encompassed by computerized, integrated information systems.

What does this mean to professional nursing? Nursing faces many challenges in professional practice in the twenty-first century. Many of these are directly related to the changing political and economic marketplace of health care. One is demonstrating that nurses provide measurable cost-effective, high-quality care. Practice in a cost-conscious environment is here to stay. Nurses will constantly challenge the current way of practice and examine each process for improvement and cost effectiveness. Accurate data must be collected to show cost containment and positive patient outcomes.

BOX 6-3	*Economic Issues and Trends*

From		To
Illness emphasis	→	Preventive emphasis
Acute care	→	Preventive, home care
Hospital/institution-based	→	Noninstitution-based (clinic/home)
Fee-for-service (cost-based)	→	Prospective payment and managed care
Physician-directed	→	Diverse decision-makers and managed care
If it helps (at all), use it (regardless of cost)	→	Outcomes measurement and cost-effectiveness
Independent decisions (practice variation)	→	Protocols/guidelines (best practice)
Local perspective (practice variation, standards/benchmarking)	→	Global perspective (protocols/guidelines/practice)
Introduce new technologies (regardless of cost)	→	Outcomes measurement and cost-effectiveness
Paper records, medical charts	→	Information systems, computer records

Change in Orientation

Illness, crisis	→	Prevention
Specific, specialist	→	Holistic
Quantity of care	→	Quality of care

Location of service

Inpatient	→	Outpatient, clinic, home

Payment mode

Retrospective	→	Prospective
Fee-for-service	→	Managed care

Outlook

Just do it	→	Outcomes measurement
Just do it	→	Quality of care; quality of life

Nurses need to assume the professional self-confidence necessary for leadership in the ever-changing economic and political environment that determines payment for services. Roles on clinical teams, in administration, and with the government hold promise for empowered change.

Nurses can accept that the job market is changing and that there will be job insecurity. However, changes in the health care marketplace will create new opportunities for health care professionals and eliminate the need for others. Professional nurses can prepare for these changes by recognizing health care trends and shifts in financing care and by educating themselves for evolving careers. This demands a commitment to lifelong learning.

Malone (1997), former president of the American Nurses Association, wrote about the "new order of health care" of the twenty-first century resulting from the many changes in the health care environment. Many of these changes are the result of economic forces and managed care and technologic innovations. Malone describes the presence of "twin sisters of excitement and anxiety" as this new order evolves. Her positive attitude is shown as she describes the twenty-first century as the "century of opportunity" for nurses.

As new systems are being designed for health care delivery models in managed care, professional nurses are uniquely qualified to play an integral role in this transformation process. The success of managed care will depend on creating healthier and better-informed consumers. The outcomes will be reduced health care costs with increased worker productivity. Nurses can position themselves to take a lead in educating consumers and encouraging personal responsibility for improved health practices. A managed care philosophy is congruent with that of professional nursing practice, bringing nurses back to the basics as society recognizes that healthy people are good business.

Critical Thinking Activities

1. The health care financing revolution has motivated important changes in the delivery of care across all health care settings. Describe the ways in which these changes are creating new or expanded opportunities for nurses. How do you expect these financing changes to affect your career?
2. Assume that you have become a nurse manager for the maternity floor of a large urban hospital. Use the concepts of a production function and a cost function to describe how you will go about making staffing decisions for your area.
3. Define ways that you, as a professional nurse, can obtain current health care economic information and trends. Why is this important? How can this knowledge add value to the practice of nursing?

REFERENCES

American Association of Managed Care Nurses, Inc., www.aamcn.org.

American Nurses Association: *Nursing's agenda for healthcare reform,* Kansas City, Mo, 1991, American Nurses Association.

Berk ML, Schur CL: Access to care: how much difference does Medicaid make? *Health Affairs* 17(3):169, 1998.

Durrer C, Wright S: Case management over the Internet, *Managed Healthcare News* 17(2):35, 2001.

Hatcher CE: Cedar-Sinai hypertension program reaches a new high in lows, *Managed Healthcare Executive* 1(2):38-41, 2001.

Health Care Financing Administration: www.hcfa.gov/stats/NHE-Proj/proj2000/default.htm, 2000.

Kaiser Family Foundation: The Medicare program: Medicare at a glance, Menlo Park, Calif, 1997, Henry J. Kaiser Family Foundation.

Komisar HJ et al: Medicare chart book, Menlo Park, Calif, 1997, Henry J. Kaiser Family Foundation.

Malone B: President's perspective *Nurse* 28(8):6, 1997.

Managed care now dominates employer health insurance markets, *The digest of managed care,* Skaneateles, NY, May, 1997, HealthCare Press, p 5.

Markus G: Medicare payment reform: implications for the nursing specialties, *Spec Nurs Forum* 2(2):2-T, 1990.

National Health Statistics Group: Office of Actuary, National Health Expenditures, 1998, Health Care Financing Review, vol 24, no 2, HCFA Publication 03420, Health Care Financing Administration, Washington, Winter 1999, US Government Printing Office, www.cdc.gov/nchs/fastats/hexpense.htm.

New patient protections in managed care rule, *Tenn Hosp Health Systems Newsletter* 6(2):5, 2001.

News Briefs: employee choice, *Managed Healthcare News* 17(2):1, 2001.

Nies M, McEwen M: *Community health nursing: promoting the health of populations,* Philadelphia, 2001, WB Saunders.

Perrin D: MSAs and the next generation of healthcare, *Managed Healthcare News* 17(2):30, 2001.

Pew Health Professions Commission: *Healthy America: practitioners for 2005,* Report of the Pew Health Professions Commission, Durham, NC, 1991, Duke University Medical Center.

Shaw G: Coronary artery disease: practicing prevention, *Managed Healthcare News* (2):18, 2001.

US Census Bureau: *Health insurance coverage 1998,* www.census.gov/hhes/www/hlthins.html.

US Department of Health and Human Services: *Health United States 1996–1997 and injury chartbook,* Washington, DC, 1997, US Government Printing Office.

US Department of Health and Human Services, Centers for Disease Control and Prevention, National Center for Health Statistics, *Health insurance coverage,* Nov. 7, 2000, www.cdc.gov/nchs/fastats/hinsure.htm. www.cdc.gov/nchs/fastats/hinsure.htm.

US Department of Labor, Bureau of Labor Statistics, Consumer Price Index, 2000, www.cdc.gov/nchs/fasts/hexpenseFeb.2001.htm

SUGGESTED READINGS

Chang CF, Price SA, Pfoutz SK: *Economics and nursing: critical professional issues,* Philadelphia, 2001, FA Davis.

Feldstein PJ: *Health care economics,* ed 4, Albany, NY, 1993, Delmar Publishers.

Phelps CE: *Health economics,* New York, 1992, HarperCollins.

Santerre RE, Neun SP: *Health economics: theories, insights, and industry studies,* New York, 1996, Irwin Publisher.

US Council of Economic Advisors: *Economic report of the President,* Washington, DC, 1997, US Government Printing Office.

The Health Care Delivery System and Managed Care

Phyllis Skorga, PhD, RN, CCM

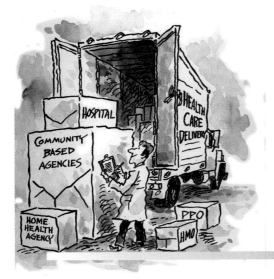

Health care delivery systems
are packaged in a wide variety of ways
and offer a wide range of services.

Vignette

Halfway through the evening shift in the emergency room, 52-year-old Lillian Baker was admitted with a hip fracture after she slipped and fell getting out of her bathtub. The emergency room nurse assessed Mrs. Baker's presenting symptoms and her relevant health history and physical status and documented her findings in the medical record. The nurse coordinated Mrs. Baker's medical and diagnostic care while she was still in the emergency room and managed her transfer to the hospital surgical orthopedic unit. In the acute care hospital unit Mrs. Baker's surgeon scheduled the operating room to repair the fracture. Because Mrs. Baker worked for an engineering firm with insurance benefits through a health maintenance organization (HMO), her physician called the preauthorization hot line to notify them of Mrs. Baker's admission and need for surgery. The HMO preauthorization nurse collected the medical information, authorized the admission for medical necessity and subsequent benefits coverage, and applied an admission length of stay according to recognized medical criteria. Her physician selected the fast track option that included surgery followed by early rehabilitation. Mrs. Baker's entire hospital stay was planned for up to 5 days, depending on her physical progress. On the second postoperative day, Mrs. Baker was recuperating well enough to move to acute level rehabilitation with active physical therapy. She was anxious to return to work and to resume her regular "life" with her children and grandchildren. After surgery, although her physical strength returned quickly, she developed an infection, necessitating a round of antibiotic treatment. Mrs. Baker's nurse case manager collaborated with her family, physician, pharmacist, and the home health provider to

133

schedule home health services. This allowed Mrs. Baker to be discharged on time as planned, with home infusion therapy for the antibiotic regimen, physical therapy for ambulation and gait training, and skilled nursing visits to provide additional needed care in the home environment. As her infection cleared and her condition warranted, the physician approved Mrs. Baker's discharge from home health services and ordered outpatient physical therapy, which was coordinated by her case manager with assistance from the social worker to identify community resources to provide Lillian's transportation to and from physical therapy. Lillian's physical functioning and health status continued to improve, and, as originally planned, Lillian Baker returned to her job and her routine interests and hobbies.

Questions to consider while reading this chapter

1. Why does Mrs. Baker's health maintenance organization (HMO) require preauthorization for hospital admission and surgery?
2. What range of services across the continuum of care contributed to Mrs. Baker's recovery and eventual return to work and normal activities?
3. Why was it important to discharge Mrs. Baker from the hospital "on time" even though she still had an infection requiring treatment with intravenous antibiotics?

Key Terms

Capitation A method of reimbursing providers (usually physicians) with a fixed payment typically expressed as a per-member-per-month payment that is paid in advance for future anticipated contracted health services.

Collaboration A method of working together on a joint project as different disciplines problem solve interdependently.

Consolidation Combination or unification of health care entities into a system or body.

Credentialing Procedures undertaken by health care organizations to ensure the competence of physicians being considered for affiliation with the organization. Credentialing procedures include, at a minimum, the careful review and verification of the physician's state licensure, education and training, board certification, disciplinary actions and malpractice experience, continuing medical education courses, references, and professional liability coverage.

Fee-for-service A method of reimbursing providers retrospectively (after care is given) for each service provided at a rate that does not exceed the billed charge for each unit of service.

Indemnity insurance Traditional insurance that provides payment for covered expenses of illness care under major medical or supplemental policies.

Integrated delivery system An organized system of health care that operates under a unified management structure and includes physician practices, hospitals, and other health agencies in a cooperative effort to accept capitation and deliver health care to a defined population. Some models of integration include physician-hospital organizations and management service organizations.

Managed care A system of health care delivery that manages or controls use and cost of services for a set fee. The goal is a system that delivers value by giving people access to quality and cost-effective health care. Examples of managed care are health maintenance organizations and preferred provided organizations.

Payer A public or private organization that pays for or underwrites coverage for health care expenses.

Peer review Evaluation of health care to determine if care meets quality standards and is provided in a reasonable, necessary manner in the most appropriate setting. The evaluation is conducted by medical staff with training equivalent to that of the provider under review.

Primary care Health care services provided by a physician, nurse practitioner, or physician's assistant that include first contact in the health care system, as well as coordination of comprehensive health care needed by an individual. Primary care addresses a person's most common health care needs and stresses prevention and disease management to maximize health and well-being.

Provider Licensed professionals such as physicians, optometrists, psychologists, and nurse practitioners, whose services under state or federal law must be included in coverage offered by a health plan.

Risk sharing A negotiated agreement between provider and payer in which both parties share in the financial risk of providing certain health care services. For example, a pool of money is budgeted by the payer to cover expected expenses for contracted health care services. If the services do not consume the entire budgeted amount, both payer and provider share in the savings; but if costs for the services exceed the budgeted amount, both parties share the additional cost.

Seamless care delivery Organized movement from one health care service to another without interference or disruption in service.

Utilization controls Procedures such as preadmission review, concurrent review, and case management used to assess medical necessity, efficiency, or appropriateness of health care services and treatment plans on a prospective, concurrent, or retrospective basis.

Learning Outcomes

After studying this chapter, the reader will be able to:

1. Analyze the effect of health care delivery systems on health care cost, quality, and access.
2. Analyze the interactive relationship between changes in the continuum of care and the reorganization of the health care delivery system.
3. Compare the defining features of the major types of managed care organizations.
4. Analyze the benefits of having accrediting agencies in health care delivery.
5. Evaluate the impact of the health care delivery system on nursing.

CHAPTER OVERVIEW

The American health care system continues to evolve as we move into the twenty-first century. The recent history of rapid and uncontrolled cost increases of the 1980s led to a health care system that attempted to resolve cost issues through managed care systems in the 1990s. Managed care is designed to contain costs and improve access to health care while maintaining quality of services. However, the health care delivery system continues to be assaulted by a new global marketplace, relentless competition, radical technical innovations, major attitudinal shifts, and work redesign. In all segments of the health care delivery system from hospitals to pharmaceutical companies to home health agencies, consolidation is paramount with mergers, acquisitions, and organizational reform among all sectors of the market (Institute for the Future, 2000).

These tumultuous changes that continue to occur in the health care delivery system are being driven by high health care costs and are resulting in the greatest reorganization in modern times. According to the Centers for Medicare and Medicaid Services (formerly the Health Care Financing Administration), health care costs increased dramatically from 5% of the gross domestic product in 1960 to nearly 14% in 1990. However, the 1990s saw annual growth in health care costs fall and health expenditures stabilize at 13.6% of the gross domestic product throughout that decade. Costs remained steady because of the influence of managed health care, but some predict cost increases for the future (McGuire, 1997). Because of efforts to limit services and reduce costs, managed care has come under intense public scrutiny. This backlash against managed care has led to court actions and state legislative mandates for longer hospital stays and more expensive procedures, thus adding to the increased cost scenario (Currents, 1997a).

Providers of health care services are being forced to continue to rein in costs of care, cut excess use of hospital care and other health care services, and improve quality and access to care. The changes to lower health care costs include:

- Health care organizations becoming part of corporations with a focus on for-profit business vs. nonprofit status (Scott, 1997)
- Mergers among organizations that were once long-standing competitors now becoming partners within the same organization
- Integrated delivery networks with a goal of seamless care delivery
- Reimbursement modifications with payment incentives to reduce the utilization of health care services (capitation)
- Movement from illness treatment to health promotion with quality and service improvements
- Increasing attention to complementary and alternative therapies (Institute for the Future, 2000).

Nurses working at this time have witnessed unprecedented change. Propelled by technologic and economic forces, health care is being reengineered and reshaped for the next century. Graduate nurses must be prepared to practice in this changing health care system by developing an understanding of the health care delivery system, managed care, and the expectations of consumers—those people for whom nurses are obligated to care.

A consumer report from the collaborative focus group of the American Hospital Association and the Picker Institute (1997) provides a long-term examination of consumer's perceptions and experiences with their health care. Results of more than 10 years of surveys and over 350,000 respondents indicate that consumers are worried about the future of health care, and that, even though they indicate satisfaction with health care delivery on surveys, their personal experiences reflect a different picture. Consumers report the following concerns about health care:

- Reduced access to health care services
- Higher out-of-pocket costs
- Questionable quality of care
- Questionable quality of caregiver competence

The report further suggests that health care organizations need to focus on the "eight dimensions of care that are most critical from the point of view of patients" (Box 7-1).

BOX 7-1   *Eight Dimensions of Care Identified by Patients As Critical*

1. Respect	5. Coordination of care
2. Access to care	6. Physical comfort
3. Emotional support	7. Involvement of family and friends
4. Information and education	8. Continuity and transition

From the American Hospital Association and Picker Institute: Eye on patients: report to the American public, 1997.

The purpose of this chapter is to describe the health care delivery system, with a focus on the continuum of care, changes in health care, and the role and contribution of nursing to the larger health care system. As issues are explained, trends affecting health care and the influence on nursing are explored.

CONTINUUM OF CARE

The health care delivery system is a continuum of care from primary preventive care to acute institutional care to postacute outpatient or freestanding facility care and ultimately to long-term care. The continuum of care involves a range of clinical services provided to an individual or group and reflects treatment given during a single hospitalization or care for multiple health problems over a lifetime (Fig. 7-1). Distinctions among the levels of care have blurred as the delivery of services provided by traditional hospitals or long-term care providers has changed. In addition, levels of care delivery have overlapped, creating confusion in terminology. For example, subacute care, a reference to an acuity level in health care, may also include care provided in skilled nursing units and rehabilitation facilities.

Primary Care

Points of contact with the physician or physician extender (nurse practitioner, physician's assistant) in the office, outpatient, or ambulatory clinical setting usually are described as primary care. Primary care addresses a person's most common health care needs and stresses prevention and disease management to maximize health and well-being. Health care delivery in the primary care setting incorporates health promotion activities such as immunizations, screening tests, and health education, as well as maintenance of acute and chronic health care needs. For example, a patient with diabetes is evaluated for status of glucose control and for chronic progression of the disease by the primary care provider, who may perform a retinal eye examination and analyze laboratory results of urine and blood tests for evidence of vascular and organ damage. During the same visit, disease management, including correct diabetic diet and foot care, are taught to prevent complications.

Another goal of primary care is to perform diagnostic testing and treatments in the outpatient community setting rather than in the acute care setting. For example, suspected medical conditions are diagnosed using computed tomography (CT) scans and magnetic resonance imaging (MRI) in outpatient testing departments or imaging centers. Walk-in clinics such as sports medicine and wellness centers, ambulatory surgery centers, freestanding urgent and emergent care centers, and psychiatric partial hospitalization facilities have also increased the availability of health care in the outpatient setting. Medical treatments for chemotherapy, hemodialysis, and lithotripsy for renal stones also are provided in the community setting.

Physician care in office and clinic settings continues in the traditional form and has expanded with the use of physician extenders such as nurse practitioners. Nurse practitioners are educated in various specialty areas such as mental health, maternal and child care, adult health, and geriatric care. Physicians and nurse practitioners have defined practice privileges, depending on state legislation, area of specialty, and organizational affiliation.

Primary care and specialty physicians are organizing in a variety of ways, which has led to increased efficiencies, changes in practice behavior, and power in the marketplace. It is now rare to see a physician in solo practice with no affiliation with a group of physicians or with a hospital system. Some physicians are selling their medical practices to practice management companies. In addition to financial incentives, practice management companies offer

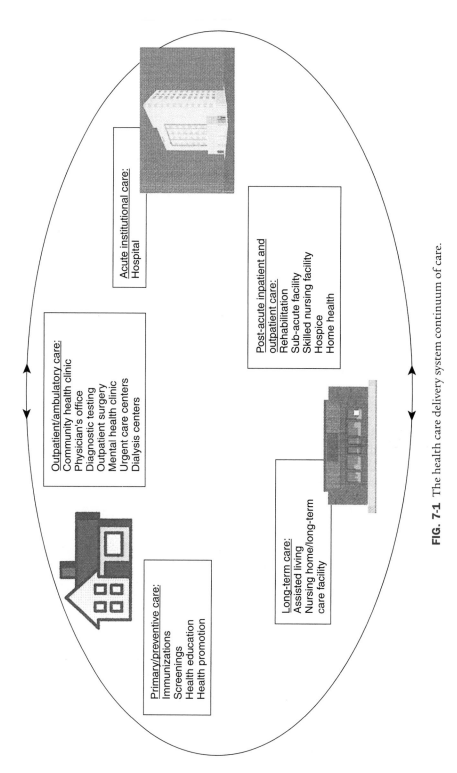

FIG. 7-1 The health care delivery system continuum of care.

Acute institutional care:
Hospital

Outpatient/ambulatory care:
Community health clinic
Physician's office
Diagnostic testing
Outpatient surgery
Mental health clinic
Urgent care centers
Dialysis centers

Post-acute inpatient and outpatient care:
Rehabilitation
Sub-acute facility
Skilled nursing facility
Hospice
Home health

Primary/preventive care:
Immunizations
Screenings
Health education
Health promotion

Long-term care:
Assisted living
Nursing home/long-term care facility

increased efficiencies in areas such as billing, contracting, and personnel management and relieve physicians of administrative duties, allowing them more time to actually provide health care to their patients.

Acute Care

In the acute care setting hospitals direct their services toward patients with either critical illness or injury or acute medical conditions. Many hospitals have developed programs to reduce the length of hospital stay and therefore health care costs. For example, some hospitals have introduced programs such as 23-hour observation, same-day surgeries, and critical pathways for the efficient treatment of illnesses.

Because of the ongoing changes in the health care delivery system and cost reduction efforts discussed previously in this chapter, many hospitals have become part of larger health care systems. These "hospital systems" are networks of affiliated health care organizations that may include other hospitals, physician practices, outpatient diagnostics, urgent care facilities, rehabilitation centers, durable medical equipment companies, home health agencies, and/or home infusion therapy services. Nationally these hospital systems account for $300 billion in revenue, more than 545 million outpatient visits, and more than 33 million inpatient admissions (Health U.S., 2000). The largest health care systems in the United States as measured by net patient revenues are HCA, The Healthcare Company (formerly Columbia/HCA), Tenet, and Kaiser Permanente (Japson and Scott, 1997).

Across the country, hospitals and doctors have formed networks known as integrated delivery systems. Integrated delivery systems are organizations of physicians, hospitals, and other health facilities that accept capitation from health insurance payers and deliver health care services to defined populations such as specific employee groups and Medicare patients. The goal of an integrated delivery system is seamless delivery of all health care needs in the "one-stop shop" method of service and convenience. An integrated delivery system is able to lower costs by eliminating duplicate services and combining other services to increase efficiencies.

However, large health systems are experiencing increased community scrutiny because of their integration efforts. They are being asked to justify the value of acquisitions and mergers. Increasing financial pressures simultaneously challenge giant health care systems to make reform efforts work. In this context the newest trend beyond the integrated delivery system is a movement "back to basics." Shrinking Medicare reimbursement, tight managed care rates, increasing costs of new technology, and escalating drug expenditures combine to make ancillary services that aren't performing up to financial expectations look less attractive. After pouring $5 billion into integrated delivery systems over the last 10 years, now some organizations are limiting integration efforts (Haugh, 2001).

Postacute Care

Postacute care represents the other side of the continuum with skilled nursing facilities, rehabilitation facilities, home health services, assisted living, and longer-term options such as nursing homes. Pressure is intense on acute care providers to offer high-quality services at lower cost. Postacute care providers offer another, and perhaps the last, chance to cut the excess out of health care cost while still keeping patients healthy and satisfied.

In postacute care the numbers of outpatient facilities and rehabilitation services continue to grow the fastest, with skilled nursing centers in steady pursuit. These providers of health care services offer lower-cost alternatives to the traditional in-hospital approach to patient care. As the market tightens on acute care facilities, these postacute centers offer options that usually are less costly and more convenient for a majority of clients.

Postacute care in the home health market boomed in the early 1990s but slowed significantly after implementation of the Balanced Budget Act of 1997, which limited Medicare payment for home health services. In 2000 $44 billion was spent on home health services; this included a 45% decline in Medicare reimbursement after the drastic cuts of the Balanced Budget Act. The Benefits Improvement and Protection Act of 2000 is poised to return some of the funds cut by the first Balanced Budget Act. Many home health agencies are owned by acute care hospitals (60%), which presents an example of the consolidation that is occurring daily (Meyer, 1997; Rauber, 2000).

Home health services are of proven benefit in postacute care, palliative care, and also in lieu of hospitalization. The role of nursing in the home setting is mushrooming with a full range of nursing services. Home health nurses provide skilled visits, educational services, and hospice care. In addition to nursing services, a range of other professional services, including physical therapy, respiratory therapy, occupational therapy, social work, and nonskilled services provided by nursing assistants and companions, are available in the home. Home care also often includes the provision of medical equipment and infusion therapy.

In addition to home health, long-term care settings are increasing in popularity and use as the population ages. Nursing homes, assisted living centers, and retirement communities or facilities offer varying levels of nursing care for disabled or older adults with minimal to severe health care needs.

MANAGED HEALTH CARE

The strongest movement in health care delivery over the past 10 years is managed health care. Eighty percent of all employed health care workers are enrolled in a managed care program (health maintenance organization [HMO], point-of-service [POS] plan, or preferred provider

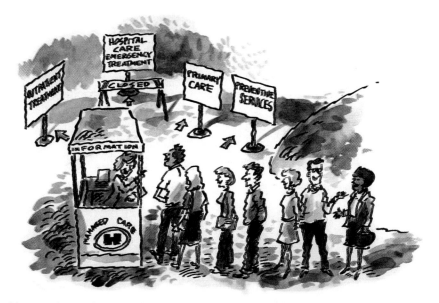

Managed care has continued to grow in response to employers' demands
for lower-cost health care institutions.

organization [PPO]), up from less than 30% a decade ago (Staff, 1997). Employers across all industries have driven the managed care movement by demanding lower health care costs. Most large employers pay a significant part of the health insurance premium for their employees. Those costs have a direct impact on business profits. Because health care costs have continued to rise, business profits have been negatively impacted. Therefore most employers are motivated to seek the lowest cost health insurance packages for their employees. Managed care has continued to grow in response to employers' demands for lower cost health insurance.

Definition of Managed Health Care

Managed health care is the principal form of health care delivery in the United States today. Most consider managed care to be a system of health care delivery that uses financial incentives and management controls to direct patients covered by the health plan to the most appropriate provider (both physician and hospital) in the most efficient treatment settings. For example, if a primary care physician in an office setting can effectively treat the problem, the patient is directed to that provider as opposed to being treated by a specialist or in a more acute-care setting such as the emergency room. Effectively managed systems control quality and use of services, as well as medical costs and administrative expenses.

Managed care can also be defined as a health care system that integrates the financing and delivery of health care services to covered individuals by arrangements with selected providers. These managed care systems offer a package of health care benefits that might include coverage for outpatient office visits, preventive care, emergency care, diagnostic and surgical procedures, hospitalizations, and prescription drug coverage. Managed care systems also offer standards for selecting health care providers, formal programs for ongoing quality improvement and utilization review, and financial incentives for their members to use providers and procedures associated with the managed care plan.

Types of Managed Care Organizations

Managed health care has evolved over the past 10 to 20 years to become a hybrid industry that includes HMOs, PPOs, and the POS plan. Historically the HMO was the model of managed health care delivery. The traditional fee-for-service (indemnity) health insurance product added management controls and specialized contracting to become the PPO, and a derivative that blurs the distinctions between these two types is the POS plan option. Each of these types of managed care will be explained in greater detail. (Refer to Box 7-2 for a summary of some of the more common managed care terms and associated acronyms.)

BOX 7-2	*Health Care Delivery Alphabet Soup*

AAHC/URAC American Accreditation Healthcare Commission/Utilization Review Accreditation Commission
HMO Health Maintenance Organization
IDS Integrated Delivery System
IPA Independent Practice Association
JCAHO Joint Commission on Accreditation of Healthcare Organizations

MCO Managed Care Organization
NCQA National Committee for Quality Assurance
POS Point of Service
PPO Preferred Provider Organization

Health Maintenance Organizations

HMOs are a form of health insurance that provides for primary care services, specialty care, emergency treatment, and hospital care to people who are members in the plan. The philosophy of HMOs is that maintenance and promotion of health will result in savings. HMOs have grown incredibly from enrolling two million Americans in 1970 to 20 million in 1985 to over 40 million by the late 1990s (Barents Group, 1996). HMOs attempt to control unnecessary medical services through (1) various forms of provider risk sharing, (2) providers acting as "gatekeepers," and (3) utilization and peer review processes.

Provider Risk Sharing. One premise of provider risk sharing is to encourage the prescription of appropriate and necessary services by paying providers a fixed payment per patient for comprehensive health services, no matter what the cost of treatment. This "one-payment-covers-all" type of reimbursement for providers discourages them from overprescribing health care services and encourages the use of health promotion activities. This payment mechanism is intended to reverse the tendency for providers to overprescribe services, which is inherent in the fee-for-service payment mechanism.

Payment to the provider from the HMO can be in the form of salary or capitated fee. With capitation the physician is paid a set payment per-member-per-month for a defined patient population to deliver specified care over a set time period. For example, a primary care physician may be paid $20 per month per individual enrolled in the managed care plan. This payment covers care needed by that individual, including office visits and other necessary services that are covered under the terms of the contract with the HMO. If an individual patient does not need or elect to use the covered health care services, the physician receives the same per month payment. However, under the capitated payment system, the physician assumes the risk because he or she receives the same payment for an individual who is very ill and needs extensive care as for the individual who never makes an office visit.

Utilization Controls. A part of the physician's capitated payment may be withheld until the end of the year to create an incentive for efficient care. If the physician exceeds utilization norms, he or she may not receive the payment that was withheld. For example, a range of in-hospital use is accepted in terms of numbers of admissions and lengths of hospital stays; if the physician regularly exceeds that range of acceptable use, he or she could be penalized by having a part of the payment withheld.

The Primary Care Provider as Gate-Keeper. The primary care provider serving as the "gatekeeper" to health care services is another method established by HMOs to encourage efficient use of services and to control costs. As the gatekeeper, the primary care provider must authorize referrals for the patient to access specialty care. If this authorization is not received, the HMO will not pay for the specialty care. As previously discussed in risk sharing, the primary care provider may have a financial incentive to effectively control specialty referrals.

Types of Health Maintenance Organizations. There are four main varieties of HMOs that are identified by their financial and organizational arrangements with the physicians who provide services. The four types of HMOs are independent practice association (IPA), staff, group, and network models and are defined as follows:

- *IPA model:* The HMO contracts with physicians who practice in their own offices or with associated independent groups of doctors in private practice to provide health care services to its covered members.
- *Staff model:* Physicians are hired as employees of the HMO and paid a salary to provide health care services to its covered members; this is considered the traditional type of HMO.
- *Group model:* The HMO contracts with a group of physicians who practice in a group setting; the physicians are paid a set amount per patient to provide a specified range of services for the HMO's covered members.
- *Network model:* An extension of the group model that is identified by contracts between the HMO and more than one group of solo practice physicians, multispecialty groups, or independent group practice physicians.

HMO Membership. The largest of the managed care organizations, ranked by total enrollment, is the Blue Cross and Blue Shield Association with 21 million members, followed by United Health Care Corporation with 11 million members, Kaiser Foundation with 9 million members, and Aetna U.S. Health Care Plan with eight million members (Managed Care Digest, 1999). Medicare and Medicaid enrollment in HMO products is increasing as well. As use of managed care increases, the number of HMOs decreases, and fewer companies control a majority of managed care enrollees. The challenge continues to be to ensure that the managed care product is evaluated on the quality of health coverage it can offer its covered members rather than solely on the price of that coverage.

Preferred Provider Organizations

A PPO is an organization of providers that contracts on a fee-for-service basis with payer groups to provide comprehensive health services to the people covered by the health plan. Insurers, employers, providers, and independent agents sponsor PPOs, and these sponsoring groups contract with physicians to provide health care services for a discount on the physicians' customary charges. In return for the discounted fee, the physician will receive an increased volume of patients from the PPO. This increased volume is achieved by the health plan providing an incentive for patients to select physicians from the panel of preferred providers. The panel of providers is the list of physicians who are contracted with the health plan to provide services at a discounted fee. Provider charges usually are 10% to 20% below customary fees. Physicians do not assume risk and are paid a fee-for-service at the discounted rate. Over 98 million workers are covered by PPOs and POS organizations in the United States (AAHP, 1998).

PPO members can receive health services from a provider not affiliated with the plan, but the rate of insurance coverage is reduced, and the patient will have a greater out-of-pocket expense. PPOs have been endorsed as an alternative to the strict use parameters and risk contracts of HMOs. However, employers are indicating that PPOs are less capable of controlling health care costs than was projected originally, and this weakness may be related to less stringent utilization review practices (Managed Care Digest, 1999).

Point-of-Service Plan

The POS plan has increased in popularity in the past few years. The POS option allows members to have a choice at the time of service delivery to use a nonmember physician or health care provider in return for reduced reimbursement, resulting in an increased out-of-pocket expense for the patient. The POS plan has grown rapidly as employees have demanded the choice of providers that it offers.

Managed Care Processes

Utilization Review. Utilization review involves screening processes undertaken by the managed care organization to ensure the medical necessity and appropriateness of health care services that are being considered. The managed care organization generally requires that authorization for certain procedures and hospital admissions be obtained in order for payment to be authorized. For example, in the vignette the surgeon had to contact Mrs. Baker's HMO to document the medical necessity of the hip repair surgery and get authorization so that the HMO would pay for the surgical procedure.

Utilization review processes also involve the managed care staff, most often a nurse with physician back-up, working with the providers to develop a treatment plan based on the patient's medical condition. Again as seen in the vignette, Mrs. Baker's treatment plan was developed by her surgeon in consultation with the HMO nurse, and this plan included early rehabilitation and a hospital stay of up to 5 days. Utilization review is an ongoing process that may occur prospectively (before the provision of health care services) or concurrently (while the patient is receiving treatment, such as during a hospitalization). Managed care systems also use case management processes to authorize and plan care for patients with costly, complex care requirements to ensure that the most efficient and appropriate health care services and treatment plans are used.

To provide safe and effective health care to its covered members, the managed care organization's utilization management program should incorporate the following components:

- Comparison of the patient's proposed plan of care to established standards
- Medical criteria based on professional standards of care and nationally recognized guidelines
- First-level review by a nurse, with second-level review from a physician if questions regarding the medical necessity or appropriateness of a planned service arise.

Utilization management programs with these components have been studied for effectiveness in reducing hospital use and decreasing overall medical expenditures (Feldstein, Wickizer, and Wheeler, 1988; Barents Group, 1996). Findings from these studies revealed that utilization management reduced admissions by 13%, inpatient days by 11%, hospital room and board expenditures by 7%, hospital ancillary service expenditures (laboratory, x-ray) by 9%, and total medical expenditures by 6%. Results support the belief in managed care cost controls as an effective means of resource allocation (Terry, 1995). Managed care systems using appropriate utilization review activities reduce the use of services by up to 6.9% compared with unmanaged care (Barents Group, 1996).

Peer Review. Peer review is another process used by managed care organizations to ensure that appropriate and high-quality care is provided. Peer review involves evaluation of health care to determine if the care meets quality standards and is provided in a reasonable, necessary manner in the most appropriate setting. The evaluation is conducted by medical staff with training equivalent to that of the provider under review. For example, a cardiologist will be involved in the review of medical care provided by another cardiologist.

Trends in Managed Care

As discussed previously, employers' demands to decrease the rate of employee medical expenses propelled the momentum toward managed care. Managed care organizations control use of health care services and cost by providing incentives to patients and providers to consider lower-cost treatment alternatives and to promote economic use of health care resources (Stano, 1996). For example, patients who belong to managed care organizations have less costly premiums and preventive care services such as immunizations that are not often covered by traditional health insurance. Primary care providers, as the gatekeepers of services, may receive incentive payments for reduced utilization of health care services, including numbers of referrals to specialists or numbers of admissions to hospitals. For example, the managed care company will set the expectation for the number of referrals to specialists that a primary care provider will make for his or her patients covered by the plan. If the number of referrals to specialists is less than the expected level, the provider could receive an incentive payment for having used fewer health care services.

Consumers have begun to demand more choice in their health care options due in part to the drastic changes in health care delivery and the information explosion in the last 20 years. Future trends include continued reduction in inpatient length of stays, growth in technologic innovations, although at a slower pace, and slower increase in life expectancy (Rubin et al., 1998).

The future development and direction of managed care depends on responsible and equitable sharing of health care risks and rewards. Risk involves exposure to a factor, element, or course of action that might incur a loss. Risk sharing in health care indicates that an agreement has been negotiated between the managed care organization and the provider of services to share risk in terms of financial payments. For example, the provider assumes the risk when he or she receives the same payment to care for a patient with multiple, complex medical problems as for a patient who only comes in for a yearly physical examination. Research in the field of managed health care indicates that costs were saved primarily by avoiding unnecessary care, reducing hospital admissions, and decreasing lengths of hospital stay. Research findings suggest that 15% to 40% of major procedures such as hip replacements and coronary artery bypass graft surgery are unnecessary (Wennberg and Gittelsohn, 1982; AAHP, 1998).

In addition to reducing unnecessary care, managed care has also saved families money. According to a study commissioned by the American Association of Health Plans and prepared by the Lewin Group, "in 1996 managed care saved families between $408 and $549, including savings in premiums, out-of-pocket health care costs and increased wages . . . Lewin said wages increased as employers passed along their health care savings to employees" (Kertesz, 1997, p. 8). This report estimates a $23.8 to $37.4 billion total health care cost savings for all payers as a result of managed care.

Ongoing assessment of managed care efforts indicates that access to medical care has not been compromised within the managed care environment. Managed care members perceive comparable or higher levels of satisfaction than their fee-for-service counterparts (Winslow, 1994; EBRI, 1999; AAHP, 1998). As managed care organizations have matured, the focus of research has moved to outcome management and demonstration of the quality of clinical care and service delivery.

However, despite cost savings and member satisfaction, there is a backlash effort directed at the managed care movement in response to perceptions of limited services and reduced access to care. National and state laws are directed at legislating health care guidelines, criteria for care, and utilization management. For example, a mandatory 48-hour length of stay in the hospital for normal infant delivery has been legislated in some states. The fact that managed care has slowed the growth of medical spending often is lost in the criticism and debate.

An alternative to managed health care is universal health care coverage, which would provide all Americans with health insurance coverage. However most analysts believe that universal health care is not a realistic option in the foreseeable future. In January 2000 the Robert Wood Johnson Foundation sponsored a conference called *Health Coverage 2000,* and eight major health care organizations and associations presented proposals to expand health insurance coverage. Some of the proposals introduced incremental reform by expanding Medicaid and the State Childrens Health Insurance Program (SCHIP), whereas other proposals included universal coverage. The Lewin Group estimated total costs for these proposals if implemented in the United States. Incremental reform costs were estimated between $15 and $59 billion and were predicted to reduce the uninsured population by approximately 40%, leaving 19 million uninsured Americans. The universal proposal to cover all Americans was estimated to cost between $324 and $454 billion per year (Sheils, 2000).

EXTERNAL OVERSIGHT: ACCREDITATION OF THE MANAGED CARE ORGANIZATION

Accreditation indicates that an independent third party completely external to the managed care organization has applied a set of accepted standards to the policies, procedures, and initiatives of the managed care organization and determined a score or rank for the organization. The process of adherence to standards provides assurance to the public that the organization provides a quality service. There is increasing evidence that consumers' levels of satisfaction with the service they receive from a managed care organization are associated with perceptions of higher-quality clinical care (Mera, 2000).

Health care systems have remained open to the need for external oversight of health care delivery. Dominance of the Joint Commission on Accreditation of Healthcare Organizations (JCAHO) is evidence of that belief. JCAHO is the national accrediting body that reviews and accredits most health care providers. Types of organizations accredited by JCAHO include hospitals and specialty acute and chronic care providers such as rehabilitation facilities, outpatient facilities, home health agencies, infusion therapy companies, and durable medical equipment companies. As managed care has evolved, external oversight in this area of health care delivery has been spearheaded by employers, who see accreditation as a safety measure to explain to employees that standards are being met as health care costs are lowered.

The most prominent accrediting bodies for managed care entities are the National Committee for Quality Assurance (NCQA), JCAHO, and the American Accreditation Healthcare Commission/Utilization Review Accreditation Commission (URAC). Information about these accrediting agencies as a current trend can help explain the overall external oversight process in health care delivery.

National Committee for Quality Assurance

Established in 1990, the NCQA typically accredits HMOs, PPOs, and POS plans. To be accredited, organizations must have provided comprehensive inpatient and outpatient care through an organized delivery system for at least 18 months and have defined administrative processes in place. Standards and substandards for NCQA address the areas of quality improvement, utilization management, provider credentialing, member rights and responsibilities, preventive health services, and medical records.

To be NCQA accredited, health plans (i.e., HMOs, PPOs) are asked to demonstrate that:

- Patients have access to care in a reasonable time period.
- Improvements in patient care and services are ongoing.
- Members with chronic or high-risk illnesses are identified and provided with effective disease management programs.
- Processes for deciding what health services are appropriate and for responding to appeals when payment for services is denied are in place and satisfy NCQA examination.
- Written policies for credentialing, recredentialing, and reappointment of physicians and other providers are in place.
- Preventive services, as well as guidelines for the use of such services, are offered (e.g., specific screening and preventive programs such as childhood and adult immunizations, prenatal care, and cholesterol, cancer, and hypertension screenings must be in place).
- Consistency and verification of compliance with established guidelines for medical records can be demonstrated (McGuire, 1996; Graham, 1996).

In addition, NCQA publishes a national comparison of health plans and has developed the Health Plan Employer Data and Information Set (HEDIS). HEDIS is a measurement system that quantifies health plan processes and outcomes of quality, enrollment, utilization, and other data (Edlin, 1996; Pallarito and Morrissey, 1996).

Joint Commission on Accreditation of Healthcare Organizations

The JCAHO, established in 1951, accredits most types of inpatient and outpatient health care facilities, hospital and health care networks, and health plans. JCAHO accreditation is voluntary for the organization but is viewed by the health care industry and the public as the "seal of approval" for the organization. The JCAHO standards address rights, responsibilities and ethics, the continuum of care, education and communication, health promotion and disease prevention, leadership, management of human resources, management of information, and improvement of network performance. To be JCAHO accredited, health plans (i.e., HMOs, health insurance companies) must demonstrate that:

- Services are integrated into a seamless continuum of care.
- Policies to address treatment decisions, privacy and confidentiality of medical records, and complaints and grievances are in place.
- Members (individuals who have health coverage through the plan) are informed of services and how to access services.
- Communication about fees, out-of-network benefits, and education on self-care and disease prevention is provided.
- Appropriate health and disease prevention services for the population served are documented.

American Accreditation Healthcare Commission/Utilization Review Accreditation Commission

The American Accreditation Healthcare Commission/URAC was established in 1990. The URAC accredits utilization review organizations, both freestanding and within managed care organizations. The URAC focuses on the policies and procedures of utilization review and is

TABLE 7-1	*Selected Measurement Initiatives*		
CATEGORY	**TITLE**	**QUALITY INDICATORS**	**WEB SITE**
Health system	Joint Commission on Accreditation of Healthcare Organizations	Performance measures in five core areas: 1. Acute myocardial infarction 2. Community acquired pneumonia 3. Pregnancy and related conditions 4. Heart failure 5. Surgical procedures and complications	www.jcaho.org
Hospital	Maryland Hospital Association	Indicators in four core areas: 1. Acute care 2. Psychiatry care 3. Long-term care 4. Home care	www.qiproject.org
Nursing	American Nurses Association	Quality report card initiative: 1. Mix of RNs, LPNs, and unlicensed staff 2. Total nursing care hours/pt day 3. Pressure ulcers 4. Patient falls 5. Patient satisfaction w/pain management 6. Patient satisfaction w/educational information 7. Patient satisfaction w/overall care 8. Patient satisfaction w/nursing care 9. Nosocomial infection rate 10. Nurse staff satisfaction	www.nursingworld.org

an operational requirement in certain states. It strives to improve quality by evaluating network participation and management standards; quality, utilization, and provider credentialing standards; member protection and participation; confidentiality of patient information; and marketing and sales standards within the managed care organization. The URAC has developed a unique area of focus in their standards to prevent misrepresentation of benefits. Networks must inform plan members of exclusions, limitations, benefit reductions, utilization management requirements, provider networks, and satisfaction statistics (McGuire, 1996; Graham, 1996).

All three of the accrediting bodies share a strong bond requiring quality improvement to achieve accreditation. Although the programs have unique features, they share many of the same objectives and standards (Berger, 1996). Beyond managed care accreditation, there are quality initiatives and outcomes measurement activities for health care organizations across the continuum of care. See Table 7-1 for examples of measurement initiatives.

NURSING'S CONTRIBUTION TO HEALTH CARE DELIVERY

Changes in the health care delivery system are aimed at reducing costs of health care and utilization of services and improving access to providers and quality of services. In addition, changing demographics have affected health care, with the aging of the baby boomers and the paradigm shifts of illness care to wellness promotion and acute hospital care to community primary care. These changes have affected nursing dramatically. With globalization of health care has come an increased need for nurses with specialized training and advanced education. In response, nursing research has produced valuable insights into the practice domain, and nursing education has produced an increasing number of nurses with advanced practice degrees and specialties in various clinical areas.

The overwhelming national movement in health care is toward health promotion, maintenance and prevention, and wellness. Nursing is poised to provide this service. "The Registered Nurse is the only health care professional who is specifically educated to: (1) assess the patient to determine health status and risks, unhealthy lifestyles, minor health problems, and health education needs of patients and families; (2) provide support and reassurance while caring for patients with current or potential health problems; and (3) advocate for primary and preventive care services" (ANA, 1995).

Nursing Roles in Managed Care Settings

Utilization Management. In current managed care settings, utilization management positions for nurses directly influence health care delivery. Utilization management nurses employed by managed care organizations evaluate treatment options to determine medical necessity and appropriateness of treatment settings without sacrificing quality in health care outcomes. The nurse in preservice review analyzes the proposed health care service, whether it is an inpatient hospitalization, outpatient procedure, ambulatory surgery, or same-day surgical admission. This analysis includes comparison with standard written screening criteria that contain rigorous utilization data. Medical criteria are based on professional standards of care and nationally recognized guidelines. If the first level reviewer (nurse) questions the medical necessity or appropriateness of a planned service, the second level reviewer, a physician, is consulted for expertise and decision making. After preservice review the nurse assesses the hospital stay to determine if the need exists for continued inpatient service delivery. The intent of this concurrent review is to determine medical necessity and appropriateness of the setting for the services ordered or anticipated. Nurses in this role have a direct impact on the quality of care received by the patient.

Quality Management. Quality management nurses are instrumental in programs that support health promotion and disease management. They develop health promotion programs and may provide services within the program. They evaluate and document the results of ongoing programs to improve the quality of health care delivery. Quality management nurses also often have responsibilities for maintenance of accreditation standards for the managed care organization.

Case Management. Case management is an area of nursing practice garnering a great deal of interest and potential for continued growth. A nurse case manager is responsible for following a selected patient through the continuum of care with a goal of maximizing appropriate care and cost efficiency. A rationale for case management is to decrease fragmentation of services to enhance the patient's quality of life and to contain costs. Case management includes discharge planning and appropriate use of home health services and medical equipment. Case management often is directed at high-cost cases or chronic or catastrophic situations. The nurse case manager explores alternative health care settings and, when appropriate, makes recommendations for alternative care instead of traditional inpatient hospitalization. Disease management programs that target patients with selected conditions for intensive education, risk assessment, and case management help to control utilization of health care services and costs. For example, programs that target patients with a diagnosis of congestive heart failure provide intensive education related to diet and medications, as well as frequent nursing assessments. These programs have been demonstrated to greatly reduce the number of hospital readmissions and therefore costs. Case management is further discussed in Chapter 19.

Primary Care Provider. A patient's first point of contact in the community setting with the health care system is called primary care. Advanced practice nurses such as nurse practitioners function in this growing collaborative health care role of primary care provider and are supported by state laws that extend practice privileges and prescriptive authority for nurses meeting specific qualifications. Nurse practitioners are responsible for identifying and managing health care problems and referring specialized problems to appropriate resources. Advanced practice nurses function in many health care areas, including mental health and family, pediatric, and geriatric care. Although the original goal was to place these skilled nurse practitioners in economically underserved areas, nurse practitioners also are available and working successfully in settings that are not underserved.

SUMMARY

As managed care helps shape the future of health care in the United States, many believe that a majority of hospitals and insurers will move to for-profit status, the majority of Americans will be covered by some form of managed care, and all parties will be striving to allocate resources in the best care scenario for the growing aging population. The continuum of health care will include long-term care as a necessity. The most important site for care will move from the hospital to the home. The drive for medical data will be commonplace; data from all avenues will be provided on-line. The next generation of health care includes health plan administrators, providers, patients, and payers as partners in developing incentives and risk-sharing arrangements designed to achieve health care objectives. The future includes managed care companies and payers reinvesting the savings gained from utilization management activities designed to improve the overall health of patients and to contain health care costs over the long term.

Policy experts recommend that any future health care system needs to include universal health care access, a transdisciplinary team approach to preventive health, emphasis on quality of care outcomes, standardized data, advanced technology incorporated into medical practice, and encouragement of educational and research efforts (Currents, 1997b). Nursing will play a pivotal role in this new system of health care delivery.

Critical Thinking Activities

1. As the health care delivery system changes, studies have identified consumers' worries about the future. Identify three issues that are propelling change in health care delivery.
2. How are clinical services in the acute and postacute care settings changing as the health care system reorganizes?

3. What are the positive features of managed health care?
4. Contrast the differences among HMO, PPO, and POS health plans.
5. How have roles in nursing such as case management and nurse practitioner responded to the needs of a changing health care delivery system?

REFERENCES

AAHP Report: Managed Care Debate: Correcting the Errors and Omissions 1998, www.aahp.org.

American Hospital Association, Picker Institute: *Eye on patients: report to the American public,* Chicago, 1997, American Hospital Publishing Co.

American Nurses Association: *Nursing facts,* Washington, DC, 1995, ANA.

Barents Group: *Characteristics of health plan choices available to employees through employer-based health benefits,* KPMG Peat Marwick LLP, 1996, American Hospital Association.

Berger D: Playing the accreditation game: strategies for networks, *Health Care Innovations* 62(2):8, 1996.

Currents: *Hosp Health Care Networks* 71(9):10-16, 1997a.

Currents: *Hosp Health Care Networks* 71(7):16-36, 1997b.

EBRI: Mathew Greenwald and Associates and Employee Benefit Research Institute: *Health confidence survey,* Washington, DC, 1999, www.ebri.org.

Edlin M: Define your health plans' value with reporting, *Health Manage Technol* 17(8):11, 1996.

Feldstein P, Wickizer T, Wheeler J: The effects of utilization review programs on health care use and expenditures, *N Engl J Med* 318(20):1310, 1988.

Graham J: *The rise of the healthcare consumer,* Montvale, NJ, 1996, Business and Health.

Haugh R: Back to basics, *Hosp Health Networks* 75(1):33-35, 2001.

Health US 2000, National Center for Health Statistics, Hyattsville, Md, www.cdc.gov/nchs/.

Institute for the Future: *Health and health care 2010: the forecast, the challenge,* Princeton, NJ, 2000, Jossey-Bass.

Japson B, Scott L: System growth a close race, *Mod Healthcare* 27(21):51-68, 1997.

Kertesz L: But managed care savings will grow—study, *Mod Healthcare* 21(23):8, 1997.

Managed Care Digest, Kansas City, 1999, Aventis Pharmaceuticals, www.managedcaredigest.com.

McGuire D: Study: media reports of renewed healthcare inflation premature, *Managed Care Outlook* 10(13):1-5, 1997.

McGuire D: NCQA unveils draft version, *Managed Care Outlook* 9(15):1996.

Mera C: Consumerism and health care quality, *J Cost Qual* 6(1):27-30, 2000, www.cost-quality.com.

Meyer H: Home health on the high wire, *Hospitals* 71(14):26, 1997.

Pallarito K, Morrissey J: The future, *Mod Healthcare* 26(35): 932, 1996.

Rauber C: Home health: light at the end of the tunnel? *Healthcare Business,* 2000, www.healthcarebusiness.com.

Rubin B et al: Tracking the system: American health care: report of the Lewin Group for the National Committee for Quality Healthcare, 1998, www.lewin.com.

Scott L: A vendor's guide to six managed care trends, *Medical Interface* 10(2):111-114, February 1997.

Sheils J: Health coverage 2000: cost and coverage analysis of eight proposals to expand health insurance coverage: report of the Lewin Group, www.lewin.com.

Staff: Data watch, *Business Health* 15(8):60, 1997.

Stano M: An alternative framework for evaluating the efficiency of managed care, *Am J Managed Care* 2(6):639, 1996.

Terry K: Disease management, *Business Health* 13(4):65, 1995.

Wennberg J, Gittelsohn A: Variations in medical care among small areas, *Scientific Am* 246(4):120, 1982.

Winslow R: Performance of HMO's is rated higher than fee for service plans in study, *Wall Street J* B7, June 23, 1994.

Legal Issues in Nursing and Health Care

Laura R. Mahlmeister, PhD, RN

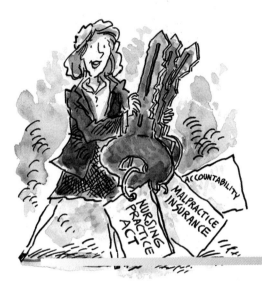

Knowledge of the law enhances
the nurse's ability to provide safe
and effective care.

Vignette

Mary Clark is a registered nurse (RN) employed in the Emergency Department of a large for-profit hospital. The facility treats clients who are privately insured and individuals with Medicare coverage. Nurse Clark is the assigned triage nurse when Mr. Jones, a 48-year-old man, walks in for evaluation. He states that he has persistent, mild substernal pain that is now radiating laterally toward both shoulders. His skin is pink and dry, and he does not appear to be in obvious distress. He reports eating half of a garlic pizza and drinking three beers 1 hour ago. "I'm pretty sure it's just indigestion. This happened before when I ate garlic." He also tells the nurse, "I know I'm supposed to go to Community Hospital; I have 'Feel-Well' insurance, but I'm miserable and don't want to drive 10 miles across town in rush hour traffic with this much pain."

Mr. Jones is enrolled in a health maintenance organization (HMO) "Feel-Well." The HMO may not reimburse the for-profit hospital for Mr. Jones' visit if it is determined that his condition was not a true emergency after review by the HMO's utilization review department. In that case, Mr. Jones will have to pay out-of-pocket for the medical evaluation and care received in the Emergency Department. In this cost-conscious health care environment, the nurses in the Emergency Department are well aware of the financial losses the hospital has recently suffered as a result of unpaid emergency services. Nurses in this facility are expected to contribute to the facility's success in reducing operating costs.

Questions to consider while reading this chapter

1. What is Nurse Clark's legal duty in this situation?
2. What legal principles underlie the nurse's obligations to the patient?
3. What laws, if any, would govern the nurse's decision-making process in this case?
4. If Mr. Jones is not evaluated or treated and suffers a myocardial infarction while driving to Community Hospital, who would be legally accountable for his injuries?
   a. The nurse?
   b. The for-profit hospital?
   c. The HMO that may not have reimbursed for services?

Key Terms

Accountability Being responsible for one's actions; a sense of duty in performing nursing tasks and activities.

Adverse event An injury caused by medical management rather than the patient's underlying condition. An adverse event attributable to error is a preventable adverse event.

Case law Body of written opinions created by judges in federal and state appellate cases; also known as judge-made law and common law.

Civil law A category of law (Tort Law) that deals with conduct considered unacceptable. It is based on societal expectations regarding interpersonal conduct. Common causes of civil litigation include professional malpractice, negligence, and assault and battery.

Common law Law that is created through the decision of judges as opposed to laws enacted by legislative bodies (i.e., Congress).

Comparative negligence A type of liability in which damages may be apportioned among two or more defendants in a malpractice case. The extent of liability depends on the defendant's relative contribution to the patient's injury.

Criminal negligence Negligence that indicates "reckless and wanton" disregard for the safety, well-being, or life of an individual; behavior that demonstrates a complete disregard for another, such that death is likely.

Damages Monetary compensation the court orders paid to a person who has sustained a loss or injury to his or her person or property through the misconduct (intentional or unintentional) of another.

Defendant The individual who is named in a person's (plaintiff's) complaint as responsible for an injury; the person who the plaintiff claims committed a negligent act or malpractice.

Durable power of attorney for health care An instrument that authorizes another person to act as one's agent in decisions regarding health care if the person becomes incompetent to make his or her own decisions.

Error A failure of a planned action to be completed as intended, or the use of a wrong plan to achieve a specific aim.

Immunity Legal doctrine by which a person is protected from a lawsuit for negligent acts or an institution is protected from a suit for the negligent acts of its employees.

Liability Being legally responsible for harm caused to another person or property as a result of one's actions; compensation for harm normally is paid in monetary damages.

Licensing laws Laws that establish the qualifications for obtaining and maintaining a license to perform particular services. Persons and institutions may be required to obtain a license to provide particular health care services.

Malpractice Failure of a professional to meet the standard of conduct that a reasonable and prudent member of his or her profession would exercise in similar circumstances that results in harm. The professional's misconduct is unintentional.

Negligence Failure to act in a manner that an ordinary, prudent person (either lay person or professional) would act in similar circumstances that results in harm. The failure to act in a reasonable and prudent manner is unintentional.

Plaintiff The complaining person in a lawsuit; the person who claims he or she was injured by the acts of another.

Res ipsa loquitur Legal doctrine applicable to cases in which the provider (i.e., the physician) had exclusive control of events that resulted in the patient's injury; the injury would not have occurred ordinarily without a negligent act; derived from a Latin phrase, "the thing speaks for itself."

Respondent superior Legal doctrine that holds an employer indirectly responsible for the negligent acts of employees carried out within the scope of employment; derived from a Latin phrase, "let the master answer."

Risk management Process of identifying, analyzing, and controlling risks posed to patients; involves human factor and incident analysis, changes in systems operations, and loss control and prevention.

Standard of care In civil cases the legal criteria against which the nurse's (and physician's) conduct is compared to determine if a negligent act or malpractice occurred; commonly defined as the knowledge and skill that an ordinary, reasonably prudent person would possess and exercise in the same or similar circumstances.

Statute or statutory law Law enacted by a legislative body; separate from judge-made or common law.

Tort Civil wrong or injury committed by one person against another person or a property. There are two types of torts—intentional and unintentional.

Vicarious liability Legal doctrine in which a person or institution is liable for the negligent acts of another because of a special relationship between the two parties; a substituted liability.

Learning Outcomes

After studying this chapter, the reader will be able to:

1. Differentiate among the three major categories of law on which nursing practice is established and governed.
2. Analyze the relationship between accountability and liability for one's actions in professional nursing practice.
3. Outline the essential elements that must be substantiated to prove a claim of negligence or malpractice.
4. Differentiate between intentional and unintentional torts in relation to nursing practice.
5. Incorporate fundamental laws and statutory regulations that establish the patient's right to self-determination in the health care setting.

CHAPTER OVERVIEW

The preceding vignette highlighted a growing clinical dilemma that nurses face in the complex, ever-changing health care system. Financial considerations may conflict with clinical concerns for patient well-being. In an increasingly complex health care environment, the nurse's ability to make appropriate decisions about the provision of patient care services is facilitated by a sound knowledge of the laws governing practice. In the case of Mr. Jones, triage, evaluation, and treatment are governed by federal law known as the Emergency Medical Treatment and Active Labor Act (EMTALA) (COBRA, 42 U.S.C. 1395dd). There also may be a specific state law regarding essential care and transport of patients in Emergency Departments. Lastly, sections of the Nursing Practice Act delineating professional conduct for the registered nurse (RN) also would assist Nurse Clark in managing this clinical problem. Financial concerns become a secondary consideration for the nurse with this baseline knowledge of the law.

Each nurse must be able to articulate his or her professional duty to the patient or client under the law and to recognize legal risks in practice. Knowledge of the law enhances the nurse's ability to provide safe and effective care in all settings. This chapter examines legal aspects of nursing practice. The concepts of law, professional accountability, legal liability, negligence, malpractice, and criminal offense are defined. Specific laws or statutes governing nursing practice are also reviewed. The reader is introduced to current, relevant information about case law, also known as common law or judge-made law, as it applies to professional nursing practice. Patients' rights are explored within the context of law and court opinions. Finally, the Institute of Medicine report on medical errors is discussed, and specific strategies to reduce errors and legal risk are elaborated.

SOURCES OF LAW AND NURSING PRACTICE

The actions of all individuals are regulated through two systems of principles known as laws and ethics. Laws enforce a minimum level of conduct by imposing penalties for violations of acceptable behavior (Rhodes, 1994). Laws are expressed in terms of "must" and "shall" and are based on a society's interest in prohibiting or controlling certain behaviors. Ethics are described in terms of "should" and "may" and address beliefs about appropriate behaviors within a societal context (Lagana, 2000). Chapter 9 presents an in-depth discussion about nursing ethics. Professional nursing conduct also is regulated by a variety of laws. There are two major sources of law:

- ■ Statutory law
- ■ Common law

The standards for professional nursing practice are in great part derived from both statutory and common law. The following section of the chapter deals with statutory law and describe how it governs and indirectly influences nursing practice.

STATUTORY LAW

Laws that are written by legislative bodies such as Congress or state legislatures are enacted as statutes. The terms law and statute will be used interchangeably in this chapter. The aforementioned EMTALA is an example of a federal statute. Violation of law is a criminal offense against the general public and is prosecuted by government authorities. Crimes are punishable by fines or imprisonment. The list of federal and state statutes that govern nursing practice has multiplied over the past 25 years. Nurses at all levels of practice must develop a greater depth and breadth of knowledge about laws related to professional practice, their specific practice setting (i.e., the Emergency Department in the case of EMTALA), and health care systems in general. Ignorance of the law is never a defense when the nurse violates a health care statute. A nurse who violates the law is subject to penalties, including monetary fines, suspension or revocation of his or her license, and even imprisonment in some instances (*Nurse's Legal Handbook*, 2000).

Federal Statutes

As I travel across the United States speaking with nurses about the rapid and often daunting changes in health care, a common question raised is, "Isn't there a law prohibiting this—reduction in RN staff? floating? the use of nurse aides in this patient care situation?" Nursing staffing is influenced to some degree by federal (and state) laws. For instance, in 1999 California became the first state to enact a law (California Assembly Bill 394) that mandates the establishment of minimum nurse-patient ratios in acute care facilities (Schreiber, 2000). The projected nursing shortage may prompt other states to follow suit. Federal laws also have a major impact on nursing practice, mandating a minimum standard of care in all settings that receive federal funds (i.e., reimbursement for treatment of Medicare patients).

Unfortunately, most nurses are unfamiliar with health care law and rely on authorities in their employment setting to know what is legal and therefore permissible. Automatically deferring to administrators or nurse managers about the legality of a particular issue is no longer acceptable behavior for the professional nurse. Each RN must take accountability for knowing the law and understanding how it relates to patient care and nursing practice. When concerns about work-related issues arise (e.g., a change in scope of practice for unlicensed staff or a reduction in RN staffing), the first question the nurse should ask and answer must be: "Is this legal?" (Mahlmeister, 1996).

Three federal statutes that nurses must be familiar with and have a clear understanding of are discussed. This list is not comprehensive, but it includes examples of federal law that directly impact nursing practice. Many federal laws are relevant to specific health care settings (i.e., mental health, Emergency Departments, maternity settings). When nurses are knowledgeable about the federal laws applicable to their area of practice, they will be able to more effectively advocate for patients in that setting.

Emergency Medical Treatment and Active Labor Law (COBRA, 42 U.S.C. 1395dd). This federal statute, often referred to as the "anti-dumping" law, was enacted in 1986 to prohibit the refusal of care for indigent and uninsured patients seeking medical assistance in the Emergency Department (Moy, 1999). This law also prohibits the transfer of unstable patients, including women in labor, from one facility to another. The law states:

- All persons presenting for care must receive the same medical screening examination and be stabilized, regardless of their financial status or insurance coverage, before discharge or transfer.

The Emergency Medical Treatment and Active Labor Law (EMTALA) is applicable to people presenting to non–Emergency Department settings such as urgent care clinics. It even governs the transfer of patients from an inpatient setting to a lower level of care in some parts of the United States (Roberts v. Galen of Virginia, Inc., 1997). Significant penalties can be levied against a facility that violates the EMTALA, including a $50,000 fine (not covered by liability insurance). The federal government also can revoke the facility's Medicare contract, and this could result in a major loss of revenue for the institution or even insolvency. Many legitimate concerns that nurses have about the discharge or transfer of patients could be promptly addressed if the nurse had a solid understanding of the EMTALA. This is not a daunting task. Nursing journals have published many articles about the EMTALA and the nurse's role in upholding this statute (Snyder, 1999; Casaubon and Sparks, 2000).

Americans With Disabilities Act of 1990 (Public Law No. 101-336), 42 U.S.C. Section 12101. The intent of this law is to end discrimination against qualified persons with disabilities by removing barriers that prevent them from enjoying the same opportunities available to persons without disabilities. Recent court cases have established that, as a place of public accommodation, a health care facility must provide reasonable accommodation to patients (and family members) with sensory disabilities such as vision and hearing impairment (Negron v. Snoqualmie Valley Hospital, 1997, and Aikins v. St. Helena Hospital, 1994).

This statute has relevance for all nurses. As patient advocates, nurses have a legal and ethical duty to provide appropriate patient and family education and to support the process of informed consent. The health care facility must have a policy that defines how it will meet the client's needs for education and information when there are vision or hearing disabilities. The policy also must delineate how the nurse can obtain translators and special types of equipment needed to facilitate communication.

Patient Self-Determination Act of 1990; Omnibus Budget Reconciliation Act of 1990 (Public Law No. 101-508, Sections 4206 and 4751). This federal statute is a Medicare/Medicaid amendment intended to support individuals in expressing their preferences about medical treatment and making decisions about end-of-life care. The law requires that all federally funded hospitals:

- Inform adult patients, in writing, about their right under state law to make treatment choices. These choices include collaborating with the physician in formulating "do not resuscitate" (DNR) orders.
- Ask patients if they either have prepared a "living will" or have executed a "durable power of attorney" for health care.

The law provides guidance to nurses who often are in the best position to discuss these issues with the patient (e.g., while completing a comprehensive admission assessment). (Legal considerations related to living wills, durable power of attorney, and DNR orders are discussed in the last section of this chapter.)

Health Insurance Portability and Accountability Act of 1996 (Public Law No. 104-191). The intent of this law is to ensure confidentiality of the patient's medical records. The introduction of electronic medical records has provided additional impetus for introduction of this legislation. The statute sets guidelines for maintaining the privacy of health data. Legitimate concerns regarding the uses of and release of medical information, particularly to private entities such as insurance companies, led to the passage of this law. It provides explicit guidelines for nurses who are in a position to release health information. To maintain confidentiality of the medical record and privacy of patients' health data, all nurses must have a basic understanding of the new rules and regulations that went into effect in 2001.

State Statutes

In addition to federal laws, nursing practice is governed by state laws that delineate the conduct of licensed nurses and define behaviors of all health care professionals in promoting public health and welfare.

| BOX 8-1 | *Common Elements Contained in Nursing Practice Acts* |

Definition of nursing
State of Nebraska: Statutes Related to Nursing
71-1,132.05. Nursing; terms, defined
The practice of nursing means the performance for compensation or gratuitously of any act expressing judgment or skill based on a systematized body of nursing knowledge. Such acts include the identification of and intervention in actual or potential health problems of individuals, families, or groups, which acts are directed toward maintaining health status, preventing illness, injury, or infirmity, improving health status, and providing care supportive to or restorative of life and well-being through nursing assessment and through the execution of nursing care and of diagnostic or therapeutic regimens prescribed by any person lawfully authorized to prescribe.

Standards of competent performance
California Code of Regulations: Title 16. Division 14. Board of Registered Nursing
California Nursing Practice Act Section 1443.5
A registered nurse shall be considered to be competent when he/she consistently demonstrates the ability to transfer scientific knowledge from social, biological, and physical sciences in applying the nursing process as follows:
1. Formulates a nursing diagnosis through observation of the client's physical condition and behavior and through interpretation of information obtained from the client and others, including the health team
2. Formulates a care plan, in collaboration with the client, that ensures that direct and indirect nursing care services provide for the client's safety, comfort, hygiene, and protection and for disease prevention and restorative measure
3. Performs skills essential to the kind of nursing action to be taken, explains the health treatment to the client and family, and teaches the client and family how to care for the client's health needs
4. Delegates tasks to subordinates based on the legal scopes of practice of the subordinates and on the preparation and capability needed in the tasks to be delegated, and effectively supervises nursing care being given by subordinates
5. Evaluates the effectiveness of the care plan through observation of the client's physical condition and behavior, signs, and symptoms of illness, and reactions to treatment and through communication with the client and health team members, and modifies the plan as needed
6. Acts as the client's advocate, as circumstances require, by initiating action to improve health care or to change decisions or activities that are against the interests or wishes of the client, and by giving the client the opportunity to make informed decisions about health care before it is provided

State Nursing Practice Act and Board of Nursing Rules and Regulations. One of the most important state laws governing nursing practice is the Nursing Practice Act. This law was enacted to define the scope and limitations of professional nursing practice. The aim of regulating practice in this manner is to protect the public and make the individual nurse accountable for his or her actions (Booth and Carruth, 1998). State legislatures authorize the nurses' licensing board to promulgate administrative rules and regulations necessary to implement the Nursing Practice Act. Once these administrative rules and regulations are formally adopted, they have the same force and effect as any other law (*Nurse's Legal Handbook,* 2000).

Although nursing practice acts vary from state to state, they usually contain the following information:
- Definition of the term *registered nurse*
- Description of professional nursing functions

BOX 8-1	*Common Elements Contained in Nursing Practice Acts—cont'd*

Grounds for disciplinary action
Texas Nursing Practice Act: Article 4525, Section (b)
The board may take disciplinary action against a registered nurse for any of the following reasons:
1. Violation of the Nursing Practice Act or Board of Nurse Examiners Rules
2. Fraud or deceit in procuring or attempting to procure a license to practice professional nursing
3. Conviction of a crime of the grade of felony, or a crime of lesser grade that involves moral turpitude or any conduct resulting in the revocation of probation pursuant to such conviction
4. Use of any nursing license, certificate, diploma, or permit, or transcript of such license, certificate, diploma, or permit that has been fraudulently purchased, issued, counterfeited, or materially altered
5. The impersonation of, or acting as a proxy for, another in any examination required by law to obtain a license to practice professional nursing
6. Aiding or abetting, directly or indirectly, or in any manner whatsoever, any unlicensed person in connection with the authorized practice of professional nursing
7. Revocation, suspension, or denial of or any other action relating to the license to practice nursing in another jurisdiction
8. Intemperate use of alcohol or drugs that the board determines endangers or could endanger patients
9. Unprofessional or dishonorable conduct which, in the opinion of the board, is likely to deceive, defraud, or injure patients or the public
10. Mental incompetency
11. Lack of fitness to practice by reason of mental or physical health that could result in injury to patients or the public
12. Failure to care adequately for patients or to conform to the minimum standards of acceptable professional nursing practice

- Standards of competent performance
- Behaviors that represent misconduct or prohibited practices
- Grounds for disciplinary action
- Fines and penalties the licensing board may levy when the Nursing Practice Act is violated

Box 8-1 provides excerpts from three separate state nursing practice acts to illustrate how the Nursing Practice Act defines the scope of practice for nurses.

Surprisingly, many nurses are not even aware that the Nursing Practice Act is a law, and they unknowingly violate aspects of this statute. They are not familiar with the administrative rules and regulations enacted by the licensing board. This is an unfortunate lapse because these administrative rules and regulations answer crucial questions that nurses have about the day-to-day aspects of practice and unusual occurrences. For example, rules promulgated by the Ohio Board of Nursing include the following section:

> At all times when a licensed nurse is providing direct nursing care to a client within the scope of the licensed nurse's practice as set forth in [the law] Section 4723.02 of the Revised Code, the licensed nurse shall display and identify applicable licensure as a registered nurse or as a licensed practical nurse (Ohio Administrative Code, Section 4723-4-03, (H), 1996).

An RN in Ohio who does not wear an identification badge that clearly displays his or her status as an "RN" is in violation of the law. In this era of health care redesign, knowledge of this administrative rule would be essential because many health care systems are attempting to remove the licensure status of health care professionals from identification badges. In these latter settings all workers (even nurses and physicians) are identified by a generic title such as "patient care team member." An increasing number of licensing boards are considering amending administrative rules to require that the nurse's licensure status (RN, licensed practical nurse [LPN], or licensed vocational nurse [LVN]) be clearly displayed on the worker's identification badge.

Each nurse should own a current copy of the Nursing Practice Act and the licensing board's administrative rules and regulations. The dramatic changes occurring in health care often lead to uncertainty among nurses about which functions constitute the exclusive practice of registered nursing and which patient care tasks may be lawfully delegated to LPNs, LVNs, or unlicensed assistive personnel. The Nursing Practice Act and licensing board rules and regulations provide essential information that clarify these important questions.

The Nursing Practice Act broadly defines the practice of registered nursing in accordance with nursing's rapidly evolving functions. In recent years, with the expansion of basic nursing functions and the development of advanced nursing practice, many states have revised their nursing practice acts (Weiss, 1995). Licensing boards also have been authorized in some states to provide guidelines for the development of "standardized procedures." Standardized procedures are a legal means by which RNs may expand their practice into areas traditionally considered to be within the realm of medicine. The standardized procedure actually is developed within the facility where the expanded nursing functions have been approved. It is developed in collaboration with nursing, medicine, and administration. An example of a standardized procedure would be a written protocol authorizing a nurse to implement a peripherally inserted venous catheter for patients in the neonatal intensive care unit.

Violations of the Nursing Practice Act. State legislatures have given licensing boards the authority to hear and decide administrative cases against nurses when there is an alleged violation of the Nursing Practice Act or the nursing board's rules and regulations. Nurses who violate the Nursing Practice Act or board's administrative rules and regulations are subject to disciplinary action by the board. Research indicates that there has been an increase in the number of consumer complaints to licensing boards related to nursing misconduct (Malugani, 2000) Table 8-1 provides a synopsis of the licensing board proceedings when a complaint is made about a nurse. Box 8-2 presents the more common grounds for disciplinary action by state boards of nursing. Penalties that licensing boards may impose for violation of the Nursing Practice Act include:

- Issuing a formal reprimand
- Establishing a period of probation
- Levying fines
- Limiting, suspending, or revoking the nurse's license

An estimated 7% of the 1.9 million RNs in the United States are chemically dependent (Bernzweig, 1996). The majority of disciplinary actions by licensing boards are related to misconduct resulting from chemical impairment, including the misappropriation of drugs for personal use and the sale of drugs and drug paraphernalia to support the nurse's addiction. When the nurse's license is limited or suspended because of problems related to chemical

TABLE 8-1	*Licensing Board Procedure When a Complaint Is Filed*
ACTION	**CONSEQUENCE**
Complaint is made (initial complaint may be lodged as a telephone call or letter mailed to the licensing board)	Sworn complaints must be filed
Consumer (patient or family member)	
Nurse's employer or nurse manager	
Professional nursing organization	
State authority (i.e., Centers for Medicare and Medicaid Services [CMS], formerly the Health Care Financing Administration [HCFA])	
Licensing board reviews complaint	Determination made by board
Examines evidence	Insufficient evidence to proceed
	Administrative review is scheduled
	Nurse is notified
	Rules of proceeding explained
	Witnesses called to testify
	Evidence is examined
Licensing board makes decision	
Nurse exonerated	Case closed
Nurse guilty of violating Nursing Practice Act	Disciplinary action
	Board issues formal reprimand
	Nurse placed on probation
	Nurse's license is not renewed
	Fines levied against nurse
	Nurse's license is suspended or revoked
Nurse may challenge licensing board decision	Nurse must file appeal in court
Court reviews case (court action dependent on jurisdiction)	
Reviews licensing board ruling and conduct of proceedings	Licensing board ruling reversed
	Licensing board can appeal ruling
or	*or*
Court reviews case	Licensing board ruling is upheld
Case scheduled for trial	Licensing board ruling overturned
	Board may appeal case to higher court
	or
	Licensing board ruling is upheld
	Nurse may appeal to a higher court

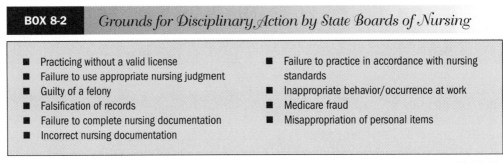

Adapted from Booth D, Carruth A: Violations of the nursing practice act: implications for nurse managers, *Nurs Manage* 29(10):35-40, 1998.

impairment, the ability to practice in the future often is predicated on successful completion of a drug rehabilitation program and evidence of abstinence. An increasing number of state licensing boards have established programs to guide nurses through the process of rehabilitation to reestablish licensure. Booth and Carruth have identified other grounds for disciplinary action in their study of Louisiana State Board of Nursing disciplinary actions for violation of the Nursing Practice Act (1998).

Reporting Statutes

In 1973 the United States Congress enacted the Child Abuse Prevention and Treatment Act. The law mandated all states to meet specific uniform guidelines to qualify for federal funding of child abuse programs. All 50 states and the District of Columbia now have created laws that mandate reporting of specific health problems and the suspected or confirmed abuse of vulnerable individuals in society. Nurses often are explicitly named within the context of these statutes as one of the groups of designated health professionals who must report the specified problems under penalty of fine or imprisonment. The following are reportable in all states:

- Infant and child abuse
- Dependent elder abuse
- Specified communicable diseases (for example, bubonic plague)

An increasing number of states also require a report of suspected or confirmed domestic violence. For example, a California law (Assembly Bill 890) enacted in 1995 requires nurses and other health care workers to recognize and report symptoms of domestic violence to local law enforcement authorities or face a misdemeanor charge.

The nurse must be familiar with these state-specific reporting statutes as they apply to his or her practice setting. For example, pediatric nurses must have in-depth knowledge regarding child abuse reporting laws. Agency policies and procedures in the nurse's work setting may provide guidance regarding reporting duties. If information is not available within the institution, the nurse may consult with the State Department of Health or the state nurses' licensing board for guidance in obtaining these reporting statutes.

Nurses need not fear legal reprisal from individuals or families who are reported to authorities in suspected cases of abuse. Most legislatures have granted immunity from suit within the context of the mandatory reporting statute. A recent court decision upheld this doctrine of immunity. In the case Heinrich v. Conemaugh Valley Memorial Hospital (1994), the family of an injured child initiated a lawsuit against a hospital that reported suspected child abuse after a state investigation found them innocent of the charge. The court ruled that the hospital and the physician who made the report in "good faith" were immune from litigation under a Pennsylvania Child Protective Service Law that required reports of suspected child abuse.

Institutional Licensing Laws

All facilities (i.e., hospitals, nursing homes, rehabilitation centers) providing health care services must comply with licensing laws promulgated by state legislatures. These laws are created to protect the public and ensure the safe and effective provision of health care services. Specific language usually is contained within health facility licensing statutes regarding the following:

- Minimum standards for the maintenance of the physical plant
- Basic operational aspects of major departments (nursing, dietary, clinical laboratories, and pharmacy)
- Essential aspects of patient rights and the informed consent process

Many state licensing laws mandate minimum levels of education, experience, or credentialing for department administrators such as nurses, anesthesia personnel, pediatricians, and obstetricians. Several states also require minimum nurse-patient ratios in critical care units and other specialty departments such as the operating room, nursery, or Emergency Department.

Health care restructuring and redesign have led to many changes in the way health care services are provided and the settings in which care is rendered. Not all change has been positive, and some redesign schemes have resulted in adverse outcomes for patients. Investigations by state authorities on report of patient injuries or death have discovered that in some cases health facilities have operated in violation of existing licensing laws (Hytha, 1997). In the past, direct-care RNs generally could rely on their nurse managers to have a comprehensive knowledge of health facility licensing law and to create policies and procedures that implement and enforce applicable aspects of the law. The trend toward flattened management and reduction in staff development personnel has altered this picture. In an increasing number of settings, nurse managers have been replaced with nonnurse administrators who may have minimal knowledge of the health facilities licensing laws.

In light of these changes, direct-care nurses should have a working knowledge of current licensing laws as they relate to nursing care and patient care services. I have found that nurses who have serious questions regarding quality of care in their employment setting have been able to resolve these concerns once they have read applicable sections of the health facility licensing law relevant to their setting. Bringing the pertinent section of the law to the attention of managers, administrators, or the risk management department often is the most effective strategy to resolve problems. In settings in which nurses are represented by union contracts, potential violations of health facility licensing laws may be most effectively addressed through union representatives (Mahlmeister, 2000a).

Nurses can obtain a copy of the health facilities licensing law for their employment setting through the State Department of Health or Public Health, Division of Licensing and Certification. Other states provide the statute and address questions through the Department of Health, Division of Facilities Regulations or Division of Health Facilities Inspection or Division of Health Quality Assurance. The telephone number for this agency can be found in the white pages of the local telephone directory under the heading "State of (for example,

Michigan)." Nurses also may call their licensing board or the state nursing association for guidance in reaching the appropriate authority to obtain a copy of the licensing law and to speak to a consultant about concerns.

COMMON LAW

In addition to statutory law, nursing practice is guided by common law, also known as decisional or judge-made law. Common law is created through cases heard and decided in federal and state appellate courts. Throughout the years judge-made law regarding nursing practice has accumulated in the form of written opinions. These opinions eventually contribute to the expected standard of nursing conduct (Trandel-Korenchuk and Trandel-Korenchuk, 1997). The body of written opinions about nurses also is known as nursing case law. The importance of nursing case law in establishing the current standard of practice cannot be overstated.

One of the most important cases to establish the expected conduct of nurses was Utter v. United Hospital Center, Inc. (1977). This West Virginia case affirmed that nurses were required to exercise independent judgments to prevent harm when caring for patients. Before the 1970s the issue of whether nurses were licensed professionals who made independent judgments was not clearly established. In the Utter case a patient whose arm was casted had signs and symptoms of compartment syndrome. The affected limb became progressively more edematous and eventually turned black. The nurses failed to activate the chain of command when the primary providers did not respond to their reports and requests for medical reevaluation. The patient's arm eventually had to be amputated. The court wrote:

> Nurses are specialists in hospital care who, in the final analysis, hold the well-being, in fact in some instances, the very lives of patients in their hands. In the dim hours of the night, as well as in the light of day, nurses are frequently charged with the duty to observe the condition of the ill and infirm in their care. If the patient, helpless and wholly dependent, shows signs of worsening, the nurse is charged with the obligation of taking some positive action . . . there was evidence that certain nurses did not fulfill their obligation.

The duty to prevent harm, known as the nurse's "affirmative duty," has been reaffirmed in numerous court decisions.

Every nurse should understand the impact that nursing case law has on his or her current practice. Case law made in appellate court decisions has addressed a range of vital issues related to professional nursing including:

- Nursing malpractice cases
- Lawsuits claiming violation of the nurse's civil rights, including free-speech issues and reasonable accommodation for nurses with disabilities
- Questions concerning labor law and collective bargaining
- Lawsuits alleging wrongful termination
- Legal challenges to state board of nursing disciplinary action against a nurse's license
- Legal actions against the nurse instituted by medical licensing boards
- "Practicing medicine without a license" claims

Efforts should be made by professional nurses to review case law as it is published and discussed in nursing journals. There has been a trend to incorporate "legal advice" columns into many practice journals, and journals often include discussions about nursing case law. There also has been a proliferation of nursing journals dedicated solely to legal issues in nursing practice. Table 8-2 lists examples of these publications.

TABLE 8-2	*Examples of Journals Dedicated to Legal Issues in Nursing Practice*
JOURNAL	**PUBLISHER**
Nursing Law's Regan Report	Medica Press Inc., Providence, RI
Journal of Nursing Law	KRM Information Services, Inc., Eau Claire, WI
Legal Eagle Eye Newsletter for the Nursing Professions	Legal Eagle Eye Newsletter, Seattle, WA
Journal of Legal Nurse Consulting	American Association of Legal Nurse Consultants, Glenview, IL

In addition to contributing to the expected standard of nursing care through court decisions, common law also provides the courts with guidelines in deciding future cases containing similar facts about nursing practice. These decisions are called "legal precedents." The reliance of judges on previous court decisions to guide current opinions is based on the legal doctrine of stare decisis ("let the decision stand"). The principle of applying previous decisions to current cases most often occurs within the same jurisdiction or state in which the legal precedent was established. However, legal precedent may influence an opinion in cases heard on appeal in other regions of the United States.

Nurse managers in particular should have knowledge regarding the disposition of cases in their jurisdiction. A risk manager or agency attorney may assist any nurse in understanding how judge-made law in his or her state relates to expectations for nursing practice in the local community. Many medical libraries also subscribe to publications that review federal or appellate court decisions in health care law that are relevant to the local community. Although local jury verdicts do not contribute to common law, it also is useful for managers and interested nurses to periodically review published reports of malpractice cases in the state and their immediate community. Medical libraries also often subscribe to a local "jury verdicts" publication.

Finding Nursing Case Law

Nurses who wish to read original case law can be guided by an increasing number of articles published in nursing journals about finding case law. Locating case law is not a difficult process, once the nurse learns how to access topics and understands how to interpret a legal citation (Rhodes, 1994). Box 8-3 describes how to decipher a legal citation and find the original case.

CIVIL LAW

Two major types of categories of law have been created to deal with conduct that is considered unacceptable—criminal law and civil law. Nurses generally are more familiar with civil law and, in particular, the branch of civil law that deals with torts. Tort law is discussed first, and a discussion of criminal law follows.

A tort is a civil wrong or injury committed by one person against another person or a property. The wrong results from a breach in one's legal duty regarding interpersonal relationships between private persons. This duty is established through societal expectations regarding interpersonal conduct (*Nurse's Legal Handbook*, 2000). Civil suits almost always are brought by one person against another and generally are based on the concept of "fault." The person who initiates the civil lawsuit, the plaintiff, seeks damages for the wrongful behavior from the

BOX 8-3	*The Process of Locating Nursing Case Law*

Pertinent case law may be found in any local law library.
Case law can be located by
 Case Name: *Francis v. Memorial General Hospital 726 P 2d 852* (NM, 1986)
 Topic: Nurses (ask assistance of librarian)
Cases are found in one of two digests
 State Digests
 Federal Practice Digests
If you have the case name, go to the appropriate digest (Federal or State).
If you do not know if it was a Federal or State case, you'll have to look in both.
 Go to the Table of Cases
 Find the case name
 Note the **full citation**
 Decipher the citation
 Francis v. Memorial General Hospital 726 P 2d 852 (NM, 1986)

Francis	**versus**	**Memorial General Hospital**	
(Name of plaintiff)		(Name of defendant)	
(Names will be reversed if case heard on appeal)			
842	**S.W.**	**2d**	**869**
Volume	Region	Series	Page on which case found
	Southwestern Reporter		
	(Region case decided in)		

(NM, 1986)
 State and year in which case decided
If state case: Go to State Reporter for region listed in citation (i.e., S.W. = Southwestern Reporter).
If federal appeals court:
 (Cited as F.2d or F.Suppl):   Go to Federal Reporter
 (Cited as F.Suppl):   Go to Federal Supplement
If U.S. Supreme Court:
 (Cited as U.S.):   Go to United States Reports
 (Cited as S. Ct)   Go to Supreme Court Reporter

offending person, known as the defendant. The determination of whether wrongful behavior has occurred usually is determined by a jury, although in certain cases the right to a trial by jury can be waived by the private parties in the suit. In that case the judge considers the facts and determines the outcome. If the plaintiff succeeds in the civil lawsuit (plaintiff verdict), damages generally are awarded in the form of monetary compensation. Damages may include "hard" damages—financial reimbursement for treatment of injuries, loss of wages, rehabilitation services, or special equipment—and "soft" damages—monetary compensation for pain and suffering, loss of companionship, or mental anguish, among other things (Aiken, 1994).

Negligence and Malpractice

There are two types of torts: an unintentional tort or wrong and an intentional tort. An unintentional tort is an unintended wrong against another person. The two most common unintentional torts are negligence and malpractice.

Negligence is defined as the failure to act in a reasonable and prudent manner. The claim of negligence is based on the accepted principle that everyone is expected to conduct themselves in a reasonable and prudent fashion. This is true of lay persons, student nurses, and licensed professionals. A more formal definition of negligence is the "failure to exercise the degree of care that a person of ordinary prudence would exercise under the same circumstances" (*Nurse's Legal Handbook,* 2000).

Malpractice is a special type of negligence—that is, the failure of a professional, a person with specialized education and training, to act in a reasonable and prudent manner. As state nurse practice acts have evolved to reflect the increasing professionalism of RNs, courts have begun to recognize the negligent acts of nurses as malpractice. Evidence of this change in perceptions is apparent in the increasing use of RNs as expert witnesses in "malpractice" cases.

In general, expert testimony is not needed in cases of "simple" negligence, when the actions of the defendant are so obviously careless that even a lay person would recognize the conduct as negligent. In contrast, if the jury does not possess the special knowledge and information that professionals ordinarily have, an expert witness is required to establish whether the person breached the expected standard of care. In that case the breach in duty is not simple negligence, but malpractice.

Elements Essential to Prove Negligence or Malpractice. Although any patient or surviving family member in the case of a patient death may sue the nurse and his or her employer, the following elements must be proved for the plaintiff to succeed in the case.
 A. The nurse owed the patient or client a special duty of care based on the establishment of a nurse-patient relationship.
    1. When the nurse accepts a patient assignment, it establishes the relationship and requires the nurse to meet his or her duty to the patient.
       a. The duty of the nurse is to possess the knowledge and skill that a reasonable and prudent nurse would possess and exercise in the same or similar patient care situation.
       b. The duty of the nurse as described is the standard of care.
    2. A nurse-patient relationship also may be established through telephone communication in the case of a nurse who performs telephone triage and advice or via computer or audio-video systems that are now being introduced in some health care settings (Mahlmeister, 2000b).
 B. The nurse has breached his or her duty to the patient or client.
    1. Evidence is presented that proves the nurse breached the standard of care.
    2. The standard of care is essentially what the nurse expert witness states that it is.
    3. The standard of care is derived from a multiplicity of sources, and they are described in Box 8-4.
 C. Actual harm or damage is suffered by the patient.
 D. There is proximate cause or a causal connection between the breach in the standard of care by the nurse and the patient's injury.
    1. No intervening event is responsible for the injury.
    2. A direct cause and effect can be demonstrated.
    3. In some jurisdictions the nurse's breach in duty must only be proven to be a "substantial cause" of the patient's injury.

BOX 8-4	*Sources That Contribute to the Standard of Nursing Care*

Federal laws
Emergency Medical Treatment and Active Labor Law
Americans with Disabilities Act
Patient Self-Determination Act
Occupational Health and Safety Law

Federal administrative rules and regulations
Rules and Regulations for Participation in Medicare

Federal guidelines
Agency for Health Care Policy and Research Clinical
    Guidelines
National Institutes of Health Publications
Centers for Disease Control and Prevention
    Publications (Morbidity and Mortality Weekly
    Reports)

Nursing case law
Appellate court decisions

Professional organizations
Standards and guidelines for practice
Nursing journals
Position statements
Technical bulletins and practice resources
Code of ethics

Manufacturer guidelines
Durable medical equipment
Drugs and solutions
Disposable equipment and supplies

Agency policies and procedures
Job descriptions
Agency-specific documents
Nursing care plans
Care maps or critical pathways
Unit- or department-based standards of practice

Medical bylaws

State laws
Nursing Practice Act
State reporting statutes
Health facility licensing laws

State administrative rules and regulations
Licensing board rules

Board of nursing licensure
Position statements
Advisories
Standardized procedures

This last element merits further discussion. The relationship between the nurse's breach in the standard of care and the patient's injury must be established by the plaintiff. To prove "proximate cause," there must be a direct causal link. For example, a patient reports that he has an allergy to penicillin and wears a MedicAlert bracelet to that effect. A physician orders penicillin to treat the patient's infection. The nurse fails to check for or ask the patient about allergies. The nurse administers the penicillin, and the patient suffers an anaphylactic reaction and dies. There is a direct connection between the nurse's actions and the patient's death. Proximate cause has been established.

In some jurisdictions it only is necessary to prove that the nurse's actions were a substantial cause of the injury or harm to prove negligence. For example, in a large teaching hospital a nurse notes a significant change in a patient's vital signs, suggesting a deterioration in his condition. A first-year resident is called to the bedside and made aware of the patient's status. The resident orders the nurse to simply continue observing the patient. The physician remains immediately available in the unit and receives repeated reports of a continued decline in the patient's condition. There is a clear chain of command policy established in the hospital to deal with unresolved disagreements between health care professionals. Despite the policy's existence, the nurse does not activate the chain of command.

The patient suffers hypovolemic shock caused by internal bleeding, and this leads to permanent anoxic brain damage. In this case the nurse's failure to obtain additional medical advice and consultation (a senior resident was physically present and available in the hospital) was a substantial cause of the patient's injury. These two examples illustrate that negligence may constitute a commission (inappropriate penicillin administration) or an omission (failure to activate chain of command) in care.

Negligence and the Doctrine of Res Ipsa Loquitur.   In the majority of cases a plaintiff must retain a nurse expert witness because the jury does not ordinarily possess the scientific and technologic knowledge necessary to determine the required standard of care. When the negligent act clearly lies within the range of a jury's common knowledge and experience, the doctrine of res ipsa loquitur ("the thing speaks for itself") may be applied. For example, leaving a surgical instrument in the patient's body after an operation is one case in which the doctrine may apply (*Nurse's Legal Handbook*, 2000). It would be obvious to any lay person that it is below that standard of care not to remove a surgical instrument.

Dickerson v. Fatehi (1997) illustrates this point. A woman who underwent neck surgery experienced severe pain in her right arm, hand, and neck after the procedure. Approximately 20 months later a second surgery was performed to determine the cause of the patient's continued pain. An 18-gauge hypodermic needle with a plastic attachment for a syringe was discovered in her neck and removed. The woman sued the surgeon and nurses involved in the original surgical procedure. The claims against the nurses included a failure to maintain a proper needle count and a failure to ensure the removal of the needle after surgery.

The court hearing this case dismissed the suit. On appeal the Supreme Court of Virginia reversed the lower court's decision and directed the case for trial. The Supreme Court held that in this particular case expert testimony was not necessary to establish the applicable standard of care and that the doctrine of res ipsa loquitur applied. A jury would be able to determine whether a reasonably prudent circulating nurse and scrub nurse should have made and reported an accurate needle count.

Gross Negligence.   In some cases the negligent act of the nurse is so reckless and reflects such a conscious disregard for the patient's welfare that it represents gross negligence. When the nurse acts with complete indifference to the consequences for his or her patient, the court may award special damages meant to punish the nurse for the outrageous conduct. These damages are referred to as punitive damages. Each state has established standards to determine when punitive damages may be awarded.

A case in point is Manning v. Twin Falls Clinic and Hospital (1992). Punitive damages in the amount of $300 were awarded against an Idaho nurse for willful disregard of a terminally ill patient's comfort and physiologic stability during transfer from one unit of the hospital to another. The patient, who suffered from severe respiratory distress, required continuous oxygen administration. Despite the family's insistent and repeated requests that the nurse administer oxygen during the transfer, the nurse transported the patient without oxygen. The patient suffered a respiratory arrest and died shortly thereafter.

Nurses should be aware that as a rule malpractice insurance policies do not provide coverage for punitive damages. The purpose of punitive damages is not only to deter such egregious behavior from occurring in the future, but also to punish the nurse by requiring an out-of-pocket payment. Although the amount awarded in the Manning case was relatively modest, courts in some cases have levied damages in the thousands of dollars against nurses.

Criminal Negligence. Criminal negligence represents a case in which the negligent acts of the nurse (normally an unintentional civil wrong) also constitute a crime. In most states a nurse can be prosecuted when the conduct is deemed so reckless that the action results in serious harm or death to the patient. In 1997 two registered nurses and an advanced practice nurse licensed in Colorado were charged with criminal negligent homicide in the death of a newborn resulting from a medication error (Kowalski and Horner, 1998). In this case an oil-based form of penicillin was erroneously administered to the infant. The drug was administered at 10 times the physician's prescribed dose. This case is detailed in the Kowalski article and should be read by every student and graduate nurse.

The Colorado case reflects the changing perspective of our justice system when negligent acts of health care professionals result in patient death. In the event of an unanticipated patient death, it is more likely that the conduct of both basic and advanced practice nurses will be scrutinized by the criminal justice system (Laughlin, 1998). This shift may in part be a result of the public's increasing awareness of the magnitude of error in health care. It also may stem from consumer demands for greater accountability by health care systems and workers when injury or death occur. Conservative estimates suggest that as many as 98,000 patients die each year as a result of the negligence and malpractice of health care providers (Institute of Medicine, 2000).

Other negative consequences that the nurse faces when criminal charges are filed include the loss of his or her job and disciplinary action by the state licensing board. Even when the criminal charges are not supported, the nurse's license can be suspended or revoked, and out-of-pocket fines levied by the board if there is evidence of violation of the Nursing Practice Act.

An attorney may have to be retained to represent the nurse at considerable personal expense when criminal charges are filed. The nurse's malpractice insurance generally does not cover the attorney's fees in this case. Neither is the nurse's employer obligated to pay the legal fees of a nurse charged with a felony. In the Colorado case the nurse practitioner was immediately terminated. The two direct care nurses were permitted to work in nonpatient care areas of the hospital. The costs of the criminal defense of all three nurses were paid by the hospital.

Defenses Against Claims of Negligence. In some cases the nurse can use certain legal doctrines as a defense against a claim of negligence. These standard defenses are discussed in the next section. In no case may a nurse provide a defense of "only following the provider's orders" against allegations of negligence (Tammelleo, 2000) The Nursing Practice Act, licensing board rules and regulations, and nursing case law have delineated the nurse's independent duty to evaluate all provider orders before implementing them. The nurse must consider two points.

- ■ Is the order lawful?
- ■ Is the order in this particular patient's best interest?

Each nurse has an absolute duty to take some positive action to prevent harm when orders are inappropriate or incomplete or when the actions of another health care provider endanger the patient's well-being. This principle of "affirmative duty" is well recognized in law and in ethics. The ANA's "Code for Nurses" (1995) and the American Medical Association's "Code of Medical Ethics" (1994) recognize the central role of nurses in preventing patient harm.

Concepts of Immunity in Claims of Negligence. Standard legal defenses used as defenses against claims of negligence include those listed in the following paragraphs.

Contributory Negligence. When the patient's own behavior contributes to worsening of an injury that has been caused by a nurse's negligence, in some jurisdictions the patient may not be permitted to recover damages. The nurse in that case is not held responsible for the patient's injury. If a patient fails to follow the provider's orders or the nurse's precautionary advisements, it would be evidence of the plaintiff's contributory negligence. To effectively use this defense, the nurse must carefully chart all efforts to warn the patient of potential adverse consequences of an act and document an assessment of the patient's ability to comprehend the warnings, as well as indicators that he or she intends to comply. In some states the plaintiff (patient) may be able to recover a part of the damages, even when he or she contributed to the negative outcome. The court in these states "apportions" liability between the patient and defendants in the case. For instance, if a jury decides a nurse is 60% negligent for the patient's injury and the patient 40% responsible for the adverse outcome, the patient would only claim 60% of the damages awarded (Trandel-Korenchuk and Trandel-Korenchuk, 1997).

Comparative Negligence. Many states permit the damages to be apportioned among multiple defendants. For example, in an obstetric case the damages may be apportioned among the obstetrician, nurse midwife, charge nurse, direct care nurse, and nurse anesthetist. Comparative negligence is illustrated in Chin v. St. Barnabas Medical Center (1996). Two nurses who participated in a hysteroscopy procedure were individually named in the lawsuit. The nurses attempted to assemble equipment used to inflate a woman's uterus during this diagnostic procedure. Lacking the requisite knowledge or skill, they negligently failed to open a gas release valve. When the procedure was started, the woman suffered a fatal pulmonary embolus. The patient's husband filed suit after her death. The jury awarded $2 million in damages. The nurses were found personally liable for their negligent conduct.

The jury was instructed to apportion liability among the hospital, its nurses, and the physician in the case. The senior nurse participating in the procedure was found liable for 25% of the damages ($500,000); a second circulating nurse who was uncertain about operating the equipment and called the senior nurse for advice was found liable for 20% of the damages ($400,000). The defendant physician was found 20% liable (the remaining $400,000). The state of New Jersey had enacted a law that limited liability of nonprofit hospitals to $250,000. Although the jury found the hospital 35% liable (700,000 dollars), it was limited to payment of the $250,000 state cap.

Emergency Situations. Nursing care rendered in a life-threatening emergency may breach the standard of care required under ordinary circumstances. For instance, a woman who is 8 months' pregnant arrives in the labor and delivery suite. She is hemorrhaging because of a premature separation of the placenta (abruptio placenta). An emergency cesarean delivery is ordered by the doctor. The woman is near death as a result of blood loss. There also are clear signs of fetal distress. To expedite the surgical delivery, the operating room team does not observe the strict aseptic technique normally required during insertion of a Foley catheter into the woman's bladder and foregoes the lengthy abdominal scrub normally performed with an iodine solution.

The mother and infant are brought through the crisis safely, although the woman develops a skin infection at the site of the abdominal incision, which causes noticeable scaring. She also must be treated for a bladder infection, which resolves by discharge on the fourth postpartum day. She sues the nurses and physician. In this case the defense could argue that, to save the life of the mother and baby, the methods used were reasonable and prudent. Even a delay of seconds could have resulted in the death of the woman or her infant. Expert witnesses are produced to support the defense assertion that it would breach the standard of care in this particular situation to follow customary procedures in preparing the woman for surgery.

Governmental Immunity. For nurses working in federal or state health care facilities, a defense of governmental immunity may be used. Laws have been enacted that shield individual health care workers employed in federal or state facilities from personal responsibility for damages awarded in malpractice cases. Nurses employed by the Department of Veteran Affairs, the U.S. Public Health Service, the National Aeronautics and Space Administration, and the Department of Defense are shielded from civil suits in the performance of professional duties. This immunity was granted through enactment of specific federal statutes, including the Federal Tort Claims Act of 1946 and the Federal Employees Liability Reform and Tort Compensation Act of 1988.

The intent of these laws was to substitute the U.S. government as the defendant in a malpractice suit. The government has waived its "sovereign immunity" against suit and pays the damages for injuries caused by the negligent acts of health care professionals employed in the aforementioned federal agencies.

State immunity statutes vary. In some instances, individual states have not waived their "sovereign immunity" from lawsuits. In those cases the state is not substituted for the individual health care provider in malpractice cases. Nurses and physicians are liable for their negligent acts in these states and are personally responsible for damages awarded. It would be imperative in this circumstance for the health care professional to have individual malpractice insurance (Bernzweig, 1996).

Good Samaritan Immunity. Good Samaritan laws may limit a nurse's liability or shield the nurse from a malpractice claim if the nurse renders assistance in an emergency that occurs outside of the employment setting. Although in most states the nurse owes no legal duty to an accident victim, once the nurse makes a decision to stop and render aid (an ethical decision), a nurse-patient relationship is established. (Some states have enacted "duty to rescue" or "compulsory assistance" laws, including Vermont, Minnesota, and Wisconsin.)

When the nurse renders care at the scene of an accident, he or she is required to render the standard of care that any reasonable and prudent nurse would render in a similar situation. To prevail in a malpractice suit under the Good Samaritan Law, the plaintiff must prove that the nurse intentionally caused the injury or was grossly negligent (*Nurse's Legal Handbook,* 2000). Therefore each nurse should be familiar with his or her state-specific Good Samaritan statute. Nurses also should be reassured by the fact that the preponderance of malpractice cases that invoke the Good Samaritan defense are settled in favor of the nurse.

Basic Phases of a Malpractice Case

The recent media attention in criminal and civil cases has educated the public to basic and more esoteric aspects of the law and court proceedings. The average citizen has been subjected to lengthy television discussions about the trial process, including jury selection, the "voir dire" process in establishing expert witness qualifications, and burden of proof. Whereas the public in general has a greater knowledge of the legal system, unfortunately for most nurses, their first encounter with the courts occurs when they receive a summons stating the plaintiff's charges in a malpractice suit.

Every nurse should take the time to become familiar with the basic aspects of a civil suit. The litigious nature of our society makes it likely that most nurses will be involved in some degree with a civil case asserting negligence. Although the nurse may have no direct involvement or may not be a target of litigation, he or she may be asked to assist in production of documents (evidence) or to testify about some aspect of the case. Box 8-5 outlines the basic sequential steps in the malpractice process. It is beyond the scope of this book to discuss the details of the trial process. The reader is referred to one of the excellent articles now published in nursing journals that describe all phases of the malpractice suit (*Nurse's Legal Handbook,* 2000; Rostant and Cady, 1999; Trandel-Korenchuk and Trandel-Korenchuk, 1997)

Statutes of Limitation in Malpractice Cases

Each state has established a time limit in which a person may initiate a lawsuit. Although many states have established a time limit of 2 or 3 years from the date of the patient's injury or death in which the plaintiff must sue, statutes of limitation vary widely from state to state. In some jurisdictions a "termination of treatment" rule exists. It is predicated on the assumption that some injuries result from a series of treatments over time (Bernzweig, 1996). In this case the statute of limitation does not begin to run until the treatment ends.

Other rules and regulations govern the "tolling" or running of the statutes of limitation. The court recognizes that an injured party cannot initiate a malpractice case until he or she discovers that some harm was done (discovery rule). This can occur when health care providers actually conceal the facts in the case of an injury through fraud, deceit, or concealment such as:

- Fraudulent or misleading entries in the medical record
- Destruction of evidence
- Destruction of the medical record
- Lying to the patient about the cause of the problems

The statute of limitation also is altered when a foreign object is left in the patient's body. Until the foreign object is discovered, the statute of limitation does not begin to run. States have rules that regulate the tolling of the statute of limitation in mentally incompetent adults and minors. In the case of an adult patient who is so severely injured that there is a loss of mental capacity, the statute of limitation may not begin to toll until mental competence is regained. The statute of limitation varies in the case of minors and may only expire when the child reaches the age of majority (age 18 or 21 years) (*Nurse's Legal Handbook,* 2000).

Each nurse should be familiar with the statute of limitation for his or her state. If the nurse suspects that some form of fraud or deceit has occurred relative to a patient's injury, the agency's risk manager or attorney should be contacted immediately. Major penalties and fines are applicable in cases in which health care providers deliberately deceive the patient or destroy evidence. These acts rise to the level of criminal misconduct and can result in loss of one's professional license.

When errors occur in practice, studies confirm that telling the patient (and family) about the mistake promptly results in far less severe ramifications for the clinicians and health care facility (When and How, 1997). The nurse should not assume responsibility for disclosure.

BOX 8-5	*Phases in a Malpractice Case: the Trial Process—Step by Step*

The chart below summarizes the basic trial process from complaint to execution of judgment. If ever involved in a lawsuit, the nurse's attorney will explain the specific procedures that the case requires.

Pretrial preparation

Complaint—Plaintiff files a complaint stating his or her charges against the defendant

Summons—Court issues defendant a summons stating plaintiff's charges

Answer or counterclaim—Defendant files an answer and may add a counterclaim to plaintiff's charges

Discovery—Plaintiff's and defendant's attorneys develop their cases by gathering information by means of depositions and interrogatories and by reviewing documents and other evidence

Pretrial hearing—Court hears statements from both parties and tries to narrow the issues

Negotiations for settlement—Both parties meet to try to resolve the case outside the court

Trial

Opening statements—Plaintiff's and defendant's attorneys present facts as they apply to their cases

Plaintiff presents case—Plaintiff's witnesses testify, explaining what they saw, heard, and know; expert witnesses review any documentation and give their opinions about specific aspects of the case

Cross-examination—Defendant's attorney questions plaintiff's witnesses

Plaintiff closes case—Defendant's attorney may make a motion to dismiss the case, claiming plaintiff's evidence is insufficient

Defendant presents case—Defendant's witnesses testify, explaining what they saw, heard, and know; expert witnesses review any documentation and give their opinions about specific aspects of the case

Cross-examination—Plaintiff's attorney questions defendant's witnesses

Defendant closes case—Plaintiff's attorney may claim defendant has not presented an issue for the jury to decide

Closing statements—Each attorney summarizes his or her case for the jury

Jury instruction—Judge instructs the jury in points of law that apply in this particular case

Jury deliberation and verdict—Jury reviews facts and votes on verdict; jury announces verdict before judge and both parties

Appeal (optional)—Attorneys review transcripts; the party against whom the court ruled may appeal if he or she believes the judge did not interpret the law properly, instruct the jury properly, or conduct the trial properly

Execution of judgment—Appeals process is completed, and the case is settled

The primary provider, the agency's administrator, and the risk manager should formulate a plan. It should be determined in advance who will speak with the patient (or family) and how questions and concerns about the patient's condition, subsequent treatment, and the cost of any required care will be addressed.

Nursing Malpractice Insurance

With more states recognizing nursing malpractice as a legitimate claim in a civil suit, the question of whether nurses should carry malpractice insurance has become increasingly important (*Nurse's Legal Handbook,* 2000). Nursing journals have published a number of articles that either address this question or describe the types of malpractice coverage the nurse should consider (Morrison et al., 1998; Tammelleo, 1997). An increasing consensus appears to recommend that all nurses purchase malpractice insurance as a result of changes in the health care system, civil law, and insurance company policies. Legal authors also are quick to note the fallacy of the assumption that having malpractice insurance increases the risk that the nurse will be targeted in a malpractice case. Lack of coverage will not discourage a lawsuit when there is a legitimate claim. Reasons given for the purchase of malpractice insurance by RNs include:

- Expanding functions of RNs and advanced practice nurses
- Floating and cross-training mandates
- Increasing responsibility for supervising subordinate staff
- Failure of some employers to initiate an adequate defense for nurses
- Insurance coverage limits that are lower than the actual judgment made against the nurse in a lawsuit

Other considerations that the nurse must take into account when considering malpractice insurance include whether he or she is employed by the federal government. In that case the nurse may be shielded from personal liability by federal tort statutes, although some states still uphold the doctrine of "sovereign immunity," making it impossible to sue a state-run medical facility for negligence. In those states it is a virtual necessity for nurses to purchase malpractice insurance because health care workers become the only available targets in a malpractice case (Bernzweig, 1996). States that uphold the doctrine of "joint and several liability," whereby nurses could be responsible not only for their own liability but also for that of another insolvent defendant, place nurses in a position in which malpractice insurance may be necessary. Texas is one such state that can require a partially negligent party to pay for 100% of the judgment (Concern in Texas, 1995).

As many malpractice carriers point out, the employer's malpractice policy does not cover the nurse for acts of negligence that occur outside the scope of the work setting. Situations that the nurse may be involved in that would not be covered include:

- Giving advice to a friend or neighbor about health care or medication
- Volunteering as a nurse at a community event
- Performing an act (even at work) that is not permitted by the Nursing Practice Act or job description

LIABILITY

Closely tied to the concepts of negligence and malpractice is that of liability. Liability asserts that every person is responsible for the wrong or injury done to another resulting from carelessness.

Personal Liability

Within the context of nursing practice, the nurse is always accountable for the outcomes of his or her actions in carrying out nursing duties. The rule of personal liability requires the professional nurse to assume responsibility for patient harm or injury that is a result of his or her negligent acts. The nurse cannot be relieved of personal liability by another professional, such as a provider or nurse manager, who asserts, "Don't worry, I'll take responsibility for the consequences" (Snyder, 2000; Gardner and Hagedorn, 1997).

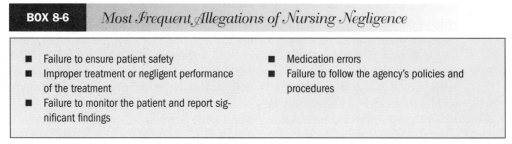

Adapted from American Nurses Association: *Liability prevention and you,* Washington, DC, 1989, American Nurses Publishing, American Nurses Foundation/American Nurses Association.

In 1989 the ANA summarized the most frequent allegations of negligence leveled against nurses in malpractice cases. They are listed in Box 8-6. These charges have not substantially changed in the past 10 years (Smith-Pittman, 1998). Nurses may be educated to implement effective risk control strategies that reduce these claims. These personal and system-wide strategies are discussed in the next section.

Many nurses practice under the misconception that they are protected from personal liability when employed by a health care entity such as a hospital. I have heard nurses say, "Why would a patient sue me personally? I don't have the financial resources of this (hospital, nursing home, home health care agency)!" Nurses can and have been individually named in lawsuits and found negligent. Damages can be levied against the nurse's current assets and future earnings for negligent acts (LaDuke, 1999). Tammelleo (1996) reports that hospitals have sued nurses to recoup financial losses suffered when they were required to pay damages for the alleged negligence of the nurses named in the malpractice case. Personal liability is illustrated in a recent case, Shelton v. Penrose/St. Francis Healthcare (1999):

> Gretchen Shelton was hospitalized for hip replacement surgery. After surgery she was fitted with a special brace to prevent posterior dislocation of her hip. Six days after surgery she was transferred to the rehabilitation unit in the hospital for daily physical therapy. During therapy her brace was removed. After the treatment, she was returned to her room and placed in a chair, where she fell asleep. Two nurses entered her room and proceeded to move her from the chair back to her bed without waking her or ascertaining if her brace was on. During the transfer, her hip was dislocated, causing extreme pain. Ms. Shelton sued, claiming the nurses were negligent for failing to waken her and determine if her brace was in place. One of the defense arguments was that the nurses would have ordinarily expected that her brace would have been on when she was returned to her room and were therefore not required to check the affected leg. The jury found the two nurses negligent, agreeing with the expert witness nurse. She concluded that, within a reasonable degree of nursing probability, the patient sustained the dislocation and pain due to a failure to assess the patient and correctly transfer her to bed. The hospital appealed, but the jury verdict was affirmed by the Supreme Court of Colorado.

Personal Liability With Floating and Cross-Training

New models of patient care often mandate floating and cross-training of patient care staff to enhance efficiency and reduce the costs of staffing. They also have increased the personal liability of nurses (Stein, 2000). Professional nurses must be cognizant of state statutes and case law when asked to perform services outside of their usual area of practice. In no case is a nurse ever permitted to perform tasks or render services when he or she lacks the requisite knowledge and skill to act competently.

The Nursing Practice Act and the administrative rules and regulations of the licensing board provide explicit statutory language regarding the nurse's duty to provide safe and competent care. For example, the Administrative Rules of the Tennessee Board of Nursing (March, 1996) state:

> Each individual is responsible for personal acts of negligence under the law. Registered nurses are liable if they perform delegated functions they are not prepared to handle by education and experience, and for which supervision is not provided. In any patient care situation, the registered nurse should perform only those acts for which each has been prepared and has demonstrated ability to perform, bearing in mind the individual persons responsibility under the law.
>
> Tennessee Rules and Regulations of Registered Nurses
> Rule 1000-1-04 (3): Responsibility.

In addition to the laws governing practice in floating and cross-training situations, an increasing body of nursing case law also defines the limitation of assignments. Appellate court decisions have addressed the issue of when a nurse may safely refuse an assignment to float without risk of job termination. In Winkelman v. Beloit Memorial Hospital (1992), the Supreme Court of Wisconsin ruled that under certain circumstances a nurse had a right to refuse floating assignments without fear of reprisal.

> Nurse Winkelman was a skilled maternity nurse who was employed for 16 years at Beloit Memorial Hospital, working exclusively in the nursery. In 1987 the hospital created a new policy that required nurses in the maternity setting to float when the patient census was low in their unit. Nurse Winkelman was asked to float to an adult floor dedicated to the care of postoperative and geriatric patients. She notified her immediate supervisor that she did not feel qualified to float to that unit and that attempting to provide care in that setting would place the patients at risk. In her testimony the nurse said that she was given three choices: float, find another nurse who would float in her place, or take an unexcused absence day. She subsequently went home, and her employer construed her actions as "voluntary resignation of her employment." Nurse Winkelman then filed a complaint for wrongful discharge and breach of contract. A jury verdict was rendered in favor of Nurse Winkelman on the charge of wrongful discharge. The case was appealed and affirmed by the Supreme Court of Wisconsin. The court found that the nurse had identified a fundamental and well-defined public policy in the Wisconsin Administrative Code, which stated that a nurse should not offer or perform services for which he or she is not qualified by education, training, or experience.

The nurse's right to refuse a floating assignment has not been supported in all cases. Courts have affirmed the right of a health care facility to redirect staff to meet the needs of patients. The New Mexico Supreme Court in Francis v. Memorial General Hospital (1986) held that the hospital was not prohibited from discharging a nurse who refused to float when the employer had made a reasonable offer to train the nurse for new responsibilities.

> Nurse Francis, a critical care nurse, refused to float to an orthopedic unit, stating he did not feel qualified to care for orthopedic patients. The hospital then offered to provide him with an

orientation to the floors where he might float in the future. When he refused the opportunity for orientation, he was terminated. The court upheld his discharge.

Although it is clear that nurses have a legal duty to refuse specific tasks that they cannot perform safely and competently, the prudent nurse should carefully consider the consequence of not floating. Careful negotiation with the nursing supervisor and the team leader making the actual assignment often can result in a satisfactory compromise. The floated nurse should clarify what aspects of professional nursing care he or she can safely carry out and which tasks are beyond his or her current capabilities. A reasonable supervisor will not insist that a nurse attempt to perform a task that he or she has no education, training, or current expertise to implement.

Another important strategy that may reduce the nurse's personal liability is to request that the team leader appoint a resource nurse who is skilled in the care of the patients on the unit. The resource nurse can assist the floatee as needed. It also is prudent practice for the floated nurse to enter a note in the medical record naming the resource or support nurse who will be available and responsible to assist with planning and evaluating care. For instance:

> Assumed care of Mrs. Jones after report completed. L. Doe, RN, will co-manage patient and assist with procedures, planning, and evaluation of care as needed.
>
> J. Smith, RN (floatee)

The Nursing Practice Act affirms that an RN ultimately is responsible for the quality of care provided to each patient, regardless of who actually is delegated the responsibility of carrying out the task. A claim of negligence may be leveled against the team leader who does not assign a competent "back-up" or resource nurse to assist the floatee. Only a nurse who is competent in the care of the patients normally treated in the setting (hospital, clinic, or home) can properly supervise a lesser skilled worker and evaluate the outcomes of care. The point is so critical that professional nursing organizations in California recently joined together to affirm this concept in law.

A section of the California Health Facilities Licensing for Hospitals (California Code of Regulations, Title 22, 1996) now mandates:

> A registered nurse who has demonstrated competency for the patient care unit shall be responsible for nursing care . . . and shall be assigned as a resource nurse for those registered nurses and licensed vocational nurses who have not completed competency validation for that unit. Registered nurses shall not be assigned total responsibility for patient care . . . until all the standards of competency for that unit have been validated.
>
> Section 70214, Nursing Staff Development: (B) and (C)

Personal Liability for Team Leaders and Managers

The concept of personal liability extends to nurses who function as team leaders, supervisors, and upper-level managers. Team leaders, charge nurses, and managers are held to the standard of care of the reasonably prudent nurse employed in that role (Mahlmeister, 1999). Claims of negligence leveled against managers generally surround: (1) triage of patients and allocation of staff and equipment; (2) delegation of patient care tasks; (3) supervision of orientees, float staff, and subordinates; (4) reporting performance deficits in team members; and (5) supporting or invoking the chain of command process when indicated.

Nurse managers and administrators at the upper end of the management ladder also may be held liable for:

- Inadequate training.
- Failure to periodically reevaluate staff competencies.
- Failure to discipline or terminate unsafe workers.
- Negligence in developing appropriate policies and procedures.

The implementation of new models of care that alter staffing patterns and mixes "may place managers at the same risk for liability as the health care providers delivering the actual bedside care . . ." (Kreplick, 1996).

The appropriate standard of care is established in the case of team leaders, charge nurses, and managers by expert nurse witnesses who function in those positions. An increasing body of case law in malpractice suits also is contributing to expectations about team leader and manager conduct. Although nurse managers and administrators generally are well aware of their particular liability risks, direct-care nurses who are relatively unfamiliar with the expanding role of team leaders or charge nurses may be particularly vulnerable to claims of negligence. Health care redesign has resulted in considerable flattening of the chain of command for nursing departments. Team leaders, regardless of their title or designation, have assumed greater responsibility for unit- or department-based functions such as those listed in Box 8-7.

BOX 8-7   *Typical Functions and Role Responsibilities of the Team Leader or Charge Nurse*

With flattened management the norm in an increasing number of redesigned health care settings, the "team leader" or "charge nurse" may be accountable for the following functions.

1. Staff assignments
2. Delegation of patient care tasks to unlicensed team members
3. Supervision of:
   a. Licensed practical or vocational nurses
   b. Unlicensed assistive personnel
   c. Temporary staff (floats, agency, or registry nurses)
4. Evaluation of the outcomes of care for licensed practical or vocational nursing staff and unlicensed team members
5. Triage of staff and equipment during acute patient events
6. Consultant for clinical problems
   a. Personal assessment or interview of patients
   b. Personal interpretation of data
   c. Advice about care or management of problems
7. Arbitrator in clinical disputes between patient care staff and primary providers
8. Traffic manager during acute patient events
9. Expert in operation of biotechnical equipment
10. Expert in unit operations
    a. Location of supplies and equipment
    b. Chain of command process
    c. Disaster plans

Any RN functioning in the role of team leader or charge nurse should review the following documents from administration.

- Detailed job description for the role, including how responsibilities are limited when the nurse is asked to team lead or serve as a charge nurse on an unfamiliar floor or department
- Job descriptions for the team members assigned delegated tasks
- Formal period of training and mentoring in the role
- Validated proof of competence before team leading independently
- Guidelines regarding personal patient care assignment when also serving as team leader
- Chain of command model for the facility, department, or unit

Administrators and nurse managers should be aware of recent case law regarding incompetent charge nurses and team leaders. A jury directed a verdict in excess of $7 million against a hospital in a 1995 Illinois case, Holston v. Sisters of the Third Order (1995).

> A charge nurse repeatedly refused a direct-care nurse's requests to personally evaluate a patient whose vital signs were rapidly deteriorating after gastric bypass surgery. The charge nurse also refused to call the patient's physician until the patient experienced cardiopulmonary collapse. Emergency surgery revealed that a central venous pressure catheter had migrated and perforated the cardiac muscle. The patient experienced cardiac tamponade and died approximately 1 week after this critical incident.

In a second case, Justin and Michelle Malovic v. Santa Monica Hospital Medical Center (1995), a California jury found a nurse manager negligent for failing to implement the chain of command. The case is described as follows:

> The nurse manager failed to summon the chief of obstetrics when the primary obstetrician was unresponsive to a nonreassuring fetal heart rate. The primary nurse asked the nurse manager to personally evaluate the electronic fetal heart rate pattern. The manager did so but decided there was no need to call the chief of the department. This case was complicated by the fact that the managing obstetrician's practice already was under investigation, and the nurse manager was aware of this fact (Freeman, 1995). The primary obstetrician eventually attempted a forceps birth over an unacceptably long period of time (1 hour). A subsequent cesarean delivery resulted in the birth of an infant who is now mentally retarded. The plaintiff's attorney successfully argued that, had the nurse manager called the chief of obstetrics, he would have effectively intervened, and the infant would have been born without damage.

This case illustrates the necessity of validating the strong clinical skill of all RNs who are being considered for a leadership role that includes clinical supervision and consultation. Effective risk management of an unresolved clinical problem requires direct-care nurses to consult early and frequently with team leaders or managers. Each consultation with the team leader or manager should be carefully documented in the patient's medical record to demonstrate that appropriate chain of command process has occurred. The employer will likely be named in any lawsuit under the rule of vicarious liability if the team leader or manager offers negligent advice. Vicarious liability is discussed in the next section of this chapter.

Personal Liability in Delegation and Supervision of Team Members

Team leaders and charge nurses who are responsible for delegation and supervision of team members must be absolutely clear about the legality of patient care assignments. He or she also must determine whether it is reasonable and prudent to delegate a particular task based on his or her knowledge of the worker, the patient's status, and the current conditions in the work setting. The determination of whether a team leader or charge nurse has been negligent in delegating any particular patient care task or supervising subordinates will be based on these aforementioned considerations. Criteria for lawful and safe delegation have been spelled out by state boards of nursing and professional organizations such as the American Nurses Association, the American Association of Critical Care Nurses, and the National Council of State Boards of Nursing (ANA, 1996; AACN, 1995; NCSBN, 1995). These guidelines and a growing body of case law assist the nurse in making decisions about safe delegation of patient care. Singleton v. AAA Home Health, Inc., (2000) illustrates the professional duties of the registered nurse, and the legal risks inherent in delegating nursing care to unlicensed assistive personnel.

> Rhea Polk, a patient with cardiac and renal disease, was released from the hospital with a discharge plan for home health care to be provided by skilled nursing staff. Orders were issued to provide treatment for a right hip decubitus, including packing with Betadine gauze. The wound did not heal, and surgical debridement was required. The surgeon discovered gauze embedded in the ulcerated wound, and this was determined to be the cause of the problem. On behalf of Ms. Polk, Ms. Singleton sued the home health agency. Evidence uncovered during the trial indicated that the RN responsible for Ms. Polk's care had instructed home health aides in packing the wound and inappropriately delegated the task to them. The expert witness in the case asserted that the failure of an RN to properly inspect, clean, and treat the wound was the cause the of the ulceration and need for surgery. The trial court rendered a verdict in favor of Ms. Singleton. The Louisiana Court of Appeal affirmed the verdict of the lower court on appeal.

It is important to note that, in addition to acting negligently in delegating the wound packing to a home health aide, the nurse had violated the Nursing Practice Act. Although this issue was not addressed in the Singleton case, courts have ruled in previous malpractice cases that a failure to adhere to the Nursing Practice Act (a law) and the administrative rules and regulations of the licensing board constitutes negligence per se (negligence as a matter of law) (Carroll, 1996).

Employer Liability

Although the nurse is never relieved of personal liability, the doctrine of vicarious or substituted liability permits a person to also sue the employer for the negligent conduct of nurses within the scope of their employment. Vicarious liability is based on the legal principle of respondent superior, a Latin term that means "let the master answer" (for the actions of his subordinates or servants). Because the employer has some control over the worker, the courts have affirmed that the employer may be held responsible for the employee's negligent acts when injury occurs.

In a Texas case, Convalescent Services, Inc. v. Schultz (1996), a nursing home was found negligent for failure of its nursing staff to provide appropriate skin care to an elderly client with Alzheimer's dementia. The patient developed severe pressure sores. He required surgery to repair the decubitus ulcers, experienced significant pain and suffering, and had a prolonged hospitalization. The suit claimed that the care provided by the staff in the nursing home was so substandard that it represented gross negligence. The jury awarded a verdict for the plaintiff and punitive damages for the gross negligence of the nursing staff. The appeals court upheld the ruling, which the nursing home had contested.

Defenses Against Claims of Vicarious Liability

The financial stakes are high in any malpractice case, and the attendant negative publicity that often ensues can adversely affect a hospital's standing in a community for years. The law permits hospitals in certain circumstances to rely on specific doctrines that absolve the hospital of its normal liability.

Charitable Immunity. In past decades nonprofit agencies that provided free care to medically indigent patients were shielded from claims of liability. The rationale for this immunity from liability was that permitting damages to be paid in malpractice actions would eliminate the funding available to provide charitable services to needy members of the community. Second, granting immunity was thought to allay the malpractice fears of otherwise willing professionals who would provide services at no cost to indigent patients. Many states have now rejected the rule, and several other states have limited its applicability.

Borrowed Servant and Captain of the Ship Doctrines. If the health care facility can prove that the nurse who normally provides services as an employee of the institution was temporarily under the control of another agent, it may use the "borrowed servant" doctrine to defend a claim of negligence. This defense has been used in cases involving intraoperative care, where it has been asserted that the nurse involved in the case was under the direct control and authority of the surgeon. This defense is closely aligned with a second doctrine known as the "captain of the ship" doctrine.

The captain of the ship doctrine states that, during an operative procedure, the surgeon is legally responsible for the actions of all other nonphysician assistants in the room. The courts have begun to severely limit the use of the borrowed servant and captain of the ship doctrines as a defense in cases of nursing negligence. As a licensed professional, the nurse is held fully accountable for his or her actions during surgery, including responsibility for instrument, needle, and sponge counts. In some instances in which the nurse may legally function as the first assistant during surgery, the borrowed servant doctrine may be successfully used as a defense by the hospital. In that case the court may decide that the nurse was under the direct control of the surgeon.

Corporate Liability

Hospitals and other health care facilities have evolved into dynamic systems that coordinate the care provided by a range of health care professionals (Smith-Pittman, 1997). As a consequence of these changes, the courts have expanded the concept of corporate negligence in verdicts rendered against health care giants (Carroll, 1996). The "standard of care" required of a health care corporation has been established through these cases but varies from state to state. Some jurisdictions have permitted Joint Commission for Accreditation Standards or State Department of Health Licensing Laws to define the "corporate standard of care" (Carroll, 1996). An agency's own medical bylaws or policies and procedures have been admitted as evidence of the appropriate corporate standard of care. In Thompson v. Nason Hospital (1991), the court elaborated four duties of a health care corporation.

1. Maintain safe and adequate physical facilities and equipment
2. Select and retain competent physicians
3. Oversee the acts of all persons who practice medicine within the facility as they relate to patient care
4. Formulate, adopt, and enforce rules and policies to ensure quality of care

In another case, Rodebush v. Oklahoma Nursing Homes, Ltd. (1993), the court found a nursing home liable for negligent hiring and supervision of a staff member, a nurse aide, who had a previous conviction of a violent felony: assault and battery with the intent to kill. The criminal record was discovered only after the family of a patient in the nursing home filed a lawsuit. The suit was initiated when the family's elderly parent was injured by the nurse aide, who was intoxicated at the time of the incident. The jury awarded $50,000 in actual damages and $1.2 million in punitive damages against the corporation for failing to follow its own policies in hiring, training, and supervising employees and in investigating employee misconduct.

Health care facilities also have been found corporately liable for failing to have adequate numbers of qualified nursing staff assigned on each shift to meet the needs of patients. In Merritt v. Karcloglu (1996), a Louisiana hospital was found negligent for failing to have sufficient nursing staff to provide essential care. The hospital had a written policy that directed a nurse in the cardiac care unit to respond to "Codes" called in other areas of the hospital. A nurse assigned exclusively to an elderly, confused patient in the critical care unit was required to respond to a code. While she was out of the unit, her patient attempted to get out of bed, fell, and fractured her hip. She subsequently died, in part because of complications of her fall (pneumonia, decubitus development, sepsis). Her family sued and was awarded $500,000. The verdict was upheld on appeal. The hospital had a policy that required a nurse to be in "two places at one time," an impossible standard to meet.

A similar finding of negligence was found in an Arkansas case when a hospital failed to have sufficient nursing staff in a nursery to monitor newborns, HCA Health Services v. National Bank (1988). An unattended infant experienced a respiratory arrest and suffered permanent anoxic brain damage. The jury awarded $2 million in compensatory damages (for the cost of ongoing care) and $2 million in punitive damages for failing to provide an adequate number of qualified staff. The current nursing shortage is anticipated to grow in the first decade of this century. Nurses must develop a clear understanding of principles of safe staffing and advocate for appropriate staffing levels. Guidelines published by the American Nurses Association (1999) can assist nurses to ensure the efficient use of human resources and the delivery of quality care.

REDUCING LEGAL LIABILITY
Risk Management Systems

One of the most powerful allies the nurse has in any health care setting to facilitate positive change and reduce personal and corporate liability is the risk manager. The risk manager is a professional who tracks accidents and injuries that occur in the facility. The job of the risk manager is to establish and strengthen systems within the agency to reduce preventable patient injuries or deaths and to eliminate the loss of revenues as fines or the payment of damages through the insurance carrier. The risk manager may assist nurse managers in the development of effective policies and procedures to improve practice. Finally, the risk manager also is knowledgeable about federal and state administrative rules and regulations affecting health care systems, health care licensing laws, and health care case law. This knowledge is essential to prevent inadvertent violation of health care laws and to reduce claims of negligence and malpractice within the institution.

The Institute of Medicine (IOM) report, "To Err is Human" (2000), recommends a "proactive" approach to risk management. Nurses are encouraged to anticipate the potential for errors, report "near misses," and work closely with the risk manager to reduce preventable adverse events. All health care providers are urged to develop "high-reliability" operating systems. This concept is derived from the airline and nuclear energy industries. Both have established excellent safety records despite the highly complex and dangerous nature of their operations. The IOM recommends creation of a nationwide mandatory reporting system for collection of information about adverse events and the development of performance standards that focus on patient safety. Nurses will play a central role in this process.

Incident Reports

Nurses are legally bound to report critical incidents to their nurse managers, agency administration, and the risk manager through a formal, intraagency document generally entitled the "Unusual Occurrence" or "Incident Report." This form often is directed to the risk management department through the nurse's immediate manager. The nurse manager has an opportunity to review the written report and begin the process of risk control in a timely fashion, depending on the nature of the incident. The report then is forwarded (usually within 24 hours) to the risk manager. If an ongoing problem does not appear to be any closer to resolution as the nurse works through the formal chain of command, the nurse may speak directly to the risk manager for guidance and advice. However, in the usual course of events, the nurse would first address concerns with his or her immediate nurse manager.

Critical incidents that result in patient injury or death eventually may lead to a malpractice claim. Because state laws vary as to whether the incident report may be "discovered" by the plaintiff's attorney in a lawsuit, it is essential that the nurse follow appropriate procedures when completing and filing this document.

1. The nurse should describe all events objectively, avoid subjective comments, personal opinions about why the incident occurred, or assumptions about events that were not witnessed. For example, if a patient was found lying on the floor at the foot of his bed, the nurse should avoid the statement, "Patient fell out of bed—found on floor." That the patient fell out of bed is an unfounded assumption. The nurse should instead state, "Entered room. Patient discovered lying prone at the foot of the bed. Both upper and lower side rails were raised."

2. The nurse should never note in the patient's medical record that an incident report has been completed and filed. This may alter the protection from discovery normally provided the document in some states. The jury also will be made aware that an incident report has been filed because they have access to nurses' notes submitted in evidence during the trial.

3. The nurse should never photocopy the incident report for his or her personal files. Photocopying an incident report generally is prohibited by agency policy and may be expressly prohibited in writing on the incident report itself. Photocopying the incident report and taking it out of the agency violates patient confidentiality. It may fall into the hands of persons who are not authorized to read any information about the patient. It may fall into the hands of the plaintiff's attorney, should a lawsuit be filed, with damaging effects on the agency's ability to defend against the claims of negligence.

4. Physicians and advanced practice nurses should not write an order for an incident report to be filed. This brings the existence of an incident report to the attention of the plaintiff's attorney.

BOX 8-8	*Circumstances Under Which the Incident Report Should Be Filed**

- Patient or client injury
- Unanticipated patient death
- Malfunction or failure of durable medical equipment
- Significant or unanticipated adverse reactions to ordered therapy or care
- Inability to meet a patient's need(s) (ordered therapy, medications, treatments) after consultation with appropriate nurse mangers or providers. This may be related to:
  System problems (e.g., pharmacy closed, drug not available)
  Unresolved problem with order (e.g., incomplete or illegible order)
  Lack of qualified staff to implement order to provide needed care (e.g., RN not available to perform task, and law stipulates that only an RN may perform)
  Patient or family refusal of care (e.g., request for DNR orders)
- Unresolved problems with physical plant that jeopardize patient well-being (i.e., crack in floor, loose carpet section, delay in repair)
- Unethical, illegal, or incompetent practice that is witnessed
- Patient complaint about provider or health care worker
- Toxic spills, fires, other environmental emergencies
- Violent behavior on part of family or patient

*This list is not comprehensive but is a representative list of occurrences that should be reported.

5. Report every unusual occurrence or incident. Do not assume that "everyone knows about the problem or event."

Box 8-8 lists circumstances under which incident reports should be filed.

INTENTIONAL TORTS IN NURSING PRACTICE

Ordinarily, in the course of carrying out one's nursing duties, breaches in the applicable standard of care are assumed to be unintentional acts. In other words, the nurse did not intend to harm the patient. As noted, this civil wrong is referred to as an unintentional tort. An intentional tort is a second category of civil wrong. It involves the direct violation of a person's legal rights. In this case the nurse intends to perform the offensive act, although normally most nurses do not mean to harm the patient. The following acts are intentional torts.

- Assault
- Battery
- Defamation of character
- False imprisonment
- Invasion of privacy
- Intentional infliction of emotional distress

In the case of intentional torts, the plaintiff does not have to prove that the nurse breached a special duty or was negligent. The duty is implied in law (e.g., the duty to respect a patient's right to privacy). Generally, legal remedies for intentional torts include fines and punitive damages, although some intentional torts rise to the level of a criminal act (such as battery) and may result in a jail sentence. Some states such as California also have enacted penalties that include a term of imprisonment for willful and malicious breach of confidentiality in releasing information about a patient's human immunodeficiency virus (HIV) status.

Assault and Battery

Patients who agree to treatment or nursing care do not surrender their rights to determine who touches them. Assault is causing the person to fear that he or she will be touched without consent. Battery is the unauthorized or the actual harmful or offensive touching of a person. It is important to note that a charge of battery does not require proof of harm or injury. Nurses engaged in therapeutic procedures may face charges of battery if they touch the patient without his or her consent. It is essential that the nurse ask the patient's permission to proceed before initiating any procedure, particularly those of an invasive nature. Nurses also should document that the patient has given his or her permission for the treatment or procedure. Consider the following situation:

A woman in active labor cries out through each contraction. The nurse has a standing order from the obstetrician for administration of an intravenous narcotic should the woman request pain relief. However, the woman refuses, being determined to experience a medication-free birth. As labor progresses, the woman's cries become so loud that other laboring women and visitors in the unit express concern and anxiety. Repeated efforts to assist the woman with breathing and relaxation exercises to reduce her vocalization have failed. The nurse finally says to the patient, "Look, if you don't stop screaming and making those horrible noises, I'm going to give you the pain medication your doctor has ordered, whether you want it or not. You're frightening the other patients!" She repeats this threat several times and in the presence of the woman's family. Although the woman continues to cry out, the nurse does not give the medication. The delivery of the infant is uneventful and without problems. After discharge from the hospital, the patient retains a lawyer, claiming she was threatened with being sedated against her will. She further asserts that the nurse's repeated threats to inject her with a narcotic created an unbearable level of anxiety that interfered with her ability to cooperate with other necessary procedures during the birth. This assertion could result in a charge of negligence or intentional infliction of emotional distress.

In this case the nurse is charged with assault (i.e., threatening the patient with unauthorized touching). Had the nurse actually carried out her threat of giving the medication, the charge could be expanded to assault and battery. Consequences for the nurse charged with assault may include:

- Imposition of fines and punitive damages
- State board of nursing disciplinary action
- Termination by the employer

When battery occurs, the nature of the touching may raise the offense to the level of a crime. In the aforementioned scenario, assume that the nurse decides to give the narcotic against the woman's will. She engages the assistance of a scrub technician to physically restrain the woman so that she can access a vein for the injection. The technician, becoming frustrated with the woman's resistance to the procedure, says, "You're going to be sorry if you don't stop struggling." The technician purposefully hyperextends the woman's arm and says, "There, maybe if it hurts enough, you'll stop this nonsense." A loud snapping sound is heard, and tests indicate that the technician has fractured the woman's arm. The charge of battery in this case may result in more serious ramifications, including punitive damages and a term of imprisonment. Both of these cases are fact-based events known to me. Unfortunately, similar cases are noted in the nursing and legal literature each month.

Defamation of Character

A person has a right to be free from attacks on his or her reputation (defamation of character). Libel is one form of defamation caused by written work. Slander refers to an injury to one's reputation caused by the spoken word. Nurses may be subject to a charge of libel for subjective comments meant to denigrate the patient that are placed in the medical record or in other written materials read by others. For example, a patient suffering from extreme pain who requested narcotics frequently was labeled as a "whiner," a "liar," and a "drug seeker" with an "addictive" personality. These comments were noted on the medical record, the nursing kardex, and in nurse's notes attached to a clipboard, which was kept on a wall peg outside of the patient's room.

The patient subsequently was found to have a severe intraabdominal infection that accounted for the intense pain he experienced. The patient sued for failure of the medical staff to identify and treat the infection. In the process of discovery, the patient, his family, and the attorney he had retained read the defamatory comments about his character. It was a distinct possibility that other family members, co-workers, and the patient's employer who visited may have read these subjective comments on the clipboard. A charge of libel was leveled against the nursing staff.

Nurses also may face charges of slander when they repeat similar types of subjective comments about patients in public places such as elevators or hospital cafeterias. All patient care staff must be extremely cautious about discussing the patient or their opinions about the patient in public places. Even in report rooms or conference rooms, nurses should consider who in the immediate vicinity could inadvertently overhear the conversation. Only objective, professional language should be used in discussing patients in all circumstances.

False Imprisonment

False imprisonment is defined as the unlawful restraint or detention of another person against his or her wishes. Actual force is not necessary to support a charge of false imprisonment. An adult of sound mind (mentally competent) has a right to refuse any treatment that has previously been agreed to (Klepatsky and Mahlmeister, 1997). If he or she refuses, the person can leave the facility (i.e., hospital, rehabilitation center, long-term care facility) whenever he or she chooses. The nurse has no authority to detain the patient, even if there is a likelihood of harm or injury as a result of discontinuing therapy.

Intentional Infliction of Emotional Distress

When the nurse's behavior is so outrageous that it leads to the emotional shock of another, the court can compensate the patient for emotional distress.

Invasion of Privacy

Another basic right is to be free from interference with one's personal life. An invasion of privacy occurs when a person's private affairs (including health history and status) is made public without consent. The nurse has a legal and ethical duty to maintain patient confidentiality, and there may be serious repercussions when the nurse breaches this duty and violates this fundamental patient right.

With the explosion in electronic information systems, issues related to patient confidentiality and invasion of privacy are now being addressed by the federal and state legislatures. Statutes have been enacted to control access to electronic health data. Nurses are given passwords to access the patient's electronic medical record. Nurses should never share passwords with colleagues because this increases the risk of unauthorized access to the patient record.

In certain circumstances the law permits divulging information contained in the patient's medical record. These situations include reporting certain communicable diseases, child abuse, and gunshot wounds to the proper authorities. If a nurse is asked to provide information to any sources, the matter should immediately be referred to the agency's administrator or risk manager. In no case should the nurse personally divulge the information or provide copies of the patient's record to another person or agency. Another fact-based case known to me illustrates the intentional torts of invasion of privacy and intentional infliction of emotional distress. Consider the following situation:

A nurse works in a physician's office in a small, semi-rural community. The majority of the town's residents know each other. A patient being treated for several opportunistic infections has an HIV test performed. The nurse also is aware that the patient has been questioned by the physician about his sexual activities and that he has divulged that he is gay and has had unprotected sex with several male partners. When the test results are reported as positive, the nurse calls several close friends (who also know the patient) and reports the finding and information about the patient's sexual conduct. Before the patient is informed about his diagnosis by the physician, the man encounters two of the people who have been told about the HIV test result. They tell him that they know he is gay and infected with the HIV virus. He then discovers that the nurse has informed them about his condition. Suffering from intense shock and emotional pain, the man unsuccessfully attempts suicide.

In this case, the nurse's actions rise to the level of willful, malicious, and intentional infliction of emotional distress. The nurse faces serious charges and, in some states with HIV confidentiality laws, could face a prison sentence for intentionally violating the patient's confidentiality in a manner meant to harm the patient. It is likely that the nurse's license also will be revoked for her actions, and the board may impose a significant fine.

THE NURSE AND CRIMINAL LAW

A crime is an offense against society, defined through written criminal statutes or codes. A criminal act is deemed to be conduct so offensive that the state is responsible for prosecuting the offending individual on behalf of society. Legal remedies for crimes include fines, imprisonment, and, in some states, execution (death penalty). Criminal acts are classified as either minor (misdemeanors) or major (felonies) offenses. Common misdemeanor offenses that nurses are charged with include:

- Illegal practice of medicine.
- Failing to report child or elder abuse.
- Falsification of the patient's medical record.
- Assault and battery and physical abuse of patients.

Felony acts may be committed against the federal government and generally involve drug trafficking offenses and, increasingly, fraud in billing for services of Medicare patients. Other serious criminal acts include theft, rape, and murder. A nurse found guilty of a felony generally serves time in prison and usually suffers the permanent revocation of his or her nursing license. Five registered nurses were indicted on 21 counts, including falsification of records, alteration of forms filed with the state department of health, and tampering with physical evidence in the death of a 97-year-old nursing home patient (Kelley, 2000). The woman died after being fed through a stomach tube attached to an enema bag. The nurses used the enema bag in lieu of the appropriate feeding receptacle because the proper receptacle was not available.

In another interesting case discussed by Fiesta (1994), an RN was charged by the state of New York with four misdemeanor counts of physically abusing residents in a nursing home. The abuse included pushing, slapping, and striking elderly residents in the facility. She subsequently was convicted on all four counts and fined $3000 by the court. She was placed on 3 years' probation, during which time she could not practice nursing. However, under federal law conviction of patient abuse results in a minimum 5-year exclusion from participating or working in Medicare and Medicaid programs. The state-imposed penalty of 3 years during which time the nurse was not permitted to work was superseded by the federal law, which extended that time to 5 years.

THE LAW AND PATIENT RIGHTS
Advance Directives

Society now recognizes the individual's right to die with dignity rather than be kept alive indefinitely by artificial life support. As a consequence, the majority of states have enacted "right-to-die" laws. These statutes grant competent adults the right to refuse extraordinary medical treatment when there is no hope of recovery. The term *advance directive* refers to an individual's desires regarding end-of-life care. These wishes generally are made through the execution of a formal document known as the "living will." Right-to-die statutes vary from state to state; therefore nurses must become familiar with their state-specific statute. Agency policies and procedures in the nurse's employment setting also will guide the nurse in an understanding of the patient's rights in this matter.

Living Wills. A living will is a formal document, a type of advance directive, in which a competent adult makes known his or her wishes regarding care that will be provided in the final stages of a terminal illness. A living will generally contains the following.
1. Designation of the individual (proxy or surrogate) who is permitted to make decisions once the patient is decisionally incapacitated
2. Specific stipulations regarding what care is acceptable and which procedures or treatments are not to be implemented
3. Authorization of the patient's physician to withhold or discontinue certain life-sustaining procedures under specific conditions

Although living wills are legal in every state, they may not be legally binding. In some cases a proxy is not recognized or sanctioned by the state statute. Living wills have been overturned, particularly when disputes arise among family members or significant others when the terminally ill patient is no longer able to make decisions. A living will may be revoked under any of the following conditions.
- Evidence that the patient was not competent when the living will was executed
- The patient's condition is not terminal
- A state-imposed time for enforcement of the will has expired, and a new living will must be executed
- The patient's condition has changed substantially, and the stipulations of the will no longer apply

A living will must be written (in some cases using a state-specific document), dated, signed, and witnessed. If asked to witness a patient's living will, the nurse should refer the matter to the agency's risk manager. It may not be lawful in a particular state for the nurse to witness this document.

Medical or Physician Directives and "Do Not Resuscitate" Orders. A more specific type of living will that the patient may execute is known as the medical or physician directive. This document lists the desire of the patient in a particular scenario, such as whether he or she would want to be resuscitated if cardiopulmonary arrest occurs. "Do Not Resuscitate" (DNR) orders would be written by the physician based on written medical directives dictated by the patient. The medical directive, if properly executed, provides the physician with immunity from claims of negligence or intentional wrong-doing in the patient's death. The physician must also follow any state-specific statute and the agency's policies and procedures before writing a DNR order.

The nurse has an absolute duty to respect the patient's wishes in the case of DNR orders. A lawfully executed DNR order must be followed. Nurses have been sued for failure to observe DNR orders (Tammelleo, 1997). Claims against the nurse include battery, negligent infliction of pain and suffering, and "wrongful life" (Anderson v. St. Francis–St. George Hospital, 1992). When questions arise regarding the appropriateness of the DNR order or if the patient or a family member wishes the DNR order rescinded, the nurse must act promptly. The nurse should document the patient's or family's comments and immediately inform the physician and nurse manager. A patient may revoke a living will, including a DNR order, at any time.

Durable Power of Attorney for Health Care. An increasing number of health care law experts recommend that persons interested in writing a living will also seek legal assistance with executing a durable power of attorney for health care. This document authorizes the patient to name the person who will make the day-to-day and final end-of-life decisions once he or she is decisionally incompetent. With the current limitations in living wills, several states have enacted a "Uniform Durable Power of Attorney Act," which sanctions a durable power of attorney for health care. Living wills always require some degree of interpretation. Naming a proxy who is intimately knowledgeable about the person's true wishes is important to ensure that one's wishes will be carried out when he or she is no longer able to make decisions.

Nurses may be asked questions about living wills and durable power of attorney for health care by patients and their families. An important aspect of speaking to the patient about these issues is to provide the written materials about advance directives that are required under the federal statute, the Patient Self-Determination Act.

Informed Consent

For any patient to make meaningful choices about a particular procedure or treatment, the provider must convey certain material information. Under the doctrine of informed consent, the physician or advanced practice nurse has a duty to disclose information so that the patient can make intelligent decisions. This duty is mandated by federal statute (in the case of Medicare and Medicaid patients) and state law and is grounded as well in common law. In the case of both routine and specialized care, the primary provider must disclose the following.

- Nature of the therapy or procedure
- Expected benefits and outcomes of the therapy or procedure
- Potential risks of the therapy or procedure
- Alternative therapies to the intended procedure and their risks and benefits
- Risks of not having the procedure

This duty to disclose rests with the provider and cannot be delegated to the RN. When the nurse has reason to believe that the patient has not given informed consent for a procedure, the provider should be immediately notified. In no case should the nurse proceed with initiating any part of the therapy that he or she is responsible for implementing. The patient's questions or concerns should be documented in the medical record to indicate why there has been a delay in carrying out the procedure (Klepatsky and Mahlmeister, 1997). If the nurse is responsible for witnessing the patient's signature on a consent form for the specified procedure, this process also should be deferred until the provider has had an opportunity to clarify the patient's questions.

A variety of negligence claims arise out of the informed consent process. The provider may be alleged negligent for failure to obtain informed consent. Court decisions generally have upheld the provider's duty to obtain informed consent and have dismissed cases that have claimed hospitals and its nurses were negligent for "failing to obtain informed consent" (Kelley v. Kitahama, 1996). With adoption in some states of the corporate negligence doctrine, an increasing number of appellate courts have ruled that hospitals and nurses may be liable for failure to obtain informed consent (Keel v. St. Elizabeth Medical Center, 1992; Karibjanian v. Thomas Jefferson University Hospital, 1989).

In all cases, the reasonable and prudent nurse would be expected to notify the provider promptly when questions arise about whether the patient has given informed consent. In no case should the nurse attempt to convey information required for informed consent. As noted, providing information about the therapy remains the responsibility of the provider. Physicians have sued nurses for attempting to give the patient information, alleging interference with the patient–physician relationship, or for giving false or misleading information to the patient.

The Right to Refuse Treatment

As noted previously, an adult of sound mind has a right to refuse any treatment that has previously been agreed to. A recent Connecticut Supreme Court decision affirmed the fundamental right of adults to refuse medical treatment. In the case, Stamford Hospital v. Vega (1996), a woman who hemorrhaged after the birth of her infant refused blood on the grounds that it violated her beliefs as a Jehovah's Witness. The hospital obtained an emergency court order authorizing the facility to administer blood. The woman survived and was discharged in good health. Although it was a moot point (the blood already had been given), the family appealed the initial court decision authorizing the blood transfusion. The Supreme Court decided to hear the case and reversed the lower court's decision, stating the hospital did not have a right to substitute its decision for that of the patient.

If a patient under the nurse's care refuses treatment, the nurse has a duty to notify the primary provider. The same principles pertaining to the informed consent process apply to situations when the patient refuses care. The physician or advanced practice nurse should provide the patient with information about the consequences, risks, and benefits of refusing therapy. The provider also must explore any alternative treatments that may be available to the patient. Hospitals have a right to seek a judicial review when patients refuse specific types of lifesaving treatments, but current case law falls squarely in favor of the patient's right to self-determination.

Leaving Against Medical Advice. If a patient intends to leave the facility without a written order, the nurse also must act promptly to notify the provider. When circumstances suggest that the person may suffer immediate physical harm, the nurse must clearly articulate the dangers inherent in leaving. In the case of a competent elder, prompt notification of the immediate family also would be a reasonable and prudent action. The nurse should document all these actions and any communication with the aforementioned parties.

Almost all health care facilities have a document commonly known as the "Against Medical Advice" (AMA) form. Patients are asked to sign the AMA form when they decide to refuse or discontinue ordered therapy or intend to leave the facility. The value of the document in countering a claim of negligence should the patient or family later sue will depend in great part on the quality of the nurse's charting. A common allegation made in this case is that the patient was not fully apprised of the risks inherent in leaving the facility. If the primary provider has not arrived before the patient leaves, the nurse's notes should reflect the specific advice given the patient. Leaving the facility could:

- Aggravate the current condition and complicate future care.
- Result in permanent physical or mental impairment or disability.
- Result in complications leading to death.

This precautionary statement is reserved for situations in which the life and limb of the patient are at risk and the appropriate providers (physicians or advanced practice nurses) are not available to address the direct and indirect consequences with the patient.

Nurses have been charged with a variety of offenses when unlawfully detaining patients, including assault, battery, and false imprisonment (Snyder, 2001). These charges generally arise when well-meaning nurses try to prevent the patient from carrying out his or her intent. Actions that lead to a claim of false imprisonment include applying restraints, refusing to give the patient his or her clothes or access to a telephone, intimidating the patient by assigning a security person to guard his or her room, and sedating the patient against his or her will. As can be expected, in addition to civil penalties, the nurse faces disciplinary action by the licensing board when charges of false imprisonment are reported to the board.

The Use of Physical Restraints

One last, but equally important, area of patient rights to be discussed in this chapter is the right of a competent adult to be free of restraint. Even patients with mental illness cannot be incarcerated or restrained without due process, and the institution must have the treatment and rehabilitation services necessary to reintegrate the individual into society (*Nurse's Legal Handbook*, 2000). Restraint of any kind is a form of imprisonment; and the reasonable and prudent nurse will closely adhere to all laws, rules, and policies pertaining to the use of restraints. The goal when restraints are clinically indicated is to use the least restrictive restraint and only when all other strategies to ensure patient safety have been exhausted. Patients may never be restrained physically or chemically because there are not enough staff to properly monitor them. Nurses have a legal and ethical duty to report institutions or individuals who violate patient rights through unlawful restraint.

As noted previously, one of the most common allegations leveled against nurses is a failure to ensure patient safety. Nurses in many practice settings must balance the right of patients to unrestricted control of their bodies and movements against the need to keep vulnerable patients safe from harm. The use of physical restraints such as vests, mittens, belts, and wrist restraints; chemical restraints; and seclusion are all governed by federal and state statutes and accrediting bodies such as the Joint Commission on Accreditation of Healthcare Organizations (JCAHO). Many nurses do not realize that even use of bed rails and chair trays falls under the category of physical restraints; these articles may not be used indiscriminately.

Violation of restraint statutes and the administrative rules and regulations promulgated to enact these laws can result in stiff penalties. The institution can lose its Medicare contract (decertification) and its JCAHO accreditation, effectively putting it out of business. Patients and family members may initiate civil suits for unlawful restraints, resulting in monetary damages if the plaintiff succeeds in the suit. Charges of assault and battery and false imprisonment may be leveled against nurses who use restraints improperly.

Based on the aforementioned information, some nurses are under the misconception that current law prohibits restraining patients until a written order is obtained. Nurses may lawfully apply restraints in an emergency, when in their independent judgment no other strategies are effective in protecting the patient from harm. The physician must be contacted promptly to discuss the patient's condition, and the need to restrain and to obtain an order for temporary continuance of restraints. The nurse is guided in the decision to restrain by knowledge of the laws, the agency's policies and procedures, qualifications of the staff, and conditions on the unit or in the department.

Careful nursing documentation is essential when restraints are applied. The patient's mental and physical status must be assessed at close and regular intervals as prescribed by law and the agency's policies. The chart must reflect these assessments and the frequency with which restraints are removed. Neurovascular and skin assessments of limbs or other body parts covered by the restraints also must be entered in the medical record. Written physician orders for restraints must be timed and dated, and renewal of orders must be accompanied by evidence of medical evaluations and nursing reassessments.

SUMMARY

Professional nursing practice is governed by an ever-widening circle of federal and state statutes and is constantly evolving in great part because of an accumulating body of nursing case law. The law provides guidance for every aspect of practice and can assist the nurse in managing the complexities of practice in a rapidly changing health care system. Knowledge is power, and the nurse who possesses a sound understanding of the law as it pertains to professional practice is empowered. Box 8-9 presents a list of Internet resources to learn more about legal issues.

This chapter has reviewed the major sources and categories of law influencing nursing practice. The reader has been introduced to the doctrines of civil and criminal law that impact all nurses. The chapter has explored issues related to the legal "rights" of the patients and clients who are served by professional nurses. As patient advocates, all nurses should keep these fundamental rights uppermost in their minds as they attempt to provide safe, effective, quality care in all settings.

BOX 8-9	*Helpful Websites*

American Association of Legal Nurse Consultants
www.aalnc.org.
Provides information about legal nurse consultants:
credentialing process, standards of practice,
publications networking opportunities, continuing
education

American Society for Healthcare Risk Management
www.ashrm.org
Provides information to consumers and members
about risk management and risk control in
health care settings; Publications; News
regarding health care laws and regulations

Federal Food and Drug Administration
www.fda.gov
Provides information about adverse events related
to medication administration and use of durable
medical equipment

Joint Commission for Accreditation of Healthcare
Organizations
www.jcaho.org
Provides information regarding health care
standards, sentinel event alerts, related health
care law

National Council of State Boards of Nursing
www.ncsbn.org
Provides general information regarding nursing
practice, nursing practice act; position
statements regarding nursing conduct such as
delegation of nursing tasks

The American Association of Nurse Attorneys
www.taana.org
Website of the association of nurse attorneys;
provides information on select laws; provides
guidance for nurses interested becoming
attorneys

Centers for Medicare and Medicaid Services (CMS)
(formerly the Health Care Financing
Administration [HCFA])
www.hcfa.gov/about/agency
Provides information a wide range of health care
law, Medicare program; offers access to other
websites in health care law

Critical Thinking Activities

1. The nurse is asked to implement a new, complex, and invasive procedure and is concerned that it may violate the state's Nursing Practice Act. What are the logical steps to take to clarify the legal scope of nursing practice in this case? In what order should the nurse proceed?

2. A nurse who works the night shift in an Emergency Department is told to prepare a pregnant woman in labor for transport to a high-risk perinatal center. The nurse is aware that there is an "anti-dumping" law governing transfer of Emergency Department patients and is unsure if this transport is lawful. How can the nurse quickly determine the lawfulness of this transport at 3 o'clock in the morning? What resources would the nurse access for information? How would the nurse prioritize the process of obtaining clarification?

3. A nurse in an ambulatory setting administers a prescribed antibiotic. The "five rights" of medication administration are observed. The patient, who has no known allergies, experiences an anaphylactic reaction. He is skillfully resuscitated and promptly transported to the nearest hospital. Unfortunately he suffers permanent hypoxic brain damage and severe disability. The family sues the clinic,

physician, and nurse. What evidence must the plaintiff's attorney provide to prove the nurse was negligent? Can it be done? Why or why not? Explore the concepts of negligence and malpractice in this case to validate your answer.

4. A home health care agency hires a pediatric nurse case manager for children with severe disabilities. They require 24-hour skilled nursing care by licensed professionals. The agency bills the insurance company (or government) for skilled nursing care. One day the case manager makes an unscheduled visit to the home of a client. She finds an unlicensed home health care aide providing technologically complex care requiring nursing judgment. She is told by the aide, "They just couldn't find a nurse today, and I've had a crash course in how to manage this child just in case we didn't have a nurse." What further information would the nurse need in this situation? What must be done, and in what order of priority? What laws must the nurse defer to in this case? What is the RN's liability in the situation? The agency's? The nurse aide's?

5. At change of shift a nurse working days in a nursing home is told by the night nurse, "Mr. Jones is always tied in a vest restraint at night, just to make sure he doesn't get out of bed and fall, but he's really upset. He just doesn't understand it's for his own good." The nurse quickly reviews Mr. Jones' record. He is noted to be a competent, compliant adult, without a psychiatric history or evidence of mental disorientation. He takes no medications that would alter his mentation. When the nurse enters the room, Mr. Jones is weeping. He states, "I feel like a criminal being tied up. I've urinated in my bed because no one answered my call light. I'm so humiliated." What is the relationship between Mr. Jones' right to self-determination in this case vs. the need to protect patients from harm? How does the law guide the nurse in this situation? Are there civil liability issues related to restraining this patient? What charges could be leveled against the nurse for restraint? Could the nurse be sued for not restraining Mr. Jones in this case? Would staffing levels influence the legal right of nurses to restrain patients?

REFERENCES

Aikin T: *Legal, ethical, and political issues in nursing,* Philadelphia, 1994, FA Davis.

Aikins v. St. Helena Hospital, 843 F. Supp. 1329 (ND Cal, 1994).

American Association of Critical Care Nurses: *Delegation: a tool for success in the changing workplace,* Aliso Viejo, CA, 1995, AACN.

American Medical Association: *Code of medical ethics,* Chicago, 1994, AMA.

American Nurses Association: *Code for nurses,* Washington, DC, 1995, ANA.

American Nurses Association: *Protect your patient—protect your license,* Washington, DC, 1995, ANA.

American Nurses Association: *Registered professional nurses and unlicensed assistive personnel,* ed 2, Washington, DC, 1996, ANA.

American Nurses Association: *Principles for nurse staffing,* Washington, DC, 1999, ANA

Anderson v. St. Francis-St. George Hospital, 614 N.E. 2d 841 (OH, 1992).

Bernzweig E: *The nurse's liability for malpractice,* ed 6, St Louis, 1996, Mosby.

Booth D, Carruth A: Violations of the nursing practice act, *Nurs Manage* 29(10):35-40, 1998.

Carroll M: Nursing malpractice and corporate negligence: how is the standard of care determined? *J Nurs Law* 3(3):53-60, 1996.

Casaubon D, Sparks R: Patient dumping and EMTALA: How does it apply to you? *J Nurs Law* 7(2):35-41, 2000.

Chin v. St. Barnabas Medical Center, No. L11457-92 (NJ Super Ct Nov. 21, 1996).

Concern in Texas: NSO Risk Advisor 2, 1995.

Convalescent Services, Inc. v. Schultz, 921 S.W. 2d 731 (Tex App, 1996).

Dickerson v. Fatehi, 84 S.E. 2d 880 (VA, 1997).

Fiesta J: Failing to act like a professional, *Nurs Manage* 25(7):15-17, 1994.

Francis v. Memorial General Hospital, 726 P 2d 852 (NM, 1986).

Freeman G: Nurse reports suspicions to manager, but no action taken on OB-GYN's care, *OB-GYN Malpractice Prevention* 2(11):84-85, 1995.

Gardner S, Hagedorn M: Holding nurses accountable, *Lifelines* 1(2):55-56, 1997.

HCA Health Services v. National Bank, 745 S.W. 2d 120 (AR, 1988).

Heinrich v. Conemaugh Valley Memorial Hospital, 648 A. 2d 53 (PA, 1994).

Holston v. Sisters of the Third Order, 650 N.E. 2d 985 (IL, 1995).

Hytha M: Nurses' strike tops long list of Kaiser woes, *San Francisco Chronicle,* July 17, 1997, pp A1, A11.

Institute of Medicine: *To err is human: building a safer health system,* Washington, DC, 2000, National Academy Press.

Justin and Michelle Malovic v. Santa Monica Hospital Medical Center, Los Angeles County Superior Court, Case No SC019 167 (CA, 1995).

Karibjanian v. Thomas Jefferson University Hospital, 717 F. Supp. 1081, 1083-84 (ED Pa, 1989).

Keel v. St. Elizabeth Medical Center, 842 S.W. 2d 869 (KY, 1992).

Kelley T: Death at a nursing home leads to indictment of five, *New York Times,* November 7, 2000, p B-1.

Kelley v. Kitahama, 675 So. 2d 1181 (La App, 1996).

Klepatsky A, Mahlmeister L: Consent and informed consent in perinatal and neonatal settings, *J Perinat Neonat Nurs* 11(1):34-51, 1997.

Kreplick J: Unlicensed hospital assistive personnel: Efficiency or liability? Part II, *J Nurs Law* 3(2):7-21, 1996.

Kowalski K, Horner M: A legal nightmare: Denver nurses indicted, *MCN* 23(3):125-129, 1998.

LaDuke S: When the blaming stops: lessons in risk management, *J Nurs Law* 6(2):23-32, 1999.

Lagana K: The "right" to a caring relationship: the law and ethic of care, *J Perinat Neonat Nurs* 14(2):12-24, 2000.

Laughlin S: Criminal charges for clinical errors: advanced practice nurse liability, *J Nurs Law* 5(2):65-74, 1998.

Mahlmeister L: A positive approach to managing short staffing, *Excellence Nurs Admin* 1(3):1-2, 2000a.

Mahlmeister L: The process of triage in perinatal settings: clinical and legal issues, *J Perinat Neonat Nurs* 13(4):13-30, 2000b.

Mahlmeister L: Professional accountability and legal liability for the team leader and charge nurse, *JOGNN* 28(3):300-309, 1999.

Mahlmeister L: When cost-saving strategies are unacceptable, *Pediatr Nurs* 22(2):130-132, 1996.

Malugani M: Nurse, interrupted, *Nurseweek,* 13(18):1, 26-27: 2000.

Manning v. Twin Falls Clinic and Hospital, 830 P. 2d 1185 (ID, 1992).

Merritt v. Karcloglu, 668 So. 2d 469 (LA, 1996).

Morrison D et al: Should nurses purchase their own professional liability insurance? *MCN* 23(3):122-123, 1998.

Moy M: *The EMTALA answer book,* Gaithersburg, Md, 1999, Aspen Publishers.

National Council of State Boards of Nursing: *Delegation: concepts and decision-making process,* Chicago, 1995, NCSBN.

Negron v. Snoqualmie Valley Hospital, 936 P. 2d 55 (Wash App, 1997).

Nurse's legal handbook, ed 2, Springhouse, Pa, 2000, Springhouse Corporation.

Rhodes A: Locating case law, *MCN* 19(2):107, 1994.

Roberts v. Galen of Virginia, Inc., 111 F. 3d 405 (6th Cir, 1997).

Rodebush v. Oklahoma Nursing Homes, Ltd., 867 P. 2d 1241 (OK, 1993).

Rostant D, Cady R: *Liability issues in perinatal nursing,* Philadelphia, 1999, JB Lippincott.

Schreiber C: Playing the numbers: effects of California nurse ratio bill are yet to be seen, *Nurseweek* 13(4):34-35, 2000.

Shelton v. Penrose/St. Francis Healthcare, 984 P.2d 623 (CO, 1999).

Singleton v. AAA Home Health, Inc., WL 1693814, So.2d (LA, 2000).

Smith-Pittman M: Nursing and the corporate negligence doctrine, *J Nurs Law* 4(2):41-50, 1997.

Smith-Pittman M: Nurses and litigation, *J Nurs Law* 5(2):7-19, 1998.

Snyder E: Automatic blood pressure cuff: Nurses ignored the patient, committed battery, *Legal Eagle Eye Newsletter for the Nursing Profession* 9(4):1, 2001.

Snyder E: Chain of command: court rules nurses should have gone over doctor's head, *Legal Eagle Eye Newsletter for the Nursing Profession* 8(2):1, 2000.

Snyder E: EMTALA: the act applies when an emergency arises in the hospital, court rules, *Legal Eagle Eye Newsletter for the Nursing Profession* 6(8):3, 1999.

Stamford Hospital v. Vega, 674 A. 2d 821 (CT, 1996).

Stein T: On the defensive: more patients are naming nurses in malpractice suits, *Nurseweek* 13(11):1, 7, 2000.

Tammelleo A: Are nurses often used as individual defendants? *Regan Report Nurs Law* 37(7):4, 1996.

Tammelleo A: Malpractice insurance: for your protection, *RN* 60(10):73, 75-77, 1997.

Tammelleo A: Nurse's failure to call for physician or supervisor, *Regan Report Nurs Law* 40(10):1, 2000

Trandel-Korenchuk D, Trandel-Korenchuk K: Gaithersburg, Md, 1997, Aspen Publishers.

Thompson v. Nason Hospital, 591 A. 2d 703, 707 (PA, 1991).

Weiss J: Nursing practice: a legal and historical perspective, *J Nurs Law* 2(1):17-36, 1995.

When and how do you tell patients about mistakes? *Healthcare Risk Manage* 19(5):54-55, 1997.

Winkelman v. Beloit Memorial Hospital, 483 N.W. 2d 211 (WI, 1992).

Utter v. United Hospital Center, Inc., 236 S.E. 2d 213 (W. Va 1977).

Ethical and Bioethical Issues in Nursing and Health Care

Carla D. Sanderson, PhD, RN

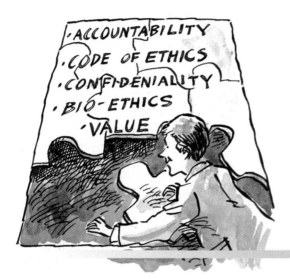

Ethical dilemmas are
the puzzles of life.

Vignette

Melinda Stone has been assigned to care for an intensive care unit (ICU) patient, an 80-year-old woman who is being sustained by mechanical ventilation after respiratory distress associated with pneumonia. Melinda and the patient formed a meaningful relationship during the patient's periods off the ventilator. Melinda now must grapple with what she knows to be her patient's wishes for end-of-life care, wishes inconsistent with those of her family.

Questions to consider while reading this chapter
1. How will ethical and bioethical issues in nursing and health care affect my professional nursing practice?
2. What ethical theories ahd principles serve as a basis for nursing practice?
3. How can I assist patients and families who face difficult ethical decisions?

Key Terms

Accountability An ethical duty stating that one should be answerable legally, morally, ethically, or socially for one's activities.

Autonomy Personal freedom and right to make choices.

Beneficence An ethical principle stating that one should do good and prevent or avoid doing harm.

Bioethics The study of ethical problems resulting from scientific advances.

Code of ethics Set of statements encompassing rules that apply to people in professional roles.

Deontology An ethical theory that states that moral rule is binding.

Ethics Science or study of moral values.

Nonmaleficence An ethical principle stating the duty not to inflict harm.

Utilitarianism An ethical theory that holds that the best decision is one that brings about the greatest good for the most people.

Values Ideas of life, customs, and ways of behaving that society regards desirable.

Veracity An ethical duty to tell the truth.

Learning Outcomes

After studying this chapter, the reader will be able to:

1. Integrate basic concepts of human valuing that are essential for ethical decision making.
2. Analyze selected ethical theories and principles as a basis for ethical decision making.
3. Analyze the relationship between ethics and morality in relation to nursing practice.
4. Use an ethical decision-making framework for resolving ethical problems in health care.
5. Apply the ethical decision-making process to specific ethical issues encountered in clinical practice.

CHAPTER OVERVIEW

In a nursing education program, educators can only begin to introduce the nursing student to the complex and dynamic profession of nursing. Prelicensure nursing education is only an introduction to a discipline in which there are no knowledge boundaries. The abundance of nursing practice information is clear from a quick glance across the nursing textbook shelves in the college bookstore.

Most of that information addresses the "how to" aspects of nursing care. The scientific aspects of nursing care are evolving more rapidly than ever as a host of nurse researchers delve into questions about the safe, competent, and therapeutic aspects of professional nursing care. As quickly as nursing science produces new nursing knowledge, "how to" information is shared through professional journals, textbooks, and electronically through on-line Internet resources. The scientific aspects of care for someone like the elderly woman described in the opening vignette are evolving constantly through "how to" research.

A myriad of potential questions that surpass the "how to" body of knowledge are inherent in the patient care situation presented in the vignette. Everywhere in today's health care delivery system are potential questions of another nature—the "how should" questions. "How should" questions sound something like this.

- How should I determine the competency of my acutely ill 80-year-old patient? Is her competency intact? How should I gain her informed consent?
- How should I act if it is determined that her wishes for aggressive care are not consistent with those of her family?
- How should I view her care? Is a resuscitation effort for an 80-year-old considered ordinary and routine, or is it considered extraordinary and heroic?
- How should I respond to her in the middle of the night when she awakens to ask me if she is dying?
- How much of the truth is warranted?

- How should I decide when the availability of ICU beds becomes threatened and the decision must be made to move someone out of ICU to make room for a new trauma patient?
- How should I make staffing assignments when the number of nurses on a given shift is insufficient to provide routine ICU care to all?
- Is the life of this 80-year-old woman any less significant than that of the 40-year-old father-of-four executive who has just been admitted after a tragic car accident?
- How should I feel when this 80-year-old patient is entered into a research study designed to test a new beta-blocker that has previously only been tested on a middle-age population?

This chapter introduces the nursing student to a different aspect of nursing care, this "how should" aspect or, as it is more appropriately called, the ethical aspect. Ethics is a system for deciding, based on principles, what should be done. Socrates once said, "The unexamined life is not worth living." Ethics is about examining life in a way that will add a dimension to the understanding that goes beyond the scientific and moves toward a more complete and whole understanding of human existence.

NURSING ETHICS

Nursing ethics is a system of principles concerning the actions of the nurse in his or her relationships with patients, patients' family members, other health care providers, policy makers, and society as a whole. A profession is characterized by its relationship to society. Codes of ethics provide implicit standards and values for the professions. A nursing code of ethics was first intro-

---

BOX 9-1	*American Nurses Association Code of Ethics*

- The nurse, in all professional relationships, practices with compassion and respect for the inherent dignity, worth, and uniqueness of every individual, unrestricted by considerations of social or economic status, personal attributes, or the nature of health problems.
- The nurse's primary commitment is to the patient, whether an individual, family, group, or community.
- The nurse promotes, advocates for, and strives to protect the health, safety, and rights of the patient.
- The nurse is responsible and accountable for individual nursing practice and determines the appropriate delegation of tasks consistent with the nurse's obligation to provide optimum patient care.
- The nurse owes the same duties to self as to others, including the responsibility to preserve integrity and safety, to maintain competence, and to continue personal and professional growth.
- The nurse participates in establishing, maintaining, and improving health care environments and conditions of employment conducive to the provision of quality health care and consistent with the values of the profession through individual and collective action.
- The nurse participates in the advancement of the profession through contributions to practice, education, administration, and knowledge development.
- The nurse collaborates with other professionals and the public in promoting community, national, and international efforts to meet health needs.
- The profession of nursing, as represented by associations and their members, is responsible for articulating nursing values, for maintaining the integrity of the profession and its practice, and for shaping social policy.

duced in the late nineteenth century and has evolved through the years as the profession itself has evolved and as changes in society and health have come about. Current dynamics such as emerging genetic interventions and new threats to the effective delivery of health care such as managed care and impending nursing shortages bring nursing's code of ethics into the forefront. Box 9-1 illustrates the American Nurses Association (ANA) nursing code of ethics, which was recently updated in 2001. Another nursing code of ethics is illustrated in Box 9-2.

BOX 9-2 | *International Council of Nurses Code for Nurses*

- The fundamental responsibility of the nurse is fourfold: to promote health, to prevent illness, to restore health, and to alleviate suffering.
- The need for nursing is universal. Inherent in nursing is respect for life, dignity, and rights of humans. It is unrestricted by considerations of nationality, race, creed, color, age, sex, politics, or social status.
- Nurses render health services to the individual, the family, and the community and coordinate their services with those of related groups.

Nurses and people
- The nurse's primary responsibility is to those people who require nursing care.
- The nurse, in providing care, promotes an environment in which the values, customs, and spiritual beliefs of the patient are respected.
- The nurse holds in confidence personal information and uses judgment in sharing this information.

Nurses and practice
- The nurse carries personal responsibility for nursing practice and for maintaining competence by continual learning. The nurse maintains the highest standards of nursing care possible within the reality of a specific situation.
- The nurse uses judgment in relation to individual competence when accepting and delegating responsibilities.
- The nurse when acting in a professional capacity should at all times maintain standards of personal conduct that reflect credit on the profession.

Nurses and society
- The nurse shares with other citizens the responsibility for initiating and supporting action to meet the health and social needs of the public.

Nurses and co-workers
- The nurse sustains a cooperative relationship with co-workers in nursing and other fields.
- The nurse takes appropriate action to safeguard the patient when his or her care is endangered by a co-worker or any other person.

Nurses and the profession
- The nurse plays a major role in determining and implementing desirable standards of nursing practice and nursing education.
- The nurse is active in developing a core of professional knowledge.
- The nurse, acting through the professional organization, participates in establishing and maintaining equitable social and economic working conditions in nursing.

From International Council of Nurses: *ICN code for nurses: ethical concepts applied to nursing,* Geneva, 1973, Imprimiéres Populaires.

BIOETHICS

Nursing ethics is a part of a broader system known as bioethics. Bioethics is an interdisciplinary field within the health care organization that has developed only in the past three decades. Bioethics can be differentiated from ethics as ethics has been discussed in the written word since there was written word, whereas bioethics has developed with the age of modern medicine. New questions surface as new science and technology produce new ways of knowing. Bioethics is a response to contemporary advances in health care.

Dilemmas for Health Professionals

Physicians, nurses, social workers, psychiatrists, clergy, philosophers, theologians, *and policy makers* are joining to address ethical questions, difficult questions, and right vs. wrong questions. As they seek to deliver quality health care, these professionals debate situations that pose dilemmas. They are confronting situations for which there are no clear right or wrong answers. Because of the diverse society in which health care is practiced, there are at least two sides to almost every issue faced.

Every specialization in health care has its own set of questions. Life and death, quality of life, right to decide, informed consent, and alternative treatment issues prevail in every field of health care from maternal-child to geriatric care, from acute episodic to intensive, highly specialized care, and from hospital-based to community-based care. In every aspect of the nursing profession lie the more subtle and intricate questions of "how should" this care be delivered and "how should" one decide when choices *are in* conflict.

Many nursing students do not consider health care and the practice of nursing in terms of the personal and subjective side; rather they look at it only in terms of the technical and objective side. Yet there most definitely are factors that influence the way patients actually are treated, or at least the way they perceive their treatment, that go beyond the technical aspect. In many ways technology has changed the face of health care and created the troubling questions that have become central in the delivery of care.

Dilemmas Created by Technology

Advances in health care through technology have created new situations for health care professionals and their patients. For the very young and old and for generations in between, illnesses once leading to mortality have now become manageable and are classified as high-risk or chronic illness. Although people can now be saved, they are not being saved readily or inexpensively. Care of the acutely or chronically ill person sometimes creates hard questions for which there are no easy or apparent answers. Mortality for most will be a long, drawn-out phenomenon, laced with a lifetime of potential conflicts about what ought to be done. Health care professionals who adhere to an exclusively scientific or technologic approach to care will be seen as insensitive and will fail to meet the genuine needs of the patient, needs that include assistance with these more subjective concerns.

ETHICAL DECISION MAKING

A professional nurse in the twenty-first century will be deemed competent only if he or she can provide the scientific and technologic aspects of care and has the ability to deal effectively with the ethical problems encountered in patient care. A competent nurse must be able to deal with the human dimensions of that care. The previously listed "how should" questions should be just as important as the "how to" questions surrounding the care of the 80-year-old patient introduced previously. As the nurse seeks to understand the "how to" aspects of the patient's care, such as comfort measures for dyspnea, pharmacologic care considering her organ dysfunction, and decubitus prevention in her immobile and malnourished state, he or she also must seek to understand more.

Answering Difficult Questions

Care combining human dimensions with scientific and technical dimensions forces some basic questions.

- What does it mean to be ill or well?
- What is the proper balance between science and technology and the good of humans?
- Where do we find balance when science will allow us to experiment with the basic origins of life?
- What happens when the proper balance is in tension?

No tension is created in the effort to save the life of a dying healthy adolescent or set the broken leg of a healthy elderly adult. Science and the human good are not in conflict here. However, what is the answer when modern medicine can save or prolong the life of an 8-year-old child but the child's parents refuse treatment based on religious reasons? Or what is the answer when modern medicine has life to offer a 30-year-old mother in need of a transplanted organ but the woman is without the financial means to cover the cost of the treatment? What is the answer when new discoveries allow some to even choose biologic characteristics of children not yet conceived? At one end of the spectrum lies the obvious; at the other there is often only uncertainty. Health care professionals in everyday practice often find themselves striving somewhere between the two.

Balancing Science and Morality

If nursing care is to be competent, the right balance between science and morality must be sought and understood. Nurses must first attempt to understand not just what they are to do for their patients but who their patients are. They must examine life and its origins, as well as its worth, usefulness, and importance. Nurses must determine their own values and seek to understand the values of others.

Health care decisions are seldom made independently of other people. Decisions are made with the patient, the family, other nurses, and other health care providers. Nurses must make a deliberate effort to recognize their own values and learn to consider and respect the values of others.

The nurse has an obligation to present himself or herself to the patient as competent. The dependent patient enters into a mutual relationship with the nurse. This exchange places a patient who is vulnerable and wounded with a nurse who is educated, licensed, and knowledgeable. The patient expects nursing actions to be thorough since total caring is the defining characteristic of the patient–nurse relationship. The nurse promises to deliver holistic care to the best of his or her ability. The patient's expectations and the nurse's promises require a commitment to develop a reasoned thought process and sound judgment in all situations that take place within this important relationship. The more personal, subjective, and value-laden situations are deemed to be among the most difficult situations for which the nurse must prepare.

VALUES FORMATION AND MORAL DEVELOPMENT

A value is a personal belief about worth that acts as a standard to guide behavior; a value system is an entire framework on which actions are based. Diane Uustal, a well-known nurse ethicist, describes values as being a basis for what a person thinks about, chooses, feels for, and acts on (1992). Perhaps many nursing students come to the educational setting with an intact value system. No doubt anyone living in these times has faced many situations in which important choices had to be made. The options available to this generation are too numerous to avoid hard choices. Values have been applied to those decisions. Yet often people do not take time to seriously contemplate their value system, the forces that shaped those values, and the life and world-view decisions that have been made based on them.

Examining Value Systems

To become a competent professional in every dimension of nursing care, nurses must examine their own system of values and commit themselves to a virtuous value system. A clear understanding of what is right and wrong is a necessary first step to a process sometimes referred to as values clarification, a process by which people attempt to examine the values they hold and how each of those values functions as part of a whole. Nurses must acknowledge their own values by considering how they would act in a particular situation.

A values clarification process (Uustal, 1992) is an important learning tool as nursing students prepare themselves to become competent professionals. The deliberate refinement of one's own personal value system leads to a clearer lens through which nurses can view ethical questions in the practice of their profession. A refined value system and world view can serve professionals as they deal with the meaning of life and its many choices. A world view provides a cohesive model for life; it encourages personal responsibility for the living of that life, and it prepares one for making ethical choices encountered throughout life.

Forming a world view and a value system is an evolving, continuous, dynamic process that moves along a continuum of development often referred to as moral development. Just as there is an orderly sequence of physical and psychologic development, there is an orderly sequence of right and wrong conduct development. Consider an adult of mighty physical prowess and strong moral character. Just as with each biologic developmental milestone there is a more mature, more expanded physical being, with each life experience that has right and wrong choices there is a more mature, more virtuous person.

Learning Right and Wrong

The process of learning to distinguish right and wrong often is described in pediatric textbooks. Donna Wong describes such development in children (1999). Infants have no concept of right or wrong. Infants hold no beliefs and no convictions, although it is known that moral development begins in infancy. If the need for basic trust is met in infancy, children can begin to develop the foundation for secure moral thought. Toddlers begin to display behavior in response to the world around them. They will imitate behavior seen in others, even though they do not comprehend the meaning of the behavior that they are imitating. Further, even though toddlers may not know what they are doing or why they are doing it, they incorporate the values and beliefs of those around them into their own behavioral code.

By the time children reach school age, they have learned that behavior has consequences and that good behavior is associated with rewards and bad behavior is associated with punishment. Through their experiences and social interactions with people outside their home or immediate surroundings, school-age children begin to make choices about how they will act based on an understanding of good and bad. Their conscience is developing, and it begins to govern those choices they make (Wong, 1999).

The adolescent questions existing moral values and his or her relevance to society. Adolescents understand duty and obligation, but they sometimes seriously question the moral codes on which society operates as they become more aware of the contradictions they see in the value systems of adults.

Adults strive to make sense of the contradictions and learn to develop their own set of morals and values as autonomous people. They begin to make choices based on an internalized set of principles that provides them with the resources they need to evaluate situations in which they find themselves (Wong et al., 1999).

Understanding Moral Development Theory

Perhaps the most widely accepted theory on moral development is Lawrence Kohlberg's theory (1971). Kohlberg theorizes a cognitive developmental process that is sequential in nature with progression through levels and stages, which vary dramatically within society. At first morality is all about rules imposed by some source of authority. Moral decisions made at this level (preconventional) are simply in response to some threat of punishment. The good-bad, right-wrong labels have meaning but are defined only in reference to a self-centered reward and punishment system. A person who is in the preconventional level has no concept of the underlying moral code informing the decision of good-bad or right-wrong.

At some point people begin to internalize their view of themselves in response to something more meaningful and interpersonal (conventional level). A desire to be viewed as a good boy or nice girl develops when the person wants to find approval from others. He or she may want to please, help others, be dutiful, and show respect for authority. Conformity to expected social and religious mores and a sense of loyalty may emerge.

Not all people develop beyond the conventional level of moral development. A morally mature individual (postconventional level), one of the few to reach moral completeness, is an autonomous thinker who strives for a moral code beyond issues of authority and reverence. The morally mature individual's actions are based on principles of justice and respect for the dignity of all humankind and not just on principles of responsibility, duty, or self-edification (Kohlberg, 1971).

Moving Toward Moral Maturity

The rightness or wrongness of the complex and confounding health care decisions that are being made today depends on the level of moral development of those professionals entrusted with the tough decisions. Moving toward the level of moral maturity required for such decision making is, for most, a learning endeavor that requires a strong commitment to the task. Nurses must commit themselves to such learning.

The American Association of Colleges of Nursing (AACN) provides the profession with the results of a study in which the essential knowledge, skilled practice, and values necessary for nursing were delineated. From a consensus-building effort across the nation, the AACN has recommended seven values that are essential for the professional nurse. These values are described in Table 9-1.

The study and examination of these nursing values is a worthwhile endeavor for the nursing student. Students who seek to become morally mature health care providers will appraise the values of the nursing profession and strive to find a comfortable union of those values

TABLE 9-1	*Essential Nursing Values and Behaviors*	
ESSENTIAL VALUES	**ATTITUDES AND PERSONAL QUALITIES**	**PROFESSIONAL BEHAVIORS**
Altruism—concern for the welfare of others	Caring, commitment, compassion, generosity, perseverance	Gives full attention to the client when giving care; assists other personnel in providing care when they are unable to do so
		Expresses concern about social trends and issues that have implications for health care
Equality—having the same rights, privileges, or status	Acceptance, assertiveness, fairness, self-esteem, tolerance	Provides nursing care based on the individual's needs irrespective of personal characteristics
		Interacts with other providers in a nondiscriminatory manner
		Expresses ideas about the improvement of access to nursing and health care
Esthetics—qualities of objects, events, and persons that provide satisfaction	Appreciation, creativity, imagination, sensitivity	Adapts the environment so that it is pleasing to the client
		Creates a pleasant work environment for self and others
		Presents self in a manner that promotes a positive image of nursing
Freedom—capacity to exercise choice	Confidence, hope, independence, openness, self-direction, self-discipline	Honors individual's right to refuse treatment
		Supports the rights of other providers to suggest alternatives to the plan of care
		Encourages open discussion of controversial issues in the profession
Human dignity—inherent worth and uniqueness of a person	Consideration, empathy, humaneness, kindness, respectfulness, trust	Safeguards the individual's right to privacy
		Addresses individuals as they prefer to be addressed
		Maintains confidentiality of clients and staff
		Treats others with respect, regardless of background
Justice—upholding moral and legal principles	Courage, integrity, morality, objectivity	Acts as a health care advocate
		Allocates resources fairly
		Reports incompetent, unethical, and illegal practices objectively and factually
Truth—faithfulness to fact or reality	Accountability, authenticity, honesty, inquisitiveness, rationality, reflectiveness	Documents nursing care accurately and honestly
		Obtains sufficient data to make sound judgments before reporting infractions of organizational policies
		Participates in professional efforts to protect the public from misinformation about nursing

From American Association of Colleges of Nursing: *Essentials of college and university education for professional nursing,* Washington, DC, 1986, American Association of Colleges of Nursing.

with their own. Further, the study of ethical theory and ethical principles can provide a basis for moving forward as a morally mature professional nurse.

ETHICAL THEORY

Ethical theory is a system of principles by which a person can determine what ought and ought not to be done. Although there are others, utilitarianism and deontology are theories that encompass modern moral thought and provide approaches for answering the question regarding what is right to do in a given ethical dilemma (Davis et al., 1997).

Utilitarianism

Utilitarianism is an approach that is rooted in the assumption that an action or practice is right if it leads to the greatest possible balance of good consequences or to the least possible balance of bad consequences. Utilitarian ethics are noted to be the strongest approach used in bioethical decision making. An attempt is made to determine which actions will lead to the greatest ratio of benefit to harm for all persons involved in the dilemma.

Deontology

Deontology is an approach that is rooted in the assumption that humans are rational and act out of principles that are consistent and objective and that compel them to do what is right. Ethics are based on a sense of universal principle to consistently act one way. In bioethical decision making, moral rightness is the act that is determined not by the consequences it produces, but by the moral qualities intrinsic to the act itself. Deontologic theory claims that a decision is right only if it conforms to an overriding moral duty and wrong only if it violates that moral duty. All decisions must be made in such a way that the decision could become universal law. Persons are to be treated as ends in themselves and never as means to the ends of others.

ETHICAL PRINCIPLES

Perhaps the most useful tool for the morally mature professional nurse is a set of principles, standards, or truths on which to base ethical actions. Common ground must be established between the nurse and the patient and the family, between fellow nurses, between the nurse and other health care providers, and between the nurse and other members of society. A set of mutually agreed on principles makes it possible for people to come together to discuss ethical questions and move toward a sense of understanding and agreement (Husted and Husted, 1995).

The practice of ethics involves applying principles to the two ethical theories described, utilitarianism and deontology, or to other theories that are described elsewhere. Principles can permit people to take a consistent position on specific or related issues. If the principles, when applied to a particular act, make the act right or wrong in one situation, it seems reasonable to assume that the same principle, when applied to a new situation, can share similar features.

Three principles have proven to be highly relevant in bioethics: (1) autonomy, (2) beneficence, nonmaleficence, and (3) veracity. These principles are not related in such a way that they jointly form a complete moral framework. One may be relevant to a situation, whereas the others are not. Yet these principles are sufficiently comprehensive to provide an analytic framework by which moral problems can be evaluated.

Autonomy

Autonomy, the principle of respect for the person, or the principle of autonomy, is sometimes labeled as the primary moral principle. The umbrella concept says that humans have incalculable worth or moral dignity not possessed by other objects or creatures. There is unconditional intrinsic value for all persons. People are free to form their own judgments and whatever actions they choose. They are self-determining agents, entitled to determine their own destiny.

If an autonomous person's actions do not infringe on the autonomous actions of others, that person should be free to decide however he or she wishes. This freedom should be applied even if the decision creates risk to his or her health and even if the decision seems unwise to others. Concepts of freedom and informed consent are grounded in the principle of autonomy.

Beneficence, Nonmaleficence

In general terms, to be beneficent is to promote goodness, kindness, and charity. On the other end of the spectrum from the beneficence principle is nonmaleficence, a principle that implies a duty not to inflict harm. In ethical terms nonmaleficence is to abstain from injuring others and to help others further their own well-being by removing harm and eliminating threats, whereas beneficence is to provide benefits to others by promoting their good. The beneficence-nonmaleficence principle is largely a balance of risk and benefit. At times the risk of harm must be weighed against possible benefits. The risk should never be greater than the importance of the problem to be solved.

Although it may seem natural to promote good at all times, the most common bioethical conflicts result from an imbalance between the demands of beneficence and those acts and decisions within the health care delivery system that might pose threats. For instance, it is not always clearly evident what is good and what is harmful. Is the resuscitation effort of the 80-year-old woman good or harmful to her overall sense of well-being? How much beneficence is there in supporting someone toward a peaceful death?

Veracity

Most contemporary professionals believe that telling the truth in personal communication is a moral and ethical requirement. If there is the belief in health care that truth-telling is always characteristic of right, then the principle of veracity can itself pose some interesting challenges.

In the past, truth-telling was sometimes viewed as inconvenient, distressing, or even harmful to patients and families. The first American Medical Association Code of Ethics in 1847 contained such a message:

> The life of a sick person can be shortened not only by the acts, but also by the words or the manner of a physician. It is, therefore, a sacred duty to guard himself carefully in this respect, and to avoid all things that have a tendency to discourage the patient and to depress his spirits.

The belief that the truth could at times be harmful was held for many years. Only recently with the shift from a provider-driven system to a consumer-driven system has the history of silence begun to break. With this shift have come interesting questions. Is the provider-patient relationship generally understood by both parties to include the right of the provider to control the truth by withholding some or all of the relevant information until an appropriate time for disclosure? How much deception with patients is morally acceptable in the communication of a poor or terminal prognosis?

Difficult questions surface, but at the heart of the principle of veracity is trust. Health care consumers today expect accurate and precise information that is revealed in an honest and respectful manner. A few generations ago the trust factor may have been such that it was acceptable for providers to share parts of truth or to distort the truth in the name of beneficence. Today, however, for trust to develop between providers and patients, there must be truthful interaction and meaningful communication. The moral conflict that results from being less than truthful to patients is too troublesome for today's practitioner. The deontologic theory of the health care provider having a duty to tell the patient the truth has taken precedence over the fear of harm that might result if the truth is revealed. The challenge today is to mesh together the need for truthful communication with the need to protect. Health care providers must lay aside fears that the truth will be harmful to patients and come to the realization that more often than not the truth can alleviate anxiety, increase pain tolerance, facilitate recovery, and enhance cooperation with treatment. With a pledge toward human decency, health care providers must commit themselves to truth-telling in all interactions and relationships.

ETHICAL DECISION-MAKING MODEL

Theories provide a cognitive plan for considering ethical issues; principles offer guiding truths on which to base ethical decisions. Using these theories and principles, it seems appropriate to consider a system for moving beyond a specific ethical dilemma toward a morally mature and reasoned ethical action.

Many ethical decision-making models exist for the purpose of defining a process by which a nurse or another health care provider actually can move through an ethical dilemma toward an informed decision. Box 9-3 depicts one ethical decision-making model.

Situation Assessment Procedure

Identify the Ethical Issues and Problems. In the first step of assessment there is an attempt to find out the technical and scientific facts and the human dimension of the situation—the feelings, emotions, attitudes, and opinions. A nurse must make an attempt to understand what values are inherent in the situation. Finally, the nurse must deliberately state the nature of the ethical dilemma. This first step is important because the issues and problems to be addressed are often complex. Trying to understand the full picture of a situation is time consuming and requires examination from many different perspectives, but it is worth the time and effort to understand an issue fully before moving forward in the assessment procedure. Wright (1987) poses some important questions that must be addressed in this first step.

1. What is the issue here?
2. What are the hidden issues?
3. What exactly are the complexities of this situation?
4. Is anything being overlooked?

BOX 9-3	*Situation Assessment Procedure*

1. Identify the ethical issues and problems.
2. Identify and analyze available alternatives for action.
3. Select one alternative.
4. Justify the selection.

Wright RA: *The practice of ethics: human values in health care,* New York, 1987, McGraw-Hill.

Identify and Analyze Available Alternatives for Action. In the second step a set of alternatives for action is established. The second step is an important step to follow. Because actions are based most commonly on a nurse's own personal value system, it is important to list all possible actions for a given situation, even actions that seem highly unlikely. Without deliberately listing possible alternatives, it is doubtful that the full consideration of all possible actions will take place. Wright's questions for the second step are:

1. What are the reasonable possibilities for action, and how do the different affected parties (patient, family, physician, nurse) want to resolve the problem?
2. What ethical principles are required for each alternative?
3. What assumptions are required for each alternative, and what are their implications for future action?
4. What, if any, are the additional ethical problems that the alternatives raise?

Select One Alternative. Multiple factors come together in the third step. After identifying the issues and analyzing all possible alternatives, the skillful decision maker steps back to consider the situation again. There is an attempt to reflect on ethical theory and to mesh that thinking with the identified ethical principles for each alternative. The decision maker's own value system is applied, along with an appraisal of the profession's values for the care of others. A reasoned and purposeful decision results from the blending of each of these factors.

Justify the Selection. The rational discourse on which the decision is based must be shared in an effort to justify the decision. The decision maker must be prepared to communicate his or her thoughts through an explanation of the reasoning process used. According to Wright (1987), the justification for a resolution to an ethical issue is an argument wherein relevant and sufficient reasons for the correctness of that resolution are presented. Defending an argument is not an easy task, but it is a necessary step to communicate the reasons or premises on which the decision is based. A systematic and logical argument will show why the particular resolution chosen is the correct one. This final step is important to advance ethical thought and to express sound judgment. Wright's formula for the justification process is as follows:

1. Specify reasons for the action.
2. Clearly present the ethical basis for these reasons.
3. Understand the shortcomings of the justification.
4. Anticipate objections to the justification.

Usefulness and Application of the Situation Assessment Procedure

A procedure or model for ethical decision making is useful for individuals and groups alike. The more subtle and tenuous issues that arise in health care often are resolved within the context of the patient-provider relationship that exists between two people. Dilemmas resulting from questions about truth-telling, acknowledging uncertainty, paternalism, privacy, and fidelity are examples of issues that may be resolved between as few as two people.

Questions that are more encompassing often are addressed in group settings. Institutional ethics committees now are common within health care agencies. The purpose of the committee is to provide ethics education, aid in ethical policy development, and serve as a consultative body when resolution of an ethical dilemma cannot be reached otherwise. Although institutional ethics committees do not make legal decisions that are the province of the patient, the family, or the health care provider, a model such as the Situation Assessment

Procedure can be a useful procedure to guide the thinking of a group that has been asked to provide counsel.

More and more nurses are finding themselves facing ethical dilemmas as members of hospital administration teams or policy-making bodies within professional organizations or governmental bodies. Nurses contribute a highly relevant perspective to discussions and decisions about safe and effective care in these times of change. The Situation Assessment Procedure can be applied to the decision-making process when procedures and policies are being developed to address conflicting variables.

Thus application of the Situation Assessment Procedure can occur on two levels. The procedure is applicable to the daily practice level of ethical decision making as patients and providers make choices between right and wrong actions. The procedure is equally applicable to the policy-making level where professionals come together to consider right and wrong choices that affect society as a whole. Professional organizations such as the ANA have established committees such as the Ethics and Human Rights Committee, which allow nurses to meet to set policy for the practice of nursing. Inherent in the policy formation are questions that affect patient care. The Situation Assessment Procedure can be applied to hard questions that arise in any setting in which the nurse is responsible for or contributes to ethical decision making.

BIOETHICAL DILEMMAS: LIFE, DEATH, AND DILEMMAS IN-BETWEEN

Bioethical dilemmas are situations that pose a choice between perplexing alternatives in the delivery of health care because of the lack of a clear sense of right or wrong. It is imperative that every nursing student consider the potential dilemmas that might arise in a given practice setting. Concepts of life and death are central to nursing's body of knowledge, but a discussion of these concepts is incomplete unless the threats of conflict also are explored. A nursing student must not assume that conflict is rare or that it is to be dealt with primarily by other professionals on the health care team. Conflict must be addressed as the concepts of life and its origins, birth, death, and dying are addressed. But conflict must also be addressed in the many varied situations that come up day after day in the practice of professional nursing.

Life

Entire textbooks are written to address the potential conflict that surrounds questions about the beginning of life. The most significant conflict that will be recorded in the historical accounts of the twentieth century will be the debate about when life begins. The abortion conflict became central in 1973 when the Roe v. Wade decision was made. Although the legal aspects of abortion have been resolved in courtrooms in the United States, the bioethical concerns are debated day-to-day 30 years later. The bioethical abortion conflict has been debated using ethical theories, ethical principles, value systems, rights issues, choice questions, and so on. Answers acceptable to society as a whole have not materialized; thus the right or wrong of abortion continues to rest with each person. Despite clear, generalizable answers to the abortion question, nurses serving in women and child health settings must be prepared to face this morally laden issue.

Closely akin to the abortion question are newer questions about reproduction. Genetic screening, genetic engineering, stem cell therapy, and cloning are newer, highly advanced, and sophisticated techniques that bring with them the most ethically entangled questions ever. Moving beyond the question about when life begins, health care providers now must address their patients' questions about the right or wrong of designing life itself. The entire human genome project with its rapidly developing advances has created a whole new dimension of bioethics.

Death

The second most important conflict in health care involves the issue of death and dying. Since the development of lifesaving procedures and mechanical ventilation, questions about quality of life and the definition of death have escalated. With the advances in health care, it has become unclear what is usual care and what is heroic care. The purpose and quality of life of a person in a vegetative state frequently is debated. Health care providers regularly contend with questions of cerebral vs. biologic death in their dealings with patients and families. The "dying with dignity" and "toward a peaceful death" concepts are examined in light of ever evolving advances in life-prolonging care. Euthanasia and assisted suicide present the newest ethical questions surrounding the dying process. Because death is universal and part of human existence, every health care provider serving in every delivery setting must address the difficult end-of-life questions.

Dilemmas In-Between

Life and death dilemmas receive the most attention in the written word through the media and in real-life drama played out on television and theater screens. But a host of other questions comprise most ethical decision-making activities for the professional nurse in the practice of today's health care. Between questions of life and death are questions of existence, reality, individual rights, responsibility, equality, justice, and fairness. Added to these are an unlimited number of other questions that arise from the human dimension of caring.

It is in these ordinary, day-to-day situations of caring that many professionals find the most important and nagging questions. Basic notions of individual and social justice are viewed in terms of fairness and what is deserved. A person has been treated justly when he or she has been given what is due or owed. Any denial of something to which a person has a right or entitlement is an act of injustice.

The Right to Health Care. Handling injustice has been a part of nursing since the days of Florence Nightingale. But as health care delivery has recently shifted to a managed care system, new questions of injustices have surfaced. The system has become more selective in the amount and type of treatment offered. A full range of diagnostic testing may not be available to every person seeking answers for perplexing illnesses. The particular benefit package offered through one insurance company may be more limited in scope of services than the benefit package offered through another company. Two families living side-by-side in a typical suburban neighborhood may be entitled to different health care services based on where they are employed. Perhaps one family has access to health care, and the other does not.

What right to health care do people have? Is each person entitled to the same health care package? Should ability to pay affect the specific level of entitlement? How ethical is the reality of gatekeeping in the new managed care system? Are employers and insurance groups removing patient autonomy by choosing the least costly insurance plans (Lee and Estes, 2001)? Resolutions to such questions have been based largely on the doctrine of justice, which states that like cases should be treated alike and equals ought to be treated equally. Some have suggested that issues such as right to health care and distribution of health care are political, not bioethical, issues (Husted and Husted, 1995), but such issues grip at the core of nursing practice wherein access to health care and a respect for human dignity are paramount. Justice becomes a bioethical issue at the point that it affects if, when, where, and how a patient will receive health care.

Allocation of Scarce Resources. The issues of organ transplantation and the allocation of scarce resources flow from the doctrine of justice. The problem of scarce medical resources is becoming more common. Which people in need of transplantation should receive organs when available organs are in shorter supply than the number of people who could benefit from them? The justice question is applicable to this situation. The utilitarians argue that the allocation decision should be framed so as to serve the greatest good for the greatest number of people affected. Should the selected recipient be the man with the largest, most loving family who does the greatest work for society? Or should a more universal law be applied? Should the people in need of organ transplantation be placed on a first-come, first-served list? Or should they be entered into a lottery? Distributive justice, or taking the needs, interests, and wishes of each patient, cannot alone answer allocation dilemmas. Who has the more meaningful life? Who has the best prognosis? Who can pay? As unjust as it may seem to some, these are the kinds of questions responsible parties must make regarding the allocation of scarce resources. And what about the fact that nurses themselves are scarce resources? What about the challenges of the nurse's autonomous right to refuse to work in understaffed settings? Whose rights come first?

ETHICAL CHALLENGES

What about the doctrines of justice and freedom and the need for human experimentation and biomedical research? It is accepted that human experimentation is necessary for the progression of health care knowledge. But what about the risk of harm and the moral imperative that providers should, above all, do no harm? What about specifically problematic aspects of research such as the use of institutionalized or imprisoned research subjects or research on a viable fetus? Memories of harmful medical research and human experimentation such as the Nazi atrocities and the Tuskegee incident have resulted in governmental regulations involving the use of human subjects in medical research (Pence, 1998). The Nuremberg Code is a set of provisions for research that must be followed for the federal government to approve research. Institutional Review Boards are established within research institutions for the purpose of overseeing that the degree of risk to the subject is minimized, if not eliminated. Human experimentation tests the principles of autonomy and respect for personhood.

The Challenge of Veracity

Everyday issues that test the principle of veracity are the issues of alternative treatment and acknowledging uncertainty. It is the nature of health science that new knowledge must come forth to abolish less effective dogma. However, new ignorance comes with these new discoveries. Which treatment among two or more is best for a patient in a specific situation? Which of the new drugs should be used? Should every patient be subjected to every possible form of diagnostic evaluation? Should this patient be treated with surgery, medication, or both? And most important, should the patient be made aware of all these questions and various options for his or her care? Can patients comprehend medicine's esoteric knowledge, in general, and its accompanying certainties and uncertainties, in particular? Is disclosure of uncertainty ultimately beneficial or detrimental?

Acknowledging uncertainty is difficult for today's health care provider. As never before it seems that providers need to present themselves as confident, knowledgeable, and sensitive to their patients, who may see them as arrogant, dogmatic, and insensitive. Acknowledging uncertainty may be worth the effort. For the diagnostician, it may lighten the burden by absolving him or her of the responsibility for implicitly making decisions for which there may be conflicting answers. For the patient, knowing about the uncertainty may give him or her a greater voice in decision making and, in the event of treatment failure, may leave him or her better informed and more trustful of the caregiver. It seems that disclosure of uncertainty is ultimately beneficial to both parties. It seems that full disclosure and open communication through a commitment to veracity could prevent many everyday ethical situations. Optimum health care results from an exchange between patient and provider with open communication about the patient's wants and needs and the provider's judgment and advice. All too often time is not taken for open communication, and the exchange becomes one of the patient listening to what the all-knowing and wise provider says about his or her needs. It is easy for the provider to assume a paternalistic attitude in the delivery of health care.

The Challenge of Paternalism

Paternalism is an action and an attitude wherein the provider tries to act on behalf of the patient and believes that his or her actions are justified because of a commitment to act in the best interest of the patient. Paternalism is a reflection of the "father knows best" way of thinking. The phenomenon of paternalism presumes, in the name of beneficence, to overlook the patient's right to autonomy. Thus, in the process of attempting to act in the best interest of the patient, paternalism involves actions not based on the patient's choices, wishes, and desires. Paternalism interferes with a patient's right to self-determination and occurs when the provider believes that he or she can make a better decision than the patient.

Paternalism erodes the patient–provider relationship. Every provider must guard against actions and attitudes that are paternalistic. Perhaps in the past paternalism was associated with the white coat image of the physician as a sovereign god. Today paternalistic actions and attitudes can be found among nurses, pharmacists, physical therapists, occupational therapists, social workers, or anyone who assumes the image of the all-knowing in the delivery of care. The healthy patient-provider relationship is based on the open communication described previously wherein patient choice and respect for personhood are deemed just as important as scientific knowledge and sound health care advice. The provider-patient relationship is built on trust when the right to confidentiality and privacy become ethical and legal obligations.

The Challenge of Autonomy

The provider-patient relationship makes way for the crucial legal concept of informed consent, which stipulates that the patient has the right to know and make decisions about his or her health. These decisions take the form of consent or refusal of treatment. Based on the principle of autonomy, the consent process must be voluntary and without coercion; the fully informed patient must clearly understand the choices being offered.

Informed consent dilemmas evolve from questions about whether patients are competent to make informed decisions and whether there are family members or surrogates to make those decisions by proxy. The need for informed consent from minors; confused elderly; people who are mentally compromised, imprisoned, inebriated, or unconscious; and people in emergency situations poses difficult questions for health care providers. The burden of informed consent lies with the physician in most circumstances, although the nurse frequently is responsible for aspects of informing and obtaining consent.

In the latter part of the twentieth century another crucial concept of consent was introduced. Advances in technology and the potential to keep people alive for extended periods have brought about legislation aimed at giving people choices about end-of-life decisions while they are still healthy and well enough to make informed decisions. The opportunity for people to make advance directives is now common and is a requirement for admission to hospitals and other health care agencies that receive federal dollars. People are not required to decide but must be given an opportunity to do so. Ideally the health care community will provide such an opportunity while the patient is well, perhaps in a community setting such as a public library or community center. Health care professionals such as nurses and other health care educators have an ethical obligation to educate the public about the use of advance directives. These opportunities can serve as excellent means of educating patients not only about advance directives but also about their rights in general, changes in health care delivery and managed care, and the role of the various health care providers. This is an excellent opportunity to educate the public about the scope of practice of today's professional nurse.

The Challenge of Accountability

A host of specific ethical issues exists within the practice of nursing itself. Professional nursing is a complex profession that is unlike most others. The accountability factor in the practice of nursing is such that a keen sense of responsibility and personal integrity are necessary qualities for every practicing nurse. It is the nurse's ethical obligation to uphold the highest standards of practice and care, assume full personal and professional responsibility for every action, and commit to maintaining quality in the skill and knowledge base of the profession.

Failure to meet such obligations places the patient-nurse relationship at risk. Failure to be accountable for one's own actions places a tremendous burden on the relationship with the patient and poses ethical dilemmas for fellow nurse professionals. In health professions in which the safety and health of society is at stake, the obligation of professionals to police the practice of their colleagues is important.

There are public and legal official policing bodies such as the State Board of Nursing for matters of public record and formal conviction. But there are countless situations in which the official policing body will never be involved, and the obligation to denounce a harmful action or potentially threatening situation falls to a fellow member of the profession. Sometimes known as "whistle blowing," the obligation to denounce is based on the fact that to remain silent is to consent to the action or threatening situation. Whether denouncing a chemical impairment, negligence, abusiveness, incompetence, or cruelty, the obligation is a moral one based at least in part on the principle of beneficence. Unless professionals of integrity blow the whistle on those whose actions are irresponsible and harmful, the wrong will continue, and the harm to others will escalate. In the end, the profession as a whole will suffer, and the well-being of society will be diminished.

SUMMARY

Professional nurses must be prepared to face any number of potential ethical conflicts in the day-to-day practice of their profession. They must realize that each situation is different and that recognizing the uniqueness demands that responsible parties seek a loving and humane solution to every situation that poses an ethical dilemma. When the answer remains clouded, the decision maker must choose the most appropriate action, given the situation, based on a variety of potentially applicable principles.

To think that dilemmas such as the ones described here are unlikely or far removed is to think that the surgery patient will not be troubled by pain or the trauma patient by anxiety or the cancer patient by fear. Ethical conflict is inherent in the practice of nursing and is played out in every practice setting every day. The challenge is not to escape the conflict but to meet it with expectancy and preparedness.

The profession of nursing often is described as a discipline of human caring. Those seeking a career in nursing must realize the multifaceted aspects of the profession. They also should appreciate the rich and diverse opportunities that will be afforded them. Braced with scientific knowledge and the resources for critical examination of health and illness, the professional nurse is provided access to life's most intimate and precious encounters. Perhaps more than any other health care provider, a sensitive and caring nurse is invited to join patients who are experiencing the most intense moments of their lives. Nurses are given the opportunity to embrace patients in their joy over the birth of a child or the good news of a successful surgery or chemotherapy treatment for cancer. They also are privileged to support patients and their families during the trials of waiting for the outcome of a tragic head injury or the last breath in a life wrecked by terminal illness. To all of this, nurses are invited.

With such privilege comes responsibility. The purpose of this chapter has been to introduce nursing students to the idea that ethical conflict in health care abounds and to increase students' awareness of their role in resolving conflict. It is important for professional nurses to have a basic knowledge of the ethical thinking enterprise that is described in this chapter and realize that there are other resources for committed professionals to draw on in an effort to stay abreast of the issues they are likely to face in their practice. There are journals such as *The Hastings Center Report* and *Ethics in Medicine* that come from centers and institutes such as the Center for Health and Human Dignity; the Institute of Society, Ethics, and the Life Sciences; the Kennedy Institute Center for Bioethics; and the ANA Committee on Ethics and Human Rights. These groups prepare position statements and white papers on specific ethical dilemmas arising from today's health care practice. Learning centers, libraries, and websites generally provide access to these resources, although individual membership and subscriptions are available. Box 9-4 presents online resources available to learn more about ethics, bioethics, and the issues nurses are likely to face in their practice.

Bioethics and ethical decision making is a philosophic enterprise, a thinking activity. Many activities in nursing practice require an actual skill that involves training, practice, and technique development. For example, nursing students are introduced to the principles of intravenous line insertion while in a campus laboratory setting. They may have an opportunity to practice starting an intravenous line in a simulated setting before actually assuming the responsibility for starting one on a "real" patient. The first few times that students insert an intravenous line, their effort is based on a deliberate thinking through of each step and each principle of asepsis, circulation and blood flow, and positioning. In time, the principles of starting an intravenous line become a well-developed technique and skill activity.

The same process can be used when developing one's capacity for a critical thinking activity. This chapter has presented a vignette describing a patient care situation laden with potential for ethical conflict. As nursing students move through their educational experience, they will be assigned to care for many patients. Each patient care situation has the potential of presenting an ethical dilemma. As students are faced with ethical decisions, they refine their

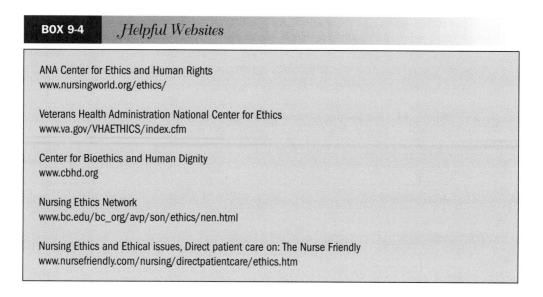

decision making. Each time they reflect on ethical theories or consider ethical principles, students develop critical thinking skills. In time the professional nurse is able to refine what he or she has learned into a morally mature personal code of ethics. At that point, there is a liberating joy that comes from knowing that competence in professional nursing practice goes beyond technique and skill to include the ability to reason life's most difficult and challenging questions, and all for the benefit of another human being! Although it is not as easy as it may sound, it is well worth the effort.

Girded with truth, nurses must commit themselves to take a bold stance for what is right and against what is wrong. Nurses should feel empowered through their role as primary patient advocates to voice their morality in the face of a new century that promises sweeping changes in health care delivery. Nurses must speak in support of patient choice and self-determination in the era of managed care. They must speak against the moral wrong of practice trends wherein patient safety is jeopardized. Nurses must monitor legislation that affects health care and study current issues such as assisted suicide and cloning. Professional nursing embodies a commitment, not just to think and act wisely in the administration of therapeutic nursing interventions, but also to think and act in accordance with specified values and basic principles of right and wrong. Nursing is making a commitment to all of the above.

Critical Thinking Activities

1. The elderly patient had not issued a legal advance directive for her care before her hospitalization. Once admitted to the Emergency Department, she was in no condition to be counseled about the advance directive concept. Plan and implement a strategy that could have prevented this ethical dilemma.

2. During a brief stable period, the patient called her nurse, Melinda Stone, to her bedside late in the night. She asked Melinda if the medication for her pneumonia was working. Melinda was fully aware that the aggressive antibiotic treatment not only was ineffective for the pneumonia but also was

causing significant adverse effects. Discuss the nurse's ethical obligation to truth-telling vs. the obligation to encourage, instill hope, and inspire a will to live.

3. Later that night, the patient expressed to her family and health care providers her desire to forego further resuscitation efforts. Her family did not agree with her decision. The health care providers believed that the patient was sufficiently competent to make her own choices. However, a second cardiac arrest occurred before legal action was taken. Discuss the issues involved when patients, their families, and health care providers disagree.

4. Late in the course of treatment, the physician was faced with a decision about whether to institute parenteral nutrition. The family asked Melinda about the choices involved in the decision. Describe how a nurse might respond to the family.

5. Given the entire scenario of this patient's care needs, describe the kind of professional nurse the patient deserves.

REFERENCES

Davis AJ et al: *Ethical dilemmas and nursing practice,* ed 4, Stamford, Conn, 1997, Appleton & Lange.

Husted GL, Husted JH: *Ethical decision making in nursing,* ed 2, St Louis, 1995, Mosby.

Kohlberg L: Stages of moral development as a basis for moral development, In *Moral interdisciplinary approaches,* Paramus, NJ, 1971, Newman.

Lee PA, Estes CL: *The nation's health,* ed 6, Boston, MA, 2001, Jones and Bartlett Publishers.

Pence GE: *Classic works in medical ethics,* New York, 1998, McGraw-Hill.

Uustal D: *Values and ethics in nursing: from theory to practice,* ed 4, Greenwich, RI, 1992, Educational Resources in Nursing and Wholistic Health.

Viens DC: A history of nursing's code of ethics, *Nurs Outlook* 37:45-49, 1989.

Wong DL et al: *Nursing care of infants and children,* ed 6, St Louis, 1999, Mosby.

Wright RA: *The practice of ethics: human values in health care,* New York, 1987, McGraw-Hill.

10

Health Policy and Politics

Virginia Trotter Betts, MSN, JD, RN, FAAN, and
Barbara Cherry, MSN, MBA, RN

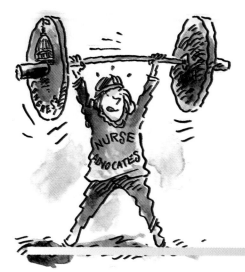

Nurses are powerful advocates for
health care.

Vignette

Juan Hernandez is one of only three registered nurses (RNs) now staffing the 7 AM to 7 PM shift in a 12-bed medical intensive care unit after unlicensed assistive personnel (UAP) have replaced two RNs on this unit. Recently a new unit policy was circulated stating, "all RNs will work overtime as necessary and determined by hospital administration." Juan was already concerned about the compromised safe delivery of patient care because of the decrease in the RN staff, the increase in UAP, and the increase in patient load and acuity. Although Juan feels a professional and moral obligation to ensure that adequate RN coverage is available for patient care, he also knows that the increased physical and mental strain of working overtime hours will be an additional detriment to quality care and patient safety. Juan also understands that by requiring mandatory overtime hospital administrators are failing to address the underlying issue of inadequate numbers of RNs to provide high-quality, safe patient care. Other RNs with whom Juan works have also voiced these same concerns.

Juan realizes that, based on the Nursing Practice Act in his state, he has a professional responsibility to his patients to "implement measures to promote a safe environment for clients." He further understands that he is professionally accountable for his daily practice with each patient. Juan calls the State Nurses Association to discuss his concerns. He then discovers that other nurses around the state and across the United States are involved in some of the same dilemmas of practice. Although he has a professional responsibility to advocate for safe care for patients, issues of working hours are not currently protected under

219

the Nursing Practice Act (NPA) or through any other state policy or regulation. Therefore Juan makes a commitment to participate in discussing political strategies for amending the NPA to protect himself and other RNs in refusing mandatory overtime assignments without being accused of unprofessional conduct.

Questions to consider while reading this chapter

1. How can Juan apply the nursing process to develop an effective plan for policy development related to mandatory overtime assignments?
2. What types of local, state, and federal health policies affect Juan's nursing practice?
3. What are the major steps in health policy development that Juan must understand?
4. What types of grassroots political strategies can Juan use to ensure that policy makers hear his interests and concerns about safe patient care?

Key Terms

Constituent A citizen who has the opportunity to vote for candidates in elections for his or her representation at the local, state, and federal government level.

Constituent member association The state professional organizational member of the American Nurses Association that represents all nurses at the state level (formerly known as the State Nurses Association).

Grassroots lobbying Advocacy by individual constituents in support of an organization's official position related to a policy issue.

Health policy A set course of action undertaken by governments or health care organizations to obtain a desired health outcome. Private health policy is made by health care organizations such as hospitals and managed care organizations, whereas public health policy refers to local, state, and federal legislation, regulation, and court rulings that govern the provision of health care services. Health policy as used in this chapter most often refers to public policies directly related to health care service delivery and reimbursement.

Lobbying An act of persuading or otherwise attempting to educate and convince policy makers to comply with a request, support a particular position on an issue, or follow a particular course of action.

Platform The statement of principles and policies of a political party, candidate, or elected official.

Regulation Rules used to implement legislation and translate concepts into legal action.

Stakeholders Individuals, groups, or organizations who have a vested interest in and may be affected by policy decisions and actions being taken and who may attempt to influence those decisions and actions.

Learning Outcomes

After studying this chapter, the reader will be able to:

1. Differentiate between policy and politics and the actions required for each one.
2. Discuss the roles of the legislative, administrative, and judicial levels of government.
3. Differentiate between federal, state, and local governments and their role in governing and influencing health care and nursing practice.
4. Identify four policy issues of significant consequences to nurses and nursing.
5. Demonstrate knowledge to be a responsible and informed politically active nurse.
6. Write an effective letter to an elected official to support a valid policy position related to a health care issue.
7. Use diverse technologic resources to obtain information about current health policy developments and political issues.

CHAPTER OVERVIEW

The ways in which nurses view their profession determines the commitment, behavior, and strategies that they use to promote and protect it. Although caring and empathy are important to the clinical practice of nursing, these attributes are not enough to sustain the nursing profession. As illustrated by the previous vignette, nurses face many issues related to delivery of patient care, including safety, quality, and availability of care. Sometimes these issues can only be resolved through the policy process. Without a doubt, legislation and health policy that result from these processes will directly affect how nursing is practiced at an individual and facility level.

This chapter explores the impact of governmental roles, structure, and action on health care policy and demonstrates how participation in the policy process can help shape health care. Local, state, and federal legislative concerns, along with the involvement of professional nursing organizations in policy and politics are discussed. The nurse's role in the policy process and involvement in political advocacy and campaigns are described. The chapter provides the reader with a basic understanding of policy development and political processes, ways to gain political savvy, and methods for getting politically involved.

NURSES' INVOLVEMENT IN HEALTH POLICY AND POLITICAL ACTION

Nurses' involvement in policy and politics has become more intense in recent years for two primary reasons:

1. State and federal governments play a major role in health care and may well be the most important shaper of the health care delivery system and nursing practice.
2. Nursing practice in various states has been directly affected by nurses' involvement in policy development and political action.

Because of these two issues, it is absolutely essential that nurses understand health policy development, legislative processes, and political action and work diligently to develop health policies that are reflective of the nursing perspective. Nurses must understand that decisions about the nursing profession will be made *with or without* the input of nurses.

Getting Involved Through the Nursing Process

The first step for nurses to get involved in health policy development and politics is to learn to recognize nursing and health care issues that require policy action. Too many nurses and nursing students have erroneously believed that their education (along with writing nursing process plans!) ended once they graduated. However, they all soon discover that the nursing process is the foundation of professional practice. It is the root of how sound clinical judgments are made and how nursing competence is obtained and maintained. Therefore use of the nursing process to identify broader professional and health care issues is no surprise to politically astute nurses (Texas Nurses Association, 1995).

As politically active nurses soon discover, effective involvement in policy development and political activities requires efforts similar to those used in the nursing process. Comparatively, the policy process and the nursing process are systematic approaches. These approaches involve:

1. Collection of information (assessment).
2. Identification of the issue (diagnosis).
3. Development of a plan.

4. Implementation of the plan.
5. Evaluation of the intervention.

Collection of Information (Assessment). Collecting information and understanding the information collected are important initial steps in determining policy issues and how to handle them. As a nurse, one would not care for a patient without first knowing the patient's health problems and other factors that may affect his or her health. Once the nurse understands the health problems and other possible influencing factors, he or she has enough information to move to the next step in the process: identifying the patient's diagnosis. This same principle applies to health policy and political action. Information and material must be gathered from as many sources as possible before the health care issues amenable to policy intervention can be identified.

An excellent example of health policy assessment is provided by the Institute of Medicine's (IOM) 2001 report on the quality of long-term care. This report presents a comprehensive review of the quality of life and long-term care provided by nursing homes, home health agencies, residential care facilities, family members, and others. This report describes the current state of long-term care, identifies problem areas, and offers recommendations to federal and state policy makers, including recommendations for setting and enforcing standards of care, strengthening the caregiving workforce, addressing reimbursement issues, and expanding the knowledge base to guide caregivers in improving the quality of care (Wunderlich and Kohler, 2001).

Identification of the Issue (Diagnosis). Once the information is gathered (system symptoms), it must be analyzed to identify the real issue or underlying problem that needs to be addressed. For a patient, the nursing diagnosis is determined after analysis of all objective and subjective data is completed. For an issue that may lend itself to a policy intervention, the collected information is analyzed, and the parameters of the issue are determined.

Development of the Plan. After collecting the information and identifying the issue, the nurse is ready to develop a plan. Generally an effective policy plan involves input from many people. It includes options and a determination of potential consequences if each is adopted.

Implementation of the Plan. Once a policy option is selected, it must be implemented. Implementing a policy plan requires political action and a set of strategies. For example, through active membership in a state nurses' association and previous close working relationships with the state nurses' association lobbyist, a member of the Association of Operating Room Nurses learned about a regulatory issue of great importance to perioperative nurses. The issue involved the state administrative code dealing with licensure of hospitals—the part regarding the RN circulator. As part of a regulation review, the state department of health and social services proposed a change that would have allowed non-RNs to circulate in selected cases. Because of development and implementation of a policy plan by the nurses in that state, the state regulation continues to require assignment of an RN to circulating duties, with other personnel allowed to only assist with circulating duties (Oxhorn and Rosen, 1992).

This example raises at least two critical issues. First is the special relationship between the nursing profession and society. Nurses have a legal obligation to provide at least a "safe" standard of care to the persons they serve. Passively allowing use of non-RNs to circulate in even selected operative cases would jeopardize nurses' commitment and obligation to safe-guard patients. Second is the connection between standards of practice and standards of education. RN circulators possess advanced skills, knowledge, and judgment that surpass the technical skills of non-RNs (Oxhorn and Rosen, 1992). This case is an excellent example (that is nearly universal) that what is good for nursing is good for patients and vice versa.

Evaluation of the Plan. After implementing the plan, evaluation of the action must occur. The Needlestick Safety and Prevention Act, which was signed into law by President Clinton on November 6, 2000, provides a current example of how evaluation will be important to demonstrate that (1) the new law is appropriately implemented and enforced, and (2) reductions in needlestick injuries and the associated savings are realized. Over 80% of the 600,000 to one million needlestick injuries that health care workers suffer annually could be prevented with the use of safer needle devices. These exposures can lead to hepatitis B, hepatitis C, and human immunodeficiency virus (HIV), the virus that causes acquired immunodeficiency syndrome (AIDS). The American Hospital Association estimates that a single case of serious infection by bloodborne pathogens can soon add up to $1 million or more in expenditures for testing follow-up, lost time, and disability payments (ANA, 1999b). The Needlestick Safety and Prevention Act requires all health care facilities to use needle systems and sharps with engineered protections such as retractable needles. As part of the legislation, employers are required to work with direct health care workers who use such devices to ensure the appropriate selection of technology (ANA, 1999a).

HEALTH POLICY: WHAT IS IT?

Health policy can be defined as a set course of action undertaken by governments or health care organizations to obtain a desired outcome. Private health policy is made by health care organizations such as hospitals and managed care organizations and includes those policies instituted to govern employee practices and health care services provided by the organization. Public health policy refers to local, state, and federal legislation, regulation, and court rulings that govern the behavior of individuals and organizations in the provision of health care services (Hanley, 1998). Examples of public policy include a state requirement for mandatory licensure to practice professional nursing and federal legislation to shape the Medicare program. There is a close link between private and public policy in that the policies of health care organizations are frequently implemented to comply with a public policy (Hanley, 1998).

Although it is absolutely essential for the RN to be involved in policy development at the health care organization in which he or she is employed, this chapter focuses on the development of public health policy and will be referred to simply as "health policy." "*Health policy* refers most often to public policies directly related to health care service delivery and reimbursement" (Hanley, 1998, p. 125).

Health Policy at the Local, State, and Federal Level

Health policies may be developed and implemented at the local, state, or federal level and are characterized by the fact that they apply to all residents under the jurisdiction of the respective government. For example, local health policy applies only to those people who are residents of that town or city, whereas health policy enacted at the federal level applies to residents in the United States.

Local Health Policy. At the local level many cities or counties offer a variety of health care services to meet the needs of their residents. For example, as part of city's health policy, free or reduced-rate immunizations may be offered to all children in the community. More controversial policies might include a requirement for tobacco-free public areas, including restaurants and entertainment establishments. Local health policy varies considerably across the United States, with some communities funding a variety of extensive health programs and others offering only limited health services. However, even the smallest communities are involved to some extent in health policy through partnerships with state government to ensure safe drinking water, the enforcement of seat belt and child restraint laws, and the provision of an emergency medical system for their residents.

State Health Policy. Health policy at the state level has a powerful influence on the health and safety of the state residents. In addition to its lead role in governing nursing practice through the Nursing Practice Act, each state also has health policies that may be invisible to the general public. These policies include maintaining a safe meat supply through livestock inspections, ensuring safe food storage and preparation in restaurants, and ensuring that health care facilities provide safe, quality care through regulatory activities. Only when these activities fail do the state's residents realize the importance of these policies.

State health policy also involves paying for some health care services. The Medicaid program, which pays for health care services for poor people and other qualified groups (as defined by the state), is funded through matching state and federal funds. More recently the State Children's Health Insurance Program (SCHIP) is being implemented in many states to provide health insurance coverage to uninsured children who do not qualify for the Medicaid program. The SCHIP is funded though a partnership between state and federal governments based on state-defined criteria and state-generated proposals. State governments are also the prime sources of funding for mental health services, long-term care services, and workforce development.

Federal Health Policy. Just as state health policies have an enormous impact on people's health and safety, the federal government plays a vitally important role in the health of Americans. The federal government's role in health care includes significant funding for health-related research; supplemental funding for education for health professionals, including nurses and physicians; and paying for health care through Medicare, Medicaid, SCHIP, and the Veteran's Administration health care system.

Federal health policies have played and continue to play a monumental role in shaping nursing practice. For example, the first federal policy to provide funding for nursing services was the Sheppard-Towner Act, enacted in 1921. This Act provided states with matching funds to establish prenatal and child health centers staffed by public health nurses with the goal of reducing the rates of maternal and infant mortality by teaching women how to care for themselves and their families. The highly successful program was discontinued in 1927 at the urging of the American Medical Association, whose membership considered it to be excessive interference in local health care concerns (Heinrich, 1998). Another example of legislation that influenced nursing practice was The Hill-Burton Act, also known as the Hospital Survey and Construction Act, passed in 1950. This Act provided federal funding for hospital construction and created a boom in the construction of hospitals across the country. As the number of hospitals increased rapidly, so did the need for nurses to staff the hospitals. Thus the nurse's role shifted from public health to the acute care setting. Today federal legislation is affecting nursing practice through expanding reimbursement for advanced practice nurses and considering policies to address the nursing shortage. Other current policy issues affecting nursing practice are addressed later in this chapter.

HEALTH POLICY: HOW IS IT DEVELOPED?

The development of health policy at the state or federal level is a complex, dynamic process that occurs in a variety of ways, including (Mason and Leavitt, 1998):

- Enactment of legislation and the accompanying rules and regulations that carry the weight of law.
- Administrative decisions made by various governmental agencies.
- Judicial decisions that interpret the law.

Health policy development usually involves numerous individuals and groups, including elected officials; officials from governmental agencies; experts in the related area; and stakeholders such as corporate representatives who may be affected by the policy, representatives from special interest groups who have a particular interest in the policy, and other affected citizens. As a special interest group, the American Nurses Association (ANA) represents nurses throughout the United States and carries a very strong voice in influencing health policy that may affect nursing practice. At the state level the constituent member associations (CMAs) of the ANA are the policy voice of the profession.

The development of health policy also involves all three branches of government: executive, legislative, and judicial. A basic understanding of the three branches of government is necessary if the reader is to understand health policy development. Table 10-1 presents a very brief review of the three branches of the federal government and their roles in health policy. Although most state governments parallel the structure and functions of the federal government, there are differences among states. The nurse is highly encouraged to learn about the government structure of his or her state. In addition to understanding the branches of government, it is also important to understand the role of legislation and regulation in the development of health policy.

Legislation and Health Policy Development

The development of health policy refers to the steps through which a policy moves from a societal problem to an actual social program that can be evaluated. The legislative process is fundamental to this movement from a public problem to a viable program. Although there are many public health problems, the only problems that will qualify as policy problems are those that are brought to the attention of a policy maker who is willing to take definitive action through the policy process (Hanley, 1998). Generally individuals or groups approach policy makers with prepared legislative solutions to problems, but policy makers may also learn of problems through their personal experiences and take action independently. At the federal level, only members of Congress can introduce legislation. The congressional member or members who introduce a specific piece of legislation become the sponsor(s) of that legislation.

Legislation is introduced by a member of Congress only after careful analysis of the problem, including:

- Public perception of the problem.
- Definition of the problem.

TABLE 10-1	*The Three Branches of the Federal Government*		
	EXECUTIVE	**LEGISLATIVE**	**JUDICIAL**
Composition	Office of the President and 14 Executive Departments (State, Treasury, Defense, Agriculture, Energy, Housing and Urban Development, Justice, Commerce, Education, Health and Human Services, Interior, Labor, Transportation, and Veteran's Affairs)	Senate and Congress	U.S. Supreme Court, federal district courts, and U.S. circuit courts of appeals
Role in health policy	Recommends legislation and promotes major policy initiatives Implements laws and manages programs after they have been passed by Congress Writes regulations that interpret statutes (laws) Has the power to veto legislation passed by Congress	Possess the sole federal power to enact legislation Able to originate and promote major policy initiatives Power to override a presidential veto	Judicial interpretations of the constitution or various laws may have a policy effect Resolve questions regarding agency regulations that may affect policy
Restrictions to power	Unable to enact a law without the approval of Congress (legislative branch)	Presidential veto; U.S. Supreme Court may invalidate legislation as unconstitutional	Unable to recommend or promote legislative initiatives

- Societal consequences and the number of people affected by the problem.
- Degree of support and opposition from other members of Congress, special interest groups, corporate supporters, and the general public.

After the problem is thoroughly analyzed and the decision is made to draft a piece of legislation, the staff members who work for the congressman translate the idea into legal, technical, and constitutional language. Only then does the problem become a bill as a proposed legislative solution.

Steps in the Legislative Process

The official legislative process at the federal level begins when a bill or resolution is introduced by the sponsoring member(s) of Congress and is numbered, referred to a committee, and printed by the U.S. Government Printing Office. Following are the basic steps a bill follows in the legislative process (ANA, 2001b).

Step 1: The bill is referred to a standing committee in the House or Senate according to carefully defined procedures.

Step 2: The bill may be referred to a subcommittee or be considered by the committee as a whole; it is examined carefully, and its chances for passage are determined. If the committee does not act on the bill, it is essentially dead.

Step 3: Bills may be referred to a subcommittee for study and hearings; hearings provide committee members with the opportunity to obtain written or oral testimony about the bill from the executive branch, experts in the related area, and supporters and proponents of the bill.

Step 4: After hearings, the subcommittee may choose to "mark up" the bill, which means to make changes or amendments before recommending the bill to the full committee. The bill dies if the subcommittee votes not to refer the bill to the full committee.

Step 5: After the full committee receives the bill from the subcommittee, the committee can conduct further hearings and study or vote on the subcommittee's recommendations. The full committee then votes on its recommendations to the House or Senate, a procedure known as "ordering a bill reported."

Step 6: The committee staff members prepare a written report about the bill that includes its intent, impact on existing laws and programs, position of the executive branch, and views of dissenting members of the committee.

Step 7: The bill is scheduled on the calendar in either the House or the Senate for floor action.

Step 8: Debate begins when the bill reaches the floor of the House or Senate; various rules govern the conditions and amount of time allowed for debate.

Step 9: After debate, the bill is passed or defeated.

Step 10: After a bill is passed by either the House or Senate, it is referred to the other chamber, where it normally follows the same process through committee and floor action; at this point the bill may be approved as received, rejected, ignored, or changed.

Step 11: If the second Chamber significantly alters the bill, a Conference Committee is formed to reconcile the differences between the House and Senate.

Step 12: After the bill is approved by both the House and Senate in identical form, it is sent to the President, who may (a) approve and sign the bill into law, (b) take no action for 10 days while Congress is in session and then the bill automatically becomes a law, (c) veto the bill, or (d) take no action after Congress has adjourned and the legislation dies.

Step 13: If the President vetoes the bill, Congress may override the veto, which requires a two-thirds roll call vote of the members who are present in sufficient numbers for a quorum.

Although this legislative process appears to be a simple, straightforward method for creating public law, it is actually very complex and convoluted, with only a fraction of the legislation introduced actually making it through the final process to become law. For example, in both sessions of the 106th U.S. Congress (January 6, 1999 through December 15, 2000) 10,840 measurers were introduced, and only 580 actually became public law (Congressional Record, 2001). In other words, only 5% of bills introduced in the 106th Congress actually became public law.

Once a bill finally becomes a law, implementation falls under the jurisdiction of one of the departments under the executive branch of government (see Table 10-1). For example, at the federal level most health-related policies fall under jurisdiction of the Department of Health and Human Services (DHHS) and its related agencies. The agency that will administer the law develops the regulations to implement the law. Implementation of new legislation can often be very different from what was intended when the bill was passed by Congress. It is important at this point that supporters of the new law take steps to ensure that it is implemented as intended by the lawmakers, which leads us into the discussion about regulation and health policy.

Regulation and Health Policy Development

The regulatory arena is an important but often overlooked area of political action that affects nursing practice. An understanding of regulatory processes provides nurses with the knowledge necessary to become involved and affect the future of nursing. Regulation refers to the written set of rules issued by the government agency that has responsibility for administering the new law. Because regulations carry the force of the law, they directly shape the implementation of health policy. Thus it is very important that the regulations reflect the intent of the law as enacted by Congress. And as stated in the previous paragraph, supporters of a new law must be vigilant and involved in the development of regulations.

As regulations are being developed by the government agency, public hearings are held to allow individuals to comment on the content of the regulations. At this stage nurses can play an influential role in the final regulations by writing to the regulatory agency or speaking at public hearings. Once the proposed regulations are developed, they must be published and open to public comment for a specified length of time before being adopted. Comment is critical for the development of administrative law. Each comment received must be considered and responded to before final regulations are issued. At the federal level the proposed (interim) regulations are published in the Federal Register. The time interval between the interim and final rules is critical for assessing the impact of the proposed rules and requires concerted nursing action in reacting to them either positively or negatively. Final published regulations carry the force of the law and will dictate how the law is actually implemented and the outcomes that will be achieved.

A great deal of effort in a complex legislative and regulatory process goes into the development of health policy, from the time a public problem is identified and a legislative solution is conceived until the health policy is actually implemented. By understanding and becoming involved in these processes, nurses can protect and influence nursing practice and create and direct change throughout the health care system.

POLITICS: WHAT IS THE CONNECTION WITH HEALTH POLICY?

Many people view politics as rather "shady" activities that occur in federal, state, and local governments to influence the outcomes of candidate elections and/or support for or against legislation. Mason and Leavitt (1998) have defined politics as a "process by which one influences the decisions of others and exerts control over situations and events." As the reader will see, "influence" is the common denominator in any definition of politics. Political influence can come in many forms, including money, knowledge, relationships, information, talent, and/or control over large groups of votes. Florence Nightingale was the consummate political nurse and understood how to influence the British Parliament to allocate funds to reform British military hospitals and substantially improve the health and sanitary conditions for the troops.

Politics are a necessary part of the policy process when multiple interest groups such as elected officials, special interest groups, and corporate leaders are all competing to achieve their individual goals. The process becomes more interesting when you add the two-party political system and the varied agendas of the Democratic and Republican parties to the mix.

Groups and individuals who have a stake in the fate of a piece of legislation or the election of a candidate can use political strategies to obtain their desired outcome. Thus it is through effective political action that nurses can positively influence legislative and regulatory decisions and health policies that will impact nursing practice and the health of Americans. A discussion of effective political strategies follows.

GRASSROOTS POLITICAL STRATEGIES

Grassroots political strategies are actions taken at the local level to influence policy makers. Nurses have a right to petition, lobby, or persuade policy makers to ensure that their interests and concerns are heard. Such actions (usually referred to as lobbying) provide those individuals and groups who are stakeholders in a particular issue an opportunity to be heard. Lobbying also provides policy makers with information on which to base their decisions. Following are various methods through which nurses can be effective grassroots players:

- Registering to vote and voting in *ALL* elections
- Joining the professional nursing organization
- Working in candidates' campaigns
- Attending "meet the candidates" town hall meetings
- Visiting personally with policy makers or their staff
- Writing letters
- Telephoning
- Sending telegrams, mailgrams, e-mail, facsimiles, and public opinion messages about issues
- Testifying at hearings

Registering To Vote and Voting in All Elections

Voting is a must for every nurse! However, voting is not enough. *Informed voting* is necessary to enhance nurses' political power to ultimately improve the health of patients and the nursing care that they receive. Nurses should become informed about the issues. Becoming informed involves reading legislative newsletters and finding out about policy makers' backgrounds, voting records, and current platform. Discussing these issues with nurse colleagues and others in the community serves to enhance everyone's understanding of candidates and their positions.

Joining a Professional Nursing Organization

Another must for the professional nurse is to join a professional nursing organization. The value of the ANA and CMAs and the specialty nursing organizations is that together the nursing profession is much more powerful than the individual RN. As professionals in a collective, nurses know more, nurses have more resources, and nurses are able to pool strengths and direct resources toward winning the health policy "game."

The ANA is the foremost recognized professional nursing organization in Washington, D.C., for federal health and public policy. This organization speaks for professional nurses, regardless of specialty. All nurses should belong as one of their basic professional responsibilities. Nurses who choose to maintain membership in the specialty organization that represents their area of nursing practice have the additional advantage of receiving both clinical and health policy information related to that specialty.

Because professional nursing organizations monitor public policy and offer avenues for their members to learn about health policy, they serve as an invaluable resource for reliable information related to policy issues and policy makers. Generally the information needed to make informed voting decisions does not come neatly packaged with the issues clearly identified. Obtaining this information and deciphering it requires skills that many nurses do not readily possess. Joining a professional nursing organization that has a political action committee (PAC) can help develop the necessary skills to understand political issues. A PAC is an arm of a corporation, association, or labor union formed to provide support either to persuade a policy maker to support a certain policy or program or, more often, to ensure that a policy maker who supports the organization's goals attains office or remains in office.

Professional nursing organizations may choose to endorse a specific candidate for office. Endorsement simply means that, in a particular political race, the nursing organization selects one candidate to support because of that candidate's platform on record supporting specific issues or goals. Although endorsement does not mean that everyone in the organization *must* vote for the selected person, it does mean that the organization has carefully screened the candidate and the nurse can be reasonably sure that the candidate will support nursing's interests.

Working in Political Candidates' Campaigns

Most political candidates are not health professionals and do not clearly understand health-related issues. By working in their campaigns, nurses can (and should) educate and inform them about health care issues. Other activities that the nurse may undertake on behalf of the candidates include assisting in writing health care position statements, working in campaign offices, attending local debates, displaying the candidates' political buttons and signs, and participating in fundraising events. Nurse supporters may also write letters to and/or call other nurses in the region to tell them about their support of the candidate and to ask for their vote.

"Meet the Candidates" Town Hall Meeting

A strategy that CMAs use to determine endorsing a candidate is to invite all candidates running for a particular office to a town hall meeting to discuss their platforms with nurses. Town hall gatherings with nurses allow the candidates to talk about their platform to a group of interested voters in a time- and cost-saving manner. A town hall meeting affords nurses an opportunity to understand the candidate's platform and to voice their opinions and concerns about health care issues.

Hosting a "Meet the Candidates" town hall meeting can be an exciting activity for student nurses and faculty. Nursing students at a hosting school should prepare for the town hall meeting as follows (TNA, 1995):

1. Before the town hall meeting, become familiar with the each candidate's background, including his or her voting record on health policy issues, major contributors, personal occupations, family information, and hobbies. This information can provide insight into the candidate's positions on issues.
2. Identify current issues that would be relevant for discussion with the candidates. Collect and review information related to the issues and then prioritize the issues. Time may not be sufficient to discuss all of the issues of interest.
3. Prepare to give concise examples of how the issue affects the individual, community, health care consumers in the district, and other members of the nursing profession. Be prepared to debate arguments that unfavorably reflect one's position.

4. Plan the agenda for the meeting to allow ample time for discussion.
5. On the day of the meeting, dress conservatively and arrive a few minutes early.
6. After introductions are made, listen carefully as each candidate presents his or her campaign platform; then be prepared to clearly and concisely discuss the issues with relevant examples as detailed in preceding paragraphs.
7. At the conclusion of the meeting, provide the candidate with your name, address, and telephone number.
8. After the town hall meeting, write a short note summarizing your understanding of each candidate's position on the issue.

Visiting With Policy Makers and Their Staff Members

Personal visits to policy makers and/or their staff members can be the most effective method of lobbying for or against a health care policy. Nothing is more effective in communicating nursing's position than face-to-face contact between a policy maker and his or her staff and a group of well-informed nurses. There also is no better way to educate a policy maker on an issue than when nurses have the opportunity to respond to his or her questions (TNA, 1995). Policy makers are very interested in information that will increase their knowledge about health care and help them plan for future health care policy. The following steps are recommended for personal visits with policy makers:

1. Prepare before the personal visit. Become familiar with the policy maker's background. Information about the policy maker's district, his or her voting record on nursing issues, major contributors, personal occupation, family information, and hobbies can provide insight into the policy maker's thinking and position on issues.
2. Identify issues of critical importance. Collect and review information related to the issue, then prioritize them. Be prepared to give concise examples of how the issue affects the individual, community, health care consumers in the district, and other members of the nursing profession. Be prepared to debate arguments that unfavorably reflect one's position.
3. Dress conservatively and arrive a few minutes early.
4. Be prepared to wait. Policy makers' schedules often are unpredictable.
5. Address the policy maker, introduce yourself and give your name and occupation. Identify yourself as a constituent. or identify the relationship to the policy maker's district. See Box 10-1 for the correct title to use when addressing a state elected official.
6. Clearly and concisely present the issue and position. Provide copies of background materials for the policy maker and his or her staff to review.
7. During discussions, if you do not know the answer to a question, admit it. However, find the information and get it to the policy maker as soon as possible.
8. If possible, talk with the policy maker's staff. Legislative staff members can be very influential in supporting your cause and promoting it the policy maker.
9. At the conclusion of the meeting, leave your name with an address and telephone number.
10. Follow up the visit with a short note thanking the policy maker and his staff members for the appointment, relating your understanding of the policy maker's position on the issue and any additional information the policy maker had requested. Always offer to provide further assistance.

BOX 10-1	*Speaking With the Governor, Lieutenant Governor, Legislators, or Staff*

Governor: Governor (last name)
Lieutenant Governor: Governor (last name)
Speaker of the House: Mr. or Madam Speaker
Senator: Senator (last name)
Representative: Representative (last name) or Mr. or Ms. (last name)
Staff: Mr. or Ms. (last name)

Ideally, for nursing students who have no political activism experience, the best time to personally visit with a policy maker is through a nursing school field trip experience. Many schools of nursing take advantage of opportunities through their state nurses' organizations planned Lobby Day to introduce students to the political process. In many states this day is called "Nurses Day on Capitol Hill."

Writing Letters

Writing letters to policy makers can be effective if properly planned and implemented. The timing of a letter is important. It should be written early, before policy makers make up their minds or commit to vote a certain way. It is easier to convince an undecided policy maker than it is to get him or her to switch positions. A second very effective step is to send a follow-up letter immediately before the vote on the bill is scheduled. Information about voting schedules can be obtained online in most states. Guidelines for writing to policy makers include:

1. Type an individualized letter. Mass-produced form letters are easy to detect, may weaken your position, and should be avoided.
2. Obtain a roster of the state legislators, which can be found online in most states. The roster contains information on each policy maker, including various committee memberships.
3. Use a proper salutation and closing (Box 10-2).
4. Keep sentences short and to the point.
5. The letter should be one page or less.
6. Address one issue per letter.
7. Include "RN" or "Senior Nursing Student" with your name.
8. Include a reference line to convey the subject (e.g., "Re: Violence in the Workplace Legislation").
9. Be clear about what is being asked of the policy maker, and be realistic.
10. Include a direct question to the policy maker. Request a written answer.
11. Thank the policy maker for his or her consideration of the issue.

Sending E-Mail

E-mail messages are quick and easy and may be helpful when speed is crucial. It is important to remember that conciseness is very valuable when sending e-mail messages. The subject of the message should contain the number of the bill to which you are referring in the message. For example, "In opposition to Senate Bill 123" immediately focuses the reader.

BOX 10-2	*Writing a Letter to the Governor, Lieutenant Governor, Members of Congress, State Legislators, or Staff*

Governor: The Honorable (full name)
Governor of Alabama
State Capitol
Montgomery, AL 36106

Lieutenant Governor: The Honorable (full name)
Lt. Governor of Tennessee
State Capitol
Nashville, TN 37243

State Senator: The Honorable (full name) or Dear Senator _____
State Senate
P. O. Box _____
Capital City, State, Zip Code

State Representative: The Honorable (last name) or Dear Representative _____
State House of Representatives
P. O. Box _____
Capital City, State, Zip Code

U.S. Senator: The Honorable (full name) or Dear Senator _____
United States Senate
Washington, DC 20510

US Representative: The Honorable (last name) or Dear Representative _____
US House of Representatives
Washington, DC 20510

Staff: Mr. (full name) or Ms. (full name)
_____ 's Office

Closing for letters to all of the above is: "Sincerely yours,".

The message itself should be just a few short lines to relay a clear and strong message related to the issue. Brief examples of how the issue affects the policy maker's constituents are often very effective.

Telephoning

Telephoning is most useful when time is crucial. It is an easy way to give the policy maker a sense of what his or her constituents believe about a certain bill. However, it is not an effective method for educating a policy maker or the legislative staff about an issue (TNA, 1995).

The following list provides guidelines to use when telephoning a policy maker.
1. Write a prepared statement or outline before calling to facilitate the call.
2. Call early in the morning.

3. Ask to speak to the staff person assigned to the bill or issue for which the call is being made.
4. If the person is not available, leave a message.
5. Give a brief and simple message.
6. Be courteous.
7. Leave name and a telephone number.
8. If time permits, follow up the telephone conversation with a letter (Box 10-3).
9. Facsimiles may also be used when time is of the essence. The message should be typed and should include the same information as a letter to the policy maker.

Testifying at Hearings

There is some debate concerning the effectiveness of testifying at hearings. Some believe (TNA, 1995), at least at the state level, that how committee members will vote is frequently, but not always, already decided before the hearing. Others believe that testifying at a public congressional hearing is an effective method of lobbying. However, both sides of the debate believe that preparation is extremely important. Usually persons request to testify before the hearing occurs. The following guidelines are for testifying at state-level hearings (TNA, 1995).

1. Prepare a written statement and have enough copies for all committee members plus the committee clerk.
2. Clearly document the facts and be brief and concise.
3. Organize testimony around key points.
4. Notify the policy maker who represents your district if testifying before a committee on which he or she is a member.

| BOX 10-3 | *Sample Telephone Call to a Policy Maker* |

"Hello, Senator (name's) office. How may I help you?"

"Hello, my name is (name) and I am a registered nurse in (city, state). May I please speak with the person who handles health care issues? (Identify yourself again if you are transferred to the health specialist.)
   I am calling because I want to let Senator (name) know that I am very concerned about (describe the issue, such as "the vote on Senate Bill 123" or "how the Violence in the Workplace Bill will affect my role in health care"). It is critical that the Senator (support or oppose issue, name, or bill description) because (give one to three brief reasons).
   More than one of every 100 adults in this country is a nurse, and one of every 44 registered female voters is a nurse. We, as nurses and voters, believe this issue to be very important."

"I appreciate your call today. I will make sure that the Senator gets your message. May I have your mailing address so that the Senator can contact you personally?"

"Yes, this is (name and address). Please make sure that the Senator knows that I (support or oppose) (issue, name, or bill description). Thank you for your time."

Substitute *Representative* for *Senator* when calling a member of the House of Representatives
(Texas Nurses Association, 1995)

5. Become familiar with the members of the committee and their hometowns.
6. Anticipate questions that may be asked. Prepare knowledgeable responses (TNA, 1995).

THE AMERICAN NURSES ASSOCIATION

The ANA is the professional nursing organization that, through its 54 CMAs (formerly known as State Nurses Associations) and 13 Organizational Affiliates, represents the nation's 2.6 million RNs. ANA advances the nursing profession by fostering high standards of nursing practice, promoting the economic and general welfare of nurses in the workplace, projecting a positive and realistic view of nursing, and lobbying the Congress and the federal regulatory agencies on health care issues affecting nurses and the public (ANA, 2001a).

The ANA is at the forefront of policy initiatives pertaining to health care reform. Its priority issues are (ANA, 2001a):

■ A restructured health care system that delivers primary health care in community-based settings.
■ An expanded role for RNs and advanced practice nurses in the delivery of basic and primary health care.
■ Obtaining federal funding for nurse education and training.
■ Helping to change and improve the health care workplace to enhance the health and safety of the patient and the nurse.

Through political and legislative activities, ANA has taken firm positions on various issues, including Medicare reform, patients' rights, the importance of safer needle devices, whistle-blower protections for health care workers, adequate reimbursement for health care services, and access to health care (ANA, 2001a).

Nurses Strategic Action Team (N-STAT)

Nurses are impressive in their collective abilities to mobilize and take effective action in shaping national health care policy through the Nurses Strategic Action Team (N-STAT). N-STAT is an ANA program that unifies nurses' political voices across the country to enact measures to benefit health care for everyone and to defeat measures that would have a serious negative impact on the health care delivery system. N-STAT is comprised of thousands of nurses around the country who stay informed on issues and contact their legislators about pending issues. Through *Legislative Updates,* N-STAT keeps members up-to-speed on key bills as they move through the legislative process. Through *Action Alerts,* members are informed about when e-mails, phone calls, and letters will make the most impact (ANA, 2001b).

N-STAT empowers nurses by encouraging them to take action and make their opinions heard and understood by Congress and the public. N-STAT provides the structure and coordination for nurses across the country to be involved in grassroots lobbying. For example, N-STAT sends notices to nurses regarding impending legislation that affects health care. Enclosed with the notices are senators' names, addresses, and phone numbers to facilitate nurses' actions in making their opinions known to the policy makers. Therefore N-STAT makes the political process less intimidating by keeping nurses informed of political issues and providing strategies for making their opinions known.

CURRENT HEALTH POLICY ISSUES

Policy issues come and go as society, health care, and public needs and wants ebb and flow. However, a few topics will bear watching over the next decade as it is unlikely that any of these will achieve a "perfect" solution. Yet the importance of these topics will keep them on the policy agenda.

Access to Care

In 2001 there were nearly 42 million uninsured Americans, and lack of insurance is the greatest barrier to access to health care. A variety of proposals have been either enacted or proposed to incrementally deal with access since the failure of the Congress to enact the Health Security Act of 1993, which would have provided universal coverage for health services. The most successful recent access policy has been the State Children's Health Insurance Program (SCHIP), which has insured three million children since its passage in 1997. Other access proposals currently under debate include:

- Tax credits for private insurance coverage.
- Expansion of Medicare to individuals between 55 and 65 years of age who lose group coverage.
- Offering family coverage for parents and siblings of SCHIP enrollees.

Prescription Drug Coverage for Medicare Beneficiaries

Medicare became the health insurance mechanism for America's seniors in the 1960s. Health care has changed dramatically over the past few decades, especially in the areas of biologics and pharmacology. The absence of a prescription drug benefit in the Medicare package of covered services is a significant problem for the elderly. The inclusiveness of such a benefit, its scope, and how to pay for it are continuing issues between the Bush White House and the 107th Congress and between Democrats and Republicans.

Health Care Workforce and the Nursing Shortage

America is aging at a very rapid rate, and this demographic profile calls for greatly increased needs for health services over the next three decades. At the same time, the U.S. economy has exploded with new fields of study and work. Thus the numbers of individuals selecting health careers has decreased just as the need for these health services is increasing. No health profession is as hard hit as professional nursing—a group who is aging faster than the population in general and whose retirees are outpacing new recruits. Both federal and state governments are currently evaluating proposals for health care professional recruitment and retention, and the nursing workforce is being given the highest priority among the health professions for policy intervention at both levels. Will any of the proposals be effective and timely? Stay tuned!

SUMMARY

Nurses are powerful advocates for health care. By understanding the policy and political processes presented in this chapter, nurses can make effective contributions to the development of health policies that promote a healthier society. Because nurses are the critical one-to-one link between organized nursing and policy makers, their basic professional responsibility is to be involved in professional nursing organizations and to be politically active in supporting meaningful health policies. Just as we learned from the first politically active nurse, Florence Nightingale, nurses can use health policy to make a difference in the lives of people we care about, as well as in our own lives and for the future of our profession.

Critical Thinking Activities

1. What statewide office is coming up for election in your state this year? Who are the candidates for the office? Do they have stated positions on health care issues? Do you agree or disagree with these positions? What questions would you ask concerning the candidates' positions on health care if given the opportunity to talk with them?
2. Identify and discuss health care issues that you perceive to be of great interest, not only to policy makers, but also to the public.
3. Identify a nursing issue that is of concern to you. What factors would help you determine if this issue is feasible for policy action?
4. Determine if your state legislature is in session. Identify a bill related to a nursing issue. Identify the benefits to you, your community, health care consumers in the district, and other members of the nursing profession that can come from enacting this bill.
5. Determine how your state board of nurse examiners interprets the scope of nursing practice.
6. Review the methods by which grassroots lobbying can and does occur. Which methods would you choose if your plan is to maintain and improve the quality of patient care as it relates to the use of mandatory overtime as a routine staffing method? Explain your answer.

REFERENCES

American Nurses Association: Health Care Worker Needlestick Prevention Act of 1999, H.R. 1899/S. 1140, 1999a, www.ana.org/gova/federal/legis/106/gndlintr.htm.

American Nurses Association: *Nursing facts: needlestick injury,* 1999b, www.ana.org/readroom/fsneedle.htm.

American Nurses Association: About us, 2001a, http://www.ana.org/about/index.htm.

American Nurses Association (2001). Hill basics: the legislative processes, 2001b, www.ana.org/gova/federal/politic/hill/glegproc.htm.

Congressional Record: 2001 Resumé of congressional activity 106th Congress, Congressional Record Daily Digest, January 30, 2001, p. D45, http://thomas.loc.gov/home/resume/106res.html.

Hanley BE: Policy development and analysis. In Mason DJ, Leavitt JK: *Policy and politics in nursing and health care,* ed 3, Philadelphia, 1998, WB Saunders.

Heinrich J: Organization and delivery of health care in the United States: the health care system that isn't. In Mason DJ, Leavitt JK: *Policy and politics in nursing and health care,* ed 3, Philadelphia, 1998, WB Saunders.

Mason DJ, Leavitt JK: Policy and politics: A framework for action. In *Policy and politics in nursing and health care,* ed 3, Philadelphia, 1998, WB Saunders.

Oxhorn V, Rosen S: Understanding the regulatory arena, *AORN J* 55(2):623-629, 1992.

Texas Nurses Association: *Lobbying handbook for nurses,* Austin, 1995, Texas Nurses Association.

Wunderlich GS, Kohler PO: *Improving the quality of long-term care,* Committee on Improving Quality in Long-Term Care, Division of Health Care Services, Institute of Medicine. Washington, DC, 2001, National Academy Press.

Cultural Competency and Social Issues in Nursing and Health Care

Susan R. Jacob, PhD, RN, and M. Elizabeth Carnegie, DPA, RN, FAAN

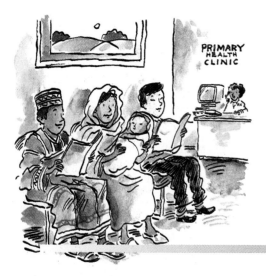

11

Clients deserve culturally competent care.

Vignette

When my instructor taught the session on cultural differences, she stressed the high alcoholism rates of Native Americans. I began to fear that my instructor and fellow classmates would stereotype me because of my Native American background. However, no one in my family drinks alcohol because we belong to the Mormon church, where drinking is not accepted. I wish the instructor had stressed the importance of not stereotyping.

Questions to consider while reading this chapter
1. What preconceived ideas do you have about the following cultural groups: Hispanic, Appalachian, Moroccan, African-American, South African, Chinese?
2. What strategies can you implement to overcome prejudice?
3. How can nurses provide effective care to different cultural groups who each have a unique set of responses to health and illness?
4. How can nursing research affect the attitudes and beliefs of health professionals in regard to minority and marginalized populations?

Key Terms

Acculturation The process of becoming adapted to a new or different culture.

Assimilation The cultural absorption of a minority group into the main cultural body.

Biculturalism Combining two distinct cultures in a single region.

Culture Shared values, beliefs, and practices of a particular group of people that are transmitted from one generation to the next and are identified as patterns that guide thinking and action.

Enculturation Adaptation to the prevailing cultural patterns in society.

Ethnicity Affiliation resulting from shared linguistic, racial, or cultural background.

Ethnocentrism Believing that one's own ethnic group, culture, or nation is best.

Marginalized population A subgroup of the population that tends to be hidden, overlooked, or on the outer edge.

Minority An ethnic group smaller than the majority group.

Prejudice Preconceived, deeply held, usually negative, judgment formed about other groups.

Stereotyping Assigning certain beliefs and behaviors to groups without recognizing individuality.

Transculturalism Being grounded in one's own culture, but having the skills to be able to work in a multicultural environment.

Worldview Perspective shared by a cultural group of general views of relationships within the universe. These broad views influence health and illness beliefs.

Learning Outcomes

After studying this chapter, the reader will be able to:

1. Integrate knowledge of demographic and sociocultural variations into culturally competent professional nursing care.
2. Provide culturally competent care to diverse client groups that incorporates variations in biologic characteristics, social organization, environmental control, communication, and other phenomena.
3. Critique education, practice, and research issues that influence culturally competent care.
4. Integrate respect for differences in beliefs and values of others as a critical component of nursing practice.

CHAPTER OVERVIEW

The United States has always been represented by a culturally diverse society. However, the volume of cultural groups entering our country is increasing rapidly. Professional nurses must provide care to persons of various cultures who have different values, beliefs, and perceptions of health and illness. This chapter explores cultural phenomena, including environmental control, biologic variations, social organization, communication, space, and time in relation to major cultural groups. It also examines different views toward health, illness, and cure. Federally defined minority groups, which include African-Americans, Asians, Hispanics, and Native Americans, are emphasized, although the needs of marginalized populations such as the homeless, refugees, and the elderly also are addressed. The need for diversity in the health care force is explored, and strategies for recruiting and retaining minorities in health care are suggested. Strategies that nurses can use to increase their own cultural competence also are given.

POPULATION TRENDS

The demographic and ethnic composition of the U.S. population has experienced marked change in the past 100 years. The United States always has been a multicultural society, although changes in immigration laws have increased the number of cultural groups entering the United States (Stanhope and Lancaster, 2000). "Federally defined minority groups have grown faster than the population as a whole" (Nies and McEwen, 2001). If migration trends continue, by mid twenty-first century the minority populations will outnumber the Caucasian population. Approximately one in every three Americans will be an ethnic minority. In some cities in the United States the number of persons from diverse cultural groups is increasing at such a rapid pace that minorities comprise more than half the population. It is predicted that at the end of this decade some states will have no majority group, only multiple minority subcultures (Meleis et al., 1995).

The aging population includes an increasing number of older adults whose age exceeds 85 years. By the year 2000 there were four million more Americans older than 65 years of age than there were in 1990. This demographic change introduces many interrelated social, economic, political, education, and health problems. The fact that people are living longer allows more opportunity for the development of chronic illness. Social isolation and depression that result from losses of friends and family will present a challenge for mental health care providers. Primary care providers will be faced with identifying risks to independence and health for the aging population (U.S. Department of Health and Human Services, *Healthy People 2010*, 2000).

Federally Defined Minority Groups

Federally defined minority groups are African-Americans, Hispanics, Native Americans, and Asians/Pacific Islanders. Although tremendous strides have been made in improving health and longevity in the United States, statistical trends show a disparity in key health indicators among certain subgroups of the population (Nies and McEwen, 2001). There is a racial gap between African-Americans and Caucasians of 5.6 years, with average life expectancy being 75.2 years for Caucasians and 69.6 years for African-Americans. The infant death rate for African-Americans is twice that of Caucasians (Nies and McEwen, 2001). Although the ranking of health problems according to excess deaths differs for minority groups, the six causes of death that are a priority are:

1. Cancer
2. Cardiovascular disease and stroke
3. Chemical dependency as measured by deaths caused by cirrhosis of the liver
4. Diabetes
5. Homicides and accidents
6. Infant mortality (Nies and McEwen, 2001)

Marginalized Populations

Not only should the concern for culturally competent care focus on ethnic minorities and populations that have a different heritage than Euro-Americans, but the needs of marginalized populations (Hall, Stevens, and Meleis, 1994), which are those populations that live on the periphery or in between, should be considered. Examples of such populations include gays and lesbians, older adults, recently arrived immigrants (e.g., from Russia, Afghanistan, and Rwanda), and groups that have been in this country for some time (e.g., from South America and the Middle East) who are less visible than the federally defined minorities (Lenburg et al., 1995). Their lives and health care needs often are kept secret and are understood only by them. Marginalized populations usually have extreme insights about their health care needs, although they often seem voiceless. This is in part a result of the different ways in which they both communicate and are silenced. It also may be because they feel even more peripheral or shut out from mainstream society when they are ill or experiencing a crisis.

ECONOMIC AND SOCIAL CHANGES

Changing world economics have had profound consequences such as increased joblessness, homelessness, poverty, and limited access to health insurance and health care. Anxiety, hopelessness, depression, and despair commonly affect the individuals in our society who find themselves suddenly without a job and sometimes even without a home as a result of downsizing. These conditions often are associated with increased stress-related symptoms, substance abuse, violence, and crime (Lenburg et al., 1995). Dramatic changes in technology and specialization in the health care field have made health care costs skyrocket. Therefore not everyone can afford health care services. More minorities lack health insurance than the general population (Nies and McEwen, 2001). Higher costs and lower wages for minority groups make it difficult to rise out of poverty (Stanhope and Lancaster, 2000).

Poverty

Most families with racially or ethnically diverse backgrounds have a lower socioeconomic status than does the population at large. African-Americans, Hispanics, and Native Americans have much higher rates of poverty than non-Hispanic Caucasians and Asians. The median family income of Asians is slightly higher than that of non-Hispanic Caucasians and is consistent with Asians' high levels of education and the higher percentage of families with two wage earners (Council of Economic Advisers, 1999). However, opportunities for education, occupation, income earning, and property ownership that are available to upper- and middle-class Americans often are not available to members of minority groups (Stanhope and Lancaster, 2000).

The poor also suffer more than the population as a whole for nearly every measure of health. Substantial disparities remain in health insurance coverage for certain populations. Among the nonelderly population, approximately 33% of Hispanic persons lacked health insurance coverage in 1998, a rate that is more than double the national average. Mexican Americans had one of the highest uninsured rates at 40%. For adults under age 65 years, 34% of those below the poverty level were uninsured. Lack of health care coverage has major implications for health (U.S. Department of Health and Human Services, 2000).

Minority members of society often live in poverty. This social stratification leads to social inequality. For instance, it is widely known that school systems and recreational facilities vary significantly between the inner city and the suburbs (Nies and McEwen, 2001). Residential segregation, substandard housing, unemployment, poor physical and mental health, and poor self-image are part of the cycle of poverty. This inequality is especially disturbing as it relates to health care. The United States has a history of providing the highest quality health care to those with the highest socioeconomic status and the worst health care to those with low socioeconomic status. Social, economic, and health problems have led to heated debates about the philosophy, scope and costs, and sources of funding for health care and insurance programs.

Violence

Changing economic and social conditions have contributed to the increasing level of violence in our society. Statistics indicate that homicide is the second leading cause of death among Americans ages 10 to 24 years and the leading cause of death among African-American males ages 15 to 34 years (Nies and McEwen, 2001). Businesses, schools, restaurants, playgrounds, and churches have become common settings for random acts of violence (Lenburg et al., 1995). Unemployment is associated with violence because it is an expectation in our society that people should be productive and gainfully employed. The inability to secure or hold a job may lead to feelings of inadequacy, guilt, and frustration, which in turn can precipitate acts of violence. Although the increasing incidence of violence affects all segments of society, women, children, the elderly population, and culturally vulnerable groups are especially at risk. "Young minority males have the highest rates of unemployment in the United States, ranging close to 50%" (Stanhope and Lancaster, 2000). This group also has the highest rate of violence, with homicide being a major problem for young African-American males. The differing rates of violence among races are more likely a result of poverty than race (Stanhope and Lancaster, 2000).

Societal changes have increased the tension between the empowered culturally dominant groups and the less visible vulnerable groups. This tension and behavioral response to tension has major implications for health care delivery and the education of nurses and other health care professionals (Lenburg et al., 1995).

ATTITUDES TOWARD CULTURALLY DIVERSE GROUPS

The range of attitudes toward culturally diverse groups can be viewed along a continuum of intensity, as illustrated in Fig. 11-1 (Lenburg et al., 1995).

The extreme negative manifestation of prejudice is hate in its many violent and nonviolent forms. Contempt is somewhat less intense but is problematic because it is so widespread and undermines many aspects of society. Tolerance reflects a more neutral attitude that accepts differences without attempting to convert them; it is the minimum-level attitude essential in democratic societies. Respect for diversity is manifested in behaviors that integrate differences into positive interactions and relationships. Respect is a demonstration of the inherent worth of the individual, regardless of differences. The most positive attitude is portrayed as a celebration (or affirmation) of the positive merits of cultural differences (i.e., of the value added to life experiences by multiple perspectives, traditions, rituals, foods, and art forms). The combination of ignorance of other cultures and arrogance about one's own culture fosters disrespect and hate. The deliberate attempt to discover and apply the positive ben-

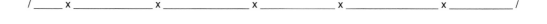

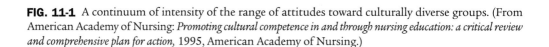

FIG. 11-1 A continuum of intensity of the range of attitudes toward culturally diverse groups. (From American Academy of Nursing: *Promoting cultural competence in and through nursing education: a critical review and comprehensive plan for action,* 1995, American Academy of Nursing.)

efits of cultural variation promotes respect and a celebration of the value of diversity, whereas perpetuating prejudice fosters narrow-mindedness and contempt. By integrating these perspectives as part of professional role behavior, educators can help students prepare for culturally competent practice in communities of diversity.

DIVERSITY IN THE HEALTH CARE WORKFORCE
Need for Diversity in the Health Care Workforce

Members of some cultural groups are demanding culturally relevant health care that incorporates their beliefs and practices (Nies and McEwen, 2001). Consumers are becoming much more aware of what constitutes culturally sensitive and competent care and are less willing to accept incompetent care (Meleis et al., 1995). There is a lack of diversity and ethnic representation of health care professionals; and there is limited knowledge about values, beliefs, experiences, and health care needs of certain populations such as immigrants, the elderly population, and gays and lesbians. Each of these groups has a unique set of responses to health and illness.

Nurses make up the largest segment of the workforce in health care delivery. Therefore they have an opportunity to be proactive in changing health care inequities and access to health care (Meleis et al., 1995). The changing health care system must reflect the community; and, as health care moves into the community, it is vital that partnerships be formed between health care providers and the community. For these partnerships to become a reality, minority representation in all health professions is vital. Factors inhibiting minority members from attaining a career in nursing include inadequate academic preparation, especially in

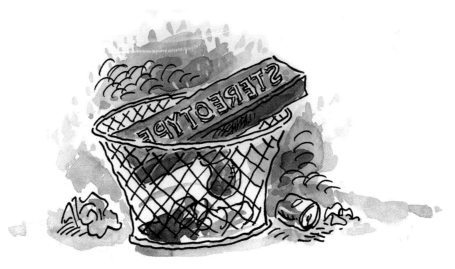

Stereotypes should be trashed.

the sciences; financial costs; inadequate career counseling; and better recruitment efforts by other disciplines (Sullivan, 1998).

Current Status of Diversity in the Health Care Workforce

Although most nurses are Caucasian women, an increasing proportion of minority students is graduating from nursing programs. In a survey conducted by the American Association of Colleges of Nursing (AACN) in 2001 (Table 11-1), minority representation was highest among those identified as black or African-American (11.4 %) and lowest among Native Americans (0.7%). Graduates from Hispanic or Latino groups totaled 4.8%; and Asian, native Hawaiian, or other Pacific Islander were 4.7% of the undergraduate students who responded to the survey. These totals lag behind the 73.55% reported Caucasian enrollment.

The number of men who graduate from basic registered nurse (RN) programs is increasing. In the AACN survey conducted in 2000, 9% of the undergraduate respondents were men (Table 11-2). Men continue to represent a minority in nursing, although geographic representation varies widely, with west Texas reporting 15% to 18% male representation in nursing. Because recruitment efforts are focused more on ethnic minorities, it is expected that the small representation from men will continue (Castiglia, 1997).

Recruitment and Retention of Minorities in Nursing

It is clear that we have been slow in preparing nurses to be reflective of our population, just as we have been unaware of the need for culturally sensitive patient care and sometimes less than welcoming to students different from the predominant population (Sullivan, 1998). Recruitment and retention of students from minority populations must not be separated. In other words, recruitment programs must have retention as their primary focus because there is no point in recruiting minorities into nursing programs and then not helping them succeed.

Before World War II the only known effort to recruit minority students into nursing on a national scale was made by the National Association of Colored Graduate Nurses (NACGN), which had had recruitment of African-Americans into nursing as one of its objectives since its inception in 1908. During World War II a mechanism was set into motion by the federal government to produce additional nursing personnel by financing basic nursing education. This was done through the Cadet Nurse Corps. The Corps had a number of recruiters, two of whom were African-American. These two African-American nurses confined their recruiting to 82 African-American colleges and universities. By the end of the war, 21 African-American nursing schools had participated in the Corps, and well over 2000 African-American nurses had acquired their basic nursing education through this mechanism.

After the war, recruitment efforts for African-Americans at the national level reverted to NACGN, an organization that voted itself out of existence in 1949 and was dissolved in 1951. However, individual African-American schools in the North and South continued to recruit. In the south law segregated the nursing schools, and in the North they were segregated by custom. In 1954 the unanimous Supreme Court decision—Brown v. the Board of education—asserted that "separate educational facilities were inherently unequal," making racial segregation in public schools unconstitutional. This decision was interpreted to mean that all kinds of educational discrimination would be considered, including nursing.

It was around the time of the Brown decision that schools of nursing were being accredited by national standards, and many schools, both African-American and Caucasian, just did

| TABLE 11-1 | *Type of Degree by Race/Ethnicity and Nonresident Alien Status of Students Enrolled (Fall 2000) and Graduates (August 1, 1999 to July 31, 2000).* |

| | UNDERGRADUATE | | | GRADUATE | | | |
| | | | | MASTER'S | DOCTORAL | POST-DOCTORAL | ND |
	GENERIC	RN	TOTAL				
Students enrolled (fall 2000)							
Race/ethnicity							
Asian, Native Hawaiian, or other Pacific Islander	3,804	963	4,767	1,457	98	1	6
(%)	(5.3)	(3.2)	(4.7)	(4.7)	(3.2)	(2.6)	(1.9)
Black or African-American	8,102	3,559	11,661	2,587	177	3	22
(%)	(11.3)	(11.7)	(11.4)	(8.3)	(5.9)	(7.9)	(7.0)
American Indian or Alaskan Native	468	226	694	217	11	1	2
(%)	(0.7)	(0.7)	(0.7)	(0.7)	(0.4)	(2.6)	(0.6)
Hispanic or Latino	3,537	1,336	4,873	1,252	56	0	12
(%)	(4.9)	(4.4)	(4.8)	(4.0)	(1.9)	(0.0)	(3.8)
White	52,524	22,568	75,092	23,997	2,260	29	264
(%)	(73.3)	(74.0)	(73.5)	(77.2)	(74.8)	(76.3)	(84.1)
Nonresident alien	1,034	222	1,256	322	338	3	7
(%)	(1.4)	(0.7)	(1.2)	(1.0)	(11.2)	(7.9)	(2.2)
Unknown	2,224	1,638	3,862	1,237	80	1	1
(%)	(3.1)	(5.4)	(3.8)	(4.0)	(2.6)	(2.6)	(0.3)
TOTAL	71,693	30,512	102,205	31,069	3,020	38	314
Schools reporting =	441	487	512	329	77	15	4
Not reported	{1,293}	{501}	{1,794}	{793}	{4}	{13}	{0}
Graduates (August 1, 1999 to July 31, 2000)							
Race/ethnicity							
Asian, Native Hawaiian, or other Pacific Islander	1,071	261	1,332	400	16		2
(%)	(4.8)	(2.4)	(4.0)	(4.1)	(3.6)		(3.3)
Black or African-American	1,984	1,141	3,125	565	21		1
(%)	(8.9)	(10.7)	(9.5)	(5.8)	(4.7)		(1.7)
American Indian or Alaskan Native	145	65	210	52	1		0
(%)	(0.6)	(0.6)	(0.6)	(0.5)	(0.2)		(0.0)
Hispanic or Latino	1,018	365	1,383	275	3		1
(%)	(4.6)	(3.4)	(4.2)	(2.8)	(0.7)		(1.7)
White	17,549	8,514	26,063	8,117	346		56
(%)	(78.4)	(79.8)	(78.9)	(83.9)	(78.1)		(93.3)
Nonresident alien	132	71	203	112	40		0
(%)	(0.6)	(0.7)	(0.6)	(1.2)	(9.0)		(0.0)
Unknown	473	253	726	151	16		0
(%)	(2.1)	(2.4)	(2.2)	(1.6)	(3.6)		(0.0)
TOTAL	22,372	10,670	33,042	9,672	443		60
Schools reporting =	431	482	502	324	77		3
Not reported	{730}	{846}	{1,576}	{600}	{1}		{0}

From American Association of Colleges of Nursing, 2001.

TABLE 11-2	*Type of Degree by Gender of Students Enrolled (Fall 2000) and Graduates (August 1, 1999 to July 31, 2000).*

| | UNDERGRADUATE | | | GRADUATE | | | |
| | | | | | | POST- | |
	GENERIC	RN	TOTAL	MASTER'S	DOCTORAL	DOCTORAL	ND
Students enrolled (fall 2000)							
Gender							
Female	64,870	27,710	92,580	28,512	2,755	45	278
(%)	(90.8)	(91.4)	(91.0)	(90.5)	(93.9)	(88.2)	(88.5)
Male	6,588	2,621	9,209	3,001	180	6	36
(%)	(9.2)	(8.6)	(9.0)	(9.5)	(6.1)	(11.8)	(11.5)
TOTAL	71,458	30,331	101,789	31,513	2,935	51	314
Schools reporting =	438	466	510	325	77	13	4
Not reported	{1,527}	{682}	{2,209}	{349}	{89}	{0}	{0}
Graduates (August 1, 1999 to July 31, 2000)							
Gender							
Female	20,324	9,819	30,143	8.844	417		29
(%)	(89.7)	(91.7)	(90.4)	(91.7)	(97.4)		(93.5)
Male	2,326	887	3,213	803	11		2
(%)	(10.3)	(8.3)	(9.6)	(8.3)	(2.6)		(6.5)
TOTAL	22,650	10,706	33,356	9,647	428		31
Schools reporting =	436	483	509	324	76		3
Not reported	{452}	{810}	{1,262}	{625}	{16}		{29}

From American Association of Colleges of Nursing, 2001.

not measure up to the standards. As a result, many schools closed. With integration permitting African-American students to be admitted to formerly all-Caucasian schools, quality African-American schools had difficulty attracting enough students, and many of the schools closed. However, the Caucasian schools that began admitting African-American students did not admit the number that would have been admitted by the African-American schools. For example, many Caucasian schools admitted only one or two African-American students per class.

In the late 1960s many efforts were made to help the economically disadvantaged in this country. Although not all people of minority groups are economically disadvantaged, the vast majority of disadvantaged people are members of ethnic minority groups. Nursing, too, became concerned about the disadvantaged and began concerted efforts to recruit more members of minority groups into nursing schools. The Sealantic Fund, one of the Rockefeller Brothers' funds, was one of the first foundations that helped minorities enter nursing school. Sealantic funded projects in 10 universities in different parts of the country to recruit students from minority groups and help them achieve success. The best example of an ongoing project, funded by the Division of Nursing since 1971, is the National Student Nurses Association's "Breakthrough to Nursing" to accelerate the recruitment of minorities, including men.

In 1997 the American Nurses Foundation published a report of a project it had funded entitled *Strategies for Recruitment, Retention and Graduation of Minority Nurses in Colleges of Nursing*. Through survey and interview analysis, Bessent and a cadre of knowledgeable leaders investigated the most effective approach to increase the nursing profession's representation of nurses of color (Bessent, 1997). Members of Chi Eta Phi, a national African-American nursing society with chapters throughout the country, serve as mentors to minority nursing students. As mentors, sorority members provide intellectual and inspirational stimulation along with counseling.

Just as contributions of diverse cultural groups are beginning to be valued, so must nursing programs value the need for diversity in their students and faculty and view this diversity as a strength. Diversity within nursing programs can increase the understanding and sensitivity of nurses and positively affect the way they provide care to their patients (Baldwin, 1997).

Strategies for Recruitment and Retention of Minorities in the Health Care Workforce

Recommendations of the American Academy of Nursing's expert panel on cultural competence (Meleis et al., 1995) include recruitment and retainment of diversity in the workforce, raising consciousness, mentoring, and consultation. There also is a need to increase the number of nurse educators and researchers who are from diverse, marginalized, and vulnerable populations. Raising consciousness involves increasing the level of awareness of nurses and other health care professionals about the issues surrounding diversity. This can be accomplished by encouraging participation in forums related to different aspects of various cultural phenomena such as environmental control, communication, and health beliefs. Such forums might be offered by state and local professional nurses' organizations and health care facilities.

Another successful strategy for recruiting and retaining minorities in education and clinical practice is matched mentoring. Matched mentoring would involve matching same-culture mentors either in the same institution or different institutions. A different mentoring strategy would involve teaching and modeling by nurses who have been trained in cross-cultural care. Cross-cultural nursing consultants in the care of specific groups are available to agencies, professional groups, licensing bodies, and individual nurses. Organizations should contact the Transcultural Nursing Society to obtain the names of consultants in the field of transcultural nursing.

Audiovisual media should be used to teach the importance of human health conditions cross-culturally. Video conferencing can provide international links for students and faculty who cannot travel. Students from various cultures can share their clinical experiences. One of the greatest benefits is the discovery that thinking, values, and decision making differ in various cultures. Collaborative arrangements should be encouraged between colleges and universities so that exchange programs can be offered to students. Such exchanges can provide firsthand, in-depth experience with a culture that is different from their own. Interactive media could be used to gain a clearer perspective than can be obtained through the print medium on particular cultures.

Strategies such as mentoring by the same culture professional are effective in recruiting and retaining minorities in nursing. In addition, the value of workshops, continuing education programs, and the use of consultants to promote culturally competent care should not be overlooked.

CULTURAL COMPETENCE

Health professionals, educators, and health care systems must all respond to the consequences of increasing cultural diversity for the future well-being of all populations. There is a shared responsibility to work collaboratively to achieve competence in nursing practice. It is evident that professional competence must incorporate cultural competence and the skillful use of knowledge and interpersonal and technical abilities (Lenburg et al., 1995). Evaluation of cultural competence in students, faculty, and staff is essential. The authors suggest that it is essential that nurses take responsibility to:

- Be sensitive to and show respect for the differences in beliefs and values of others.
- Take responsibility to inquire, learn about, and integrate beliefs and values of others in professional encounters.
- Take responsibility to try to change negative and prejudicial behaviors in themselves and others.

In light of societal changes, responsible persons at all levels in education and health care delivery systems acknowledge the need to reassess the influence of culture on achieving expected health outcomes. There is an imperative need for nurse educators, administrators, students, and others to promote sensitivity to, acceptance of, and respect for the rights and mores of all individuals within the context of their cultural orientation and society as a whole. Nurses must be culturally competent because:

- The nurse's culture often is different from the client's culture.
- Care that is not culturally competent may be more costly.
- Care that is not culturally competent may be ineffective.
- Specific objectives for persons in different cultures need to be met as outlined in *Healthy People 2000* (Stanhope and Lancaster, 2000).

For this reason the expert panels of the American Academy of Nursing (AAN) were developed in 1992 and 1995 to draft proposals for promoting cultural competence in nursing.

Principles for Culturally Competent Care

The goal of culturally competent nursing care is to provide care that is consistent with the client's cultural needs. The AAN Expert Panel Report (1992) on culturally competent nursing care suggested the following four principles:

1. Care is designed for the specific client.
2. Care is based on the uniqueness of the person's culture and includes cultural norms and values.
3. Care includes empowerment strategies to facilitate client decision making in health behavior.
4. Care is provided with sensitivity to the cultural uniqueness of the client.

Nurses have a responsibility to become knowledgeable about the values, beliefs, and health care practices of the culturally diverse groups that are dominant in the nurse's particular practice area or region of the country. For example, nurses who work for the Indian Health Service must be culturally competent to care for Native Americans. Nurses who practice in California should strive to increase knowledge and understanding of Asian and Hispanic populations. In south Texas, where 70% of the population is Hispanic, cultural competence also might include the ability to speak Spanish.

Cultural Competence in Nursing Education

Since the 1960s there has been a united effort to include concepts sensitive to cultural diversity in nursing education. The National League for Nursing (NLN) has made this requirement mandatory for accreditation. The NLN specifies that the nursing curriculum should provide "learning experiences in health promotion and maintenance, illness care and rehabilitation for clients from diverse and multicultural populations throughout the life span" (NLN, 1996). Transcultural nursing was first introduced in the 1960s (Nies and McEwen, 2001). Since then some progress has been made, but only recently have nursing programs been systematically incorporating culturally diverse nursing care concepts into the curricula. Content about the health beliefs and practices of individuals from various cultural groups is essential. Information about the prevalence of health problems and disease incidence mortality rates, cultural factors related to situations such as birth and death, and specific culture-bound syndromes such as anorexia and bulimia should be essential content in nursing curricula and in continuing education programs for practicing nurses. The cross-cultural similarities and differences of roles and responsibilities of family members should be addressed, particularly in terms of support and health care functions of family members.

The AAN Panel (1992) also recommended the following principles to be used in preparing nursing graduates who are sensitive to cultural diversity and global health care needs and able to provide culturally competent care.

- Nurses must learn to appreciate intergroup and intragroup cultural diversity and commonalities in racial/ethnic minority populations.
- Nurses must understand how social structural factors shape health behaviors and practices in racial/ethnic minorities (e.g., nurses must avoid a "blaming" and "victim" pattern).
- Nurses must understand the dynamics and challenges of biculturalism and bilingualism.
- Nurses must confront their own ethnocentrism and racism.
- Nurses must begin implementing and evaluating service provided to cross-cultural populations.

CULTURAL BELIEF SYSTEMS

A value is a standard that people use to assess themselves and others. It is a belief about what is worthwhile or important for well-being. There is a tendency for people to be "culture bound" (i.e., to assume that their values are superior, sensible, or right). Cross-cultural health promotion requires the nurse to work with clients without making judgments as to the superiority of one set of values over another. Box 11-1 provides a comparison of Anglo-American values and those of more tradition-bound countries.

Each culture has a value system that dictates behavior directly or indirectly by setting norms and teaching that those norms are right. Health beliefs and practices tend to reflect a culture's value system. Nurses must understand the patient's value system to foster health promotion.

BOX 11-1	*Anglo-American and Other Cultural Values*

Anglo-American	Other cultural values
Personal control over the environment	Fate
Change	Tradition
Time dominates	Human interaction dominates
Human equality	Hierarchy, rank, status
Individualism, privacy	Group welfare
Self-help	Birthright inheritance
Competition	Cooperation
Future orientation	Past orientation
"Action–goal," work orientation	"Being" orientation
Informality	Formality
Directness, openness, honesty	Indirectness, ritual, "face"
Practicality, efficiency	Idealism, theory
Materialism	Spiritualism, detachment

CULTURAL PHENOMENA

Giger and Davidhizar (1999) have identified six cultural phenomena that vary among cultural groups and affect health care. These phenomena are environmental control, biologic variations, social organization, communication, space, and time orientation.

Environmental Control

Environmental control is the ability of members of a particular culture to control nature or environmental factors. Some groups perceive humans as having mastery over nature; others perceive humans to be dominated by nature, and still other groups see humans as having a harmonious relationship with nature (Spector, 2000a). People who perceive that they have mastery over nature believe that they can overcome the natural forces of nature. Such individuals would expect positive results from medications, surgery, and other treatment modalities. Persons who believe that they are subject to the forces of nature or that they have little control over what happens to them may not be compliant with treatments because they believe that whatever happens to them is part of their destiny. African-Americans and Mexican-Americans are most likely to subscribe to this view. Persons who hold the harmony with nature view, such as Asians and Native Americans, believe that illness represents a disharmony with nature. These clients may see medication as relieving only the symptoms and not curing the disease. Therefore they are more likely to rely on naturalistic remedies such as herbs or hot and cold treatments to effect a cure (Stanhope and Lancaster, 2000). Included in this concept are the traditional health and illness beliefs, the practice of folk medicine, and the use of traditional and nontraditional healers. Environmental control plays an important role in the way clients respond to health-related experiences and use health resources (Spector, 2000a).

Biologic Variations

Biologic variations such as body build and structure, genetic variations, skin characteristics, susceptibility to disease, and nutritional variations exist among different cultures. For example, babies who are born in Western culture weigh more than non-Western babies. Other common variations include skin color, eye shape, hair texture, adipose tissue deposits, shape of ear lobes, and body configuration (Stanhope and Lancaster, 2000). For example, African-Americans have denser bones than Caucasians, which may account for the low incidence of osteoporosis in the African-American population. The size of teeth varies among cultures, with Caucasians having the smallest, followed by African-Americans, Asians, and Native Americans. Larger teeth can cause protruding jaws, a condition common in African-Americans, which does not represent an orthodontic problem (Nies and McEwen, 2001).

Laboratory values for some tests also vary among cultural groups. For example, serum cholesterol levels essentially are the same for African-Americans and Caucasians at birth. During childhood the levels are higher in African-Americans, but they are lower than in Caucasians in adulthood. This finding is interesting because of the high morbidity and mortality from cardiovascular disease in African-Americans (Nies and Mcewen, 2001). The maternal mortality rate of African-Americans is three times that of Caucasians; occurrence of stomach cancer is twice as high among African-American men as Caucasian men; and occurrence of esophageal cancer is three times more common among African-Americans than the general population. Japanese-Americans have a lower incidence of cardiovascular and renal disease than the general population but a higher incidence of stress-related diseases such as ulcers, colitis, psoriasis, and depression. Native Americans have a higher incidence of streptococcal sore throat and gastroenteritis than the general population (Medcom, 1997). Native American women have the highest incidence of diabetes (Nies and McEwen, 2001).

Mexican-Americans have higher rates of obesity and diabetes than the general population, although they have lower rates of cardiovascular disease. The Mexican-American population has a pattern of less use of preventive services, including prenatal care; immunizations for children, and vision, hearing, and dental care (Nies and McEwen, 2001).

Social Organization

Social organization refers to the family unit (nuclear, single-parent, or extended family) and the religious or ethnic groups with which families identify. Family is defined differently across cultures. For instance, in the African-American culture, family often includes people who are unrelated or distantly related. Families depend on the extended family for emotional and financial support in times of crisis. Mothers and grandmothers play important roles in African-American families and are involved in decision making, especially as it relates to health (Stanhope and Lancaster, 2000).

Communication

Communication differences include language differences, verbal and nonverbal behaviors, and silence. Language can be the greatest obstacle to providing multicultural care. If the client does not speak the same language as the nurse, a skilled interpreter is mandatory (Giger and Davidhizar, 1999). Comfort with direct eye contact during communication is an area that varies among cultures. Although some cultures such as the Euro-American value direct eye contact as a sign of attention, other cultures such as African-American or Native American may view direct eye contact as rude behavior.

In the Asian culture it is considered important behavior to agree with those in authority. This aspect of the Asian culture has important implications for the nurse who is involved in patient education. The patient may seem compliant and nod his or her head as in agreement with the nurse's instruction even when the instruction is not clear or when the patient has no intention of carrying out the instruction (Stanhope and Lancaster, 2000).

Anglo-Americans tend to be informal in their style of communication, whereas other cultures may prefer a more formal style. Health professionals should not assume that a first name basis is appropriate for client relationships. With any client, terms of endearment such as "honey" or "dear" are unacceptable and can be interpreted as disrespectful, derogatory, or condescending. The best solution to the challenge of different communication styles and preferences is always to ask the client how he or she prefers to be addressed.

If the nurse and the client do not speak the same language, an interpreter should be consulted. An interpreter can help the nurse establish rapport with the client and explain concepts to the patient that are foreign to the nurse. When interpreters are needed, they should be selected carefully. Adult family members or friends are possible choices, as are bilingual staff and community volunteers. Nurses should be aware that some ethnic groups consider it a breach of confidentiality to have a stranger interpret, whereas certain individuals may not want other family members or friends to know the specifics of their medical condition.

The nurse also should be careful to consider the different dialects spoken in the same country and the culture's view of women and children. Children should not be used as interpreters because of the subject matter and because of certain cultural views of authority. Many cultures view adults as having more authority than children. In many cultures women would not be acceptable interpreters because of the cultural view of women.

Nurses should be aware that AT&T has an interpreter service. A two-way calling system is arranged in which the nurse, the interpreter, and the client are on the telephone at the same time. This service is available in many hospitals, although many nurses and other health care professionals are unaware of this resource.

Space

Space refers to people's attitudes and comfort level regarding the personal space around them. There are vast cultural differences in the comfort level associated with the distance between persons. Anglo-American nurses tend to feel comfortable with an intimate zone of 0 to 18 inches. This usually is the distance between the nurse and the patient when the nurse performs certain parts of a physical assessment such as an eye or ear examination. Entering this zone could be uncomfortable for clients and nurses who have not had time to establish a trusting relationship. This discomfort would be increased for persons whose culture is not comfortable at all with such a limited space. For instance, Asians frequently believe that touching strangers is inappropriate; therefore they have a tendency to prefer more distance between themselves and others, particularly health professionals whom they have not previously known. On the other hand, Mexican-Americans tend to be comfortable with less space because they like to touch persons with whom they are talking (Stanhope and Lancaster, 2000).

Time

Time orientation is the view of time in the present, past, or future. Present-oriented persons enjoy what they are experiencing at the moment and only move on to the next event or activity "when the time is right." Punctuality and "watching the clock" are definitely part of Western culture, but many cultural groups, such as Native Americans, do not view time in the same way. This difference in time orientation can have implications for the present-oriented professional in the work setting, who may always be late for work without thinking it is an important issue. In addition, there are implications for health teaching. For example, when teaching medication schedules to a patient, it would be important to consider how that individual views time.

Clients who view the past as more important than the present or the future may focus on memories of the past. For instance, the Vietnamese may take actions that they believe are consistent with the views of their ancestors and look to their ancestors for guidance (Giger and Davidhizar, 1999). In the Asian culture time is viewed as being more flexible than in the Western culture and being on time or late for appointments is not a priority (Stanhope and Lancaster, 2000).

People who are future-oriented are concerned with long-range goals and health care measures that can be taken in the present to prevent illness in the future. These persons plan ahead in scheduling appointments and organizing activities. They may be seen as having "distant" or "cold" personalities because they are not always engaged in communication at the moment because they may be thinking about their plans for the future. Persons who are oriented more to the present may be late for appointments because they are less concerned with planning ahead (Table 11-3).

PRACTICE ISSUES RELATED TO CULTURAL COMPETENCE
Health Information and Education

According to the Task Force on Black and Minority Health, minority populations are less knowledgeable about specific health problems than are Caucasians. African-Americans and Hispanics receive less information about cancer and heart disease than do nonminority groups. African-Americans tend to underestimate the prevalence of cancer, give less credence to the warning signs, obtain fewer screening tests, and are diagnosed at later stages of cancer than are Caucasians. Hispanic women receive less information about breast cancer than do Caucasian women. Hispanic women are less aware that family history is a risk for breast cancer, and only 29% have heard of breast self-examination. Successful programs to increase public awareness about health problems are being offered to minority groups, but efforts must be continued to reach more of the population. Families, churches, employers, and community organizations need to be involved in facilitating behavior changes that will result in healthier lifestyles. Education programs have the greatest impact on diseases that are affected by lifestyle such as hypertension, obesity, and diabetes. For example, if patients with diabetes could improve their self-management skills, 70% of complications could be prevented, saving human suffering and health care dollars (Nies and McEwen, 2001).

Education and Certification

Increasingly more universities and colleges offer graduate programs in transcultural, cross-cultural, and international nursing. Many nurses have not been exposed to transcultural nursing in their basic education program. Therefore the availability of graduate study in this area often is an unrecognized possibility.

Transcultural nursing is the study of differences and similarities of various cultural health values and beliefs among different ethnic and minority groups (Medcom, 1997). The Transcultural Nursing Society has been certifying nurses in transcultural nursing since 1988. Certification as a certified transcultural nurse is based on oral and written examinations and evaluation of the nurse's educational and experiential background. Certification has increased recognition of transcultural nursing as a legitimate nursing specialty. Transcultural nurses

TABLE 11-3	*Variations Among Selected Cultural Groups*			
	AFRICAN-AMERICANS	**ASIANS**	**HISPANICS**	**NATIVE AMERICANS**
Verbal communication	Asking personal questions of someone met for the first time is seen as improper and intrusive	High respect for others, especially those in positions of authority	Expression of negative feelings is considered impolite	Speaks in a low tone of voice and expects that the listener will be attentive
Nonverbal communication	Direct eye contact in conversation often is considered rude	Direct eye contact among superiors may be considered disrespectful	Avoidance of eye contact usually is a sign of attentiveness and respect	Direct eye contact often is considered disrespectful
Touch	Touching another's hair often is considered offensive	It is not customary to shake hands with persons of the opposite sex	Touching often is observed between two persons in conversion	A light touch of the person's hand instead of a firm handshake often is used when greeting a person
Family organization	Usually have close, extended family networks; women play key roles in healthcare decisions	Usually have close, extended family ties; emphasis may be on family needs rather than individual needs	Usually have close, extended family ties; all members of the family may be involved in healthcare decisions	Usually have close, extended family ties; emphasis tends to be on family rather than on individual needs
Time	Often present-oriented	Often present-oriented	Often present-oriented	Often present-oriented
Alternative healers	"Granny," "root doctor," voodoo priest, spiritualist	Acupuncturist, acupressurist, herbalist	Curandero, espiritualista, yerbo	Medicine man, shaman
Self-care practices	Poultices, herbs, oils, roots	Hot and cold foods, herbs, teas, soups, cupping, burning, rubbing, pinching	Hot and cold foods, herbs	Herbs, corn meal, medicine bundle
Biologic variations	Sickle cell anemia, mongolian spots, keloid formation, inverted T waves, lactose intolerance, skin color	Thalassemia, drug interactions, mongolian spots, lactose intolerance, skin color	Mongolian spots, lactose intolerance, skin color	Cleft uvula, lactose intolerance, skin color

Data from Giger JN, Davidhizar, RE: *Transcultural nursing,* ed 3, St. Louis, 1999, Mosby; Spector RE: *Cultural diversity in health and illness,* ed 5, Upper Saddle River, NJ, 2000, Prentice Hall; Payne KT: In Taylor OL, editor: *Nature of communication disorders in culturally and linguistically diverse populations,* San Diego, 1986, College Hill Press.

are interested in finding a universal care for clients that will improve, maintain, and restore health and improve client satisfaction.

International Marketplace

Nurses trained in the United States work, teach, and consult in hundreds of foreign countries on every continent. They often are recognized as international pacesetters and are viewed as "commodities for import" by both the more developed countries and the less developed third- or fourth-world nations. Nurses can make a difference in the health outcomes of people all over the world. Technology has enhanced global communication and facilitated travel. As nurses help solve emerging health problems in countries throughout the world, they are the most valuable assets of the health care system. They will be called on to design, implement, and evaluate international projects, educational endeavors, and research with an intercultural focus. Therefore it is important that nurses understand the intercultural issues related to our global society (Nies and McEwen, 2001).

Nursing Literature

The number of journal articles about culturally diverse clients, transcultural nursing research, international nursing, and the inclusion of transcultural concepts in nursing curricula has increased considerably since the 1950s. *The Journal of Transcultural Nursing* is a refereed journal that was first published in 1989. This journal was created to advance transcultural nursing knowledge and practices. *The Journal of Transcultural Nursing* focuses on theory, research, and practice dimensions of transcultural nursing and provides a forum for researchers. Other journals that address cultural issues include the *Western Journal of Medicine: Cross Cultural Issues,* the *Journal of Cultural Diversity,* the *Journal of Multicultural Nursing,* the *International Journal of Nursing Studies,* the *International Nursing Review,* and the *Journal of Holistic Nursing.* Nurse authors also need to be encouraged to publish articles related to clients' cultural views and health care needs in nursing specialty and practice journals that are more widely read by nurses who actually are providing care on a daily basis to clients from diverse cultures.

Although research articles on transcultural issues are becoming a common feature in health care journals, there is a need for additional research that examines individual behavioral responses to normal life processes such as pregnancy, birth, death, and human growth and development. There also is a need for well-designed studies that explore the biologic, psychologic, sociologic, and spiritual differences within, between, and among cultural groups (Purnell and Paulanka, 1998). Even though there have been numerous research studies conducted on cultural diversity issues, a significant time gap often exists between the identification of findings and publication of results. The limited dissemination of research findings inhibits widespread acceptance of new interventions that could potentially improve health care practices of culturally diverse populations. Computer information technology and online networks help to narrow this gap and distribute research findings in a timely manner (Purnell and Paulanka, 1998).

Responsibility of Health Care Facilities for Cultural Care

Nursing policies should reflect an openness to including extended family members and folk healers in the nursing care plan, provided their presence is not harmful to the client's well-being. For example, Hispanic clients may want the support of a curandero, espiritualista (spiritualist), yerbo (herbalist), or sabador (equal to a chiropractor). African-Americans may turn to a hougan (voodoo priest or priestess) or "old lady." Native Americans may seek assistance from a shaman or medicine man. Clients of Asian descent may want the services of an acupuncturist or bonesetter. In some religions spiritual healers may be found among the ranks of the ordained and may be called priest, bishop, elder, deacon, rabbi, brother, or sister (Nies and McEwen, 2001). Most hospital chaplaincy programs have access to religious representatives available for patients of various religions.

Clients may need to consult with their support persons and folk healers before making medical decisions. Nurses must respect the client's right to privacy and allow time for the client to interact with his or her spiritual or cultural healers. Nurses must respect unconventional beliefs and health practices and work with clients to develop a plan of care that builds on their beliefs and incorporates nontraditional health practices that are not harmful. These nontraditional healers should be received with respect and provided privacy to enable the healers to interact with their patients (Nies and McEwen, 2001).

Health care facilities should provide resources for nurses and other health care professionals to assist with culture-specific needs of clients. Health care facilities should have a list of interpreters fluent in the major languages spoken by persons typically using the organization. Translators who have knowledge of health-related terminology would be more effective than those who do not. Gender, birth origin, and socioeconomic class need to be considered when selecting a translator. Gender is an important consideration because many cultures prohibit discussion of intimate matters between women and men. Birth origin of the client and translator should be determined because often there are many dialects spoken within the same country, depending on the particular region (Stanhope and Lancaster, 2000). Differences in socioeconomic class between client and interpreter can lead to problems of interpretation.

Clinical nurse specialists (CNSs) in transcultural nursing should be added to the staff of institutions serving large numbers of culturally diverse persons. The transcultural CNS could be a role model to the staff in delivery of culturally sensitive and competent care, provide inservice education to staff related to cultural differences, and conduct research related to cultural and social issues. In addition, consultants should be used to deal with specific cultural issues.

Continuing education programs for nurses should be offered by health care institutions. Programs should focus on promoting awareness of the nurses' own culturally based values, beliefs and attitudes, cultural assessment, biological variations of cultural groups, cross-cultural communication, and culture-specific beliefs and practices related to childbearing and childrearing, death and dying, issues of mental health, and cultural aspects of aging.

CULTURAL ASSESSMENT
Cultural Self-Assessment

The first step to becoming a culturally sensitive and competent health provider is to conduct a cultural self-assessment. The nurse should engage in a cultural self-assessment to identify individual culturally based attitudes about clients who are from a different culture. Cultural self-assessment requires self-honesty and sincerity and reflection on attitudes of parents, grandparents, and close friends in terms of their attitudes toward different cultures. Through identification of health-related attitudes, values, beliefs, and practices the nurse can better understand the cultural aspects of health care from the client's perspective. Everyone has ethnocentric tendencies that must be brought to a level of consciousness so that efforts can be made to temper the feeling that one's own culture is "best." Box 11-2 shows a cultural self-assessment guide adapted from Swanson and Nies (1997) for the nurse who is not African-American but is caring for an African-American client.

Cultural Client Assessment

After the nurse performs a cultural self-assessment, he or she should obtain a cultural assessment for the client. Nursing assessments in institutional and community settings should include the gathering of data pertinent to cultural beliefs and practices. Cultural assessments lead to culturally relevant nursing diagnoses and give direction to effective nursing intervention. Basic cultural data include ethnic affiliation, religious preference, family patterns, food patterns, and ethnic health care practices. Cultural assessments should be used as an adjunct to other patient assessments. These data will give the nurse sufficient information to determine if a more in-depth assessment of cultural factors is needed. A major reason that cultural assessments are performed is to identify patterns that may assist or interfere with a nursing intervention or treatment regimen (Giger and Davidhizer, 1999).

The nurse needs to find out if the client's beliefs, customs, values, and self-care practices are adaptive (beneficial), neutral, or maladaptive (harmful) in relation to nursing interventions. For example, if a Mexican-American client who is diagnosed with hypertension insists on taking garlic instead of an antihypertensive, this could be harmful. If the client agrees to take the garlic in addition to the antihypertensive, this would be a neutral practice. An adaptive or beneficial practice would include daily exercise in addition to the garlic and antihypertensive.

In the case of Southeast Asians, dermal practices such as cupping, pinching, rubbing, and burning are a common part of self-care. The dermal methods are perceived as ways to relieve

---

| **BOX 11-2** | *Cultural Self-Assessment* |

- How do your parents, grandparents, other family members, and close friends view people from racially diverse groups?
- What is the cultural stereotype of African-Americans?
- Does the cultural stereotype allow for socioeconomic differences?
- Have your interactions with African-Americans been positive? Negative? Neutral?
- How do you feel about going into a predominantly African-American neighborhood or into the home of an African-American family? Are you afraid, anxious, curious, or ambivalent?
- What stereotypes do you have about African-American men, women, and children?
- What culturally based health beliefs and practices do you think characterize African-Americans? How are these different from your own culturally based health beliefs and practices?

From Swanson J, Nies M: *Community health nursing: promoting the health of aggregates,* ed. 2, Philadelphia, 1997, WB Saunders.

headaches, muscle pains, sinusitis, colds, sore throats, diarrhea, or fever. Cupping involves placing a heated cup on the skin; as it cools it contracts, drawing what is believed to be toxicity into the cup. A circular ecchymosis is left on the skin. Pinching may be at the base of the nose or between the eyes. Bruises or welts are left at the site of treatment. Rubbing or "coining" involves rubbing lubricated skin with a spoon or a coin to bring toxic "wind" to the body surface. A similar practice is burning, which involves touching a burning cigarette or piece of cotton to the skin, usually the abdomen, to compensate for "heat" lost through diarrhea (Nies and McEwen, 2001). These practices nurture the client's sense of well-being and security in being able to do something to correct disturbing symptoms. In most cases the practice would be considered adaptive (beneficial) or neutral. However, if the client had a clotting disorder, the practices would pose a threat to physical integrity and therefore be considered maladaptive (harmful) (Nies and McEwen, 2001).

Cultural Client Nutrition Assessment

A cultural nutrition assessment should be obtained for clients who are minorities. It is necessary to assess the client's cultural definition of food. For example, certain Latin American groups do not consider greens to be food. Therefore when asked to keep a food diary, these individuals would not list greens, which are an important source of vitamins and iron. Frequency and number of meals, amount and types of food eaten, and regularity of food consumption are other important factors that should be considered.

Among Asian-Americans dietary intake of calcium may appear inadequate because this group usually has a low rate of consumption of dairy products. However, they commonly consume pork bone and shells, thus taking in adequate quantities of calcium to meet minimum daily requirements. In cultures in which obesity is a problem, it is helpful for the nurse to have an idea of food preferences to help the client select low-calorie, low-fat foods. Asians tend to prefer spicy foods that may lead to the high incidence of stomach cancer, ulcers, and gastrointestinal bleeding (Purnell and Paulanka, 1998).

Nurses should avoid cultural stereotyping as it relates to food because all Italians do not necessarily like spaghetti, nor do all Chinese like rice. However, knowing the clients' food preferences makes it possible to develop therapeutic interventions that do not conflict with their cultural food practices (Stanhope and Lancaster, 2000). Food preferences of aggregate groups are described in Table 11-4.

Cultural Beliefs About Sickness and Cures

It also is important for the nurse to consider the nontraditional beliefs of sickness and cure of various cultures. For example, there are diseases that are not classified as Western culture diseases. For different cultural groups they are real diseases for which the group has medicines and treatments. Examples of such diseases include mal ojo, susto, bilis, and empacho.

Mal ojo, also called "evil eye," is thought to be caused by persons giving admiration. "According to this belief, some people are born with 'vista fuerte' (strong vision) with which they unwittingly harm others with a mere glance" (Nies and McEwen, 2001). For example, a stranger who lovingly admires a Mexican-American baby by looking into the baby's face actually can cause mal ojo. An infant who has mal ojo sleeps restlessly, has fever and diarrhea, and may ultimately die. Treatment consists of rubbing the body with an egg for three consecutive nights. The egg is broken and left under the bed overnight. In the morning if the egg appears to be cooked, then mal ojo was definitely the cause of the illness. For protections

TABLE 11-4	*Selected Food Preferences and Associated Risk Factors Among Selected Cultural Groups*		
CULTURAL GROUP	**FOOD PREFERENCES**	**NUTRITIONAL EXCESS**	**RISK FACTORS**
African-Americans	Fried foods, greens, bread, lard, pork, and rice	Cholesterol, fat, sodium, carbohydrates, and calories	Coronary heart disease and obesity
Asians	Soy sauce, rice, pickled dishes, and raw fish	Cholesterol, fat sodium, carbohydrates, and calories	Coronary heart disease, liver disease, cancer of the stomach, and ulcers
Hispanics	Fried foods, beans and rice, chili, carbonated beverages	Cholesterol, fat, sodium, carbohydrates, and calories	Coronary heart disease, and obesity
Native Americans	Blue cornmeal, fruits, game, and fish	Carbohydrates and calories	Diabetes, malnutrition, tuberculosis, infant and maternal mortality

Data from Andrews M, Boyle J: *Transcultural concepts in nursing,* ed 3, Philadelphia, 1998, JB Lippincott; Giger JN, Davidhizar RE: *Transcultural nursing,* ed 3, St. Louis, 1999, Mosby; Jackson, Broussard: Cultural challenges in nutrition education among American Indians, *Diabetic Educ* 13(11):47-50, 1987.

mothers often adorn their children with red yarn around their wrists or amulets that usually are a deer's eyes (Nies and McEwen, 2001).

Susto, or fright sickness, is an emotion-based illness that is common among Mexicans. An unexpected fall, a barking dog, or a car accident could cause susto. Symptoms include colic, diarrhea, high temperature, and vomiting. Treatment involves brushing the body with "ruda" for nine consecutive nights. The brushing is performed to allow the spirit that has been removed by the disease to return to the body. The treatment often is accompanied by burning candles and prayers in home or church (Nies and McEwen, 2001).

Bilis is a disease brought on by anger. It primarily affects adults and commonly occurs a day or two after a fit of rage. If untreated, bilis can cause acute nervous tension and chronic fatigue, although herbal remedies usually are effective (Giger and Davidhizer, 1999).

Empacho is a disease that can affect children or adults and is caused by food particles becoming lodged in the intestinal tract, causing sharp pains. To manage this illness, the afflicted person lies face down on the bed with his or her back bared. The curer pinches a piece of skin at the waist, listening for a snap from the abdominal region. This is repeated several times in hope of dislodging the material. Empacho usually is not a serious disease (Nies and McEwen, 2001).

It is important to determine how culturally diverse clients define health and illness and whether their health beliefs and practices differ from the norm in the Western health care delivery system (Spector, 2000a). For example, the Chinese often find many aspects of Western medicine distasteful. They cannot understand why so many diagnostic tests are necessary and tend to believe that a "good" physician has the ability to diagnose by thoroughly examining the client's body. Chinese clients dislike painful procedures such as the practice of drawing blood. In their culture blood is seen as the source of life for the entire body, and the Chinese believe that it is not regenerated. They have a deep respect for their bodies and prefer to die

BOX 11-3	*Health Traditions Assessment Model*

Maintaining health

Physical Are there special clothes one must wear; foods one must eat, not eat, or combinations to avoid; exercises one must do?

Mental Are there special sources of entertainment; games or other ways of concentrating; traditional "rules of behavior?"

Spiritual Are there special religious customs; prayers; meditations?

Protecting health and preventing illness

Physical Are there special foods that must be eaten after certain life events such as childbirth; dietary taboos that must be adhered to; symbolic clothes that must be worn?

Mental Are there special people who must be avoided, rituals for self-protection, familial roles?

Spiritual Are there special religious customs, superstitions, amulets, oils or waters?

Restoring health

Physical Are there special folk remedies; liniments; procedures such as cupping, acupuncture, and moxibustion?

Mental Are there special healers such as curanderos available, rituals, folk medicines?

Spiritual Are there special rituals and prayers, meditations, healers?

From Spector RE: *Cultural diversity in health and illness,* ed 5, Upper Saddle River, NJ, 2000a, Prentice Hall.

with their bodies intact. Therefore it is not uncommon for the Chinese to refuse surgery that would be mutilating to the body (Spector, 2000a). Health represents a balance within the body, mind, and spirit. It is strongly affected by the family and community. Spector (2000b) suggests a model for assessing health traditions (Box 11-3).

Spector (2000b) also has developed a guide that can be used to assess clients' personal methods for maintaining health, protecting (preventing) illness, and restoring health (Table 11-5).

SUMMARY

In a society as diverse as the United States, health care cannot come in one form to fit the needs of everyone. Culture has a powerful influence on one's interpretation of health and illness and response to health care. All clients have the right to be understood and respected, despite their differences. They have the right to expect health care providers to acknowledge that their perspectives on and interpretations of health are legitimate. Health care professionals must make a commitment to increase their knowledge, sensitivity, and competence in cultural concepts and care. Perhaps no other group in the health profession has recognized the impact of cultural diversity on outcomes of health care more than nursing. Nurses always have supported the concept of holistic care. By understanding the client's perspective, the nurse can be a better advocate for the client. With increased knowledge, sensitivity, respect, and understanding, therapeutic interventions can be maximized to promote the highest quality of health for clients in our multicultural society. Additional information can be found in the websites listed in Box 11-4.

	PHYSICAL	MENTAL	SPIRITUAL
TABLE 11-5 *Assessment Guide for Personal Methods to Maintain, Protect (Prevent Illness), and Restore Health*			
Maintain health	Are there special clothes you must wear at certain times of the day, week, year?	What do you do for activities, such as reading, sports, games?	Do you practice your religion and attend church or other communal activities?
	Are there special foods you must eat at certain times?	Do you have hobbies?	Do you pray or meditate?
	Do you have any dietary restrictions?	Do you visit family often?	Do you observe religious customs?
	Are there any foods that you cannot eat?	Do you visit friends often?	Do you belong to fraternal organizations?
Protect health or prevent illness	Are there foods that you cannot eat together?	Are there people or situations that you have been taught to avoid?	Do you observe religious customs?
	Are there special foods that you must eat?	Do you take extraordinary precautions under certain circumstances?	Do you wear any amulets or hang them in your house?
	Are there any types of clothing that you are not allowed to wear?	Do you take time for yourself?	Do you have any practices, such as always opening the window when you sleep?
			Do you have any other practices to protect yourself from "harm?"
Restore health	What kinds of medicines do you take before you see a doctor or nurse?	Do you know of any specific practices your mother or grandmother may use to relax?	Do you know any healers?
	Are there herbs that you take?	Do you know how big problems can be cared for in your community?	Do you know of any religious rituals that help to restore health?
	Are there special treatments that you use?	Do you drink special teas to help you unwind or relax?	Do you meditate?
			Do you ever go to a healing service?
			Do you know about exorcism?

From Spector RE: *Cultural diversity in health and illness,* ed 5, Upper Saddle River, NJ, 2000a, Prentice Hall.

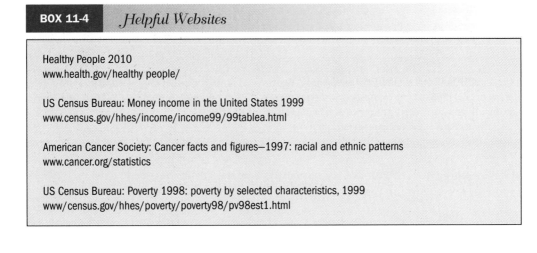

BOX 11-4 *Helpful Websites*

Healthy People 2010
www.health.gov/healthy people/

US Census Bureau: Money income in the United States 1999
www.census.gov/hhes/income/income99/99tablea.html

American Cancer Society: Cancer facts and figures—1997: racial and ethnic patterns
www.cancer.org/statistics

US Census Bureau: Poverty 1998: poverty by selected characteristics, 1999
www/census.gov/hhes/poverty/poverty98/pv98est1.html

Critical Thinking Activities

1. What principles and actions must a staff nurse apply to provide culturally competent care?
2. What factors should a community nurse educator consider when planning a health promotion program for a minority group who does not speak English?
3. How can health care organizations promote the cultural competence of nursing staff?
4. What strategies can be used to recruit and retain minorities in nursing?

REFERENCES

AAN Expert Panel on Culturally Competent Health Care: Culturally competent health care, *Nurs Outlook* 40(6):277-283, 1992.

Baldwin D: Recruitment and retention of minorities in nursing. In Strickland O, Fishman D, editors: *Nursing issues in the 1990s,* Albany, NY, 1997, Delmar Publishers.

Bessent H: *Strategies for recruitment, retention and graduation of minority nurses in colleges of nursing,* Washington, DC, 1997, American Nurses Foundation.

Castiglia P: Minority representation in nursing education programs: increasing cultural awareness. In McClosky J, Grace H, editors: *Current issues in nursing,* St Louis, 1997, Mosby.

Council of Economic Advisers for the President's Initiative on Race: *Changing America: indicators of social and economic well-being by race and Hispanic origin,* Washington, DC, 1999, US Government Printing Office.

Giger JN, Davidhizer RE: *Transcultural nursing,* ed 3, St Louis, 1999, Mosby.

Hall J, Stevens P, Meleis A: Marginalization: a guiding concept for valuing diversity in nursing knowledge development, *Adv Nurs Sci* 16(4):23-24, 1994.

Lenburg C et al: *Promoting cultural competence in and through nursing education; a critical review and comprehensive plan for action,* Washington, DC, 1995, American Academy of Nursing.

Medcom: *Cultural assessment* (film), Cypress, Calif, 1997, Medcom.

Meleis A et al: *Diversity, marginalization, and culturally competent healthcare issues in knowledge development,* Washington, DC, 1995, American Academy of Nursing.

National League for Nursing: *Criteria for the evaluation of baccalaureate and higher degree programs in nursing,* New York, 1996, National League for Nursing.

Nies M, McEwen M: *Community health nursing: promoting the health of populations,* Philadelphia: 2001, WB Saunders.

Purnell L Paulanka B: *Transcultural health care,* Philadelphia, 1998, FA Davis.

Spector R: *Cultural diversity in health and illness,* ed 5, Upper Saddle River, NJ, 2000a, Prentice Hall.

Spector R: *Guide to heritage assessment and health traditions,* Upper Saddle River, NJ, 2000b, Prentice Hall.

Stanhope M, Lancaster J: *Community health and public health nursing,* ed 5, St Louis, 2000, Mosby.

Sullivan EJ: Differences. *Reflections,* Second quarter 1998, Sigma Theta Tau.

Swanson J, Nies M: *Community health nursing: promoting the health of aggregates,* ed 2, Philadelphia, 1997, WB Saunders.

US Department of Health and Human Services, Public Health Service: *Healthy people 2000,* Washington, DC, 1990, US Government Printing Office.

US Department of Health and Human Services: *Healthy people 2010: national health promotion and disease prevention objectives—public health service,* Washington, DC, 2000, US Government Printing Office.

SUGGESTED READINGS

Andrews M, Boyle J: *Transcultural concepts in nursing care,* ed 3, Philadelphia, 1999, JB Lippincott.

Huff RM: *Promoting health in multicultural populations: a handbook for practitioners,* Thousand Oaks, Calif, 1999, Sage.

Leininger M: Transcultural nursing education: a worldwide imperative, *Nurs Health Care* 15(5):254-257, 1994.

Workplace Advocacy and Workplace Issues

Alexia Green, PhD, RN, and Clair B. Jordan, MSN, RN

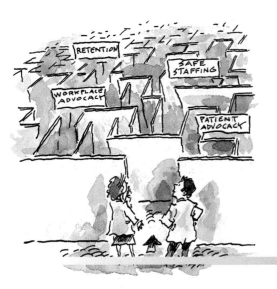

A changing workplace requires nurses to use workplace advocacy to ensure quality health care delivery.

Vignette

As a new graduate, Ellena Gonzalez is searching for her first position as a registered nurse (RN) in a large metropolitan city in the Southwest. As part of her education, she learns about the importance of the nurses' role in advocating for a workplace conducive to delivering safe and effective quality health care. She also understands that the workplace is filled with complex issues—nursing shortages, staffing issues, potential exposure to blood-borne diseases—affecting not only the nurse, but also the patient, the organization, and the profession. As a result of the nursing shortage, Ellena receives many offers from various organizations with promises of sign-on bonuses and other incentives. But she wisely chooses to not accept a job on its "face value" and decides to investigate her opportunities more thoroughly. Questions that come to her mind include: Have any organizations within my area received Magnet Hospital status? Which organizations have shared governance models? Are nurses encouraged to participate in shared governance? What is the content and length of orientation for new nurses? What is the organization's philosophy regarding staff mix designations? Does the organization have a conflict resolution process? What is the organization's turnover rate, and what is the average longevity of staff nurses? Armed with answers to these and other questions, Ellena decides to accept a position with a large tertiary care center that she believes has created an environment most supportive of ensuring the delivery of quality patient care. However, she knows that with the acceptance of this position her role as a workplace and patient advocate has not ended; rather, it has only just begun.

263

Questions to consider while reading this chapter

1. What workplace advocacy strategies can Ellena use to promote quality patient care and a safe work environment?
2. What is the value of shared governance to Ellena's individual nursing practice?
3. If Ellena becomes concerned about floating assignments, what questions can help guide her decision about accepting such assignments?
4. What online resources are available to help Ellena learn more about important workplace issues and workplace advocacy?

Key Terms

Professional practice advocacy Professional activities that encompass two primary mechanisms to promote and maintain a professional practice environment: workplace advocacy and collective bargaining.

Workplace advocacy An array of activities that promote power bases that afford nurses an optimal professional work environment. The objective is to equip nurses to skillfully use a range of external and internal workplace strategies that are complimentary in nature, focus on strengthening nursing's voice, and ensure nurse involvement in workplace decisions affecting nursing care. Workplace advocacy uses universally empowering strategies while supporting effective and efficient patient care.

Workplace issues An array of complex issues that confront nurses in the workplace on a daily basis. These complex issues not only affect the nurse, but also the patient, the organization, and the profession. Examples include the nursing shortage, adequate staffing levels, errors in health care delivery, and violence in the workplace.

Patient advocacy The nurse and the nursing profession's powerful voice at the local, state, and national levels in supporting policies that protect consumers and enhance accountability for quality by promoting safer health care systems. Patient advocacy is a cornerstone of the nursing profession, and patients depend on nurses to ensure that they receive quality care. Workplace advocacy is a component of patient advocacy.

Learning Outcomes

After studying this chapter, the reader will be able to:

1. Describe workplace advocacy as a means of improving the quality of health care delivery.
2. Identify issues that are affecting the practice of professional nursing in the health care workplace.
3. Identify available resources to assist in improving the workplace environment.
4. Define the role of nurses in advocating for safe and effective workplace environments.
5. Describe both internal and external workplace strategies that support efficient and effective quality patient care.

CHAPTER OVERVIEW

In today's modern health care system, nurses are faced with many workplace issues. These complex issues affect not only the nurse, but also the patient, the organization, and the profession. This chapter attempts to identify a few select critical issues currently facing nurses and the nursing profession, all of which affect the workplace, including the nursing shortage, appropriate staffing, patient safety and advocacy, and workplace rights and safety. Professional practice advocacy is defined, and specific strategies under the domain of workplace advocacy are highlighted. To be a successful and accountable professional, it is essential that nurses recognize current issues and know where to seek support for workplace advocacy.

WORKPLACE ADVOCACY

Professional nurses throughout the nation are struggling to deliver patient care against all kinds of barriers and with dwindling resources. Nurses' strong concern and commitment to patient care and their role as patient advocates often places them in direct conflict with administrators of health care organizations. How the nurse reacts to this conflict, how the nurse continues to advocate for patients in this environment, and what powers the nurse can call on to improve care for patients has become a new focus for the profession as we enter the twenty-first century—a focus called "professional practice advocacy." Professional practice advocacy has been described as an umbrella of professional activities that encompasses two primary mechanisms to promote and maintain a professional practice environment: workplace advocacy and collective bargaining (see Chapter 13 for a detailed discussion of Collective Bargaining).

Professional practice advocacy, as defined by the American Nurses Association (ANA) in 1999, encompasses the programs and services intended to promote and support professional practice standards in the workplace. Included are those activities supportive of nurses' advocacy for their patients and professional practice self-determination and the exercise of their employment rights and responsibilities. As we visit Ellena Gonzalez 6 months after she assumed her new position, we find that she has become involved in advocating for a safe work environment. Ellena and the other nurses working on the medical unit are concerned because retractable needle devices are not available on their unit. The patients on the medical unit often have diagnoses of hepatitis B infection, and the nurses are worried about needlestick injuries. Where will they find information about needlestick safety and other workplace safety issues? Are there laws that require hospitals to implement safety measures to protect their staff against blood-borne pathogens? What rights do nurses have to demand safe needle devices? All of these questions are related to professional practice advocacy, specifically workplace advocacy. Examples of professional practice advocacy are included in Box 12-1.

| **BOX 12-1** | *Examples of Professional Practice Advocacy* |

Promoting and protecting the occupational safety and health of nurses

Using nurse practice acts and other legislative and regulatory protections

Using the political process to influence legislative and regulatory agencies for protections of nurses and patients

Providing education regarding employment rights and responsibilities

Developing skills related to public reactions, media presentations and conflict resolution

Building coalitions and support groups to enable nurses to speak and advocate for their professional practices

Negotiating and administering strong and effective employment contracts

---

Adapted from American Nurses Association: *Definition of professional practice advocacy adopted by House of Delegates (internal document),* Washington, DC, 1999, Author.

As a component of professional practice advocacy, workplace advocacy promotes power bases that afford nurses optimal work environments. The objective is to equip nurses to skillfully use a range of external and internal workplace strategies. These strategies are to be complimentary in nature, focusing on strengthening nursing's voice and ensuring nurses' involvement in workplace decisions affecting nursing care. ANA defined workplace advocacy in 1993 as: "an array of activities which are initiated to address the many and varied employment and workplace challenges nurses face on a daily basis. As the definition of advocacy implies, these activities range from supporting and sustaining efforts to more innovative and assertive measures. Workplace advocacy is inherent in the role and responsibility of each professional nurse" (Young, Hayes, and Morin, 1993, p. 1). Workplace advocacy uses universally empowering strategies while supporting effective and efficient patient care. Ellena and her colleagues will be empowered to improve the workplace when they find the answers to their questions. By knowing where to seek information and other resources to solve workplace problems, nurses promote safe and effective workplaces.

Developing an effective workplace advocacy strategy or program is a complex multifaceted role for the individual nurse and professional organizations such as the national and state

---

BOX 12-2	*Five Opportunities/Challenges for Workplace Advocacy Programs*

1. Identify mechanisms within health care systems that provide opportunities for RNs to affect institutional policies.
   - Shared governance
   - Participatory management models
   - Magnet hospital identification
   - Statewide staffing regulations
2. Develop conflict resolution models for use within organizations that address RNs' concerns about patient care and delivery issues.
3. Seek legislative solutions for workplace problems by reviewing issues of concern to nurses in employment settings and introducing appropriate legislation, such as:
   - Whistle-blower protection
   - Safe Harbor peer review
   - Support for rules outlining strong nursing practice standards
4. Develop legal centers for nurses, which could provide legal support and decision-making advice as a last recourse to resolve workplace issues.
   - Provide fast and efficient legal assistance to nurses
   - Earmark precedent setting cases that could impact case law and health care policy
5. Provide RNs in practice with self advocacy and patient advocacy information such as:
   - Laws and regulations governing practice
   - Use of applicable nursing practice standards
   - Conflict resolution and negotiation techniques
   - Identifying state/national reporting mechanisms that allow RNs to report concerns about health care organizations and/or professionals

Adapted from Texas Nurses Association: *Workplace advocacy program*, Austin, Tx, 2001, Author, www.texanurses.org.

nurses associations. In 2000 the ANA committed to supporting the profession through workplace advocacy strategies with the formation of the Commission on Workplace Advocacy (202-651-7047 or www.nursingworld.org; or wpa@ana.org). The Texas Nurses Association (TNA), a leader in workplace advocacy, identified five opportunities and challenges for workplace advocacy programs (Box 12-2). Other examples of workplace and patient advocacy will be discussed in conjunction with specific workplace issues.

AN OVERVIEW OF WORKPLACE ISSUES

The ushering in of the twenty-first century brought with it a period of chaos in the health care arena, especially as it relates to the workplace. Of particular concern is the shortage of professional nurses and the impact the shortage is currently having and will continue to have on the quality of health care delivery. As a result of the shortage and other complex issues, identifying adequate and appropriate professional nurse staffing levels has become a major professional and public health concern. The relationship of the workplace environment to the incidence of errors in health care has recently come under increased scrutiny. In addition, nurses are also being faced with significant workplace safety issues such as ergonomic injuries and violence occurring in the workplace.

NURSING SHORTAGE

The nursing profession has a long history of cyclic shortages, which have been documented since World War II (Minnick, 2000). The acute cyclic shortage impacting the nation during the

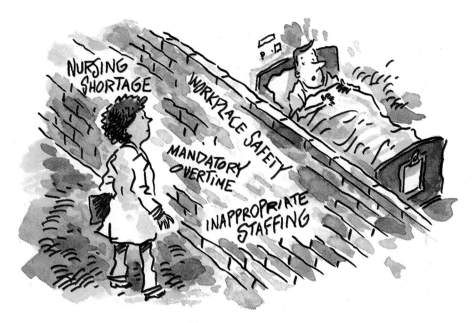

Professional nurses are struggling to deliver patient care against all kinds of barriers and with dwindling resources.

late 1990s and the early 2000s was a direct result of the struggle to implement managed care as a means of controlling the escalating cost of health care. As we move further into the twenty-first century, the profession faces another shortage, one which promises to be much more complex and long lasting and will dwarf all shortages to date (Nevidjon and Erickson, 2001). While the U.S. nursing population is aging and more nurses are moving into primary care settings, there are a multitude of aging baby boomers, resulting in an increasing demand for quality health care. As a result, there is a need for more nurses, especially those who deliver specialized care. Professional nursing is the largest U.S. health care occupation, and, according to the Bureau of Labor Statistics (1999), employment opportunities for professional nurses will grow more rapidly than all other U.S. occupations through 2008. Planning for an adequate workforce will be one of the most critical challenges of the new century. Although the current nursing shortage is related to both supply and demand issues, a closer look at several confounding variables provides an insight into the complexity of the shortage and to the need for an array of actions.

Health Care Is No Longer a Favored Employer

In examining the shortage of nurses, which is also accompanied by a shortage of other health care workers, the attractiveness of careers in health care, especially hospital care, has changed over the last two decades (American Hospital Association, 2001). In a single generation health care has moved from a favored to a less favored employment sector. The American Hospital Association (2001) framed this insight by five observations:

1. In a manufacturing economy, health care was high tech, but in an information economy, young people view health care as low tech.
2. In the 1960s, 1970s, and 1980s health care was safe, secure, and prestigious employment; but in today's labor market health care is seen as chaotic and unstable.
3. In a traditional society, health care was one of only a few employment options for women, but in contemporary society health care is one of many choices.
4. In a long-stay hospital system, such as that of the 1960s, 1970s, and 1980s, nurses had strong, supportive relationships with patients; but in today's short-stay hospital system nurses are focused on disease protocols, regulatory compliance, and documentation.
5. In a mass-production society in which production schedules controlled work hours, the 24-hour/7-days-a-week demands of hospitals were seen as unattractive; but in an information society in which people schedule work to their own convenience, these demands are unacceptable. The impact of this routine is heightened by the presence of short hospital stays and high-acuity patients who place continuous demands on nurses and other health care workers for care and support.

The identification and recognition of these changes, along with the other changes identified in the following paragraphs provide hospitals and health care systems with the unavoidable requirement to redesign work and workplace environments so that they are able to attract, retain, and develop the best RN workforce.

Decline in Nursing School Enrollments and Recruitment

One factor in the aging of the nursing workforce is that younger birth cohorts (i.e., those born after 1955) are smaller in population size, as well as significantly less likely to choose nursing as a career (Buerhaus, Staiger, and Auerbach, 2000). Evidence of this trend is seen in the decline in nursing school enrollments. Overall nursing school enrollments dropped by 20.9% between

1995 and 1998 (Carpenter, 2000). Since many young nurses are attracted to the excitement of a critical care setting, acute care settings in particular have been hit hard by this decline in younger nurses entering the workforce. The declining size of graduating classes of professional nurses has resulted in a shrinking supply of RNs wanting to work in critical care settings (Buerhaus, Staiger, and Auerbach, 2000). The shrinking workforce is primarily related to two factors: an overall smaller number of younger individuals available to enter the workforce and expanded career opportunities for women outside of nursing. Women currently make up 90% of the professional nursing workforce (Bednash, 2000). The first factor is beyond the control of the profession; however, we are challenged to make our profession attractive to young men and women as a viable career alternative.

Numerous efforts are presently underway to recruit more students into nursing. Twenty-one of the nation's leading nursing and health care organizations have formed a coalition, *Nurses for a Healthier Tomorrow,* in an attempt to provide long-term help (Sigma Theta Tau International, 2000). According to the coalition, highly visible patient and professional complaints about managed care in the early 1990s have discouraged young people from entering the nursing profession. The first phase of the coalition's work also reveals that students from second through tenth grades are confused about the training involved to become a nurse, are unsure of job security and career advancement possibilities, and voice a lack of compelling reasons to become a nurse. Another group working on recruitment into nursing is the National Student Nurses' Association, which has produced a video, *Nursing: The Ultimate Adventure,* targeted at junior and senior high school students.

Along with the need to recruit into the profession, nursing must continue to examine the ways in which new nurses are introduced into the nursing work culture. Adequate orientation and mentoring and preceptor programs are absolutely essential to both introducing and retaining new nurses. Many health care organizations eliminated these programs during the 1990s for reasons associated with cost reduction during reorganization efforts. This has proven to be a very shortsighted strategy, as many health care organizations are now working to rebuild these programs (ANA, 2000a).

Education

During past shortages, employers have hired RNs, regardless of their degree preparation (American Association of Colleges of Nursing [AACN], 2001). The current and projected demands for RNs requires not simply more RNs, but more RNs of the right type and right educational and skill mix to handle increasingly complex care demands. Demand has intensified for more baccalaureate-prepared nurses with critical thinking, leadership, case management, and health promotion skills who are capable of delivering care across a variety of structured and unstructured health care settings. Demand has also increased for experienced RNs; for nurses in key clinical specialties such as critical care, emergency room, operating room, and neonatal intensive care; and for master's- and doctoral-prepared RNs in advanced clinical specialties, teaching and research.

Although health care organizations increasingly are looking for nurses with at least a baccalaureate degree, enrollment in baccalaureate programs is on the decline. Entry level–BSN enrollment has fallen 4.6% during 2000, dropping for the fifth consecutive year (AACN, 2000). Historically nursing has sought to educate its way out of a nursing shortage, primarily by producing more associate degree graduates. According to Bednash (2000), one challenge is to overcome perceptions that nursing is not intellectually stimulating by rewarding advanced education such as a baccalaureate degree over an associate degree or diploma. Currently few health care organizations differentiate practice or provide significant financial differentials based on educational preparation of the professional nurse.

Faculty Shortage

Presently, one of the most critical problems facing nursing and nursing workforce planning is the aging of nursing faculty (AACN, 1998). According to the AACN, nursing school associate professors and assistant professors are an average age of 52.1 and 48.5 years. This problem is even more acute at the doctoral level, where in 1996 the average age of new doctoral recipients was 45 years. Both the aging of nursing faculty and overall flat enrollment in doctoral programs that produce nurse educators has impacted the capacity of nursing schools to educate sufficient numbers of RNs to meet the future demand (ANA, 2000b). In 1998 the AACN reported that more than a third of schools (37%) cited faculty shortages as the reason for not accepting all qualified applicants into entry-level baccalaureate nursing programs (AACN, 2001).

Faculty salaries continue to be a major contributor to the faculty shortage. According to the AACN (2001), doctorally prepared nursing professors at 4-year colleges and universities earned an average of $68,779 in the 1999-2000 academic year, up by just 3.8% over 1998-1999. Most schools point to budget constraints when reporting too few faculty. However, 30% said faculty shortages were due to increasing job competition from higher-paying clinical sites (AACN, 2001).

Retention

Past nursing shortages have proven that the retention of professional nurses is a key to any organization's success. As shortages occur, nurses are often enticed away from one organization to another with lucrative sign-on bonuses, shift differentials, and promises of a work environment that promotes professional autonomy. Once a shortage has abated, the monetary rewards of joining a particular organization quickly fade. The ability of an organization to retain nurses primarily depends on the creation of an environment conducive to professional autonomy. The importance of autonomy in professional practice is a critical issue for nurses. Nurses want to work in an environment that supports decision making and effective nurse-physician relationships as interdependent and essential concepts of nursing practice (Gleason, Sochalski, and Aiken, 1999).

One of the most successful retention models developed focuses on promoting standards for professional nursing practice and recognizing quality, excellence and service. In 1980, recognizing a critical and widespread national shortage of nurses, the American Academy of Nurses undertook a study to identify a national sample of what are referred to as *magnet hospitals* (i.e., those that attract and retain professional nurses in their employment) and to identify the factors that seem to be associated with their success in doing so (McClure et al., 1983). This landmark study, entitled *Magnet Hospitals: Attraction and Retention of Professional Nurses,* identified workplace factors such as management style, nursing autonomy, quality of leadership, organizational structure, professional practice, career development, and quality of patient care as influencing nurse job satisfaction and low turnover rates in the acute care setting. As a result, the ANA began a program recognizing hospitals with excellent nursing recruitment and high retention rates. Out of 165 hospitals initially participating, only 41 were deemed "magnet hospitals" for their ability to support nurse autonomy and decision making in the workplace.

In the 1990s, faced with a dramatically changing health care environment and armed with substantive data about the nursing profession, the American Academy of Nurses and the ANA joined forces to support the creation of an ongoing magnet program to recognize not only workplace environments that attract nurses, but also, nursing excellence and the role professional nurses play in the delivery of quality patient care. The new program found its home within the American Nurses Credentialing Center (ANCC), a subsidiary of ANA. The ANCC is the nation's center for nursing certification that increasingly plays a greater role in defining nursing competency.

As the magnet hospital program evolved, it sought to combine the strengths of the original study with quality indicators identified by ANA and the standards of nursing practice as defined in ANA's *Scope and Standards for Nurse Administrators* so that both quantitative and qualitative factors of nursing services were measured. With its link between quality patient care and nursing excellence, the *Magnet Recognition Program for Nursing Excellence* has reached a coveted level of prestige within the nursing community and among acute care facilities. In spring 2001 the program recognized 23 hospitals (Newscaps, 2001) and with its increasing stature, many hospitals are striving to improve the workplace environment through the empowerment of nurses. Magnet status is now seen as the single most effective mechanism for providing consumers and nurses with comparative information, a seal of approval for quality nursing care. Research has shown (Aiken, Havens, and Sloane, 2000) that magnet hospital nurses have higher levels of autonomy, more control over the practice setting, and better relationships with physicians. Nurses advocating for a strong workplace should advocate for their hospital to achieve magnet hospital status.

Aging Workforce and Retention

As the nation works to increase the supply of professional nurses through education, nursing and the health care system must develop strategies that will retain the older, expert professional nurse within the nursing workforce. In 2000, the national average age of professional nurses was 44.3 years, with RNs under 30 years of age only representing 10% of the total nurse population. An aging nursing workforce is related to the large cohorts of baby boomer RNs who in 2005 will begin to reach the age (55 years) at which RNs have historically begun to reduce their labor participation (Minnick, 2000). Professional nurses over the age of 40 now represent nearly 60% of the workforce (Buerhaus, Staiger, and Auerbach, 2000). The shortage will worsen by 2010 when almost all of these RNs will have reached retirement years. A review of the literature shows that very little research has been done, particularly within nursing, about the impact of the aging workforce and potential accommodations that may need to be made to retain the experienced nurse (ANA, 2000b).

For hospitals and other health care organizations, the challenge in helping nurses achieve long-term careers and retaining an aging nursing population is to create an environment in which both baby boomer nurses and generation X nurses can thrive (Ulrich, 2001). Many organizations have added on-site day and sick care for children of younger nurses. Because of the aging workforce, organizations will need to consider adding adult day care to assist older nurses who are caring for aging parents. Ergonomic issues are important for staff of any age, but additional attention will be needed as the workforce ages. Organizations that strategically plan for an aging workforce will be best positioned to deliver quality health care to their customers.

Foreign Nurse Recruitment

Long relied on as a remedy for nursing shortages has been the recruitment of foreign nurses. The recruitment of foreign nurses is particularly problematic as a method of resolving the U.S. shortage for two reasons. First, the current shortage is worldwide; therefore recruitment of foreign nurses results in an intensified shortage in the country from which the nurses were recruited. Second, the recognized status of RNs as a permanent shortage profession combined with the rules surrounding the granting of visas make foreign nurse recruitment open to abuse (Tabone, 2000).

Investigations into the abuse of foreign nurses have been well documented in many states, especially Texas. Foreign nurses are granted visa status, a complicated process that is under the auspices of the U.S. Immigration and Naturalization Service (INS). There are currently two mechanisms by which foreign nurses can obtain work visas. The first is by H1B visa, which allows recruitment of shortage professionals into jobs that require a university degree. Of particular interest is the fact that, unlike scientists and computer professionals currently being recruited into the U.S. workforce under H1B status, RNs are not being recruited under this visa status because the 5th Circuit Court ruled in 2000 that RN hospital jobs do not currently require a baccalaureate credential, regardless of recruiter requirements (Tabone, 2000). The second way nurses can get work visas in the United States is by seeking permanent residence. In this case, professional nurses are brought into the country and become permanent residents through petition to the INS. A problem with this visa status is that it does not require labor certification; thus the Department of Labor does not have to certify that the wage being offered nurses is prevailing (Tabone, 2000). However, the law does state that foreign nurses entering under this status cannot have a negative impact on domestic wages. Monitoring of foreign nurses' employment falls under the authority of the U.S. Department of Labor.

A primary example of foreign nurse abuse occurred in Texas during the 1990s, when many foreign nurses were employed in the state and the prevailing wage fell $3 per hour. In addition, many foreign nurses suffered abuses in living conditions, as well as sexual harassment (Tabone, 2000). An investigation conducted by the U.S. Departments of Labor, Justice, and Immigration resulted in the conviction of the owner of multiple long-term care facilities (Tabone, 1998). The owner was convicted of operating an alien-smuggling ring that exploited foreign nurses and jeopardized fair labor standards in Texas. He was found guilty of obtaining fraudulent visas; recruiting nurses from the Philippines, Jamaica, and Korea; and paying them substandard wages in Texas- and Oklahoma-based long-term care facilities. The fraud was uncovered by an investigation instigated by the TNA who advocated on behalf of the foreign nurses and nurses living in West Texas. Back wages totaling approximately $1.5 million were awarded to the foreign RNs (Tabone, 2000). State nurses' associations such as the TNA are committed to preventing foreign nurse abuse and related wage abuses of RNs, both foreign and domestic.

Compensation

A leading nursing workforce researcher, Buerhaus (1998), found that during the 1980s professional nursing hourly wages increased by approximately 3% each year. Unfortunately, during the 1990s nursing salaries remained flat as hospitals dealt with mounting financial pressures from Medicare cuts and managed care belt tightening. Low compensation levels during the 1990s have definitely contributed to the current shortage. In 1996 the national average annual salary of an RN in a staff nurse position was $38,567 (Moses, 1998). Salary compression has long plagued the nursing profession, with little opportunity for extended growth of salary as a nurse gains more experience. Again, as in past nursing shortages, health care agencies are moving to offer relocation bonuses and other financial and fringe benefits to attract nurses. To ease the shortage, hospitals and other health care employers are using sign-on bonuses of up to $10,000, increased recruitment of foreign nurses, new concessions in flexible scheduling, and a growing reliance on "traveling nurses" (Carpenter, 2000). All of these mechanisms result in considerable expenditures by health care organizations. Many believe that these costs could be better expended by increasing compensation levels of professional nurses. As past shortages have abated, so to has the offering of financial bonuses and differential pay scales. Based on market demand, compensation began to increase in the late 1990s, with the average salary rising to $45,000 in 1998 (Carpenter, 2000). Unfortunately, professional nurses continue to show increasing dissatisfaction with their jobs. A survey released by the ANA in spring 2001 indicated that RNs believe that deteriorating working conditions have led to a decline in the quality of nursing care (ANA, 2001).

Work Environment

According to the ANA (2000b), one of the most significant factors that contributes to the difficulty in both recruiting and retaining RNs is the care environment. Although pay rates continue to be a problem, the care environment is a primary motivator for individual professional nurses making employment choices. Several studies have shown that one of the primary factors for the increasing nurse turnover rate is workload and staffing patterns. In a 1998 study by the Hay Group (Healthcare, 1998) examining the nursing shortage, nurse managers, RNs, and licensed practical nurses all cited "insufficient supply of qualified managers and experienced staff" as the most likely reason for the current and growing shortage. Other studies indicate that the primary reason for nurse turnover is increased market demand (Mercer, 1999). Thus the primary causes underlying turnover are career prospects or dissatisfaction with the job or the supervisor. The second most cited reason for turnover was workload and appropriate staffing. These issues are fundamental problems that stand separate from the issues related to the supply of and demand for nursing services. Unless issues related to the work environment are addressed, strategies to increase the overall supply of nurses are unlikely to be successful (ANA, 2000b).

APPROPRIATE STAFFING AND MANDATORY OVERTIME

Appropriate staffing levels and the increased requirement for mandatory overtime are the two largest contributing factors to dissatisfaction within the workplace. The two primary factors contributing to issues and concerns about the adequacy of nurse staffing levels are the nursing shortage and the evolution of managed health care. An understanding of how managed health care has impacted our delivery systems provides a background as to why nurses have major concerns about adequacy of staffing levels. During the 1990s health care systems eagerly sought and implemented the advice of consulting firms to reduce the cost of health care. These consultants brought with them accounting expertise and new models for care delivery that would decentralize the bulk of diagnostic and support services to patient care units and then cross-train the unit staff to provide those services. A perceived outcome of decentralizing services and cross-training unit staff was that patients would have exposure to fewer personnel, personnel could spend less time off their units, and employers could reconfigure staff and eliminate unnecessary positions. Consequently, during the 1990s nursing positions, particularly experienced, higher paid nursing positions, were eliminated or downgraded, whereas lesser-skilled, lower-salaried unlicensed personnel were hired as replacements to function as part of the team under the direction of an RN.

Appropriate Staffing

During this tumultuous time frame of downsizing, cross-training, and cost-cutting, nurses and other health professionals challenged the efficacy of using unlicensed personnel to deliver care to patient populations who were more acutely ill and required high tech care and whose length of stay was being ratcheted downward to keep costs in check. The mix of staff continued to be diluted with increasing numbers of unlicensed personnel and elimination of nursing middle managers and executive level staff. These factors further decreased the support, advocacy, and resources necessary to ensure that nurses could provide optimum care. The absence of standardized, mandatory public reporting of data that could objectively quantify the effects of these staffing changes on the safety and quality of care for patients, as well as the safety and quality of work life for nurses and other health care workers, resulted in dramatic changes in staffing patterns.

Floating/Mandatory Overtime

By the late 1990s an emerging shortage of professional nurses began to further complicate staffing levels. The shortage resulted in (1) professional nurses being required to float to other patient care units for which they had little or no orientation, experience, or support; and (2) the implementation of mandatory overtime and/or mandatory on-call requirements by some employers. The practice of requiring nurses to work mandatory overtime spread across the United States as we moved to the year 2000. In studies of mandatory overtime in other industries, the U.S. Department of Labor found that increasing scheduled work time increased time lost to absenteeism, increased injuries in absolute numbers and rate of incidence, and usually required 3 hours of work to produce an additional two hours of productivity (Thomas, 1990). In the health care sector mandatory overtime by medical residents is implied to be linked to significant numbers of patient deaths as a result of care delivery by exhausted residents (Worth, 1999).

Nurses believe employer dependence on the capacity to mandate last-minute overtime or to use peer pressure as a negative motivator alleviates the employer's sense of urgency or necessity to proactively find safer and more appropriate staffing. Although nurses are fully cognizant and concerned about inadequate staffing, they are also resentful that they bear the personal, professional, and legal burden for this problem that is in large part a direct result of earlier changes in skill mix and care delivery models made acceptable by national imperatives to work swiftly to reduce the cost of health care delivery (ANA, 2000a). By the late 1990s many nurses began to unite to push mandatory overtime and inadequate staffing to the forefront through professional practice advocacy mechanisms.

Advocating for Safe Staffing

Many nurses across the country are concerned about the inadequacies of staffing and are struggling with excessive and unsafe overtime work to meet patient care needs. Health care delivery systems underwent significant changes during the 1990s as the nation moved toward managed care. Many believe that the vigorous downsizing and layoffs of professional nursing staff during the 1990s speak volumes about how nursing judgment and nursing's contribution to safe, accessible, quality care have been valued (ANA, 2000b). Before accepting a position with an organization, professional nurses should ask the questions identified in Box 12-3 regarding safe staffing. Resources to help professional nurse decision making relative to adequate staffing and mandatory overtime are included in Box 12-4.

BOX 12-3	*Questions to Ask About Safe Staffing Before Accepting Employment*

1. Who is the chief nursing officer, to whom does she or he report, and does she or he have authority over staffing?
2. Who controls the staffing budget?
3. Is the level of staffing an active and ongoing discussion in the organization and do staff nurses have input?
4. Does the organization have a shared governance model?
5. When, where, and how is staffing input obtained from staff nurses?
6. How do ratios in the organization compare to national/regional organizations' recommendations such as the American Organization of Nurse Executives and the Association of Critical Care Nurses?
7. What is the content and length of orientation for new nurses?
8. What is the philosophy regarding staff mix designations?
9. What is the frequency of floating to other nursing units?
10. What are the criteria used by the organization in determining competency of cross-trained staff?
11. What resources does the organization use to supplement staff during peak census?
12. If concerns arise about the adequacy of staffing, where and to whom is it appropriate to voice those concerns?
13. How is overtime, on-call time, and cancellation of regularly scheduled shifts handled?
14. Does the organization mandate overtime? If so, can the staff nurse refuse to participate without repercussions?
15. What is the turnover rate and what is the average longevity of staff nurses?
16. What opportunities for advancement exist in the organization such as clinical ladders or other systems of recognition?
17. Where does the organization expect discussions about staffing or practice issues to take place?
18. Is there a conflict resolution process in place?

Adapted from Texas Nurses Association: *Nurse staffing task force document (internal document)*, Austin, Tx, 1999, Author, www.texanurses.org.

BOX 12-4	*Resources for Decision Making Related to Adequacy of Staffing and Mandatory Overtime*

Principles of nurse staffing
Outlines the critical considerations needed to determine appropriate staffing. Single copies are free to members of ANA's constituent member associations by calling 1-800-274-4ANA and asking for PNS-1. Multiple copies can be ordered from 1-800-637-0323 or www.nursesbooks.org.

ANA consumer alert
"ANA Calls Hospital Staffing Practices Unsafe": www.nursingworld.org/pressrel/2000/pr0420b.htm

Nursing quality indicators: Definitions and implications; Nursing quality indicators: Guide for implementation
1-800-637-0323
www.nursesbooks.org

State nurses association
ANA's Constituent Member Associations www.nursingworld.org

| BOX 12-5 | *Questions To Ask In Making the Decision To Accept a Staffing Assignment* |

1. What is the assignment?

Clarify the assignment. Do not assume. Be certain that what you believe is the assignment is indeed correct.

2. What are the characteristics of the patients being assigned?

Don't just respond to the number of patients; make a critical assessment of the needs of each patient, his or her age, condition, other factors that contribute to special needs, and the resources available to meet those needs. Who else is on the unit or within the facility that might be a resource for the assignment? Do nurses on the unit have access to those resources? How stable are the patients, and for what period of time have they been stable? Do any patients have communication and/or physical limitations that will require accommodation and extra supervision during the shift? Will there be discharges to offset the load? If there are discharges, will there be admissions, which require extra time and energy?

3. Do I have the expertise to care for the patients?

Am I familiar with caring for the types of patients assigned? If this is a "float assignment," am I crossed-trained to care for these patients? Is there a "buddy system" in place with staff familiar with the unit? If there is no cross-training or "buddy system," has the patient load been modified accordingly?

4. Do I have the experience and knowledge to manage the patients for whom I am being assigned care?

If the answer to the question is no, you have an obligation to articulate limitations. Limitations in experience and knowledge may not require refusal of the assignment but rather an agreement regarding supervision or a modification of the assignment to ensure patient safety. If no accommodation for limitations is considered, the nurse has an obligation to refuse an assignment for which she or he lacks education or experience.

5. What is the geography of the assignment?

Am I being asked to care for patients who are in close proximity for efficient management, or are the patients at opposite ends of the hall or on different units? If there are geographic difficulties, what resources are available to manage the situation? If my patients are on more than one unit and I must go to another unit to provide care, who will monitor patients out of my immediate attention?

Adapted from Texas Nurses Association: *Workplace advocacy program*, Austin, Tx, 2001, Author, www.texasnurses.org.

The immediate concern for most nurses in a staffing conflict is whether or not to accept an assignment. Many times this comes down to a disagreement between the nurse manager making the assignment and the staff nurse asked to accept the assignment. Box 12-5 identifies a set of questions to help the staff nurse in making a decision to accept or not accept an assignment. These questions are designed to help the staff nurse think critically about the assignment so that, if there is a problem, the nurse can be clear in telling the manager what makes her or him uncomfortable with the assignment.

Mandatory overtime and adequate staffing levels have become a legislative issue at both the national and state levels of government (Jordan and Tabone, 2000). The first state to pass legislation addressing nurse staffing levels was California in 1999. The California bill

BOX 12-5	*Questions to Ask in Making the Decision to Accept a Staffing Assignment—cont'd*

6. Is this a temporary assignment?

When other staff are located to assist, will I be relieved? If the assignment is temporary, it may be possible to accept a difficult assignment, knowing that there will soon be reinforcements. Is there a pattern of short staffing or is this truly an emergency?

7. Is this a crisis or an ongoing staffing pattern?

If the assignment is being made because of an immediate need on the unit, a crisis, the decision to accept the assignment may be based on that immediate need. However, if the staffing pattern is an ongoing problem, the nurse has the obligation to identify unmet standards of care that are occurring as a result of ongoing staffing inadequacies. This may result in a request for safe harbor and/or peer review.

8. Can I take the assignment in good faith? If not the nurse will have to get the assignment modified or refuse the assignment.

Consult your individual state's nursing practice act regarding clarification of accepting an assignment in good faith. In understanding good faith, it is sometimes easier to identify what would constitute bad faith. For example, if you had not taken care of pediatric patients since nursing school and you were asked to take charge of a pediatric unit, unless this were an extreme emergency such as a disaster (in which case you would need to let people know your limitations, but you might be the best person, given all factors for the assignment), it would be bad faith to take the assignment. It is always your responsibility to articulate your limitations and to get an adjustment to the assignment that acknowledges the limitations you have articulated. Good faith acceptance of the assignment means that you are concerned about the situation and believe that a different pattern of care or policy should be considered. However, you acknowledge the difference of opinion on the subject between you and your supervisor and are willing to take the assignment and await the judgment of other peers/supervisors.

requires all acute care facilities to provide minimum nurse-to-patient ratios and to adopt written policies and procedures for training and orientation of nursing staff (ANA, 1998c). Although the California bill passed in 1999, implementation has been delayed until 2001. Federal legislation was introduced in the fall of 2000 that would limit the number of hours licensed health care workers, including RNs, are forced to work. The bill was intended to amend the Fair Labor Standards Act so that no RN would be required to work beyond 8 hours in any workday or 80 hours in any 14-day work period (Price, 2000). Realistic concerns about nurses' ability to provide safe care were amplified by the release of the two Institute of Medicine (IOM) documents: *The Adequacy of Nurse Staffing in Hospitals and Nursing Homes* (Wunderlich, Sloan, and Davis, 1996) and *To Err is Human* (Kohn, Corrigan, and Donaldson, 1999).

Shared Governance As a Method of Advocating for Excellence in Nursing Practice

Introduced in the 1970s, shared governance has been identified by RNs as a key indicator of excellence in nursing practice. The concept of professional practice models such as shared governance has attracted the attention of nursing over the last decade in response to maintaining nursing job satisfaction, quality care, and fiscal viability. During the past 15 years, there has been proliferation of such models to redesign care delivery roles and systems and restructure the governance of professional nursing.

The importance of shared governance is that such models provide an organizational framework for nurses in direct care to become committed to nursing practice within their organizations. The implementation of such models allows nurses to have an active role in decision making by providing maximum participation and accountability for the outcomes of those decisions. Shared governance models render both a structure and an environment that empowers staff to make care decisions. Attributes of shared governance include independence, accountability, and autonomy over nursing practice. These attributes are identified as important factors in nursing job satisfaction. Shared governance results in more than job satisfaction; it includes as equally important increased efficiency and better patient outcomes.

The delegation of decision making to the professional doing the work is often referred to as participatory management and may be the first level of nursing governance in a regular hierarchic organization. However, self-governance goes beyond participatory management through the creation of organizational structures that allow nursing staff to govern issues of nursing practice and nursing service delivery. An example would be the Safety Committee that Ellena was elected to by her colleagues after she initiated inquiries as to why safe needle devices were not available on her nursing unit.

Accountability forms the foundation for designing self-governance models. To be accountable, authority to make decisions concerning all aspects of responsibilities is essential. Shared governance or self-governance structure designs go beyond decentralizing and diminishing hierarchies. Accountability is determined by needs arising from the services provided to clients. Authority, control, and autonomy are placed in specifically defined areas of accountability, which are generally those areas that are related to nursing service and patient care.

The major cause of nurses' dissatisfaction with their work revolves around the absence of autonomy and accountability for nursing practice. The magnet hospital study, which identified characteristics of hospitals with stable nursing staff, found that nursing departments with structures that provide nurses the opportunity to be accountable for their own practice was the major contributing characteristic to their success in recruiting and retaining nurses (Gleason, Sochalski, and Aiken, 1999).

Shared governance of the delivery of nursing services often develops in phases. These phases offer organizations the opportunity to adjust to the changing roles and decision-making authority of nurses. Each phase provides greater autonomy to practicing nurses in determining practice policy. However, the structure allows nursing delivery decisions to be integrated with other policy needs of the organization. Box 12-6 provides an overview of potential developmental phases for shared governance. As a shared governance model is developed in the health care organization, it is important that it does not become isolated from other organizational problem-solving and policy-making bodies such as quality improvement, ethics, and risk management.

BOX 12-6	*Three Developmental Phases of Shared Governance*

Phase 1

- Staff Nurse Representatives—members of clinical forums, have authority for designated practice issues and some authority for determining roles, functions, and processes.
- Managers—members of management forums, responsible for facilitation of practice through resource management and allocation.
- Executive Committee—administrative and staff membership, often in disproportionate numbers, accept recommendations from staff nurses and managers.
- Chief Nurse Executive—retains final decision-making authority.

Phase 2

- Staff Nurse Representatives—members of nursing committees that are designated for specific management and/or clinical functions.
- Managers—serve on same committees with staff nurses.
- Committee Chairs—appointed by chief nurse executive.
- Nursing Cabinet—composed of multiple committee chairs who make final decisions on recommendations from the committees.

Phase 3

- Staff Nurse Representatives—belong to councils with authority for specific functions.
- Council Chairs—make up management committee charged with making all final operational decisions.

Adapted from Texas Nurses Association: *Workplace advocacy program,* Austin, Tex, 2001, Author, www.texasnurses.org.

Not all health care organizations place quality patient care at the top of their agenda; rather they focus more on bottom-line profits. In these situations nurses may find themselves challenged to provide quality care. Therefore it is important that nurses have access and input to the various organizational structures in place whose decisions affect the nurse and patient. Nurses need to be integral members of such organizational structures as quality improvement and ethics committees. Staff nurses need to know who their representatives are and how to access such committees. Box 12-7 identifies questions that should be asked about shared governance or participatory management models when nurses are trying to identify the organization that would be most conducive to the delivery of quality nursing care.

Nurses working under shared governance models should have access to conflict resolution procedures that define the processes they should follow if they are in disagreement with the organization. However, organizations without shared governance models may also have systems in place that could be of assistance. Examples of these are open-door policies, ombudsman programs, or dispute-resolution processes. When seeking dispute resolution, the nurse may use a third party or resources internal to the organization to assist in the resolution. Some states such as Texas have several processes that can assist in resolving patient care or professional issues. These processes include peer review, safe harbor, and mandatory reporting.

BOX 12-7	*Questions to Ask About Shared Governance Models*

Access to the process
- Are nurses encouraged to participate in shared governance?
- How do nurses become involved in the shared governance process?
- What is the ratio of staff nurses to managers involved in shared governance within the organization?
- Is adequate work time allowed to participate in governance councils?

Implementation and communication of action
- How does the organization communicate shared governance decisions with staff nurses?

Effectiveness of the process
- How did shared governance improve nursing care delivery in the organization?
- Do nurses feel shared governance within their organization is beneficial to their practice?

Outcomes of the process
- Does the organization have outcomes data related to shared governance?
- If so, how have that data impacted changes in nursing practice

Adapted from Texas Nurses Association: *Workplace advocacy program,* Austin, Tx, 2001, Author, www.texasnurses.org.

PATIENT ADVOCACY/SAFETY

Patient advocacy is a cornerstone of the nursing profession, and patients depend on nurses to ensure that they receive proper care. Although nurses have always advocated for their patients, it has only been during the last 25 years that the role of the nurse as "patient advocate" has begun to clearly emerge. The evolution of the nurse's role in patient advocacy has changed from a vague assertion of ethic-legal responsibility in the mid 1970s to a "rights" framework in the 1980s (Mallik and Rafferty, 2000). This "rights" framework has only intensified in the 1990s and will continue to do so as we move through the new century.

Today's health care systems have created an environment in which errors and adverse events are attributed to complex systems and complicated uses of technology. This environment demands that the nursing profession assert its powerful voice in the role of patient advocate by supporting public policies that protect consumers and enhance accountability for quality by promoting safer health care systems.

Errors in Health Care

Errors in the health care system carry a high cost for all involved. Based on findings of two major studies, errors in health care delivery kill approximately 44,000 people in U.S. hospitals (Cook, Woods, and Miller, 1998; Brennan et al., 1991). Another study estimates the number higher, at 98,000 (American Medical Association, 1999). Even using the lower figures, more people supposedly die from health care errors each year than from highway accidents, breast cancer, or acquired immune deficiency syndrome (Centers for Disease Control and Prevention, 1999). No health care setting is immune from errors, including hospitals, outpatient clinics, retail pharmacies, long-term care facilities, and the home. Over 7000 deaths that occur in multiple settings annually are attributed to medication errors alone (Occupational Safety and Health Administration, 1998; Phillips, Christenfeld, and Glynn, 1998).

During late 1999 a major policy paper was issued by the IOM, entitled *To Err is Human: Building a Safer Health System* (Kohn, Corrigan, Donaldson, 1999). This document quickly seized the attention of the entire health care delivery system, providers, policy makers, and the public on the seriousness of errors in health care. It described a fragmented health care system that is prone to errors and detrimental to the goal of safe patient care. The IOM report concentrated on those errors (acknowledged to be the vast majority) that result from mistakes rather than those caused by incompetence of the health care provider. The IOM report recommended a variety of legislative, regulatory, and voluntary corrective actions designed to improve the safety of health care delivery systems (Swankin and LeBuhn, 2000). Since the release of the reports, many nursing organizations have attempted to demonstrate the linkage between nurse staffing and the prevention of patient adverse events and errors. Health care errors and adverse patient incidents include:

- Transfusion and medication errors
- Equipment or device failure
- Wrong site surgery
- Preventable suicides
- Falls
- Burns
- Mistaken identity

In another report, the IOM focused on the quality of care in the long-term care industry. This report cited a need for effective government oversight and ample nurse staffing to boost the quality of care provided in long-term care (Hallam and Lovern, 2000). The IOM made sweeping recommendations intended to improve the long-term care workforce, such as improving the work environment through competitive wages, career development, work design, and better supervision. The report also outlines a role for federal and state governments in establishing minimum staffing levels and competency standards. In a separate IOM report on the quality of health care in America, scheduled to be released during spring 2001, the IOM will follow up on the 1999 *To Err is Human* report. The upcoming IOM health care quality report will expand on the patient safety focus to include areas such as efficiency, effectiveness, and timeliness within the health care system.

Whistle-Blower Protection

Nurses want the assurance that, if they are acting within the scope of their expertise, they will be able to speak up for their patients through appropriate channels without fear of retaliation. Whistle-blower legislation has been advocated for at the federal level and has actually passed in some states. Whistle-blower protection basically prohibits health care organizations from retaliating against nurses when the professional nurse in good faith discloses information or participates in agency investigations. Whistle-blower protection protects nurses who speak out about unsafe situations from being fired or subjected to other disciplinary actions by their employers.

An example of how whistle-blower protection promotes workplace advocacy is illustrated by a recent case in Texas. A Texas jury awarded a nurse formerly employed by a large health science center $810,000 in her lawsuit filed under the Texas Whistle-Blower Act (Tabone, 2000). She witnessed patients, who in her assessment were not in imminent danger of death, having their rights to informed consent disregarded. Patients refusing treatment were treated despite

BOX 12-8	*Things To Know About Whistle-Blowing*

If you identify an illegal or unethical practice, reserve judgment until you have adequate documentation to establish wrongdoing.

Do not expect those that are engaged in unethical or illegal conduct to welcome your questions or concerns about this practice.

Seek the counsel of someone you trust outside of the situation to provide you with an objective perspective.

Consult with your state nurses association or legal counsel if possible before taking action to determine how best to document your concerns.

Remember, you are not protected in a whistle-blower situation from retaliation by your employer until you blow the whistle.

Blowing the whistle means that you report your concern to the national and/or state agency responsible for regulation of the organization for which you work, or in the case of criminal activity to law enforcement agencies as well.

Private groups such as the Joint Commission on Accreditation of Healthcare Organizations or the National Committee for Quality Assurance do not confirm protection. You must report to a state or national regulator.

Although it is not required by every regulatory agency, it is a good rule of thumb to put your complaint in writing.

Document all interactions related to the whistle-blowing situation and keep copies for your personal file.

Keep documentation and interactions objective.

Remain calm and do not lose your temper, as those who learn of your actions attempt to provoke you.

Remember that blowing the whistle is a very serious matter; do not blow the whistle frivolously. Make sure you have the facts straight before taking action.

Adapted from Tabone S: 2000 update: foreign nurse recruitment, *Texas Nurs* 74(8):9, 15, 2000.

their protests to doctors. This nurse sought counsel from her state nurses association and, based on their recommendations, documented her concerns about these incidents according to the hospital's policies and tried to work within the system to stop what she believed to be serious patient rights violations. She further protected herself by documenting her interactions with those who were retaliating against her for speaking out and reported the situation to the State Board of Nurse Examiners, the Texas Department of Health, and the local police department. She was eventually terminated by the employing hospital. The jury found that she acted in accordance with the state nursing practice act in reporting her concerns about patient care practices and upheld her suit for defamation and wrongful termination (Tabone, 2000). Box 12-8 provides an overview of "Things To Know About Whistle-Blowing." Nurses should check with their state nurses association to assess the status of whistle-blower protection in their state.

Nursing Quality Indicators

Major changes in systems of care and nurse staffing are occurring with little data to justify or demonstrate the potential effects on safety and quality of patient care. Many organizations, including the National Nursing Research Roundtable, the National Institute of Nursing Research, and the major federal supporter of health systems and health outcomes research, the Agency for Healthcare Quality and Research, are working collaboratively to promote collection and publication of data that link nurse staffing mix with patient outcomes. A critical and pioneering component of this work has been the initiation of research to examine linkages between

BOX 12-9	*Ten Nursing-Sensitive Quality Indicators for Acute Care Settings*

Mix of RNs, LPNs, and unlicensed staff caring for patients
Total nursing care hours provided per patient day
Pressure ulcers
Patient falls
Patient satisfaction with pain management
Patient satisfaction with educational information
Patient satisfaction with overall care
Patient satisfaction with nursing care
Nosocomial infection rate
Nurse staff satisfaction

Adapted from American Nurses Association: *Quality indicators for acute care settings*, Washington, DC, 2001, Author, www.nursingworld.org.

professional nurse staffing, processes of care, and patient outcomes in acute care settings. Because of limited research in this area, the ANA took the lead in the design and implementation of ongoing, comprehensive, broad-based research efforts to establish and quantify the impact of professional nurse staffing on processes of care and patient outcomes. The initial step in the identification of nursing-sensitive indicators focused on the acute care setting. However, the work has now moved into testing of quality indicators appropriate for community-based non-acute health care settings. Box 12-9 lists the nursing-sensitive quality indicators for acute settings. The National Database of Nursing Quality Indicators, established in late 1997, continues to receive data and issue reports about the data analyses of participating facilities (ANA, 1998b).

Numerous states have introduced and passed legislation that calls for states to collect and disseminate nursing data to the public, including nurse staffing patterns and patient outcomes such as nosocomial infections, patient fall rates, decubitus ulcers, and patient satisfaction (ANA, 1998c). This information provides an important guide to consumers, providers, and institutions when making purchasing decisions about health care services.

WORKPLACE SAFETY

Nurses are battling to provide safe, quality care for patients in an environment that is becoming increasingly dangerous. The occupational safety and health of nurses continues to be an ongoing concern for both individual nurses and professional nursing associations. Workplace injuries for all industries cost Americans $125.1 billion, the equivalent to nearly triple the combined profits reported by the top five Fortune 500 companies during the same year (Texas Tech University Health Sciences Center, 2001). There were 5100 workplace fatalities in 1999, and for women workers homicides were the leading cause of workplace deaths. Box 12-10 describes categories of health hazards in the health care workplace.

Needlesticks

Of particular concern are the growing phenomena of exposure to blood-borne diseases. Health care workers in the United States experience at least 800,000 needlestick injuries annually. These injuries account for the majority of all exposures to blood-borne pathogens (ANA, 1998a). The Centers for Disease Control and Prevention (1997) reported results of research

| **BOX 12-10** | *Categories of Health Hazards in the Health Care Workplace* |

Biologic hazards
Bacteria, viruses, fungi, or parasites that may be transmitted by contact with infected patients or contaminated body secretions/fluids. Examples include human immunodeficiency virus, hepatitis B and C, tuberculosis, and varicella

Ergonomic hazards
Musculoskeletal injury to the back and extremities resulting from lifting, standing for long periods, and repeated hand motions

Chemical hazards
Medications, solutions, gases (such as ethylene oxide, formaldehyde, glutaraldehyde, waste anesthetic and laser gases), cytotoxic agents, pentamidine, latex, PVC plastics, Di-ethylhexyl phthalate (DEHP)

Psychologic hazards
Stress, shiftwork, mandatory overtime, verbal abuse by patients and other health care providers

Physical hazards
Radiation, lasers, noise, electricity, violence

Adapted from American Nurses Association: *Occupational safety and health: 1998 ANA House of Delegates Status Reports,* Washington, DC, 1998a, Author.

showing that the use of safer needlestick devices (including blunting intravenous catheters and retractable needles) reduced worker injuries by up to 76% without significant patient complications and that health care workers generally accepted the safer devices.

Legislative initiatives at the federal and state levels are being passed to ensure that nurses and other health care workers are protected from blood-borne diseases in the workplace. The most significant piece of legislation passed to date occurred at the federal level during fall 2000 when the Needlestick Safety and Prevention Act was signed into law (The American Nurse, 2000). The ANA was instrumental in advocating for passage of this legislation. The Needlestick Safety and Prevention Act amends the existing Blood-Borne Pathogen Standard administered by the Occupational Safety and Health Administration to require the use of safer devices to protect from sharps injuries. It also requires employers to solicit the input of nonmanagerial employees responsible for direct patient care who are potentially exposed to sharps injuries in the identification, evaluation, and selection of effective engineering and work-practice controls. This bill also requires employers to maintain a sharps injury log to contain, at a minimum, the brand of device involved in the incident, the department or work area where the exposure incident occurred, and an explanation of how the incident occurred. The log will become an important source of data for researchers to determine the relative effectiveness and safety of devices now on the market and those that may be developed in the future (The American Nurse, 2000).

Ergonomic Injuries

Although nurses have suffered from back and other musculoskeletal disorders for decades, it is only during the last decade that they are being directly attributed to the workplace. There are strong data demonstrating the problem of overexertion injuries in hospitals, nursing homes, and home care settings over the last decade. Sixty-seven percent of the disabling injuries in nursing were caused by sprains and strains, mostly overexertion injuries to the back or trunk from lifting patients (The American Nurse, 2000). Back injuries are particularly troublesome for nurses, impacting 38% of all nurses. New ergonomic standards were released in fall 2000 by the National Institute of Occupational Safety and Health and should help protect nurses from disabling back injuries and musculoskeletal disorders. The ANA was instrumental in advocating for the passage of this legislation. The standard includes work restriction protections, and the "action trigger" in the standard focuses on identification of hazards, which is crucial in preventing back injuries and musculoskeletal disorders.

Workplace Violence

Workplace violence has become a major societal issue. The National Institute for Occupational Safety and Health estimates that, for all businesses across the United States, two million workers are attacked annually in the workplace and a more alarming six million are threatened (Antai-Otong, 1998). One-sixth of all violent crimes occur in the workplace, including 8% of all rapes, 7% of all robberies, and 16% of all assaults; and 10% of all workplace violence involves handguns. Causative factors of workplace violence are multivariate (Antai-Otong, 1998). However, it is known that, as health care continues to move from primarily acute care settings to outpatient, community, and home-based settings, the risk of workplace violence remains a threat to health care workers. The continuing pressures in health care delivery to contain cost have resulted in shortened hospital stays, with many patients being discharged with unstable medical and psychiatric conditions that pose even greater dangers for nurses in all practice settings (Antai-Otong, 1998). The frequency with which health care organizations reorganize is also on the increase, resulting in job insecurity, disloyalty, apathy, stress, tension, and feelings of helplessness and devaluation. Settings where these factors seem to be the most amplified occur in high-stress practice areas, including Emergency Departments, acute care such as psychiatry and intensive care units, and long-term care. These factors, along with increased workloads and dwindling resources, further heighten the incidence of violence in the health care workplace (Antai-Otong, 1998).

An example of workplace violence can be illustrated by an incident that occurred in early 2001 in a West Texas hospital. A prison inmate with complaints of gastrointestinal bleeding was accompanied to the Emergency Department of a large hospital by two prison guards (Queen, 2001). The inmate managed to confiscate the keys to his handcuffs, becoming free and brandishing a gun while threatening the guards, emergency staff, and other patients. He then barricaded himself and two nurses in a room, where he sexually assaulted the nurses and held a SWAT team at bay for nearly 2 hours. Apparently the guards responsible for the inmate did not follow many routine safety procedures; the gun turned out to be fake.

Nurses must proactively advocate for safe workplaces. This should occur through a comprehensive organizational assessment to identify high-risk environments and psychologic conditions and populations that threaten workplace safety (Antai-Otong, 1998). Failure to recognize behavioral cues such as pacing, yelling, and verbal and physical threats further compromises the safety of nurses and patients. Staff education is essential to proactively address the identification and response to high-risk behaviors, which can lead to violence. Nursing safety is imperative and includes adequate staffing levels, adequate staff training, and environmental safeguards.

BOX 12-11	*Helpful Websites/Resources*

American Nurses Association—Occupational Safety and Health
www.nursingworld.org

American Nurses Association—Safe Needles Save Lives Campaign
www.needlestick.org

American Nurses Association—Pollution Prevention Kit for Nurses
www.nurses-books.org or 1-800-637-0323 to request publication 9811LA

Citizens Advocacy Center—unique support program for pubic members who serve on health care regulatory
   boards and governing bodies as representatives of consumer interest
www.cacenter.org

FDA MedWatch Program—report reactions to latex products and other chemical exposures
1-800-FDA-1088 (fax 1-800-FDA-0178)

Health Care Without Harm—neonatal exposure to DEHP and opportunities for prevention
Educational brochure—click on library
www.noharm.org

Information on mercury
www.epa.gov/seahome/mercury/src/mercmed.htm or www.nwf.org/greatlakes/resources/mercury.html

National Institute of Occupational Safety and Health
www.cdc.gov/niosh/publistd.html

National Institute of Occupational Safety and Health—Ergonomics Standards
www.cdc.gov/niosh/publistd.html

National Institute of Occupational Safety and Health—Latex Allergy Alert
Education information on identifying latex allergy
1-800-45-NIOSH to request publication No. 97-195

National Institute of Occupational Safety and Health—What Every Worker Should Know: How to Protect
   Yourself from Needlestick Injuries
Educational brochure on needlestick prevention
1-800-35-NIOSH to publication No. 000-135

National Institute of Occupational Safety and Health—Health Hazard Evaluation
Demonstrates the problem of indoor air causing illness to hundreds of health care workers
1-800-35-NIOSH to request report HETA 96-0012-2652

Nightingale Institute for Health and the Environment
www.nihe.org

The Environmentally Preferable Purchasing (EPP) Work Group—resources for healthy hospitals
www.geocities.com/EPP_how_to_guide/

Advocating for a Safer Workplace

The ANA has emerged as a leader in health care worker health and safety, working in collaboration with other nursing organizations, including the American Association of Occupational Health Nurses, Association of Operating Room Nurses, the Emergency Nurses Association, and other labor unions representing health care workers (ANA, 1998a). Through the ANA's Workplace Advocacy Program, the ANA advocates for administrative controls such as adequate staffing and health and safety committees, engineering controls such as ventilation and safer needle stick devices, and personal protective equipment such as respirators and synthetic gloves that will prevent exposure to hazardous substances and/or prevent illness or injury from unavoidable exposure. Although the health care industry is a dangerous place to work, many of the risks are avoidable, and dangerous exposures preventable. Box 12-11 identifies resources to improve the safety of the workplace for both nurses and patients.

SUMMARY

This chapter has covered a variety of significant workplace issues and identified professional practice strategies for the nurse to use to improve the workplace environment and quality of patient care. A rapidly changing health care environment, significantly impacted by an aging workforce and shortage of nurses, creates a challenge for all nurses. Nurses must be aware of the issues facing the profession and know where to seek assistance, information, and resources to address workplace issues. Working together with the resources of such organizations as the ANA, nurses can create a workplace that is conducive to career satisfaction and quality patient care.

Critical Thinking Activities

1. How will the nursing shortage affect you as an individual? How will the shortage affect the profession of nursing and health care delivery?
2. What activities can health care organizations undertake to promote retention of nurses? How can health care organizations retain the older, more experienced nurse?
3. Determine if your clinical practice site has a conflict resolution process. Does your state provide whistle-blower protection? How would you proceed if you believed there was cause for concern about patient safety in your clinical practice site?
4. Is your clinical practice site in compliance with the Needlestick Safety and Prevention Act (2000)?
5. Does your clinical practice site have a plan for handling workplace violence? Have nurses and other health care providers been educated on the use of the plan?

REFERENCES

Aiken L, Havens D, Sloane D: The magnet nursing services recognition program: a comparison of two groups of magnet hospitals, *Am J Nurs* 100(3):26-34, 2000.

American Association of Colleges of Nursing: *As RNs age, nursing schools seek to expand the pool of younger faculty,* Issue Bulletin, Washington, DC, June, 1998, Author.

American Association of Colleges of Nursing: *Nursing school enrollments decline as demand for RNs continues to climb,* 2000, www.aacn.nche.edu/Media/NewsReleases/2000Feb17.htm.

American Association of Colleges of Nursing: *Media talking points: the emerging nursing shortage,* 2001, www.aacn.nche.edu/MembersOnly.

American Hospital Association: *Workforce supply for hospitals and health systems issues and recommendations,* American Hospital Association Policy Forum, 2001, http://www.ahapolicyforum.org/policyresources/WorkforceB0123.asp.

American Medical Association: *Hospital statistics,* Chicago, 1999, American Medical Association.

American Nurses Association: Occupational safety and health. *1998 ANA House of Delegates Status Reports.* Washington, DC, 1998a, Author.

American Nurses Association: *Nursing facts: nursing's quality indicators for acute care settings and ANA's safety and quality initiative,* Washington, DC, 1998b, Author.

American Nurses Association: *Safety and quality initiatives: state legislative trends and analysis: special report to the 1998 House of Delegates,* Washington, DC, 1998c, Author.

American Nurses Association: *Definition of professional practice advocacy adopted by House of Delegates (Internal Document),* Washington, DC, 1999, Author.

American Nurses Association: *Opposing the use of mandatory overtime as a staffing solution: summary of proceedings: American Nurses Association 2000 House of Delegates,* Washington, DC, 2000a, Author.

American Nurses Association: *Nursing workforce and the environment of care: status report 2000 ANA House of Delegates,* Washington, DC, 2000b, Author.

American Nurses Association: 2001, http://www.nursingworld.org/pressrel/2001/pr0206.htm.

Antai-Otong D: Proactive responses to workplace violence: nurses' roles in health promotion. *Tex Nurs* 72(7):4-7, 1998.

Bednash G: The decreasing supply of registered nurses: inevitable future or call to action, *JAMA* 283(22): 2985-2987, June 14, 2000.

Brennan T et al: Incidence of adverse events and negligence in hospitalized patients: results of the Harvard medical Practice Study I, *N Engl J Med* 324:370-376, 1991.

Bureau of Labor Statistics: Occupational outlook handbook, 1999, www.bls.gov/ocohome.htm?H2.

Buerhaus P: Is another RN shortage looming? *Nurs Outlook* 46:103-108, 1998.

Buerhaus P, Staiger D, Auerbach D: Implications of an aging registered nurse workforce, *JAMA* 283(22): 2948-2954, June 14, 2000.

Carpenter D: Going . . . going . . . gone? *Hosp Health Networks* 74(6):32-36, 38, 40-42, June 2000.

Centers for Disease Control and Prevention: Evaluation of safety devices for preventing percutaneous injuries among health-care workers during phlebotomy procedures—Minneapolis-St. Paul, New York City, and San Francisco, 1993-1995, *MMWR* 46(2):21-25, 1997.

Centers for Disease Control and Prevention National Center for Health Statistics: Births and deaths: preliminary data for 1998, *National Vital Statistics Rep* 47(25):6, 1999.

Cook R, Woods D, Miller C: *A tale of two stories: contrasting views of patient safety,* Chicago, 1998, National Patient Safety Foundation.

Gleason S, Sochalski J, Aiken L: Review of magnet hospital research: findings and implications for professional nursing practice, *J Nurs Admin* 29(1):9-19, 1999.

Hallam K, Lovern E: IOM sets sights on long-term care, *Mod Healthcare* 30(22):32-33, Dec. 18-25, 2000.

Healthcare Information Resource Center: *1998 Nursing shortage study,* Walnut Creek, Calif, 1998, Hay Group.

Jordan C, Tabone S: Mandatory overtime and on call: growing concerns for nurses, *Tex Nurs* 74(8):4-6, 2000.

Kohn L, Corrigan J, Donaldson M: *To err is human: building a safer health system,* Washington, DC, 1999, Institute of Medicine, National Academy Press.

Mallik M, Rafferty A: Diffusion of the concept of patient advocacy, *J Nurs Scholarship* 32(4):399-404, 2000.

McClure M et al: *Magnet hospitals: attraction and retention of professional nurses: American Academy of Nursing Task Force on Nursing Practice in Hospitals,* Kansas City, Mo, 1983, American Nurses Association.

Mercer W: *Attracting and retaining registered nurses—survey results,* Chicago, 1999, William M Mercer.

Minnick A: Retirement, the nursing workforce, and the year 2005, *Nurs Outlook* 48:211-217, 2000.

Moses E: *The registered nurse population,* Rockville, Md, 1998, US Dept. of Health and Human Services.

Nevidjon B, Erickson J: The nursing shortage: solutions for the short and long term, *Online J Issues Nurs* 6(1):Manuscript 4, 2001, www.nursingworld.org/ojin/topic14/tpc14_4.htm.

Newscaps: the 23rd hospital to attain magnet status . . . , *Am J Nurs* 101(2):20, 2001.

Occupational Safety and Health Administration: *The new OSHA: reinventing worker safety and health.* 1998, www.OSHA.gov/oshinfo/reinvent.html.

Phillips D, Christenfeld N, Glynn L: Increase in US medication-error deaths between 1983-1993, *Lancet* 351(43):644, 1998.

Price C: A national uprising, *Am J Nurs* 100(12):75-76, 2000.

Queen S: Inmate charged in UMC sex assaults: fake gun used to hold two nurses hostage, *Lubbock Avalance-J,* January 5, 2001, p 1A.

Sigma Theta Tau International: *Nurses for a healthier tomorrow,* 2000, www.nursesource.org.

Swankin D, LeBuhn R: *Promoting patient safety: collaboration between regulators and health care organizations,* Washington, DC, 2000, Citizen Advocacy Center.

Tabone S: TNA advocates for fair labor: smuggler is sentenced, *Tex Nurs* 72(6):3, 1998.

Tabone S: 2000 update: foreign nurse recruitment, *Tex Nurs* 74(8):9, 15, 2000.

Thomas H: Effects of scheduled overtime on labor productivity: a literature review and analysis, *Construction Industry Institute Document 60,* November 1990.

The American Nurse: New federal measure protects nurses from needlesticks, *Am Nurse* 32(6):1, 8, 2000.

Texas Tech University Health Sciences Center: Worker's comp fast facts, *Safety Reporter* 47(3):4, Lubbock, Tex, 2001, Texas Tech University Health Sciences Center.

Ulrich B: Editors note: Generation RN: organizations, nurses of all ages work together to achieve professional longevity, *NurseWeek* 6(2):4: 2001, www.nurseweek.com/ednote/01/012201b.asp.

Worth R: Exhaustion that kills, *Washington Monthly* 31(1): 25-20, 1999.

Wunderlich G, Sloan F, Davis C: *Nursing staff in hospitals and nursing homes: Is it adequate? Committee on the Adequacy of Nurse Staffing in Hospitals and Nursing Homes.* Washington, DC, 1996, Institute of Medicine, National Academy Press.

Young S, Hayes E, Morin K: Developing workplace advocacy behaviors, *J Nurs Staff Dev* 11(5):265-269, 1993.

Collective Bargaining

13

Corinne Grimes, MSN, DNSc, RN

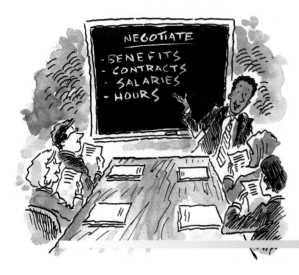

Collective bargaining: labor and management sharing a degree of power to determine selected conditions of employment.

Vignette

Jack Perkins graduated in June from nursing school. He has passed his NCLEX examination and can call himself a registered nurse (RN). His folks tried to talk him into going to medical school with what they thought were good arguments: more money, more prestige, and greater independence. But he has always admired the nurses involved in emergency care ever since he broke his arm at age 10 when he fell from a tree.

As he drives to the hospital on the first day of his new job, he is feeling a sense of pride, mixed with sheer fright, as he realizes that this is the world-class place he had chosen for his first interview. He had always dreamed of working at this hospital. It was the hospital he had always heard about from his family and the one that the press always headed for when a local comment on health care trends or events was needed as background for a news story.

When he heard he had the job, Jack was overjoyed. He would have a chance to become a seasoned nurse at one of the finest hospitals in the country. The agency had waived the typical internship period for Jack, since he had years of experience as an emergency medical technician. He would receive full salary and, he believed, the immediate respect of his peers.

Jack knows that his feelings of confidence and joy cannot last, but he is unaware that he is on the verge of walking into a battleground. As he enters the drive leading to the hospital parking area, there are picketers shouting about unfair working conditions and patient deaths. Signs tell of cruelty to nurses. As Jack starts to walk to the building, with his new name tag that reads "Registered Nurse," he is approached by a person asking him to sign a card. Jack states, "I'm sorry. I'm new around here. Just let me get my feet on the ground. I'll catch you later."

During nursing school Jack was concerned about being a male in the traditional female world of the hospital's nursing service. Now he is afraid that feelings of insecurity and alienation will engulf him again and that, because of union organizing efforts, his heady experiences of learning a new job from a base of comfort will be destroyed. He will be approached many times in the coming days by co-workers who will tell him how he should feel and what he should do. He will be left with having to make an immediate choice between two unacceptable alternatives. Jack fears that, if he fails whatever this test is, he will not be happy in this organization.

Questions to consider while reading this chapter
1. What does signing a card mean and what questions should Jack ask about this?
2. How can Jack establish good relationships with both nurse managers and staff nurses in an atmosphere in which collective bargaining has put these two groups in adversarial positions?
3. What skills and information will Jack need to navigate and make effective decisions in this hospital?
4. What resources are available to Jack to help him learn more about the labor and management issues occurring in the hospital?

Key Terms

Arbitration The process of negotiation sanctioned in the United States by the National Labor Relations Board. It is the method used for formal talks between management and labor within modern business, industry, or service organizations. Binding arbitration means that all parties must obey the arbitrator's recommendations.

Collective bargaining The process of establishing and being represented by a union in order to share a degree of power with management in determining selected aspects of the conditions of employment.

Encroachment A term applied to expanding job responsibilities for nonnursing health care providers that may appear to threaten the integrity of nursing practice. Some of the health professions, which may have encroached on nursing practice in the past, include respiratory therapists and pharmacists. Union activists often use concerns related to encroachment to initiate or sustain union-organizing activity among nurses.

Grievance A term associated with negative workplace occurrences. A grievance generally arises when two parties, such as an employee and a manager, interpret contract provisions differently. Grievances often involve job security or safety, which is a union priority, or job performance or discipline, which is a management priority.

Industrial unionism Occurs when there is a single union for all workers in a corporation. For example, all people who work in computer companies could be grouped together under one vast computer worker umbrella organization. It is possible that the industrial union, with its massive numbers of union members, is the strongest possible collective group.

Labor A group composed of those who work for others to receive a salary.

Management The group of people within a business or company who plan, organize, lead, or control the activities of employees who have agreed to work to receive a salary.

Mediation A form of settling disputes that involves a trained person who listens to all parties and makes recommendations. Such mediation is not legally binding.

Occupational unionism Means that there are separate unions for each occupation within a given company and that these occupational groups might join others of like work across boundaries and across the country. White-collar workers coming from a background of higher education and some measure of job security tend to prefer occupational unionism and organizing with like-minded professionals. In general, nurses prefer occupational unionism.

Unfair labor practices Actions that interfere with the rights of employees or employers as identified under the National Labor Relations Act. An unfair labor practice can be something as simple as a suspicion by an employee that he or she was assigned to an unpopular task unfairly, or it can be as complex as the identification of a pattern of many employees receiving discriminatory treatment in the workplace because of being union supporters. Unfair labor practices are a frequent source of either strikes or the initiation of union activity within a setting.

Union A group of workers who band together to accomplish goals related to conditions of employment.

Learning Outcomes

After studying this chapter, the reader will be able to:

1. Use terms associated with collective bargaining correctly in written and oral communications.
2. Identify questionable labor or management practices in the workplace.
3. Analyze strengths and weaknesses of collective bargaining as a method for achieving power sharing in the workplace.
4. Compare the major types of trade unions.
5. Discuss current conflicts and controversies associated with collective bargaining by professional nurses.

CHAPTER OVERVIEW

Collective bargaining is a very complex and often emotional issue. This chapter attempts to present a balanced view of collective bargaining in the hope that students, staff nurses, and nurses in managerial positions will be able to use the information to make effective decisions when confronted with collective bargaining issues. The chapter presents collective bargaining efforts in modern health care institutions, including recent history, trends, and issues. The process of certifying and decertifying a collective bargaining agent is detailed. Industrial relations studies are used to illustrate recent trends in the American workplace, particularly those with potential impact for nursing. Current characteristics of collective bargaining in nursing and some of the workplace issues that may be brought about by collective efforts are described. Finally, a special point will be made about the American Nurses Association (ANA) as the parent organization for a new form of collective bargaining.

DEVELOPMENT OF COLLECTIVE BARGAINING IN AMERICA
Early Activities

During the late nineteenth century, when the Industrial Revolution was a force throughout North America, a cadre of thinkers arose who believed that, to protect workers from circumstances such as long work hours, child labor, and unhealthy factory conditions, there needed to be collectivization of workers. These early groups sought such basic conditions as safety in work situations, adequate pay for hours worked, and the right not to be arbitrarily dismissed. This banding together of workers to accomplish goals was termed trade unionism. This technique was successful in many instances and remains with us today.

Federal Legislation

As a result of these early efforts at unionization, in 1935 Congress passed the National Labor Relations Act (NLRA). Under the terms of the NLRA, employees were given the right to self-organize, to form labor unions, and to bargain collectively. As part of the 1935 NLRA, the National Labor Relations Board (NLRB) was established to implement provisions of the NLRA. The NLRB continues to play a vital role in labor-management relations and, working through 52 regional and field offices in major U.S. cities, they conduct union elections and prosecute unfair labor practices.

With employees' rights protected by federal legislation, collective bargaining now could occur in companies across the country. Employees could organize themselves into a unit recognized under terms of the NLRA without fear of being fired for belonging to the union or for participating in union activities, such as collective bargaining. Typical goals in collective bargaining activities were to establish reasonable working conditions and formal agreements between employees and management for wages and health and retirement benefits.

However, exemptions to the NLRA were established for nonprofit companies. This meant that employees of nonprofit hospitals such as nurses were not protected under the NLRA and therefore were not legally protected for participation in collective bargaining activities. Hospitals' employees may have been excluded from protection by the NLRA because it was believed that services provided were so essential that organizing activities would be contrary to the public's interest. Eventually in 1974 legislation allowed for the inclusion of nonprofit hospitals in coverage under provisions of the NLRA. Nurses could form collective bargaining units. The 1974 amendments also included the requirement for a 10-day written notice of the intent to picket or to strike. This notice would allow the health care agency time to prepare and would protect the relative health and safety of the public.

Current Status

Conflict currently characterizes the American experience with trade unionism. Even recent reports of events seem to give conflicting answers about where we stand today with this important issue. Statistics indicate that union collective bargaining units are present in fewer than 10% of businesses within the private sector (Kaufman, 2000). This implies an erosion of union influence. It is reported that, since traditional blue-collar union influence is eroding, the trade unions are weaker than ever before. Therefore the unions are attempting to attract professionals such as nurses and physicians to keep their membership growing (Newkirk, 1999).

On the other hand, it is reported that unions are becoming stronger than ever before. For example, health care mega-unions such as the Service Employees International Union (SEIU) are becoming ever larger because of mergers and acquisitions among health care organizations, which result in more potential members. Thus it would seem that these health care unions are becoming more powerful because of increasing numbers of members (Greenhouse, 1998). Another indication of union strength is that certain powerful corporate groups are factoring unions into future plans. For example, national hospital networks such as the Catholic Hospital Association are instituting formal contracts with unions, implying that health care unionization is a potent force and that health care corporations are paying attention (Moore, 1999a). One might wonder whether unions are growing or diminishing as a force in the United States.

Since the future of nursing may be influenced by our collective and individual efforts to be fairly represented and to have a voice in the conditions of our work, it is important to understand the costs and benefits of collective action, as well as the motives of those who would represent nursing. In recent years there has been a battle between traditional large, mixed unions such as the American Federation of Labor-Congress of Industrial Organization (AFL-CIO) and the ANA bargaining arm. However, more recently there has been formalization of the relationship between the ANA and what has been termed "big labor." The collective bargaining arm of the ANA is now called the United American Nurses, or UAN. Will this arrangement change the path of nursing, or will it be of little consequence?

THE COLLECTIVE BARGAINING PROCESS

Since it is important for nurses to understand what a union organizing effort at a particular facility might mean to them, a review of collective bargaining processes and labor and management tactics and consequences will be instructive. Whether one works at a health care facility or is a bystander observing what may seem to be unusual activities during union organizing, it is useful to know what is involved with statements or actions, particularly during times of unrest.

Collective bargaining is a method of equalizing power. As such, it involves negotiation and administrative agreements between employees and employers. Since the individual employee, or even a small group of employees, has limited power to bargain with the employer, the idea of banding together in a union enhances the position of employees in situations calling for negotiation. The goals of collective bargaining are achieved by imposing rules on employers about how to treat employees represented by a union. The union movement in the United States is involved with strengthening the workers' position in the relationship between management and labor.

Nurses and nurse managers need to understand the steps involved in the union organizing and election process, as well as what are considered appropriate or inappropriate management responses. Since union organizing involves power sharing and sometimes a temporary sense of distrust between bedside nurses and management, it can become a nerve-racking and emotional process. Knowing allowable patterns for the process of union organizing can help alleviate unnecessary distress.

The following discussion of steps in the union organizing process is based on information taken from the NLRB *Guide to Basic Law and Procedures* (1997). The reader will see that careful attention is given to ensuring fairness for employer, employees, and the unions that may be involved in an election that is held to determine if employees agree to unionize.

The Preformal Period in Union Organizing

The goal of collective bargaining is the equalization of power between labor and management. To initiate collective bargaining activities, an organizing drive is instituted by union forces who attempt to create an official, NLRB-sanctioned bargaining unit in a particular institution. The bargaining unit is either accepted or rejected through an election process in which nonmanagement employees vote. If accepted, the bargaining unit will be made up of union members who are workers at the unionized facility and will be designed to protect the workers against arbitrary treatment and unfair labor practices.

A union organizing drive may be initiated when nurses in a particular health care agency contact a union because they feel a need for help in negotiating with their employer. The stimulus for this initial contact is usually not frivolous. There is typically a pervasive feeling among the nurses on a particular unit or in the health care organization as a whole that working conditions are unsatisfactory and that there is no possibility of making improvements under conventional existing circumstances.

It is helpful at this point to examine what is to be gained by those petitioning the NLRB for an election. For a group of workers a newly formed union will:

- Have the power to make certain demands of the employer.
- Provide some degree of political power on a local level.

For the union organization, a newly formed union will:

- Gain additional power for the union by adding more bargaining units, especially if the union is part of a larger national union.
- Increase monetary support for the union through contributions from workers' paychecks. The additional money can be used to pay salaries, organize other bargaining units, or contribute to political causes or candidates.

Once a union has been contacted by nurses and told that there is some interest in establishing a collective bargaining unit, union forces try to determine whether efforts to organize the majority of nurses in a health care agency will be successful. This determination is made through a process of "signing cards." These cards help the union organizer, a professional who works for the union, to decide whether there is enough interest in unionization on the part of nurses employed in the health care agency. Such cards are simply index cards that help union organizers keep track of the numbers of workers who are interested in information about the union or in joining or otherwise supporting the union. Box 13-1 presents important information about types of cards and the implications for signing a card.

If 30% of employed nurses sign cards, signaling an interest in representation by the union, the employer and NLRB are officially notified, and the employer must refrain from antilabor action such as firing those favoring the union (NLRB, 1997). If 50% plus one of eligible voters respond in the affirmative for union representation, the collective bargaining agent is considered to be officially selected, and the union has won the election.

To follow the process effectively, the nurse should be aware of details of what is and is not allowed and what is and is not likely to occur during union organizing efforts. When a specific union, such as the Teamsters, the UAN, or the Service Employees International Union, initiates organizing activities in a particular facility, an organizer goes to the facility. The organizer, who may also be called a business agent or field representative, is then responsible for making well–thought out plans and recommendations.

BOX 13-1 | *Union Authorization Cards*

The single-purpose authorization card:
- Requests a signature, date, the name and address of the person signing, and a brief description of the person's job (department, shift, and type of work).
- Does not indicate that the person is requesting union membership or asking for a union election.
- Only requests information to assist union forces with identifying total numbers of employed nurses and whether their status would permit them to take part in union-organizing efforts.
- Allows accurate counting and updating of information about potential union members.

The dual-purpose authorization card:
- Calls for the same background information as the single-purpose authorization card.
- Also contains a statement that, when signed by a nurse, indicates a request for an election and that the person is applying for union membership.

Questions to ask before signing a card:
- Is the card merely asking for information about the nurse's employment status?
- Does signing the card indicate the nurse is applying for actual union membership?

To form a core support group in the facility, the organizer locates respected leaders in the workplace. Meetings are then planned and held at nonwork settings such as homes or restaurants to gain initial information on grievances and workplace inequities. These will later be used as a basis for campaign literature.

To gain additional supporters, discussion and card-signing will take place in areas in the actual facility: locker rooms, bathrooms, lunch areas, lounges, and less visible work areas. As the drive surfaces and to gain management's attention, organizers begin to distribute cards more openly. At this point the union organizer sends a registered letter to the employer with the names of employees on the organizing committee. Management will probably have already become aware of organizing activities through clues such as employee behavior changes during this period. There will be times when individuals seem distracted or when there is an increase in the number or vociferous quality of complaints about workplace conditions. Conversely, there may be a feeling of distancing between labor and management and an air of unnatural silence among employees.

Although peaceful strikes and picketing may occur for the purpose of publicity or seeking recognition, the NLRB prohibits certain behaviors during the preelection period. The union may not:

- Inflame racial prejudices.
- Lie about loss of jobs if the union loses the election.
- Forge documents or signatures.
- Meet or distribute literature in work areas during work times.
- Hold meetings within 24 hours of an election.

During the preelection period, management may not:

- Solicit spying.
- Photograph employees engaged in union activities.
- Visit employees in their homes.
- Lie about what will happen if the union is the victor in an election.
- Question employees about their preferences regarding union activity.

The Election Process

There are several steps in the election process. Either the union or the employer must petition the NLRB for an election. Once this petition is made, the request is passed along to the regional NLRB director. Within 48 hours the union must submit proof of its claim that 30% of eligible nurses are interested in forming a collective bargaining unit. Eligible nurses are generally considered to be those nurses who are engaged in patient care. Normally, for a 10-day period literature will be mailed to eligible employees. The union and the employer may circulate literature. However, both sides must cease activities within 24 hours of the election.

On the day actually designated for the election, the three parties (NLRB, union representatives, and employer representatives) meet to review the list of those eligible to vote. The three parties then count ballots and, in case of a true tie, a victory for the employer is declared. However, any votes in dispute will be set aside for a later recount. Objections must be made within 5 working days after the election and may be made on the grounds of problems with the conduct of the election or unfair labor practices.

Postelection

After the election, in the case of a union victory, federal law guarantees workers the right to collectively bargain and strike. Nurses may subsequently drop or change a bargaining agent by having 30% of nurses sign cards. An election would follow, requiring a vote of 50% plus one in favor of the change (NLRB, 1997).

The NLRA mandates that, under the rules of collective bargaining, meetings between management and labor will be held at reasonable times for the purpose of conferring in good faith. Mandatory topics include wages; the establishment of rules about the use of labor (such as hours of work and worker safety); individual workers' rights; resolution of grievances; and methods of enforcement, interpretation, and administration of the union agreement. Negotiations between union and management occur in cycles following the initial year of collective bargaining. Negotiations are held before a contract being ratified (approved) by both union and management and again just before the contract expires.

Certain patterns will follow the initial ratification of a union contract within a facility. Following a 1991 Supreme Court decision, the NLRB established the "Eight Unit Rule," which identified the eight bargaining units in hospitals. These units are listed in Box 13-2.

If more than eight bargaining units were allowed in a health care facility, a different contract might expire each month. This would lead to a situation in which there would be year-round strike possibilities and a patchwork of rules, regulations, payment systems, and employee benefit plans in place during contract negotiations. This could eventually incapacitate the leadership of the organization. Both union and corporate leaders are committed to maintaining strength in leadership, including smooth negotiating processes.

Although there is a long tradition of union activism in the United States, nursing is a relatively new player in this arena. Following is a review of studies that relate to the workplace and may hold lessons for the nursing profession as it comes to grips with such a dramatic change in the ways in which business is conducted.

CORPORATE AMERICA AND INDUSTRIAL RELATIONS STUDIES

To make decisions about whether collective bargaining is right for nursing, lessons may be learned from the field of study known as industrial relations. Myths and negative images of unions abound as frequently as tales of corporate misconduct. Neither side tends to purposely try to create negative conditions for work, but both seek power in the workplace and control over working conditions. Since nurses tend to prefer well-thought out decisions, current studies about the realities of union representation and collective bargaining will provide information for the nursing profession to use when considering future unionizing efforts.

BOX 13-2	*The Eight Sanctioned Hospital Bargaining Units*

Registered nurses
Physicians
All other professionals
Technical employees
Skilled maintenance employees
Business office/clerical employees
All other nonprofessional employees
Guards

From the National Labor Relations Board: *A guide to basic law and procedures under the National Labor Relations Act,* Washington, DC, 1997, U.S. Government Printing Office.

Economic Consequences of Collective Bargaining

Many Americans fear that the presence of unions may precipitate bankruptcy for individual companies. Americans have a lingering sense that traditional blue-collar unions "go too far" (Freeman, 1999; Kaufman, 2000). The phrase "deadweight loss" has been used to describe the dire events involving the ability of unions to raise wages above what is considered safe for a company's continued functioning (Fisher and Waschik, 2000). Samuel Gompers, the great union activist, noted that, "The worst crime against working people is a company which fails to operate at a profit" (White, 1986, p. 52). It is obviously to the advantage of all stakeholders to have workers fairly paid for their labors, work under decent conditions, and have a measure of security stemming from their attachment to the workplace. But it is undesirable to have forces that are responsible for securing these benefits at the expense of a company's viability. Unions realize this. This self-control is particularly important in the case of nursing with its large labor costs, particularly since we live in a time of government controls over what may be charged for health care services.

Is there truly evidence that the presence of collective bargaining units is associated with dire economic consequences? Freeman (1999) finds little support for this assumption. Using a careful analysis of the large data sets of existing labor and corporate statistics, Freeman presents evidence that unions tend to behave in a fiscally responsible fashion, increasing wages and benefits for workers but not to an extent likely to do more than diminish higher levels of corporate profits. Union wages tend to come out of what would otherwise be excess profits. However, sometimes unions inadvertently misjudge and may indeed contribute to corporate insolvency. A union may make a mistake in judging how profitable a company truly is.

High-Performance Work Organizations and Collective Bargaining

Another consideration for American workers is the great success of other countries' styles of conducting business. Following upheaval in Europe and Asia after World War II, there was a period of recovery leading to new work patterns known as high-performance work organizations (HPWOs). They were so successful that, in the latter part of the twentieth century, the productivity of foreign workplaces was held up as a new paradigm for corporate America. HPWOs were touted as feel-good, gain-sharing innovations that could decentralize decision making, improve the quality and quantity of work, and take full advantage of worker creativity at the point of contact: the assembly line or customer-contact point in the case of a service-based business (Osterman, 2000).

However, problems arose as a result of shifting economic forces. As America came to grips with such things as dramatically rising costs of health insurance and other benefits for workers, management began hiring workers who would not be entitled to full-time employee status or expensive benefits. Other shifts in work patterns included an increase in the number of mobile workers who might change employers or career paths many times throughout a lifetime of work.

Motivation in the workplace has also recently become a problem. In the past, when job security seemed certain, workers would offer creative suggestions to enhance productivity and quality. But as companies began to close, restructure, or merge, employees were reluctant to offer suggestions that might mean a reduction in the workforce. The reasoning was that, if the suggestion resulted in increased productivity on the part of workers, an employer might decrease the workforce. Studies have shown that this can, indeed, happen. This would naturally make workers reluctant to make suggestions for work redesign.

However, the presence of a collective bargaining agreement would seem to be a hedge against such workforce reduction moves. Studies have shown that the worker who is part of a collective bargaining agreement has less to fear. When HPWO initiatives are undertaken in the presence of existing labor unions within a company, there is no reduction in the workforce. Worker numbers remain the same. Without union presence there can be problems (Osterman, 2000).

Power Sharing in the Boardroom

Rubinstein (2000) speaks of the Saturn experiment as a model of what can occur when trade unionism and corporate goals merge on both the shop floor and in the corporate boardroom. A successful model of power sharing in the boardroom, pioneered in Japanese factories after World War II, was implemented at the Saturn automobile plant founded in Tennessee late in the twentieth century. The Saturn model involved inviting worker representatives into the corporate boardroom. The model was built on a foundation of trust, an open atmosphere of sharing financial information, and open communication channels that fostered rapid responses to threats to productivity or quality.

In the Saturn model high quality is borne out by customer surveys, which indicate that the company was a winner in quality, reliability, and satisfaction for most of the 1990s. Self-managed work teams and the cross communication unique to union-organized enterprises are credited with some of Saturn's success. High-level leaders met twice a month with workers to share key elements of data. Quality depended not only on spotting and fixing flaws, but also on off-line meetings designed to identify causes of flaws.

Hunter (1998) believes that union representatives can be on corporate boards if the numbers are sufficient, personal characteristics of the union-selected board members are right, and communication and power sharing is open and honest. But Bruder (1999) notes that the idea of power sharing is not always going to be successful. Corporate executives see unions as a perceived threat to their control. Bruder feels that this perceived threat is at the heart of the matter and will result in an attempt to bypass such power sharing between labor and management.

But despite these problems with implementing and sustaining a power-sharing team within a unionized company, there is evidence that unions may be right for nursing. Unions are healthy in the public sector. Professors who study labor are prounion and believe that unions will make a comeback (Seligman, 1999). There is talk of the evolution of small bargaining units and increased cooperation between labor and management. Smaller units and the move to nontraditional forms of representation are believed to result in fewer situations in which labor and management reach a state of impasse (Hebdon, Hyatt, and Mazerolle, 1999). This would fit with the nursing's tradition of peaceful problem solving.

UNIONS AND PROFESSIONAL NURSING
Professionalism vs. Unionization

Nurses in the workplace are being buffeted by cost cutting, nursing shortages, shuffled duties, substitution of unlicensed personnel in place of nurses, and hospital reorganizations that bring job insecurity and uncertainty. Despite these difficult working conditions, it is often problematic for the nurse to come to grips with her own feelings related to the emotionally charged issues associated with unionization. Many nurses may be reluctant to become

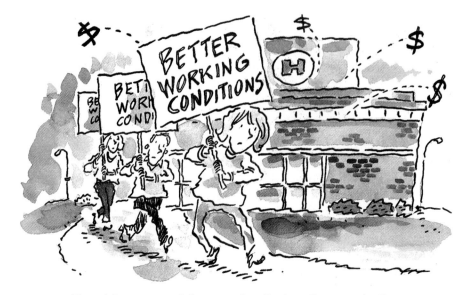

The strike: a powerful economic effect on the organization
but a complex issue for nursing.

involved with what they view as trouble-making groups who exaggerate the issues just to win the contest against the adversary, management. It is difficult to reconcile feelings of professionalism and service with the perceived union connotations of strife and discord.

In addition, when nurses try to update their thoughts about unionization through reading, it becomes difficult to find objective reading material. Few experienced authorities on collective bargaining can remain neutral or objective. It is difficult to read about unionization without encountering biased language and the attempt to paint one side or the other in extremely unflattering terms. This doesn't help in clearing away the fog of conflict surrounding unionization decisions for nurses.

Another problem with unionization being a comfortable fit for the nursing profession is that nurses have traditionally been somewhat independent thinkers. Nurses as a group are perhaps reluctant to commit to long-term joint and binding decisions. In addition, mustering the energy for the prolonged periods involved in exercising the power of the strike is difficult. And the strike, after all, is the ultimate weapon in collective bargaining.

Trends Toward Collective Bargaining

Bruder (1999) discusses the need for nurses to follow the American Medical Association (AMA) into union activities at a time when the American public supports the nursing profession and may have sympathy for nursing's efforts. In this era of mergers and fiscal belt tightening on the part of hospitals and others who employ nurses, there may be a need to assert the right to maintain quality of care in stronger ways than have been traditional for nurses. Quality of care and retaining nurses at the bedside are important. In Bruder's view (1999), a unionized workforce will result in improved quality of care, increased productivity, employee loyalty, adequate benefits, and job stability.

In response to physician concerns about the managed care environment, the AMA is becoming involved in collective bargaining (Anonymous, 2000). In February 2000 the AMA received approval from the NLRB to form its first local bargaining unit, or union. For the first time in history, physicians believed it to be necessary to collectively respond to the managed care movement to control conditions of medical practice.

Physician incomes are in the top 2% in the nation and the top 1% in the world (Newkirk, 1999). Although wages and benefits are typically at the forefront of union negotiations, in the case of doctors this is obviously not why they felt the need to form bargaining units. Patient advocacy, coupled with a sense of loss of control in the workplace, may be a very real reason for this drastic measure.

Just days before the AMA agreed to form a union, the ANA approved a structural change that would lead to creation of a bargaining unit known as the UAN (Moore, 1999b). Given the history, philosophy of caring, and traditions of fiscal sacrifice of nursing, this may seem difficult to understand; and, of course, the move was not without opposition.

Questions To Answer

Three major questions need to be answered before nursing is totally ready to accept unionization and collective bargaining:

1. Should nurses, who frequently are called on to supervise the work of others, be classified for collective bargaining purposes as management or labor? The answer to this question will determine the ultimate success of collective bargaining efforts for nurses.
2. Will nurses be too reluctant to strike, which is one of the most powerful tools that a union has at its disposal? There is concern that strikes by nurses could destroy the public's image of nursing.
3. Are there relevant gains to be made for the nursing profession through collective bargaining or is this a myth?

Management or Staff.   One of the difficult issues for nursing in relation to collective bargaining is that in the eyes of the NLRB certain nurses are singled out as management or supervisory personnel and are not allowed NLRA protection, which applies only to nonmanagement employees. Head nurses and shift supervisors have traditionally been considered part of management rather than labor. But what about nurses who routinely supervise others who act merely as extenders of care, such as in nursing homes? Are these nurses acting exclusively on behalf of the company that employs them or are they routinely carrying out their responsibilities as a professional nurse?

The definition of manager or supervisor is problematic even in nonhealth care settings. In nursing things become even more complicated. Most experienced RNs are involved in some type of supervisory or management work. For example, most staff nurses who ordinarily provide bedside care have been called on to be in charge of a particular nursing unit for a particular working shift. Does this mean that the nurse should no longer be considered nonmanagement?

Another trend that has an impact on decisions about supervisory status is the increasing use of unlicensed personnel in health care workplaces. More nurses could now be classified as supervisory because they direct the activities of these unlicensed workers. In 1994 in NLRB v.

the Health Care and Retirement Corporation, the Supreme Court ruled that nurses do indeed direct the work of others and therefore are not eligible for protection under the NLRB. This case was important to the nursing profession because, had the ruling been upheld, it would have dramatically lowered the numbers of nurses who could act as "laborers" and engage in collective bargaining. However, in 1997 the decision of the U.S. Court of Appeals for the Ninth Circuit helped clarify this point. The Court ruled that RNs who performed charge nurse duties were not management and therefore were eligible for collective bargaining protection. In another case, Providence Alaska Medical Center v. NLRB, the ruling recognized that the judgment used by RNs in assigning patients and coordinating patient care was part of their professional role rather than part of any statutory supervision as defined by the NLRB (Nguyen, 1997).

There is evidence that the ANA must continue to walk a fine line in relation to separating or insulating workplace leaders who are ANA members from any participation in the arm of the organization that takes part in collective bargaining efforts. And beyond this issue from a bargaining standpoint is the uncomfortable prospect of pitting nurse managers against their colleagues in the workplace. A definite schism occurs when supervisors and staff are placed on opposite sides of the table. Bad feelings arise. For example, a supervisor nurse represents management but is not insulated in an executive office. In addition, the supervisor nurse or nurse manager must often assume duties routinely performed by staff nurses in the event of a strike. This can lead to lingering negative feelings even after the strike is resolved.

Techniques frequently used by nurse managers to maintain smooth and efficient job performance in their work settings may be relatively ineffective when unionization or collective bargaining initiatives are occurring. For example, the nurse supervisor who believes that open communication in both upward and downward directions is useful for problem solving may become frustrated during unionization initiatives. Union tactics may involve coaching nurses at staff levels to use the "silent treatment" and not cooperate with nurse managers' attempts to communicate.

It will be interesting to see how the problems that arise from the supervisor-vs.-staff issue are ultimately resolved. It is clear that there will be turmoil in the workplace should the us-against-them model become necessary throughout the country's health care agencies.

The Strike. Strikes can have very powerful effects. The economic effect of a strike can best be understood by noting that hospitals become concerned over lost revenues when the average daily census drops only a few percentage points.

Nursing is a trusted profession, and to many nurses to strike is a symbol of negative behavior. To safeguard nursing's image and allow for hospitals to react effectively in safeguarding patient care, a 10-day notice of intent to strike is required. On receipt of such notice, the NLRB attempts to mediate, and the hospital is encouraged to decrease census and halt elective admissions. Schedules are developed for covering the Emergency Department, operating room, and intensive care areas.

It is probable that nurses will lose their reluctance to strike should the practice become widespread, particularly if there are no direct and adverse consequences involving patient care. If nurses are concerned about the effect on their public image, they should remember that airline pilots and screen actors have engaged in such actions from time to time with no lasting deleterious effect involving their overall public image. This does not mean that nurses will warmly accept such tactics, but it does mean there are possibilities.

BOX 13-3	*Helpful Websites*

For data on costs of patient care, quality of care, payment for care, patient demographics, and diagnoses, contact the website for The U.S. Agency for Health Care Research and Quality.
www.ahcpr.gov

To communicate with the California Nurses Association, a group that recently separated from traditional ANA linkage, visit:
www.igc.org/cna

To express views on unions and whether they serve the nursing profession, visit:
www.nurseweek.com

For a site listing salaries, visit:
www.forbes.com/forbes/98/0518/6110234a.htm

For codes and federal regulations, contact the Office of Labor-Management Standards, U.S. Department of Labor, Washington, D.C. 20210, or visit:
www.dol.gov/dol/esa/public/olms_org.htm

Wage Questions. In general, union efforts have resulted in only modest wage improvements in the health care sector. Over the last two decades, health care wage gains have been less than wage gains in other fields (Hirsch and Schumaker, 1998). Workforce data indicate that this lower-than-average wage gain includes effects resulting from union efforts. Nurses will need to examine this fact before pinning hopes on unionization as a moving force in overall wage gains.

The role of unions in the future of health care may hinge on cooperation versus conflict, on relative productivity gains in union versus nonunion facilities, and on success of human relations practices in both union and nonunion workplaces. Nurses live in a new era in health care. Change is happening rapidly. Box 13-3 offers some interesting websites where nurses can get more information about collective bargaining.

THE AMERICAN NURSES ASSOCIATION

In 1997 the ANA Board of Directors approved a multimillion dollar allocation to strengthen labor relations and organizing activities at the national and state levels (ANA, 1997). In 1998 additional funding led to the creation of a new ANA department in support of organizing efforts and a national labor agenda. As a result of this national labor agenda, the ANA and state nurses' associations agreed to the development of the UAN, a new national labor entity and to affiliation with the powerful labor organization, the AFL-CIO (ANA, 1998). Affiliation with the AFL-CIO was an unprecedented step for American nurses. Never before had the ANA, an organization that represents all categories of RNs, considered an affiliation that had such widespread political and economic ramifications. The national labor agenda formulated by this group involved increasing funding for state nursing associations to (ANA, 1999):

■ Organize collective bargaining units
■ Increase staff and training in relation to union organizing efforts

- Build a solid public relations base
- Upgrade legal support services

The large mixed unions with national influence have continued their campaigns to organize nurses. Just to keep union ranks steady, at least 300,000 new members must be added each year (Greene, 1998). There are 2.2 million RNs in the United States, and only 17% are unionized. Some of the larger unions have a long history of expertise in collective bargaining and possess legal knowledge that is useful in organizing situations. They have not been hesitant about recruiting nurses to bolster their dwindling ranks. Larger mixed unions promise more aggressive tactics than the ANA might be likely to use. A few unions that have been interested in organizing nurses are the Teamsters and the SEIU. The SEIU boasts that it represents more nurses than any other mixed union: 100,000 RNs and LPNs. By comparison, state affiliates of the ANA have 200,000 members in collective bargaining units (Greene, 1998).

Those who would represent nurses in collective bargaining efforts have formidable corporate opponents. Nurses engaged in collective bargaining in the future will often be dealing with multihospital systems: groups that are able to sustain operations for almost any length of time in any specific location despite slowdowns or work stoppages. Even if an RN collective bargaining group is part of a national nursing organization or large mixed union, nurses cannot necessarily sustain the vigor needed to pursue collective action over perhaps years in any one particular hospital.

The ANA and its bargaining affiliate, the UAN, will also face the problem of trying to serve all nurses in collective bargaining situations, regardless of the size of the health care agency or the likelihood of a win. Union organizers representing larger mixed unions seek out conditions likely to foster success. They pick and choose their sites carefully. UAN may not always have this luxury.

However, UAN will be interested in serving the needs of nurses and only nurses, in both a traditional wage-benefit way and in a way likely to foster gains in a professional sense. The ANA represents the interests of the profession and has done so for a very long time. This professional group has experience and knows the profession inside and out. As the parent organization for the UAN, the ANA has a history of allegiance to nurses and an awareness of public good.

A Final Word About the Future

There is an old saying that, if something can be imagined, it will someday come true. The reader is invited to picture Hunter's world (1998) in which American nurses will have seats on corporate boards in sufficient numbers to be able to maintain energies and influence directions. Picture nurse board members backed up by shareholding interests and voting blocks of stocks. Picture specialized training for nurses in how to build alliances and how to share information with constituents outside the boardroom. In such a world, nurses would have enough information about future developments to know what to ask for and how to operate in employment situations. Nurses would be able to blend the good of the company with public good.

Meanwhile, professional nurses should continue in their attempts to control practice at the level of the work setting. The question will revolve around how this is to be accomplished.

Critical Thinking Questions

1. Think of the opening vignette about Jack Perkins, the newly employed staff nurse. Assume that Jack wants to remain uncommitted during his initial 6 months of employment with the agency. In light of knowledge gained through reading this chapter, what should be Jack's responses as prounion and antiunion forces try to solicit his loyalties in the coming days?

2. Some authors believe that voluntary power sharing between corporate board members and labor is impossible. However, the Saturn Model of power sharing has proven successful in the automotive industry. Can nursing representation on the corporate board ever be achieved? If so, how? What types of leverage does nursing have, short of the ultimate power of the strike?

3. You are a nurse manager in a hospital in which organizing activity for the purposes of establishing a collective bargaining unit for nurses is occurring. You notice that the nursing personnel on your unit are behaving oddly: not speaking at unit meetings, suddenly walking away as you approach them in the mornings, and generally using a vocabulary that is odd for nurses. What should you do? Should you do anything? What actions would be considered wrong, or coercive, in view of the NLRB regulations?

REFERENCES

American Nurses Association: Are you protected under the NLRA? *Nurs Trends Issues* 2 (7):1-9, 1997.

American Nurses Association: Physicians and unions: implications for registered nurses, *Nurs Trends Issues* 3(9):1-13, 1998.

American Nurses Association: *Status report to the ANA House of Delegates,* 1999 [unpublished report].

Anonymous: Detroit doctors are first to enlist help of AMA union, *Best's Rev* 101(4):18, 2000.

Bruder P: Nursing unions: the prime time for organizing is now, *Hosp Topics* 77(2):36-39, 1999.

Fisher TGC, Waschik RG: Union bargaining power, relative wages, and efficiency in Canada, *Can J Econ* 33(3):742-765, 2000.

Freeman RB: Do unions make enterprises insolvent? *Industrial Labor Relations Rev* 52(4):510-528, 1999.

Greene J: Nurses' aid, *Hosp Health Networks* 72(12):38-40, 1998.

Greenhouse S: Health care union votes to merge, creating giant, *New York Times* 147(51090):37, March 8, 1998.

Hebdon R, Hyatt D, Mazerolle M: Implications of small bargaining units and enterprise unions on bargaining disputes: a look into the future? *Relations Industrielles-Industrial Relations* 54(3):503-524, 1999.

Hirsch BT, Schumaker EJ: Union wages, rents, and skills in health care labor markets, *J Labor Res* 19(1):125-148, 1998.

Hunter L: Can strategic participation be institutionalized? *Industrial Labor Relations Rev* 51(4):557-579, 1998.

Kaufman BE: Beyond unions and collective bargaining, *Industrial Labor Relations Rev* 54(1):182-184, 2000.

Moore JD: Catholic and labor leaders develop pact, *Mod Healthcare* 29(39):10, 1999a.

Moore JD: ANA to form collective bargaining unit, *Mod Healthcare* 29(26):3-12, 1999b.

National Labor Relations Board: *A guide to basic law and procedures under the National Labor Relations Act,* Washington, DC, 1997, US Government Printing Office.

Newkirk G: Physician union: a naked promise, *Mod Med* 67(9):8-11, 1999.

Nguyen BC: Long-awaited Providence ruling upholds right of charge nurses to bargain, *Am Nurse* 1, 14, September/October, 1997.

Osterman P: Work reorganization in an era of restructuring: trends in diffusion and effects on employee welfare, *Industrial Labor Relations Rev* 53(2):179-197, 2000.

Rubinstein SA: The impact of co-management on quality performance: the case of the Saturn Corporation, *Industrial Labor Relations Rev* 53(2):197-219, 2000.

Seligman D: Driving the AFL-CIO crazy, *Forbes* 164(11):102-108, 1999.

White RB: *The great business quotations,* Secacus, NJ, 1986, Lyle Stuart Publisher.

14

Computers, Informatics, Clinical Information, and the Professional Nurse

Leslie H. Nicoll, PhD, MBA, RN

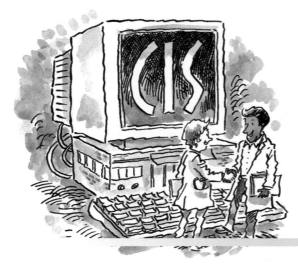

Clinical Information Systems offer nurses and other team members information when, where, and how they need it.

Vignette

The certified informatics nurse welcomed everyone to the committee meeting. She was chairing the group that would have responsibility for selecting, implementing, and evaluating the nursing service module of the new Clinical Information System (CIS) for the institution. "We have a big job ahead of us," she told the group, "but I know we are up to it."

Two years later the system was online. The group looked back on 24 months of hard work: developing specifications for the system, putting out a request for proposals to meet the specifications, reviewing bids and selecting a vendor, installing the equipment, training the staff, and finally going live. They felt enormously rewarded for all their hard work. They all knew that the new system would decrease nursing costs, help save nurses' time, and ultimately benefit their patients. It was a proud moment.

Questions to consider while reading this chapter

1. What strategies could the certified informatics nurse use to help the nursing staff adjust to the new CIS system?
2. How will the new CIS decrease nursing costs? Save nursing time? Benefit patients?

Key Terms

Clinical Information System The software and associated hardware that supports the entry, retrieval, update, and analysis of patient care information and associated clinical information related to patient care.

Computer-based patient record All information about an individual's lifetime health status maintained electronically.

Computer literacy The knowledge and understanding of computers combined with the ability to use them effectively.

Data capture The collection and entry of data into a computer system.

Hardware The physical computer and its components, such as the central processing unit (CPU), the monitor, and the screen.

Internet (1) With a lower case "i," any collection of distinct networks working together as one. (2) With an upper case "I," the worldwide "network of networks" that are connected to each other, using specific protocols.

Software Programs that run the computer; programs that perform different tasks, such as statistics or word processing, are known as applications.

Three waves of computing The three eras in the development of modern computing: Phase I, the mainframe era; Phase II, the personal computer (PC) era; and Phase III, ubiquitous computing.

URL Universal resource locator; the system of addresses used on the Internet.

Virtual reality An artificial environment created with computer hardware and software and presented to the user in such a way that it appears and feels like a real environment.

Worldwide web (www) The graphic part of the Internet. The www is based on hypertext and allows the creation and transfer of multimedia objects.

Learning Outcomes

After studying this chapter, the reader will be able to:

1. List the components that are integral to a nursing specialty and discuss how nursing informatics meets these requirements.
2. Describe educational pathways that exist for nurses interested in pursuing nursing informatics as a specialty.
3. Summarize the major points in the evolution of computer technology.
4. Predict future trends in computing as they relate to health care and nursing practice.
5. Use established criteria to evaluate the content of health-related sites found on the Internet.

NURSING INFORMATICS

The prevalence of computers in society has made it imperative for nurses to integrate the use of computers into professional practice. Because it is no longer an option, nurses must make good use of computer technology to work toward the goal of improved patient care and positive patient outcomes. Students, clinical nurses, educators, researchers, and administrators are all benefiting from computer technology. Students are using word processing programs to prepare course assignments and accessing course assignments via the Internet; they also learn nursing skills using computer-assisted instruction (CAI) programs. Educators use computers to post course assignments for access via the Internet and to prepare audiovisual materials for class presentations, papers for publication, and posters for display at professional conferences. Administrators plan their budgets with spreadsheet programs to manage costs for sound financial management. Researchers are collecting data via the Internet and then analyzing the data with statistics programs. Nurses in clinical settings retrieve patient data, document their interventions, and view laboratory and other results through electronic patient records. These are just a few examples of how computers and their associated technology are influencing nursing practice.

Although all nurses are involved with computers to some degree, there are nurses who have chosen to specialize in the area of nursing practice that relates to computers. This field is known as nursing informatics. This is a new specialty within the profession of nursing. It is only within the past 10 years that it has been named, recognized as a specialty, and defined by the nursing profession. Academic programs to prepare nurses with expertise in informatics have been established; the American Nurses Credentialing Center (ANCC) has developed a certification examination to allow nurses who demonstrate beginning levels of competency to be certified as an informatics nurse (IN) (Gassert, 2000; Newbold, 1996). There is tremendous potential for nurses within this specialty to have a major impact on the way care is planned and delivered in the current tumultuous health care environment.

What Is Nursing Informatics?

Informatics was coined from the French word *informatique*. It was first defined by Gorn (1983) as computer science plus information science. Informatics is more than just computers—it includes all aspects of technology and science, from the theoretic to the applied. Learning how to use new tools and building on capabilities provided by computers and related information technologies also are important parts of the field of informatics (Ball, Hannah, and Douglas, 2000).

Nursing informatics refers to that component of informatics designed for and relevant to nurses. Several definitions of nursing informatics have been developed since 1984, but the one that generally is accepted has been set forth by the American Nurses Association (ANA), which states:

> Nursing informatics is the specialty that integrates nursing science, computer science, and information science in identifying, collecting, processing, and managing data and information to support nursing practice, administration, education, research, and the expansion of nursing knowledge (ANA, 1994).

Embedded in this definition are the many components of nursing informatics: information processing, language development, applications of the system's life cycle, and human–computer interface issues. In addition, the definition provides guidance for content that is relevant to curricula for nurses studying to become informatics specialists (Gassert, 2000).

The Specialty of Nursing Informatics

There are many specialties in nursing that cover a range of interests and clinical domains, such as perioperative nursing, community health nursing, and administration. What makes a practice area a specialty? According to Styles (1989) the following attributes are necessary.
- Differentiated practice
- A research program
- Representation of the specialty by at least one organized body
- A mechanism for credentialing nurses in the specialty
- Educational programs for preparing nurses to practice in the specialty

In 1992 the ANA acknowledged that nursing informatics possessed these attributes and designated nursing informatics as an area of specialty practice.

Differentiated Practice. For more than two decades nurses have been working in hospitals and other settings to help with the selection, development, installation, and evaluation of information systems. This early role function of the IN continues to be important, but with the constant changes in health care, the scope of practice has expanded, and job opportunities are increasing rapidly. Hersher (2000) describes several current and future roles for nurses in informatics, both traditional and nontraditional. Some of these include:

- User liaison: A nurse in this role is involved in the installation of a CIS and interfaces with the system vendors, the users, and management of the health care institution. Generally the nurse working in this role is employed by the health care institution.
- Clinical systems installation: In this role the nurse works for the vendor who has developed and sold the CIS to a health care institution. The nurse-installer helps train the users of the system and troubleshoots problems during the conversion to the new system. The nurse-installer often serves as the liaison between the health care institution and the vendor and in most cases works closely with the system coordinator for the health care institution, who may very well be a nurse.
- Product manager: A nurse in this role is responsible for constantly updating a current product and keeping abreast of new developments in the field. Product managers interface with marketing staff, clients, technical staff, and management. Applications that nurse product managers have developed include decision-support systems, nurse staffing systems, scheduling systems, acuity systems, and bedside and handheld terminals. Although product managers typically have been employed by vendors, many health care institutions are starting to develop this role.
- Systems analyst/programmer: In this role the nurse works in the information systems department, helping analyze and maintain the system or programming. To be effective in this role, the nurse needs a strong working knowledge of the CIS. In many cases the nurse will work on all aspects of the CIS, not just the nursing applications.

These are just a few examples of the types of roles nurses in informatics are filling. Other examples that Hersher (2000) describes include chief information officer, consultant, network administrator, data repository specialist, and clinical information liaison. Settings also vary, as nurses move from the hospital-based acute care sites to community-based sites that include insurance companies, utilization review organizations, integrated health networks, and health care associations. Clearly nurses working in informatics have met the criterion of differentiated practice.

Research Program. In 1986 Schwirian proposed a framework for research in nursing informatics. At that time research in the field was practically nonexistent. Since then, however, there has been rapid development; researchers have reported their studies at national and international conferences and published in a variety of peer-reviewed journals. In nursing the peer-reviewed journal *Computers in Nursing* serves as the premier source of published research in nursing informatics, as it has since its inception in 1984.

The National Institute of Nursing Research (NINR) has provided direction for much of the research that is ongoing in nursing; informatics is no exception. In 1988 a panel of experts was convened to establish broad priorities for the NINR; this ultimately led to the development of the National Nursing Research Agenda (NNRA). Seven specific broad priorities were identified within the NNRA, with number six being "Information Systems." Subsequent Priority Expert Panels were called together to further develop each priority area and make recommendations for future research. The Priority Expert Panel on Nursing Informatics published the results of its deliberations in *Nursing Informatics: Enhancing Patient Care* in 1993 (NINR, 1993). The six goals identified by the panel included:

1. Establish nursing languages, including lexicons, classification systems and taxonomies, and standards for nursing data.
2. Develop methods to build databases of clinical information (including clinical data, diagnoses, objectives, interventions, and outcomes) and management information (including staffing, charge capture, turnover, and vacancy rates) and analyze relationships among them.
3. Determine how nurses use data, information, and knowledge to give patient care and how care is affected by differing levels of expertise and by organizational factors and working conditions. Determine how to design information systems accordingly.
4. Develop and test patient care decision support systems and knowledge delivery systems that are appropriate for nurses' needs, with consideration for expertise, organizational factors, and working conditions.
5. Develop prototypes and eventually working models of nurse workstations equipped with tools to provide nurses with all the information needed for patient care, research, and education at the point of use and linked to an integrated information system.
6. Develop and implement appropriate methods to evaluate nursing information systems and applications, particularly as to their effects on patient care (NINR, 1993).

Research is ongoing in each of these priority areas. In particular, great strides have been made in the area of developing and testing standardized languages. Both the ANA and the National League for Nursing (NLN) have provided leadership and support for these efforts. In addition, the ANA has established criteria for recognizing nursing classifications and standardized nursing languages. These criteria are promulgated through the ANA Committee for Nursing Practice Information Infrastructure, which recognizes languages that have met the criteria. Currently there are 12 standardized languages that have been recognized by the ANA, including:

- North American Nursing Diagnosis Association (NANDA) Taxonomy
- Omaha System
- Home Health Care Classification
- Nursing Interventions Classification (NIC)
- Nursing Outcomes Classification (NOC)
- Patient Care Data Set (PCDS)
- Perioperative Nursing Data Set (PNDS)
- Nursing Management Minimum Data Set (NMMDS)
- SNOMED RT
- Nursing Minimum Data Set (NMDS)
- International Classification for Nursing Practice (ICNP)
- Alternative Link

These 12 languages were uniquely developed to document nursing care. They were designed to record and track the clinical care process for an entire episode of care for patients in the acute, home, and/or ambulatory care settings (ANA, 2000). Research is underway to continue to test and refine the languages so that they fulfill their stated goal of capturing nursing practice to promote positive patient outcomes.

Representation of the Specialty by an Organized Body. There are many organizations devoted to nursing informatics at the local, regional, national, international, and even virtual level. These range from small, grassroots efforts in local communities to large, formal organizations with thousands of members. No matter what the size or geographic location, these groups provide education, networking, and support for nurses interested in informatics. Annual conferences provide the opportunity for members to share their research and innovations and to meet with informatics colleagues from around the world (Newbold, 1997; Newbold, 2000).

The American Nurses Informatics Association (ANIA) was established in 1992 to serve the needs of informatics nurses in southern California. It has since grown and expanded and become a national organization with members throughout the United States. You can learn more about the ANIA at www.ania.org.

Several nursing organizations, such as the Council on Nursing Services and Informatics of the ANA and the Council on Nursing Informatics of the NLN, have established informatic work groups. In addition, nonnursing associations such as the American Medical Informatics Association (AMIA) have nursing informatics work groups. In many of these organizations, INs have taken a leadership role. For example, Dr. Patricia Flatley Brennan has served on the Board of Directors of the AMIA and is currently serving as President. Nurses are also well represented on all of the committees of the AMIA.

Credentialing Nurses in the Specialty. When nursing informatics was recognized as a specialty by the ANA in 1992, work began to establish a process by which nurses could be credentialed in informatics. The ANCC, which offers certification examinations for a variety of specialties in nursing, describes certification as a formal, systematic mechanism whereby nurses can voluntarily seek a credential that recognizes their quality and excellence in professional practice and continuing education (ANCC, 1993). For many nurses becoming certified is a professional milestone and validation of their qualifications, knowledge, and skills in a defined area of nursing practice.

To be eligible for the nursing informatics examination, which was first offered in 1995, a nurse must meet the following requirements:

- Possess an active registered nursing license in the United States or its territories
- Have earned a baccalaureate or higher nursing degree
- Practiced actively as a registered nurse for at least 2 years
- Practiced at least 2000 hours in the field of nursing informatics within the past 5 years or completed at least 12 semester hours of academic credits in informatics in a graduate program in nursing and a minimum of 1000 hours in informatics within the past 5 years
- Earned 20 contact hours of continuing education credit applicable to the specialty area within the past 2 years (ANCC, 2001)

The nurse who successfully passes the examination is certified as a generalist in informatics nursing. The ANCC is planning to offer an examination for a specialist in informatics nursing in the future. Once certified, the nurse must be recertified every 5 years. In the first year the examination was offered, 83 nurses became certified in informatics (Newbold, 1996).

Since then, more than 200 additional nurses have become certified in the specialty (ANCC, 2000).

Education in Informatics. There are both formal and informal opportunities for education in informatics. The first formal educational programs that offered specific degrees in nursing informatics were established within the past decade, and the number of programs has been increasing steadily. However, because educational options were limited, many nurses are currently practicing in informatics who have been prepared for their role through on-the-job training or by receiving education for the role outside of nursing. For example, a nurse may have a bachelor of science degree in nursing (BSN) plus a second degree in computer science or information technology. Nurses have been successful in educating themselves using formal and informal resources. Nurses considering a career in informatics need to carefully consider options that are available and plan their educational programs accordingly.

Formal Programs. The Nursing Working Informatics Group of the AMIA (NWIG-AMIA) describes formal educational programs in nursing informatics as Category I, Category II, and Category III. Category I programs are those graduate programs with a specialist nursing informatics focus. There are currently eight Category I programs, based at the following institutions of higher learning: Excelsior College, New York University, St. Louis University, Columbia University, Loyola University-Chicago, University of Colorado Health Sciences Center, University of Maryland, and University of Utah. Although each program is unique, there are similarities. For example, students pursuing master's level education will take approximately 42 semester credit hours of course work, which are divided among core courses (such as theory, research, policy, and advanced nursing), courses in nursing informatics (such as programming, database design, systems analysis and design, clinical decision-making, informatics models, and practice activities), and support courses. Similarly, students at the University of Utah and the University of Maryland may pursue doctoral study with substantive course work in nursing informatics. Again courses are taken in nursing theory, research, statistics, and nursing informatics. As with any doctoral degree, a dissertation is required.

Category II programs are graduate and undergraduate programs and courses that allow a student to pursue a concentration (or minor) in nursing informatics. In these programs students take 6 to 12 credit hours of course work in informatics. Category II programs are available at Case Western Reserve University; Duke School of Nursing; Loyola of Chicago; Northeastern University; Slippery Rock University; and the Universities of Arizona, Iowa, Pennsylvania, and Phoenix.

Category III programs offer individual courses in nursing informatics at both the graduate and undergraduate level. The NWIG-AMIA has identified eight such programs (Georgia College and State University, Lewis University, Lewis-Clark State College, Oregon Health Sciences University, Western Michigan University, Wichita State University, University of North Carolina and University of Vermont) although it is likely that this list is incomplete. If you are interested in formal study in informatics, check with schools and colleges of nursing in your locale to see what is available.

Although these are the only formal programs available at this time, many universities have courses in computer science and information technology. Interested students are able to self-design programs that meet their individual learning needs. Programs at the University of Texas at Austin, University of California San Francisco, and the University of Wisconsin at

Madison have been identified as having particularly strong concentrations of courses available in informatics (Gassert, 2000).

Informal Education. For many nurses graduate education is not an option or personal choice, but they still desire to become more knowledgeable about informatics. In this case many informal opportunities exist, including networking through professional organizations, keeping abreast of the literature by reading journals, and attending professional conferences.

Organizations vary in their scope, services offered to members, and the types of educational programs offered. Nelson and Joos (1992) describe five types of organizations.

1. Special interest groups such as the councils of the ANA and NLN. Nonnursing organizations that have special interest groups of interest to nurses include the American Hospital Association and the Healthcare Financial Management Association.

2. Information science and computer organizations such as the Association for Computing Machinery. There also are specialty organizations within this category, such as the Health Science Communications Association.

3. Health computing organizations such as the AMIA and the International Medical Informatics Association. Other organizations in this category include the Medical Records Institute and the Computer-Based Patient Record Institute (CPRI).

4. User groups, which consist of individuals working with a specific language, software, or vendor. One such group of interest to nurses is the Microsoft Healthcare Users Group (MS-HUG), which focuses on applications of Microsoft products in health care environments.

5. Local groups such as the Capital Area Roundtable on Informatics in Nursing (CARING), located in Washington, DC, or the Tri-State Nursing Computer Network, located in Pittsburgh, Pa. These groups provide local contacts, opportunities for networking, and education. CARING, for example, offers a popular review course for people preparing to take the nursing informatics certification examination.

Anyone interested in learning more about informatics should become active in at least one related organization. As a member a nurse has access to the meetings, publications, and educational offerings that the organization provides. Getting on mailing lists or visiting organizational sites on the www also allows a nurse to keep abreast of different opportunities available through each organization. Box 14-1 provides a listing of Internet addresses for some of the larger organizations.

Reading journals and newsletters is another way to become more knowledgeable about informatics. Offerings range from trade magazines that are not related to health but are important sources of information, such as *PC Magazine* or *Byte,* to specialized journals in nursing such as *Computers in Nursing.* Since 1995 *Computers in Nursing* has offered continuing education credit for articles published in the journal. The AMIA publishes the *Journal of the American Medical Informatics Association,* a publication source for much of the research that has been conducted related to informatics. A nurse interested in informatics should become familiar with the journals that are available, subscribe to those that are most interesting, and read others in the library. Unfortunately more information is published every month than anyone could possibly hope to keep abreast of—thus the need for networking! Colleagues can alert others to articles of interest that are in journals they might not regularly read.

Finally, conferences provide an excellent source of education. At a conference the nurse is able to hear the latest information directly from experts in the field. Larger conferences

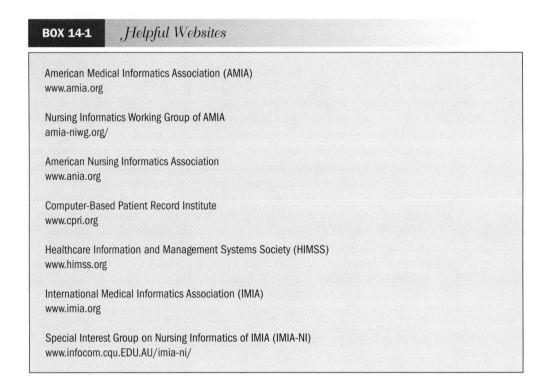

BOX 14-1   *Helpful Websites*

American Medical Informatics Association (AMIA)
www.amia.org

Nursing Informatics Working Group of AMIA
amia-niwg.org/

American Nursing Informatics Association
www.ania.org

Computer-Based Patient Record Institute
www.cpri.org

Healthcare Information and Management Systems Society (HIMSS)
www.himss.org

International Medical Informatics Association (IMIA)
www.imia.org

Special Interest Group on Nursing Informatics of IMIA (IMIA-NI)
www.infocom.cqu.EDU.AU/imia-ni/

usually have vendor exhibits that provide the opportunity for hands-on demonstrations for a variety of commercial products. Conferences vary in size, focus, location, and cost. For those interested in nursing informatics, nursing conferences especially are helpful. Local organizations, such as CARING, sponsor a variety of half-day or 1-day conferences. Rutgers, the State University of New Jersey, has an annual informatics conference; in 2001 they celebrated their nineteenth year of successful implementation. The University of Maryland hosts a week-long institute on informatics every summer at the Baltimore campus. In addition, nonnursing organizations such as the Health Information Management Systems Society and the AMIA have nursing sessions at their annual meetings. Nonnursing sessions also are often of great interest to nurse attendees.

CLINICAL INFORMATION
Clinical Information Systems

CISs are changing the way that health care is delivered, whether in the hospital, the clinic, the provider's office, or the patient's home. With capabilities ranging from advanced instrumentation to high-level decision support, CISs offer nurses and other clinicians information when, where, and how they need it. Increasingly CIS applications function as the mechanisms for delivering patient-centered care and for supporting the move toward the computer-based patient record (CPR).

What exactly is a CIS? Definitions vary, often from organization to organization. Semancik (1997) describes a CIS as a collection of software programs and associated hardware that supports the entry, retrieval, update, and analysis of patient care information and associated clinical information related to patient care. The CIS is primarily a computer system used to provide clinical information for the care of a patient.

A CIS can be patient-focused or departmental. In patient-focused systems, automation supports patient care processes. Typical applications found in a patient-focused system include order entry, results reporting, clinical documentation, care planning, and clinical pathways. As data are entered into the system, data repositories are established that can be accessed to look for trends in patient care. Departmental systems evolved to meet the operational needs of a particular department, such as the laboratory, radiology, pharmacy, medical records, or billing. Early systems often were stand-alone systems designed for an individual department. A major challenge facing CIS developers is to integrate these stand-alone systems to work with each other and with the newer patient-focused systems.

Computerized Patient Records

A CIS is not the same as a CPR or an electronic patient record. Ideally the CPR will include all information about an individual's lifetime health status and health care maintained electronically. The CPR is a replacement for the paper medical record as the primary source of information for health care, meeting all clinical, legal, and administrative requirements. However, the CPR is more than today's medical record. Information technology permits much more data to be captured, processed, and integrated, which results in information that is broader than that found in a linear paper record.

The CPR is not a record in the traditional sense of the term. "Record" connotes a repository with limitations of size, content, and location. The term traditionally has suggested that the sole purpose for maintaining health data is to document events. Although this is an important purpose, the CPR permits health information to be used to support the generation and communication of knowledge.

The health care delivery system is dramatically changing, with a strong emphasis on improving outcomes of care and maintaining health. The CPR needs to be considered in a broader context and is not applicable only to patients (i.e., individuals with the presence of an illness or disease). Rather in the CPR the focus is on the individual's health, encompassing both wellness and illness.

As a result of this focus on the individual, the CPR is a virtual compilation of nonredundant health data about the person across his or her lifetime, including facts, observations, interpretations, plans, actions, and outcomes. Health data include information on allergies, history of illness and injury, functional status, diagnostic studies, assessments, orders, consultation reports, and treatment records. Health data also include wellness information such as immunization history, behavioral data, environmental information, demographics, health insurance, administrative data for care delivery processes, and legal data such as informed consents. The who, what, when, and where of data capture are also identified. The structure of the data includes text, numbers, sounds, images, and full-motion video. These are thoroughly integrated so that any given view of health data may incorporate one or more structural elements.

Within a CPR, an individual's health data are maintained and distributed over different systems in different locations, such as a hospital, clinic, physician's office, and pharmacy. Intelligent software agents with appropriate security measures are necessary to access data across these distributed systems. The nurse or other user who is retrieving these data must be able to assemble it in such a way as to provide a chronology of health information about the individual.

The CPR is maintained in a system that captures, processes, communicates, secures, and presents the data about the patient. This system may include the CIS. Other components of the CPR system include clinical rules, literature for patient education, expert opinions, and payer rules related to reimbursement. When these elements work together in an integrated fashion, the CPR becomes much more than a patient record—it becomes a knowledge tool. The system is able to integrate information from multiple sources and provides decision support; thus the CPR serves as the primary source of information for patient care.

A fully functional CPR is a complex system. Consider a single data element (datum), such as a person's weight. The system must be able to capture, or record the weight; store it, process it, communicate it to others, and present it in a different format such as a bar graph or chart. All of this must be done in a secure environment that protects the patient's confidentiality and privacy. The complexity of these issues and the development of the necessary systems helps to explain why few fully functional CPR systems are in place today.

Data Capture. Data capture refers to the collection and entry of data into a computer system. The origin of the data may be local or remote from patient-monitoring devices, from telemedicine applications, directly from the individual recipient of health care, and even from others who have information about the recipient's health or environment, such as relatives and friends and public health agencies. Data may be captured by multiple means, including key entry, pattern recognition (voice, handwriting, or biologic characteristics), and medical device transmission.

All data entered into a computer are not necessarily structured for subsequent processing. For example, document imaging systems provide for creation of electronically stored text but have limitations on the ability to process that text. Data capture includes the use of controlled vocabularies and code systems to ensure common meaning for terminology and the ability to process units of information. As noted earlier, great strides have been made in the development of standardized nursing languages. These languages provide structured data entry and text processing, which result in common meaning and processing.

Data capture also encompasses authentication to identify the author of an entry and to ensure that the author has been granted permission to access the system and change the CPR.

Storage. Storage refers to the physical location of data. In CPR systems health data are distributed across multiple systems at different sites. For this reason, common access protocols, retention schedules, and universal identification are necessary.

Access protocols permit only authorized users to obtain data for legitimate uses. The systems must have backup and recovery mechanisms in the event of failure. Retention schedules address the maintenance of the data in active and inactive form and the permanence of the storage medium.

A person's identity can be determined by many types of data in addition to common identifiers such as name and number. Universal identifiers or other methods are required for integrating health data of an individual distributed across multiple systems at different sites.

Information Processing. Application functions provide for effective retrieval and processing of data into useful information. These include decision support tools such as alerts and alarms for drug interactions, allergies, and abnormal laboratory results. Reminders can be provided for appointments, critical path actions, medication administration, and other activities. The systems also may provide access to consensus- and evidence-driven diagnostic and treatment guidelines and protocols. The nurse could integrate a standard guideline, protocol, or critical path into a specific individual's CPR, modify it to meet unique circumstances, and use it as a basis for managing and documenting care. Outcome data communicated from various caregivers and health care recipients themselves also may be analyzed and used for continual improvement of the guidelines and protocols.

Information Communication. Information communication refers to the interoperability of systems and linkages for exchange of data across disparate systems. To integrate health data across multiple systems at different sites, identifier systems (unique numbers or other methodology) for health care recipients, caregivers, providers, payers, and sites are essential. Local, regional, and national health information infrastructures that tie all participants together using standard data communication protocols are key to the linkage function. There are hundreds of types of transactions or messages that must be defined and agreed to by the participating stakeholders. Vocabulary and code systems must permit the exchange and processing of data into meaningful information. CPR systems must provide access to point-of-care information databases and knowledge sources such as pharmaceutic formularies, referral databases, and reference literature.

Security. Computer-based patient record systems provide better protection of confidential health information than paper-based systems because such systems support controls that ensure that only authorized users with legitimate uses have access to health information. Security functions address the confidentiality of private health information and the integrity of the data. Security functions must be designed to ensure compliance with applicable laws, regulations, and standards. Security systems must ensure that access to data is provided only to those who are authorized and have a legitimate purpose for its use. Security functions also must provide a means to audit for inappropriate access.

Three important terms are used when discussing security: privacy, confidentiality, and security. It is important to understand the differences between these concepts.

- Privacy refers to the right of an individual to keep information about himself or herself from being disclosed to anyone. If a patient has had an abortion and chose not to tell a health care provider this fact, the patient would be keeping that information private.
- Confidentiality refers to the act of limiting disclosure of private matters. Once a patient has disclosed private information to a health care provider, that provider has a responsibility to maintain the confidentiality of that information.
- Security refers to the means to control access and protect information from accidental or intentional disclosure to unauthorized persons and from alteration, destruction, or loss. When private information is placed in a confidential CPR, the system must have controls in place to maintain the security of the system and not allow unauthorized persons access to the data (CPRI, 1995).

Information Presentation. The wealth of information available through CPR systems must be managed to ensure that authorized caregivers, including nurses, and others with legitimate uses have the information they need in their preferred presentation form. For example, a nurse may want to see data organized by source, caregiver, encounter, problem, or date. Data can be presented in detail or summary form. Tables, graphs, narrative, and other forms of information presentation must be accommodated. Some users may need only to know of the presence or absence of certain data, not the nature of the data itself. For example, blood donation centers draw blood for testing for human immunodeficiency virus, hepatitis, and other conditions. If a donor has a positive test result, the center may not be given the specific information regarding the test, but just general information that a test result was abnormal and that the patient should be referred to an appropriate health care provider.

Interface Between the Informatics Nurse and the Clinical Information System

Information demands in health care systems are pushing the development of CISs and CPRs. The ongoing development of computer technology—smaller, faster machines with extensive storage capabilities and the ability for cross-platform communication—is making the goal of an integrated electronic system a realistic option, not just a long-term dream. As these systems evolve, INs will play an important role in their development, implementation, and evaluation.

Because of their expertise, INs are in an ideal position to assist with the development, implementation, and evaluation of CISs. Their knowledge of policies, procedures, and clinical care is essential as workflow systems are redesigned within a CIS. It is not unusual for nurses within an institution to have more hands-on interaction with and knowledge of different departments than any other group of employees in an institution. Jenkins (2000) suggests that the process model of nursing (assessment, planning, implementation, and evaluation) works well during a CIS implementation; thus nurses have a familiar framework from which to understand the complexity of a major system change.

TRENDS IN COMPUTING: PAST, PRESENT, AND FUTURE

As noted earlier, computers have moved from the realm of a "nice to know" luxury item to a "need to know" essential resource for professional practice. Nurses are knowledge workers who require accurate and up-to-date information for their professional work. The explosion in information—some estimate that all information is replaced every 9 to 12 months—requires nurses to be on the cutting edge of knowledge to practice ethically and safely. Trends in computing will also impact the work of professional nurses and not just through the development of CISs and CPRs. Research advances, new devices, monitoring equipment, sensors, and "smart body parts" will all change the way that health care is conceptualized, practiced, and delivered.

Within this context, not every nurse will need to be an informatics specialist, but every nurse must be computer literate. Computer literacy is defined as the knowledge and understanding of computers, combined with the ability to use them effectively (Joos et al, 1996). Computer literacy may be interpreted as different levels of expertise for different people in various roles. On the least specialized level, computer literacy involves knowing how to turn on a computer, start and stop simple application programs, and save and print information. For health care professionals computer literacy requires having an understanding of systems used in clinical practice, education, and research settings. For example, in clinical practice electronic patient records and clinical information systems are becoming more widely used. The computer literate nurse is able to use these systems effectively and can address issues discussed earlier, such as confidentiality, security, and privacy. At the same time, the nurse must be able to effectively use applications typically found on personal computers (PCs), such as word processing software, spreadsheets, presentation graphics, and statistics for research. Finally, the computer-literate nurse must know how to access information from a variety of electronic sources and how to evaluate the appropriateness of the information at both the professional and patient level. The remainder of this chapter is designed to help you gain a broader understanding of computer literacy and the computing environment of PCs and the online world, along with a discussion of future trends.

The Past and Future

Weiser and Brown (1996) have characterized the history and future of computing in three phases. The first phase is known as the "mainframe era," in which many people share one computer. Computers were found behind closed doors and run by experts with specialized knowledge and skills. Although we have mostly moved beyond the mainframe era, it still exists in CISs (hence some of the problems discussed previously) or other situations with large mainframe systems, such as banking, weather forecasting, and legacy systems in academic institutions.

The archetypal computer of the mainframe era must be the Electronic Numerical Integrator and Computer (ENIAC), developed at the University of Pennsylvania in 1945. This was proposed by John Mauchly, an American physicist, and built at the Moore School of Engineering by Mauchly and J. Presper Eckert, an engineer. It is regarded as the first successful digital computer. It weighed more than 60,000 pounds and contained more than 18,000 vacuum tubes. Roughly 2000 of the computer's vacuum tubes were replaced each month by a team of six technicians. Even though one vacuum tube blew approximately every 15 minutes, the functioning of the ENIAC was still considered to be reliable! Many of the first tasks of the ENIAC were for military purposes, such as calculating ballistic firing tables and designing atomic weapons. Because ENIAC was initially not a stored program machine, it had to be reprogrammed for each task.

Phase II in modern computing is the PC era, which is characterized by one person to one computer. In this era the computing relationship is personal and intimate. Similar to a car, the computer is seen as a special, relatively expensive item that requires attention but provides a very valuable service in one's life.

The first harbinger of the PC era was in 1948 with the development of the transistor at Bell Telephone Laboratories. The transistor, which could act as an electric switch, replaced the costly, energy-inefficient, and unreliable vacuum tubes in computers and other devices, including televisions. By the late 1960s integrated circuits, tiny transistors, and other electrical components arranged on a single chip of silicon replaced individual transistors in computers. Integrated circuits became miniaturized, enabling more components to be designed into a single computer circuit. In the 1970s refinements in integrated circuit technology led to the development of the modern microprocessor, integrated circuits that contained thousands of transistors. Weiser and Brown (1996) date the true start of Phase II as 1984, when the number of people using PCs surpassed the number of people using shared computers.

Manufacturers used integrated circuit technology to build smaller and cheaper computers. The first PCs were sold by Instrumentation Telemetry Systems. The Altair 8800 appeared in 1975. Graphic user interfaces were first designed by the Xerox corporation in a prototype computer, the Alto, developed in 1974. The corporate decision to not pursue commercial development of the PC (Xerox identified its core business strategy as copiers, not computers) has become a bit of a computer history legend (Hiltzik, 2000; Smith and Alexander, 1988). Continuing development of sophisticated operating systems and miniaturization of components (modern microprocessors contain as many as 10 million transistors) have enabled computers to be developed that can run programs and manipulate data in ways that were unimaginable in the era of the ENIAC.

Phase III has been dubbed the era of ubiquitous computing (UC), in which there will be many computers to each person. Weiser and Brown (1996) estimate that the crossover with the PC era will be between 2005 to 2020. In this phase computers will be everywhere: in walls, chairs, clothing, light switches, cars, appliances, and so on. Computers will become so fundamental to our human experience that they will "disappear" and we will cease to be aware of them. For those who are skeptical that this will come to pass, consider two other ubiquitous technologies: writing and electricity. In Egyptian times writing was a secret art, known and performed only by specially trained scribes who lived on a level close to royalty. Clay tablets and later papyrus were precious commodities. Many people died without ever having seen a piece of paper in their lives! Now paper and writing are everywhere. Within the course of an average day, most people use and discard hundreds of pieces of paper, never giving them a second thought. Electricity has a similar history. When electricity was first invented in the nineteenth century, entire factories were designed to accommodate the presence of light bulbs and bulky motors. The placement of workers, machines, and parts were all designed around the need of electricity and motors. Today electricity is everywhere. It is hidden in the walls and stored in tiny batteries. The average car has more than 22 motors and 25 solenoids.

One only has to look around a typical house to see how UC is becoming part of our lives. Microprocessors exist in every room: appliances in the kitchen, remote controls for television and stereo in the den, and clock radios and cordless phones in the bedroom. And the bathroom? Matsushita of Japan has developed a prototype toilet (dubbed the "smart toilet") that includes an online, real-time health monitoring system. It measures the user's weight, fat content, and urine sugar level; plots the recorded data on a graph; and sends it instantaneously to a health care provider for monitoring (Watts, 1999).

Another dimension of UC is the Internet. Each time you connect to the Internet, you are connecting with millions of information resources and hundreds of information delivery systems. A person truly does become one person to hundreds of computers. It is ironic that the interface to the UC world of the Internet is still through a PC. But this is changing. Wireless infrared connections will eliminate wires; handheld devices will eliminate the bulky PC. Once we become wireless and mobile, UC will become a reality.*

The Present: PCs and the Internet

Although UC is exciting, the current reality is we are firmly entrenched in the PC era. The Internet is driving many changes, but the computer-literate nurse still needs a working familiarity with the basics of a PC.

Hardware. The physical computer and its components are known as hardware. Computer hardware includes the memory that stores data and instructions; the CPU that carries out in-

---

*To consider the freedom of becoming wireless, think of the modern telephone. With wireless (portable) phones, it is possible to walk around the room, fold laundry, make the bed, straighten up a room, and, yes, even go to the bathroom, all while talking on the phone. Remember being tethered by a phone cord. It amazes me how many businesses (my own included) still provide this almost obsolete technology to their workers.

structions; the bus that connects the various computer components; the input devices such as a keyboard or mouse that allow the user to communicate with the computer, and the output devices such as printers and video display monitors that enable the computer to present information to the user.

Software. Software contains the instructions that cause the hardware to work. Software as a whole can be divided into categories based on the types of work done by programs. The two primary software categories are operating systems, which control the workings of the computer, and application software, which controls the multitude of tasks for which people use computers. System software thus handles such essential, but often invisible, chores as maintaining disk files and managing the screen, whereas application software programs perform tasks such as word processing and database management. Two additional categories that are neither system nor application software, although they contain elements of both, are network software, which enables groups of computers to communicate, and language software, which provides programmers with the necessary tools to write programs.

In addition to these task-based categories, software may be described on the basis of the method of distribution. These methods include packaged software, developed and sold primarily through retail outlets; freeware and public-domain software, which is made available without cost by its developer; and shareware, which is similar to freeware but usually carries a small fee for those who like the program. Some people also include vaporware in this classification, which is software that either does not reach the market or appears much later than promised.

Nurses interact with and primarily use application programs. Software in this category can be further subdivided on the basis of its purpose and includes:

- General purpose programs, which include communications, database, desktop publishing, graphics, spreadsheets, statistics, and word processing applications.
- Educational programs, which include CAI and computer-aided learning applications
- Utilities (i.e., programs that help manage the functioning of the computers).
- Personal applications such as calendars and appointment books.
- Entertainment and simulations, such as games. Not all games are just for fun; sophisticated simulations such as "SimCity" allow the user to run a small city and deal with crises of weather, nature, and person-made disasters. This latter program has been used in nursing programs to simulate environmental issues in the real world (Bareford, 2001).

The Internet. Applications such as word processing and database management typically reside on a stand-alone PC and are under the purview of one user. However, this is only one dimension of PC use. The other major component is the online world, commonly called the Internet (with a capital I) and its graphic component, the www. The exponential growth of the Internet makes it an essential item for the computer-literate nurse to master. Information and professional resources that cannot be found anywhere else are available on the Internet; this trend shows no sign of slowing. Most people use the Internet for two broad purposes: to communicate with others, either individually or in groups, and to find information. Nurses are no exception, and as knowledge workers they must do both for their professional work.

The Development of the Internet. Many mistakenly believe that the Internet is a recent development. Rather, it has been around for more than three decades. The modern Internet started out in 1969 as a U.S. Defense Department network called ARPAnet. Scientists built ARPAnet with the intention of creating a network that would still be able to function efficiently if part of the network were damaged. This concept was important to military organizations, which were studying ways to maintain a working communications network in the event of nuclear war. Since then the Internet has grown, changed, matured, and mutated, but the essential structure of interconnected domains randomly distributed throughout the world has remained the same. ARPAnet no longer exists, but many of the standards established for that first network still govern the communication and structure of the modern Internet.

For many years the Internet was more or less the private domain of scientists, researchers, and university professors who used the Internet to communicate and exchange files and software. A number of events transpired in the 1980s and early 1990s that resulted in the enormous growth of the Internet and its ensuing popularity.

In 1989 English computer scientist Timothy Berners-Lee introduced the www. Berners-Less initially designed the www to aid communication between physicists who were working in different parts of the world for the European Laboratory for Particle Physics (CERN). However, as it grew, the www revolutionized the use of the Internet. During the early 1990s increasingly large numbers of users who were not part of the scientific or academic communities began to use the Internet, in large part because of the ability of the www to easily handle multimedia documents. Other changes have also influenced the growth of the Internet, such as the High-Performance Computing Act of 1991, the decision to allow computers other than those used for research and military purposes to connect to the network, and the development of "user-friendly" software and tools that allowed less experienced computer users to obtain information quickly and easily.

Going Online.   To access the Internet, the user needs hardware, software, and a means of access. Hardware includes the computer (such as a PC or Macintosh); and some sort of device to make a connection such as a modem (which uses a phone line), a cable modem (which connects through a cable television line), or a local area network such as might be found in a workplace setting. Newer options include handheld cellular phones with wireless modems, but the vast majority of those online are still connecting with a wire-based computer system. Necessary software includes a browser, which is used to view pages on the www, and an e-mail program, which is necessary for sending and receiving mail. Finally, a way to access the Internet, which is typically through an Internet Service Provider (ISP) is needed to make the connection between the hardware and online world. Again, there are several options, including large commercial services such as America Online or online access through a college or university. Detailed descriptions of all of these options (hardware, software, and ISPs) are beyond the scope of this chapter; one useful resource for more information is *The Nurses' Guide to the Internet* (Nicoll, 2001).

Online Activities: Communicating With Others

Individual E-Mail.   By far the most common use of the Internet is to send electronic mail (e-mail). It is also very easy. The fact that it is so easy is a major driving force behind the phenomenal growth of e-mail. In 1999 there were 569 million mailboxes, an increase of 84% over 1998 (Year End, 1999). Analysts estimate that in less than 2 years there will be one billion online mailboxes, outnumbering both televisions and phone lines. Even with this growth, every e-mail journey begins with a single message. For many people, exchanging e-mail with colleagues is their first introduction to the Internet. Since the interaction is limited and often with someone who is known, it is usually a nonthreatening experience.

E-mail tends to be informal, and most recipients are tolerant of "less-than-perfect" communications. Even so, if your mail program includes features such as a spellchecker, it is wise to use it. Another useful feature is to create a signature file. With a signature file, certain information, such as your name, e-mail address, and phone number will be appended to every message you send.

A few words of warning about e-mail:

- TYPING IN CAPITALS IS NOT A GOOD IDEA. In popular netiquette (etiquette for the Internet) terms, typing exclusively in capital letters is considered shouting and very rude.
- Just because e-mail is simple and informal, do not forget rules of common courtesy. If you are writing to someone you don't know to request information, include a brief introduction and explanation of why you need the material. Similarly, if you request information, be reasonable in your request. A two-sentence e-mail message may take the respondent an hour to answer. If you want someone to send you hard copy of protocols, guidelines or procedures, offer to reimburse for mailing or copying. Do not use e-mail as a substitute for doing your own work. I get a surprising number of requests from people asking for literature searches on nursing informatics, which I deal with quickly and completely by using the delete key.
- Be careful with attachments. Attachments are appended to e-mail messages and contain files or pictures. Although attachments are a necessary way to send files, it is possible to send a virus to someone via an attachment.
- Another problem is spam: junk e-mail. Junk e-mail can fill up your electronic mailbox just as quickly as traditional junk fills your home mailbox. There are many different types of spam: messages selling goods and services, get-rich-quick schemes, chain letters, and hoaxes. My advice for all of these is simple: HIT THE DELETE KEY. Many spam messages include a line that says, "Reply to this message to be removed from the mailing list." This is the worst thing you can do. By replying to the message you confirm your e-mail address and in so doing, run the risk of exponentially increasing the spam e-mail that you receive.

Group E-Mail: Mailing Lists.   Another popular feature of the Internet is mailing lists, which provide a forum for groups of people with similar interests to get together and share their information through a mail-based discussion group. These lists can range in size from a few dozen people to thousands, and they can generate anywhere from a few messages a week to a hundred or more in a day. Being on a mailing list can put information and resources literally at your fingertips. Imagine asking 900 fellow students around the world a question concerning a clinical problem and receiving multiple answers within minutes.

To find out about mailing lists, talk to others and find out if they subscribe. Actual subscribers are the most reliable source of information regarding a list (e.g., how active it is, whether the discussions are valuable). Another option is to visit http://www.ualberta.ca/~jrnorris/nursenet/nurlists.html. This is a "list of lists" specific to nursing and was created by Judy Norris, who is a faculty member at the University of Alberta. Dr. Norris is also the founder of NURSENET, one of the oldest mailing lists in nursing. At this site there is an alphabetized list with information about each one of the nursing lists and individual instructions on how to subscribe. Finally, another option is to visit www.liszt.com which is a list of lists in all areas, not just nursing.

Although there are hundreds of mailing lists on the Internet, they all work in a similar fashion. As noted above, each list is developed around a particular topic or interest area. One subscribes to a list, but unlike subscribing to a magazine, there is no charge for the service. Once you are subscribed to a list, you will receive messages that you can read, reply to, or delete. The communications are asynchronous (i.e., the discussions are not occurring in real time, such as you would have with a conversation). Instead the discussions occur via e-mail, with one person asking a question or posing a comment and other members on the list replying. Even though the discussions are not synchronous, they are real discussions with sometimes heated debates.

Although all mailing lists work in a similar fashion, each list has its own quirks. Typically, when you successfully subscribe to a mailing list, you will receive a welcome message from the list owner. Print this message and save it, because it will contain useful information about how to manage your subscription: how to unsubscribe, how to temporarily stop the mail, and how to receive the list in different formats such as digest.

As with individual e-mail, there are some mailing list courtesies to keep in mind. Mailing lists are not anonymous; there are real people behind the messages. These people give the list its personality, and you will get to know the other list members through their discussions and comments. Many people choose to "lurk," that is, read messages but not post, when they first subscribe to a list. This gives you a chance to get a feel for the members of the community. When you do decide to post a message, a short introduction is a good idea. Keep it simple: "Hi, my name is . . . I subscribed to this list because I am interested in . . . ."

When you post a question, be clear and to the point. Tell people what information you want and how you want it. Do you want people to post their replies to the list or reply to you privately? Similarly, if you are replying to a message, know to whom you are replying. By default, all responses go to the whole list.

If the nature of the topic changes, change the subject line. This allows the list members to quickly scan and delete messages that are not of interest.

Flaming is not a good idea. A *flame* is when someone attacks another person, usually in a virulent and violent manner. Remember that the whole point of a list is to have a discussion; it is possible to disagree with someone's ideas, but that does not mean you have to denigrate the person in the process.

Finally, *newbies* (newcomers) are afforded a wide degree of latitude, and mistakes are expected and accepted, but do your best to learn the ropes and manage your subscription in a responsible and professional manner. Although list owners are loathe to do this, they can unsubscribe people who repeatedly post off topic, flame others, send viruses, or mismanage their account. Keep these points in mind when you join a list.

Chatting Online. Mailing lists are extremely useful, but what if you want to have a synchronous (real time) conversation with someone else? To do this you need to find a way to chat, which is not too hard to do as Internet chatting is becoming as popular as e-mail. There are literally hundreds of chat rooms, scattered all over the Internet, with people talking on every imaginable topic. Chat rooms appeal to some people but not others. The only way to find out if this is a communication medium that suits you is to dive in and try it.

To get started, you have two major options: the first is to find a chat room that exists on the Internet. With that, you simply "enter the room" and begin conversing. The second option is to download software that allows you to chat, such as Internet relay chat (IRC) or ICQ ("I-seek-you"). Many people use both options. People tend to have favorites, so you may find certain friends in ICQ, others on IRC, and yet others in chat rooms on America Online.

No matter which option you choose, certain rules of etiquette govern chatting. You should also observe certain precautions to protect yourself. One important rule: never give out personal information in a chat room. Do not give out credit card information or passwords, no matter how the request is made. You might want to investigate using moderated chat rooms. Moderators are there to keep an eye on the content and flow of conversation. They also have the authority to kick people who are misbehaving out of the chats. As with mailing lists, rules of common courtesy prevail in chat rooms. Do not harass others, do not flame, and avoid obscene and suggestive language.

If you chat regularly, you may begin to see familiar names and become friends with your fellow chatters. You may fall in love. You may meet someone and get married. I know people who have done all three. You also may find yourself in a difficult and potentially dangerous situation. As with anything in life, be careful. The Internet does have a dark side.

That said, I have met some great people on the Internet, and we have met in person and become good friends. The Internet is making our world smaller and giving all of us the opportunity to meet people we might never have met otherwise. But I used caution and common sense in allowing these friendships to develop. If you do the same, you will do much to guarantee that your Internet interactive experiences are pleasant and rewarding.

Online Activities: Finding Information

The other major use of the Internet is finding information. To do so, it is important to develop skills for searching quickly and efficiently. There are a variety of strategies you can use for searching, including quick and dirty searching, links, and brute force. Keep in mind that you must be persistent: no one search strategy is going to work all the time, nor is any one search engine more effective than any other. A study published in *Science* in 1998 (Lawrence and Giles, 1998) revealed that the best search engines found approximately 33% of the information available on the Internet. That means, of course, that 67% of useful information is being missed. Search engines are good starting points, but you can augment their effectiveness by adding a few other strategies to your Web exploration toolkit.

First, you should target your search by conducting a "Purpose—Focus—Approach" (PFA) assessment. To determine your purpose, ask yourself why you are doing the search and why you need the information. Consider questions such as the following:

- Is it for personal interest?
- Do you want to obtain information to share with co-workers or a client?
- Are you verifying information given to you by someone else?
- Are you preparing a report or writing a paper for a class or project?

Based on your purpose, your focus may be:

- Broad and general (basic information for yourself).
- Lay oriented (to give information to a patient) or professionally oriented (for colleagues).
- Narrow and technical with a research orientation.

Purpose combined with focus determines your approach. For example, information that is broad and general can be found using brute force methods or quick and dirty searching. Lay information can be quickly accessed at a few key sites, including MEDLINEplus and consumer health organizations. Similarly, professional associations and societies are a good starting point for professionally oriented information. Scientific and research information usually requires literature resources that can be found in databases such as MEDLINE or CINAHL.

Quick and Dirty Searching. Quick and dirty searching is a very simple but surprisingly effective search strategy. First, start with a search engine such as AltaVista (www.altavista.com). Next type in the term of interest. At this point, do not worry about being overly broad or general. You will retrieve an enormous number of found references (called "hits") but you are only interested in the first ten to twenty. Look at the URLs and try to decipher what they mean. URLs usually start with www (for World Wide Web). Then there is the "thing in the middle" followed by a domain. Pay attention to the domains: .com is commercial; .edu is an educational institution; .gov is the government. Quickly visit a few sites. Look for the information you need, or useful links. If a site is not relevant, use the back button to return to your search results and go to the next site. Once you find a site that appears to be useful, begin to explore the site. If there are links, use the links to connect to other relevant sites. This process: quick search, quick review, clicking and linking, can provide a starting point for useful information in a relatively short period of time.

Brute Force. Brute force searching is another alternative. To do this, type in an address and see what happens. The worst outcome is an annoying error message, but you may land on a site that is exactly what you want. Perhaps you are trying to find a school of nursing at a certain university. What is the common name for the university? www.unh.edu is the very logical URL for the University of New Hampshire. Organizations are also quite logical in their URLs: www.aorn.org is AORN (the Association of periOperative Registered Nurses); www.aone.org is the American Organization of Nurse Executives.

Take Advantage of Links and Use the Bookmark Feature. Every website has links to other websites of related interest. Take advantage of these links because the site developer has already done some of the work of finding other useful resources. Combine quick and dirty searching or brute force with links to get the information you need. Each site you visit will have more links, and in this way the resources keep building. Visiting a variety of sites will open up the vistas of information that are available. When you find a site of interest, "bookmark" it or add it to your list of favorites. This guarantees you will be able to return to the site in the future.

Resources for Professionals and Consumers. The preceding discussion has focused on strategies to use when you are faced with a "needle in a haystack" searching situation—just dive in and see what you find. The advantage of this method is that it is fast and easy. The disadvantages are that sites of dubious quality may be obtained and the process, although fast, is not terribly efficient.

Another approach is to develop a "short list" of well-known, well-researched sites that can be used as starting points for further exploration. Such a list is useful to share with others so that they can begin their own exploration. These should be sites that you have determined are trustworthy and reliable. Examples of such sites include organizations and associations with which we are all familiar such as the American Cancer Society (ACS). They have patient education and consumer information materials, which can be obtained by a virtual visit to www.cancer.org. In addition to the traditional types of resources available from the ACS, at the website it is also possible to send an e-mail requesting more information, sign up for regular updates and news, read news items, and obtain updated statistical information. The website is truly a "value-added" version of the ACS. Practically any health organization you can think of has created a virtual storefront on the Internet. Professional associations in nursing, medicine, and other disciplines are also becoming comprehensive resource sites on the Internet. www.nursingcenter.com has a handy list of associations in nursing and related disciplines. Use the "AssociationLink" button on the home page to go to the complete listing.

Other resources are U.S. government agencies such as the Agency for Healthcare Research and Quality (www.ahrq.gov) and the National Institutes of Health (www.nih.gov). Once again, all of these agencies have been busy creating virtual institutes on the Internet. A useful resource is Healthfinder (www.healthfinder.gov), which can point you to news, information, tools, and databases.

Although these resources are the Internet versions of known and useful organizations, there are also virtual resources that exist only on the Internet. One such site that is particularly impressive is MEDLINEplus (http://medlineplus.gov), developed by the National Library of Medicine. A similar resource, specific to oncology, is OncoLink at the University of Pennsylvania (www.oncolink.org). OncoLink was created in 1994 and was the first multimedia oncology information resource placed on the Internet. They continue to be true to their original mission to "help cancer patients, families, health care professionals and the general public get accurate cancer-related information at no charge" (About OncoLink, 1999).

Literature Resources. Thinking back to PFA, if you are searching for scientific, technical, or research oriented information, you must search literature databases. In this case, the first place to turn is to the National Library of Medicine (NLM), which is the home of the MEDLARS (Medical Literature Analysis and Retrieval System), a computerized system of databases and databanks offered by the NLM. A person may search the computer files either to produce a list of publications (bibliographic citations) or to retrieve factual information on a specific question. The most well known of all the databases in the MEDLARS system is MEDLINE, NLM's premier bibliographic database covering the fields of medicine, nursing, dentistry, veterinary medicine, and the preclinical sciences. Journal articles are indexed for MEDLINE, and their citations are searchable, using NLM's controlled vocabulary, MeSH (Medical Subject Headings). MEDLINE contains all citations published in Index Medicus and corresponds in part to the International Nursing Index and the Index to Dental Literature. Citations include the English abstract when published with the article (approximately 76% of the current file). MEDLINE contains over 11 million records from 4000 health science journals. The file is updated weekly. An individual can search MEDLINE for free, using one of two available search engines: PubMed (http://www.ncbi.nlm.nih.gov/entrez/query.fcgi) or Internet GratefulMed (http://igm.nlm.nih.gov/). Whichever search engine is used, there are no fees to the user to access the MEDLINE database.

Another literature resource to investigate is the National Guideline Clearinghouse (NCG) (www.ngc.gov). Whereas MEDLINE includes citations to articles in professional journals, the

NGC is a comprehensive database of evidence-based clinical practice guidelines and related documents produced by the Agency for Healthcare Research and Quality in partnership with the American Medical Association and the American Association of Health Plans. The NGC mission is to provide physicians, nurses, other health professionals, health care providers, health plans, integrated delivery systems, and purchasers an accessible mechanism for obtaining objective, detailed information on clinical practice guidelines and to further their dissemination, implementation, and use.

There are also a variety of other literature resources available on the Internet, some of which have fees attached. However, do not automatically assume that you must pay the fee. Your workplace or school may have licensing agreements in place with different vendors, and as an employee or student you may have access to the literature resources. Check with your library or information services department to see if this applies to you.

The final element of literature searching online is finding full text of articles. The databases so far discussed (MEDLINE and others) do not contain full text; they just include literature citations. Finding full text online at the present time is an unorganized situation. Options range from journals that have full text available either for free or for a fee, to forcing you to do things the old-fashioned way, that is, a trip to the library and photocopying articles by hand. Given the present state of confusion that exists, my best advice is to begin exploring, using quick and dirty or brute force methods. You can also visit the publisher's website to see if access to the journal is available. A final option is to use a document delivery service, such as UnCover (http://uncweb.carl.org/). This resource allows you to conduct a search. It identifies which articles can be sent to you, and what the fees will be (including article fees, service charges, and copyright fees). If you elect to order the article, you can identify how you want to have it sent to you (mail, fax, or other).

Evaluating Information Found on the Internet

Traveling through the Internet, one must always use critical thinking skills to evaluate the information that is found. The "wide open" nature of the Internet means that just about anyone with a computer and online access can create a home page and post it for the world to see. Although there are many excellent health- and nursing-related sites, there are others that just do not measure up in terms of accuracy, content, or currency.

In recent years criteria for website evaluation have proliferated. They range from the simple and cursory to the elaborate and expansive. I have found a simple mnemonic, "Are you PLEASED with the site?" to be very helpful.* The mnemonic makes the seven criteria very easy to remember, but I have found, in hundreds of hours of surfing and evaluating, they are extremely comprehensive (Nicoll, 2000). To determine if you are PLEASED, consider the following:

P: Purpose. What is the author's purpose in developing the site? Are the author's objectives clear? Many people will develop a website as a hobby or way of sharing information they have gathered. It should be immediately evident to you what the true purpose of the site is. At the same time, consider your purpose (i.e., think back to your PFA assessment). There should be congruence between the author's purpose and yours.

---

*Thanks to Linda Johnson of Excelsior University (formerly Regents College), Albany, NY, for her original suggestion of this mnemonic.

L: Links. Evaluate the links at the site. Are they working? (Links that do not take you anywhere are called "dead links.") Do they link to reliable sites? It is important to critically evaluate the links at sites hosted by organizations, businesses, or institutions because these entities are usually presenting themselves as authorities for the subject at hand. Some pages, such as those created by individuals, are really nothing more than a collection of links. These can be useful as a starting point for a search, but it is still important to evaluate the links that are provided at the site.

E: Editorial (site content). Is the information contained in the site accurate, comprehensive, and current? Is there a particular bias or is the information presented in an objective way? Who is the consumer of the site: is it designed for health professionals, patients, consumers, or other audiences? Is the information presented in an appropriate format for the intended audience? Look at details, too. Are there misspellings and grammatical errors? "Under construction" banners that have been there forever? I find that these types of errors can be very telling about the overall quality of the site.

A: Author. Who is the author of the site? Does that person or persons have the appropriate credentials? Is the author clearly identified by name and is contact information provided? Many times I will double-check an author's credentials by doing a literature search in MEDLINE. When people advertise themselves as "the leading worldwide authority" on such-and-such topic, I figure they should have a few publications to their credit that establish their reputations. It is surprising how many times this search brings up nothing.

Be wary of how a person presents his or her credentials, too. I have seen many sites where "Dr. X" is touted as an expert. On further exploration, I verify that, in fact, Dr. X does have a PhD (or MD or EdD), but the discipline in which this degree was obtained has nothing to do with the subject matter of the site. Remember that there is no universal process of peer review on the Internet and anyone can present himself or herself in any way that he or she wants. Be suspicious.

Keep in mind that the webmaster and the author may be two (or more) different people. The webmaster is the person who designed the site and is responsible for its upkeep. The author is the person who is responsible for the content and is the expert in the subject matter provided. In your evaluation, make sure to determine who these people are.

S: Site. Is the site easy to navigate? Is it attractive? Does it download quickly or have too many graphics and other features that make it inefficient? A site that is pleasing to the eye will invite you to return. Sites that cause my computer to crash go on the "never visit again" list. I am also not fond of sites that have annoying music that cannot be turned off.

E: Ethical. Is there contact information for the site developer and author? Is there full disclosure of who the author is and the purpose of the site? Is this information easy to find or is it buried deep in the website? There are many commercial services, particularly pharmaceutical companies, that have excellent websites with very useful information. But some of them exist only to sell their product, although this is not immediately evident on evaluation.

D: Date. When was the site last updated? Is it current? Is the information something that needs to be updated regularly? Generally, with health and nursing information, the answer to that last question is yes. I become concerned with sites that have not been updated within 12 to 18 months. The date the site was last updated should be prominently displayed on the site. Keep in mind that different pages within the site may be updated at different times. Be sure to check the date on each of the pages that you visit.

As you become more proficient at website evaluation, you may have additional criteria that you would add to this list or criteria that are important to you for a specific purpose. But

I have found that this simple group of seven has served me well on countless Internet journeys. Test them for yourself. Do a quick search on a topic of interest, visit a number of sites, and determine just how PLEASED you are with what you find.

SUMMARY

Computers have opened a world of information; at the same time, they have given us the responsibility to learn how to use them and use them well. As a nurse, you have the opportunity to specialize in the expanding field of nursing informatics. Within this role, you will provide a vital link between the world of information science and clinical nursing practice. Even if you choose not to specialize in informatics, you will still be using computers on a day-to-day basis and thus must be computer literate. To be computer literate, it is not enough to know how to turn on the computer and to complete a few simple tasks. A nurse must know generalized applications such as word processing, as well as specialized applications such as clinical information systems. The nurse must also know how to access the online world of information and resources and how to critically evaluate the information that is found. None of this is going to change. As the Internet continues to grow and as computers become smaller and more powerful, they will undoubtedly continue to have a major impact on how health is conceptualized and delivered.

Critical Thinking Activities

1. Some institutions are reluctant to issue nursing students passwords to the CIS, fearing that having the students able to access the CIS could compromise its security. Is this a legitimate concern? Do you agree with this position? Why or why not?

2. A lifetime patient record, such as the type envisioned in a CPR, would include all health information from a person's life. Some people have questioned the necessity of this amount of detail. They also are concerned that it will limit the information that a person is able to keep private. Health care providers, on the other hand, argue that they need access to all information to provide appropriate care. Is this always true? Give three examples of health information from the past that might not be relevant to a current problem. What strategies could be used to help patients maintain the privacy of sensitive health data in a lifetime electronic record?

3. A major issue facing the developers of CPR systems is the patient identifier. Some have suggested using a modified version of the social security number; others have advocated developing a unique patient identifier. In your opinion, why is this a major issue? What suggestions do you have for a patient identifier?

4. Go online on the Internet and find four different types of health-related sites on similar topics, including a nurse's personal home page, a patient's home page, one from a pharmaceutical company, and one from a news agency that reports on health. Using the PLEASED criteria, evaluate the sites. Which sites would you return to for professional information? Which sites would you recommend to a patient? Which sites would you never visit again? Discuss your answers.

5. Interview a person who did a major project (e.g., thesis or dissertation) in the "precomputer" days. What resources did the person use to prepare the project? If data needed to be analyzed, how was that done? How did the person write the final version of the project? Would availability of computers have made the project easier? Why or why not?

6. Identify a listserv of interest. Subscribe and "lurk" for 3 to 5 days. What type of information is discussed? How active is the list? Is the information that is provided accurate? What is the signal-to-noise ratio?

REFERENCES

About OncoLink: Philadelphia, December 28, 1999, The Trustees of the University of Pennsylvania, www.oncolink.org/about_oncolink/.

American Nurses' Association: *Scope of practice for nursing informatics,* Washington, DC, 1994, ANA.

American Nurses' Association: *NIDSEC: recognized languages for nursing,* Washington, DC, 2000, ANA, www.nursingworld.org/nidsec/classlst.htm.

American Nurses Credentialing Center: *Statement of philosophy,* Washington, DC, 1993, ANA.

American Nurses Credentialing Center: *Examination results, generalist programs,* Washington, DC, 2000, ANA, www.nursingworld.org/sean/ancc/certify/cert/exams.htm#25.

American Nurses Credentialing Center: Informatics nurse certification: basic eligibility requirements, Washington, DC, 2001, ANA, http://www.nursingworld.org/ancc/certify/cert/catalogs/2000/cbt/infonurs.htm.

Ball MJ, Hannah KJ, Douglas JV: Nursing and informatics. In Ball MJ et al, editors: *Nursing informatics: where caring and technology meet,* ed 3, New York, 2000, Springer-Verlag.

Bareford CG: Community as client: environmental issues in the real world, a SimCity computer simulation, *Computer Nurs* 19(1):11-16, 2001.

Computer-Based Patient Record Institute: *Guidelines for establishing information security policies at organizations using computer-based patient records: work group on confidentiality, privacy and security,* Schaumburg, Ill, 1995, CPRI.

Gassert CA: Academic preparation in nursing informatics. In Ball MJ et al, editors: *Nursing informatics: where caring and technology meet,* ed 3, New York, 2000, Springer-Verlag.

Gorn S: Informatics (computer and information science): its ideology, methodology, and sociology. In Machlup F, Mansfield U, editors: *The study of information: interdisciplinary messages,* New York, 1983, John Wiley & Sons.

Hersher BS: New roles for nurses in healthcare information systems. In Ball MJ et al, editors: *Nursing informatics: where caring and technology meet,* ed 3, New York, 2000, Springer-Verlag.

Hiltzik M: Dealers of lightning: *Xerox PARC and the dawn of the computer age,* New York, 2000, Harper Business.

Jenkins S: Nurses' responsibilities in the implementation of information systems. In Ball MJ et al, editors: *Nursing informatics: where caring and technology meet,* ed 3, New York, 2000, Springer-Verlag.

Joos I et al: *Computers in small bytes: the computer workbook,* ed 2, New York, 1996, National League for Nursing Press.

Lawrence S, Giles CL: Searching the world wide web, *Science* 280:98-100, April 3, 1998.

National Institute of Nursing Research: *Nursing informatics: enhancing patient care,* Bethesda, Md, 1993, US Department of Health and Human Services.

Nelson R, Joos I: Strategies and resources for self-education in nursing informatics. In Arnold JM, Pearson GA, editors: *Computer applications in nursing education and practice,* New York, 1992, National League for Nursing.

Newbold SK: The informatics nurse and the certification process, *Computer Nurs* 14(2):84-85, 88, 1996.

Newbold SK: Update on virtual nursing informatics organizations, *Computer Nurs* 15(3):122-125, 1997.

Newbold SK: Electronic resources for nursing. In Ball MJ et al, editors: *Nursing informatics: where caring and technology meet,* ed 3, New York, 2000, Springer-Verlag.

Nicoll LH: Quick and effective website evaluation, *CIN Plus* 3(3):9, 12, 2000.

Nicoll LH: *Nurses' guide to the Internet,* ed 3, Philadelphia, 2001, JB Lippincott.

Schwirian PM: The NI pyramid—a model for research in nursing informatics, *Computer Nurs* 4(3):134-136, 1986.

Semancik M: *The history of clinical information systems: legacy systems, computer-based patient record and point of care, Clinical Information Systems,* Seattle, 1997, Space-Labs Medical.

Smith DK, Alexander RC: *Fumbling the future: how Xerox invented, then ignored, the first personal computer,* New York, 1988, W. Morrow.

Styles MM: *On specialization in nursing: toward a new empowerment,* Kansas City, Mo, 1989, American Nurses Foundation.

Watts J: The healthy home of the future comes to Japan, *Lancet* 353(9164):1597-1600, 1999.

Weiser M, Brown JS: *The coming age of calm technology,* October 5, 1996, http://www.ubiq.com/hypertext/weiser/acmfuture2endnote.htm.

Year-End 1999 mailbox report, www.messagingonline.net.

15

Alternative Healing

Charlotte Eliopoulos, RNC, MPH, PhD

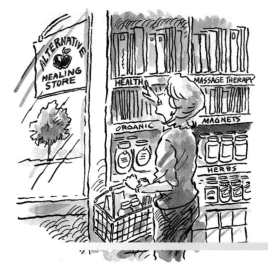

Consumers are seeking natural
remedies; nurses have a responsibility
to be aware of the potential effects.

Vignette

Ruth Jeffers is a registered nurse (RN) who works in a rehabilitation unit of a community hospital. Many of the clients on this unit suffer from chronic musculoskeletal pain. Nurse Jeffers has noted that a growing number of clients offer a history of independently using acupuncture, nutritional supplements, and other alternative healing therapies to improve their symptoms. Although they report beneficial results, most do not advise their physicians that they are using alternative therapies.

Last year, Nurse Jeffers completed a course in the use of therapeutic touch and has used this therapy to promote relaxation and pain control with friends and family with considerable success. She is aware of many positive reports on the benefits of these unconventional approaches. She believes therapeutic touch and some other alternative healing therapies could benefit clients on the rehabilitation unit and informally introduces the topic to the team with whom she works. With the exception of one nurse who states that she believes these therapies are associated with the occult and wants no part of them, the nursing staff is enthusiastic and eager to implement alternative therapies. The physical and occupational therapists believe that alternative therapies could prove helpful to clients but that only therapists within their departments, not nursing, should provide these. The physician on the team opposes the use of all alternative therapies, claiming he "isn't about to put his license on the line for these unproven ideas."

Questions to consider while reading this chapter

1. What is the best course of action for Nurse Jeffers if she really believes that alternative therapies could benefit clients on the unit?

2. What would a hospital need to do to prepare for the inclusion of alternative therapies in its existing services?
3. What are some of the obstacles that could be anticipated when introducing alternative therapies into a conventional setting?
4. What discipline(s) should be responsible for providing and/or coordinating/supervising the practitioners who provide alternative therapies in the hospital?

Key Terms

Complementary and alternative medicine Healing philosophies, practices, and products that fall outside what Western society considers mainstream medicine and that are not typically taught in the educational programs of physicians, nurses, and other health professionals.

Alternative medical systems Acupuncture, anthroposophic, Ayurvedic medicine, community-based health care practices (e.g., Native American, shamans), environmental medicine, homeopathy, naturopathy, traditional Oriental medicine.

Mind/body interventions Aromatherapy, art therapy, biofeedback, dance therapy, hypnosis, imagery, meditation, music therapy, prayer, relaxation, self-help support groups, tai chi, yoga.

Biologically based treatments Herbal therapies, individual and orthomolecular biologic therapies, special diets.

Manipulative and body-based methods Chiropracty, massage and related techniques (e.g., manual lymph drainage, Alexander technique, Feldenkrais method, pressure point therapies, Trager psychophysical integration), osteopathy.

Energy therapies Qigong, reiki, therapeutic touch, bioelectromagnetic-based therapies.

Learning Outcomes

After studying this chapter, the reader will be able to:
1. Describe various complementary and alternative healing practices.
2. Effectively incorporate pertinent alternative therapies into patient care.
3. Provide patient education regarding uses, limitations, and precautions associated with alternative healing practices and products.

CHAPTER OVERVIEW

This chapter presents an overview of complementary and alternative medicine (CAM) and products, which are rapidly gaining in popularity in Western society. As increasing numbers of consumers and clinical settings become interested in and actually use CAM therapies, nurses must become knowledgeable about the uses, limitations, and precautions associated with these new practices and products. Professional nurses have an obligation to understand such practices and products in order to advise patients and effectively incorporate pertinent therapies into the patient's care. Nurses who have knowledge and skills in this area are in key positions to empower patients for self-care that complements traditional medicine.

USE OF ALTERNATIVE HEALING METHODS

CAM includes healing philosophies, practices, and products that fall outside what Western society considers mainstream medicine and that are not typically taught in the educational programs of physicians, nurses, and other health professionals.

The past few decades have witnessed CAM progress from a fringe movement to a highly popular, widely used group of therapies. Recent surveys reveal that more than 4 out of every 10 Americans have visited an alternative health care practitioner and most are paying for these services out of their own pockets (Eisenberg et al., 1998).

Rather than emerging from the leadership of health care professionals, the growing popularity of CAM has been consumer driven. Several factors contribute to consumers' desire for CAM:

- *Dissatisfaction with the conventional health care system.* The impersonal nature of health care has grown with costs. Shorter hospital stays, several months' waiting periods to see a physician, hurried staff that barely have time to provide basic care, and horror stories of the adverse effects of medications are causing consumers to look for alternative approaches that are safer, less costly, and more responsive and personalized than conventional health care.
- *Unwillingness to grin and bear the effects of diseases.* Today's consumers are less willing than their parents to live with symptoms that alter their lifestyles or to passively accept a terminal diagnosis and wait to die. They want options and to be empowered to do everything possible to promote the best possible quality and quantity of their lives, and they are willing to look to alternative healing measures to do so.
- *Shrinking world.* The rapid pace and ease of information sharing has enabled individuals to learn about practices of people throughout the world.
- *Growing evidence of effectiveness.* The body of research supporting the effectiveness of alternative therapies increases almost daily. People are hearing testimonials from friends and family about the way they have been helped by acupuncture, herbs, and other forms of CAM. In addition, the media regularly reports these findings, contributing to consumers' awareness of the body of evidence.

CAM practices and products are consistent with the values, beliefs, and philosophic orientations toward health held by many people (Astin, 1998). With rare exceptions, consumers prefer natural approaches that afford them an active role in their care over high-tech interventions that relegate them to a passive, obedient role. They want to connect with their health care providers, have their individuality recognized, and gain education and skills to effectively make decisions and direct their care. Increasingly consumers are seeking measures to enhance not just their bodies, but also their minds and spirits. The quality of their lives is equally, if not more, important to the quantity of years they live. Consumers often discover that CAM promotes many principles of holistic care that they value, such as individual empowerment, self-care, and a high quality of life.

PRINCIPLES UNDERLYING ALTERNATIVE HEALING

A wide range of healing therapies are encompassed in CAM, yet most share some common principles at their core (Eliopoulos, 1999):

- *The body has the ability to heal itself.* Most conventional medicine works from the premise that the elimination of sickness requires an intervention "done to" the body (e.g., giving medications, surgery). In CAM there is the assumption that the body heals itself. Alternative healing therapies enhance the body's ability to self-heal.
- *Health and healing are related to a harmony of mind, body, and spirit.* The mind, body, and spirit are inseparable; what affects one affects all. Healing and the improvement of health demand that all of the facets of a person be addressed, not merely a single symptom or system.
- *Basic, positive health practices build the foundation for healing.* Good nutrition, exercise, rest, stress management, and avoidance of harmful habits (e.g., smoking) are essential in-

gredients to health maintenance and the improvement of health conditions. Practitioners of healing therapies are more likely than conventional practitioners to look at total lifestyle practices rather than the diseased body part.

■ *Approaches to healing are individualized.* The unique composition and dynamics of each person are recognized in CAM. Practitioners of healing therapies explore the underlying cause of a problem and customize approaches accordingly. It is rare in CAM to find a standing protocol that treats all persons with similar conditions similarly.

■ *Individuals are responsible for their own healing.* People can use a wide range of therapies, from conventional prescription drugs or herbal remedies, to treat illness. However, it is the responsibility of competent adults to seek health advice, make informed choices, gain necessary knowledge and skills for self-care, engage in practices that promote health and healing, and seek help when needed. Clients are responsible for getting their minds, bodies, and spirits in optimal condition to heal rather than look externally for a doctor or nurse to heal them.

A holistic philosophy, promotion of positive health habits, and the client's responsibility for facilitating his or her own health and healing are common threads among healing therapies.

Overview of Popular Alternative Healing Therapies

Hundreds of healing therapies are practiced throughout the world, with varying degrees of evidence to support their effectiveness. As the use of these therapies grew in the United States, the National Institutes of Health (NIH) established the Office of Alternative Medicine in 1992 to evaluate these complementary and alternative practices and products. In 1998 the Office of Alternative Medicine became a freestanding center within NIH and was named the *National Center for Complementary and Alternative Medicine (NCCAM)*. NCCAM has categorized CAM into five fields of practice (Box 15-1); the Center supports research and serves as a clearinghouse for information on alternative practices and products.

Consumers' growing use and the increased integration of CAM therapies into conventional care place a demand on nurses to become familiar with these therapies. Some of the frequently used CAM therapies are discussed below.

BOX 15-1   *Categories of Alternative and Complementary Therapies With Examples*

Alternative medical systems Acupuncture, anthroposophic, Ayurvedic medicine, community-based health care practices (e.g., Native American, shamans), environmental medicine, homeopathy, naturopathy, traditional Oriental medicine

Mind/body interventions Aromatherapy, art therapy, biofeedback, dance therapy, hypnosis, imagery, meditation, music therapy, prayer, relaxation, self-help support groups, t'ai chi, yoga

Biologically based treatments Herbal therapies, individual and orthomolecular biologic therapies, special diets

Manipulative and body based methods Chiropracty, massage and related techniques (e.g., manual lymph drainage, Alexander technique, Feldenkrais method, pressure point therapies, Trager psychophysical integration), osteopathy

Energy therapies Qigong, reiki, therapeutic touch, bioelectromagnetic-based therapies

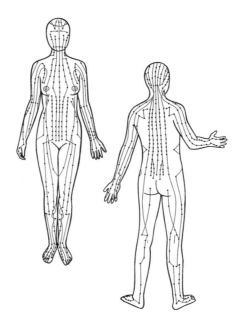

FIG. 15-1 Acupuncture meridians. (From Eliopoulos C: *Integrating alternative and conventional therapies,* St. Louis, 1999, Mosby.)

Acupuncture

Practiced in China for over 2000 years, acupuncture is a major therapy within traditional Chinese medicine. It is based on the belief that there are invisible channels throughout the body called meridians through which energy flows. This energy is called *Qi* (pronounced chee) and is considered the vital life force. It is believed that illness and symptoms develop when the flow of energy becomes blocked or imbalanced. Health is restored when the energy becomes unblocked; this is achieved by stimulating acupuncture points on the meridian(s) affected (Fig. 15-1).

The acupuncturist typically begins the treatment by taking a history, examining the tongue, and evaluating pulses. Based on where the acupuncturist assesses the energy imbalance to be, he or she places needles at specific points. The placement of the needles may have no relationship to the area of the body that is symptomatic. Sometimes the acupuncturist applies heat to the acupoints by burning a dried herb on the top of the needle or skin; this procedure is known as *moxibustion.* Electro-acupuncture, a process in which a small current of electricity is applied to the tip of the needle, is another means of stimulating acupoints.

Pain relief is the most common reason people seek acupuncture treatment, and research supports its effectiveness for this problem. The use of acupuncture for dental pain and chemotherapy-induced nausea and vomiting also has been supported by research. There is some evidence that acupuncture can be of help for nicotine withdrawal, asthma, stroke rehabilitation, carpal tunnel syndrome, and a growing list of other conditions.

Insurance companies vary in their coverage of acupuncture, so it is best for clients to call their individual insurer for determination of benefits. State health departments can be consulted for licensing requirements for acupuncturists in a given state.

TABLE 15-1	*Ayurvedic Metabolic Body Types*
TYPE	**CHARACTERISTICS**
Vata	Unpredictable, moody, vivacious, hyperactive, imaginative, intuitive, impulsive, fluctuating energy levels, slender, prominent features and joints, eats and sleeps at varying times throughout day, prone to insomnia, PMS, cramps, and constipation
Pitta	Predictable, orderly, efficient, perfectionist, intense, passionate, short-tempered, medium build, follows routine schedule, warm skin, prone to heavy perspiration, thirst, acne, ulcers, hemorrhoids, and stomach problems
Kapha	Relaxed, graceful, tendency toward procrastination, affectionate, forgiving, compassionate, sleeps long and deeply, cool, pale and oily skin, eats slowly, prone to high cholesterol, obesity, allergies, sinusitis

Ayurveda

Although it recently has gained popularity because of the writings and lectures of Deepak Chopra (1993), Ayurveda has existed in India for over 5000 years. Ayurveda means "the science of life" and is a system of care that promotes spiritual, mental, and physical balance. Noninvasive approaches are used to achieve balance and include yoga, massage, diet, purification regimens, breathing exercises, meditation, and herbs.

Individuals are believed to have distinct metabolic body types called *doshas, which* are *vata, pitta,* and *kapha* (Table 15-1). Signs of illness occur when the delicate balance of the doshas is disturbed. The treatment to restore balance is influenced by the body type a client possesses and could include:

- Cleansing and detoxification
- Palliation
- Rejuvenation through special herbs and minerals
- Mental hygiene and spiritual healing

Currently there is no process for licensing or certifying Ayurvedic practitioners. As some of the treatments could subject clients to complications (e.g., dehydration from cleansing enemas, herb-drug interactions), finding a reputable trained practitioner is important. The Ayurveda websites listed in Box 15-2 can assist in locating qualified practitioners.

Biofeedback

Biofeedback is a technique in which the client is taught to alter specific bodily functions (e.g., heart rate, blood pressure, muscle tension). The client uses various relaxation and imagery exercises to affect desired responses. Machinery such as electroencephalograms, electromyelograms, and thermistors are used to measure and offer feedback about the function that one is trying to alter. As the client becomes familiar with ways to successfully alter bodily responses, the equipment may no longer be necessary.

There are many conditions for which biofeedback can offer benefit, including urinary incontinence, anxiety, stress, irritable bowel syndrome, neck and back pain, and cardiac arrhythmias.

BOX 15-2	*Helpful Websites*

Acupuncture
American Academy of Medical Acupuncture
www.medicalacupuncture.org

National Commission for the Certification of Acupuncturists
www/acupuncture.com/Refferals/Ref.htm

Ayurveda
Ayurvedic Institute
www.ayurveda.com

Ayurveda Holistic Center
http://ayurvedahc.com/index.htm

Biofeedback
Biofeedback Webzine
www.webideas.com/biofeedback/

Biofeedback Certification Institute
www.bcia.org/

Chiropractic Medicine
American Chiropractic Association
www.amerchiro.org

International Chiropractors' Association
www.chiropractice.org

Dietary Supplements
NIH Health Office of Dietary Supplements
http://dietary-supplements.info.nih.gov/

FDA Guide to Dietary Supplements
www.vm.cfsan.fda.gov/~dms/supplement.html

Herbs
American Botanical Council
www.herbs.org

FDA's website on recent warnings on herbal products
http://www.cfsan.fda.gov/~dms/aems.html

Herb Net
www.herbnet.com

BOX 15-2	*Helpful Websites—cont'd*

Homeopathy
National Center for Homeopathy
www.healthy.net/nch

Hypnotherapy
American Institute of Hypnotherapy
www.hypnosis.com/aih

National Guild of Hypnotists
www.ngh.net

Massage
American Massge Therapy Association
www.amtamassage.org

Naturopathy
American Association of Naturopathic Physicians
www.naturopathic.org

Reflexology
Association of Reflexology
www.reflexology.org

Tai Chi
Qi Journal
www.qi-journal.com/

Touch Therapies
Healing Touch International
www.healingtouch.net

Nurse Healers Professional Associations
www.therapeutic-touch.org

Yoga
American Yoga Association
www.americanyogaasociation.org

Yoga Site
www.yogasite.com

Chiropractic Medicine

Chiropractic medicine is a popular and widely accepted CAM therapy in the United States, perhaps because it was developed and practiced here for over a century. Chiropractors are licensed in every state, and most insurance companies will pay for chiropractic treatments.

Chiropractic medicine is based on the belief that misalignments of the spine, called *subluxations,* put pressure on the nerves leading to pain and disruptions in normal bodily function. The misalignment is treated by manipulation and adjustment of the spine. Typically the chiropractor's hands do the alignment, although increasingly chiropractors are using heat, electrical stimulation, and other treatments.

Dietary Supplements

The past advice that vitamin and mineral supplements are unnecessary if one is eating well has been replaced with the recommendation that everyone should take a daily vitamin and mineral supplement. This shift in thinking has resulted from the realization that many people do not consume the proper nutrients through their diets. Pollutants, stress, and other factors that are more common today than in previous generations heighten the body's need for added protection. Also, unlike our ancestors who consumed produce that was picked the same day, we tend to eat more processed foods and produce that could have been in transit for several days before reaching us; therefore the foods we consume contain fewer vitamins and minerals. In fact, the Recommended Daily Allowances (RDAs) for vitamins and minerals are being reevaluated and increased.

Specific dietary supplements are believed to be beneficial for specific health conditions (e.g., vitamin E to improve arthritis and heart disease). However, too much of a good thing could prove harmful, as high doses of vitamins and minerals can lead to serious complications. For example, high doses of folic acid can mask a vitamin B_{12} deficiency (a cause of dementia), and calcium in excess of 2500 mg/day can cause kidney stones and impair the body's ability to absorb other minerals.

Herbs

Plants have been used for medicinal purposes for nearly as long as humans have inhabited the earth. Botanical medicine was a mainstream practice in the United States until the early nineteenth century, when medicine's shift toward a more scientific approach caused drugs to be viewed more favorably than herbs. But in the 1960s when the movement toward natural health began to swell, interest in herbal products increased. The use and sales of herbal remedies have grown significantly since.

In reality, herbs are not that foreign to conventional medicine. Thirty percent of all modern drugs are derived from plants (Kleiner, 1995), including:

- Atropine from atropa belladona.
- Digoxin from digitalis purpurea.
- Ipecac from Cephaelis ipecacuanha.
- Reserpine from Rauwolfia serpentina.

With more than 20,000 herbs and related products on the market (Herbal roulette, 1995) staying current of uses, dosage, interactions, and adverse effects is a near impossibility. Nurses would be wise to become familiar with some of the most commonly used herbs (Box 15-3) and know where to obtain information on other herbs when needed (see Box 15-2). Because of consumers' widespread use of herbs, questions regarding use of all supplements and education to ensure safe use are significant nursing responsibilities.

BOX 15-3 *Facts About Commonly Used Herbs*

Chamomile

Uses: sedative effect, calm upset digestive tract

Cautions: because it contains coumarin it could affect coagulation, although clinical studies have not proven this to date; if client is using an anticoagulant and chamomile, monitor

Echinacea

Uses: antimicrobial; stimulates immune system; useful in prevention and treatment of upper respiratory infections

Cautions: some persons with ragweed and other environmental allergies may have sensitivity; although immunosuppressive effects with long-term use are inconclusive at present, best to limit to short-term use

Feverfew

Use: relief of migraines

Cautions: contraindicated for clients with allergies to ragweed and other members of Compositae family; can affect coagulation so contraindicated in persons on anticoagulant therapy

Garlic

Uses: lowers blood pressure; reduces "bad" cholesterol; stimulates immune system; cancer preventive; antioxidant

Cautions: close monitoring necessary if taken by person using anticoagulant as it can prolong bleeding time; can potentiate action of hypoglycemic drugs

Ginger

Use: antiemetic

Caution: regular use can prolong bleeding time, monitor if used with an anticoagulant

Ginkgo biloba

Use: improves cognitive performance in persons with dementia

Cautions: close monitoring necessary if taken by person using anticoagulant as it can prolong bleeding time; can reduce effectiveness of anticonvulsants

Ginseng

Uses: improves resistance to stress, immune stimulant; general stimulant

Cautions: raises blood pressure; close monitoring necessary if taken by person using anticoagulant as it can prolong bleeding time; may increase digoxin levels; contraindicated when other stimulants are used; can cause insomnia, headache, epistaxis, vomiting

Saw palmetto

Uses: improve symptoms with benign prostatic hypertrophy; diuretic; urinary antiseptic

Caution: do not take with hormonal therapies

St. John wort

Uses: antidepressant; antianxiety

Cautions: can cause photosensitivity, particularly in fair-skinned individuals; contraindicated when other antidepressants are used

Valerian

Use: sedative

Caution: do not use with barbiturates

Homeopathy

Homeopathy is a branch of medicine developed in the late eighteenth century by Samuel Hahnemann. It was widely practiced in the United States until the early 1900s when modern (i.e., conventional) medicine discredited it as being unscientific and ineffective. Homeopathy remained popular in other parts of the world, however, and recently has become popular again in our country.

The origin of the word homeopathy helps to understand this therapy. In Greek the word *homios* means similar, and *pathos* means suffering. The foundation of homeopathy is the *Law of Similars* and builds on the belief that remedies are prescribed that produce symptoms similar to those of the illness being treated. Before judging this theory to be outrageous, it should be noted that this is the same principle on which vaccines are based. In homeopathy a dilute preparation is made from a plant or other biologic material; the more dilute the preparation, the higher its potency. The solution typically is added to a sugar tablet or powder for oral use or to a lotion or ointment for external use.

The *Law of Cure* in homeopathy is used to evaluate the effectiveness of a remedy. If the treatment is successful, symptoms should travel from vital to less vital organs of the body, move from within the body outward, and disappear in reverse order of appearance. If symptoms do not follow this sequence, a new or additional treatment is used. In homeopathic medicine a worsening of symptoms after a remedy is given is considered a positive sign that healing is taking place.

Although the reason for their effectiveness is not fully understood, homeopathic remedies have been shown to be effective for a variety of conditions; some of the most common conditions for which people use homeopathic medicine are listed in Box 15-4.

The ideal way to use homeopathic remedies is to have a homeopath prescribe a customized remedy based on individual characteristics and symptoms. However, homeopathic practitioners are not plentiful, so the next best thing is to buy over-the-counter preparations that are labeled for their intended purpose (e.g., arthritis, headache, hayfever, cold).

BOX 15-4	*Ten Most Common Conditions For Which People Use Homeopathic Medicine*

Asthma
Depression
Otitis media
Allergic rhinitis
Headache/migraine
Neurotic disorders
Allergy (nonspecific)
Dermatitis
Arthritis
Hypertension

From Jacobs J, Chapman EH, Crothers D: Patient characteristics and practice patterns of physicians using homeopathy. In Fontanarosa PB, editor: *Alternative medicine: an objective assessment,* Dover, Del, 2000, American Medical Association, pp 422-426.

Hypnotherapy

Although the use of trance states for healing purposes dates back to primitive cultures, hypnotherapy was not approved as a valid medical treatment until the 1950s. This mind-body therapy is now widely and successfully used for a wide range of conditions, including chronic pain, migraines, asthma, smoking cessation, and irritable bowel syndrome.

The process of hypnosis begins by the therapist guiding the client into a relaxed state and then creating an image that focuses attention to the specific symptom or problem that needs to be improved. The client must be in a state of deep relaxation to be receptive to a posthypnotic suggestion. Most people are capable of being hypnotized if they are willing.

Imagery

Imagery is the process of creating an image in the mind that can cause a specific bodily response. Although imagery is used in hypnosis, in hypnosis an image and suggestion are presented to the person, whereas in imagery the person creates an image on his or her own. The process of imagery begins by the client establishing a desired outcome (e.g., to relieve stress, enhance circulation, reduce blood pressure). The nurse or other practitioner assists the client in creating an image that helps to achieve the outcome (e.g., the nurse may describe how the blood circulates through the body, help the client develop an image of how cancer cells can be eliminated, or suggest that the client think of a peaceful place where cares can melt away), and guides the client in reaching a relaxed state. In addition to having someone guide him or her through an imagery exercise, a client can learn the process from books or use commercially prepared audiotapes.

Imagery is not a difficult mind-body healing therapy to master and can be easily implemented in virtually every practice setting.

Magnet Therapy

Although a mainstream therapy in Germany and Japan, magnets have only recently become popular in the United States. The major uses of magnet therapy are for pain and wound healing.

The mechanism by which magnets work is not completely understood and is being investigated at present. It is believed that magnets relieve pain by creating a slight electrical current that stimulates the nervous system and consequently blocks nerve sensations. Magnets are hypothesized to speed wound healing by dilating vessels and increasing circulation to an area. Distributors of magnet products make additional claims about the health benefits of magnets, ranging from improving attention deficit disorder to boosting the immune system, although these benefits are yet to be proven.

Magnets come in a variety of forms, strengths, and prices. There are magnet disks that can be strapped to limbs, magnet mattresses that one can sleep on, and magnet jewelry. To be effective for therapeutic purposes, the magnet should be at least 500 Gauss (which is about eight times stronger than the magnets used for attaching things to your refrigerator door).

Persons with pacemakers should not use magnets, and they should not be applied to the abdomen of a pregnant woman.

Massage, Bodywork, and Touch Therapies

Massage for healing purposes has been used for thousands of years to maintain health. Many people today receive regular massages as an important component of their self-care to aid in stress management. In addition to promoting relaxation, massage can be beneficial for reducing edema, promoting circulation and respirations, and relieving pain, anxiety, and depression.

Massage is the manipulation of soft tissue by rubbing, kneading, rolling, pressing, slapping, and tapping movements. The term *bodywork* is applied to the combination of massage with deep tissue manipulation, movement awareness, and energy balancing. Touch therapies include techniques in which the hands of the nurse/therapist are near the body, in the client's energy field. Examples of various types of massage, bodywork, and touch therapies are described in Box 15-5.

Because therapeutic touch (TT) is a popular alternative healing therapy among nurses, it deserves some discussion. TT became popular in nursing in the 1970s with the work and research of Delores Krieger (Krieger, 1979; 1997). Krieger advanced the theory that people are energy fields and that obstructed energy could be responsible for unhealthy states. She proposed that the nurse could draw on the universal field of energy and transfer this energy to the client. This incoming energy could help the client mobilize his or her own inner resources for healing and help unblock the client's obstructed energy.

BOX 15-5 *Types of Massage, Bodywork, and Touch Therapies*

Alexander technique
Teaches improved balanced, posture, and coordination by using gentle hands-on guidance and verbal instruction

Feldenkrais method
Teaches movement reeducation using gentle manipulations to heighten awareness of the body; believes each person has an individualized optimum style of movement

Healing touch
A multilevel energy healing program that incorporates aspects of therapeutic touch with other healing measures

Reflexology
Application of pressure to pressure points on the hands and feet that correspond to various parts of the body

Reiki
A therapy that uses techniques to direct universal life energy to specific sites

Rolfing (structural integration)
Use of manual manipulation and stretching of body's fascial tissues to establish balance and symmetry

Swedish massage
Most prevalent form of massage that uses long strokes, friction, and kneading of muscles

Trager approach
Use of gentle, rhythmic rocking and touch to promote relaxation and energy flow

In TT there is little direct physical contact between the practitioner and the individual being treated. Rather, TT is an energy-based therapy; the nurse enters the client's energy field to assess and treat energy imbalances.

In the first step of TT, the nurse centers herself or himself and focuses on the intent to heal (this is sometimes referred to as healing meditation). During this phase the nurse quiets the mind and prepares physically and psychologically to connect with the client. This is considered a crucial step in the process to enable the nurse to be fully present in the moment with the client. This is followed by the nurse passing his or her hands over the client's body to assess the energy field and mobilizing areas in which energy is blocked or sluggish by directing energies to that area. TT is used to reduce anxiety, relieve pain, and enhance immune function.

Meditation and Progressive Relaxation

Meditation, the act of focusing on the present moment, has been used for centuries throughout the world. This practice gained considerable attention in the United States in the 1970s when Harvard Medical School cardiologist Herbert Benson published research on the "Relaxation Response" (Benson and Beary, 1974). Benson reported that after 20 minutes of meditation, participants' heart rate, respirations, blood pressure, oxygen consumption, carbon dioxide production, and serum lactic acid levels decreased. This led to meditation being used for a variety of conditions, including stress, anxiety, pain, and high blood pressure.

Progressive relaxation is another exercise that shares some of the same benefits as meditation. Typically a person learns to guide himself or herself through a series of exercises that relax the body, such as tightening and relaxing various muscle groups. Many audiotapes are available in bookstores and health food stores that offer scripts to guide meditation and progressive relaxation exercises.

Naturopathy

An intense interest in natural cures in Europe during the nineteenth century led to the development of spas that offered natural treatments to promote health and healing. Soon the movement spread to the United States, and in 1896 the American School of Naturopathy was founded. Naturopathic physicians and treatment facilities using natural cures became popular in the early part of the twentieth century. For example, John Kellogg ran such a facility in Battle Creek in which he became famous for the natural breakfast cereals that he used. As time progressed, medications and high-tech interventions caused naturopathy to pale by comparison; however, as consumers are seeking approaches that are more natural, this form of alternative medicine is making a comeback.

Naturopathy is built on the principle that the body has inherent healing abilities that can be stimulated to treat disease. Naturopathic doctors assess and treat the cause of the disease rather than merely alleviate symptoms. They help clients identify unhealthy practices, encourage healthy lifestyle habits, and guide them in managing health problems using natural approaches such as herbs, homeopathic remedies, diet modifications, dietary supplements, and exercise.

There are a limited number of accredited schools of naturopathic medicine (e.g., Bastyr University, Southwest College of Naturopathic Medicine and Health Sciences, and National College of Naturopathic Medicine). A handful of states license naturopaths and require that they must have graduated from an accredited program. However, there are many individuals practicing as naturopaths who have obtained their education and experience through other means or who practice in states that do not require licensure; thus learning about the credentials of naturopath before receiving services is beneficial for clients.

Prayer and Faith

Many people consider their faith to be an integral part of their total being rather than a therapy, but now there is scientific evidence supporting the therapeutic benefits of faith and prayer in health and healing. Hundreds of well-conducted studies have revealed that people who profess a faith, pray, and attend religious services are healthier, live longer, have lower rates of disability, recover faster, have lower rates of emotional disorders, and otherwise enjoy better health states than those who do not (Larson, Sawyers, and McCullough, 1998). Not only do the faith and religious practices of individuals themselves affect health and healing, but research also supports the benefit of intercessory prayer.

Nurses need to appreciate that most people believe in the healing power of prayer and think that their health care providers should join them in prayer if requested. This does not suggest that nurses or other health professionals should be forced into prayer if it is contrary to their beliefs; but rather, if there is no objection from either party, prayer by the client and health care provider can be used as a valuable healing measure.

Tai Chi

Tai chi is another practice from Traditional Chinese Medicine that is used to stimulate the flow of *Qi,* the life energy. It is a combination of exercise and energy work that looks like a slow, graceful dance using continuous, controlled movements of the arms and legs. There is a specific sequence of steps to follow in doing tai chi, but fortunately there are many inexpensive videos that can be used, in addition to classes that are offered to aid people in learning this practice.

Tai chi has some proven benefits, including reducing falls and improving coordination in older adults (Province, 1995) and improving function in persons with arthritis (Horstman, 1999). Many people find that tai chi helps to reduce stress and promote a general sense of well-being.

Yoga

Yoga has changed from a mystical form of Hindu worship practiced more than 5000 years ago to what is now known as a system of exercises involving various postures, meditation, and deep breathing. The word *yoga* means union; union of body, mind, and spirit is achieved through yoga. This exercise has been found helpful for pain, anxiety, stress, high blood pressure, poor circulation, respiratory and digestive disorders, and carpal tunnel syndrome (Garfinkel et al., 2000). Yoga can be adapted to any level and capability so it can be easily used.

There are many other alternative healing modalities and new ones appearing with regularity. Some may be safe and effective but lack sufficient experience or clinical research to support their claims; others may be worthless and merely an attempt to sell a product or service. Discretion is needed. Assistance in gaining objective information regarding CAM therapies can be obtained from the National Center for Complementary and Alternative Medicine at 888-644-6226, nccam.nih.gov/.

NURSING AND COMPLEMENTARY AND ALTERNATIVE MEDICINE THERAPIES
A Holistic Approach

The use of natural or "alternative" healing measures is hardly new to nursing. From Florence Nightingale (1860) who wrote about the importance of creating an environment in which natural healing could occur through contemporary nurse theorists who discuss human and environmental energy fields (Rogers, 1970), nurses have long realized that healing quite ef-

BOX 15-6	*Beliefs Guiding Holistic Nursing Practice*

- The uniqueness of each individual is honored.
- Health is a harmonious balance of body, mind, and spirit.
- The needs of individuals' bodies, minds, and spirits are assessed and addressed in the caregiving process.
- Health and disease are natural parts of the human experience.
- Disease is an opportunity for increased awareness of the interconnectiveness of body, mind, and spirit.
- Individuals have the capacity for self-healing; the nurse facilitates this process.
- Nurses empower individuals for self-care.
- Individuals' cultural values, beliefs, and practices are honored and incorporated into the caregiving process.
- Individuals have a dynamic relationship with their environment; the environment is part of the healing process.
- Nurses, through their presence and being, are tools of the healing process.
- Nurses engage in self-care and an ongoing process of unfolding inner wisdom.

Nurses can learn about holistic nursing and network with holistic nurses through involvement in the American Holistic Nurses' Association; learn more by visiting the AHNA website at www.ahna.org.

fectively occurs in ways not encompassed within the conventional biomedical system. Nursing also has promoted many of the same principles evident in CAM, particularly care of the body, mind, and spirit. In fact, this is what holistic nursing is all about (Box 15-6). Nurses must ensure that the integration of CAM into their practice is done within a holistic paradigm to truly make them healing therapies and not merely disconnected procedures within an already fragmented health care system.

Facilitating Clients' Use of Complementary and Alternative Medicine

Nurses need to incorporate CAM into their nursing practice. This begins during the assessment process by exploring clients' use of CAM practices and products. As it is not unusual for clients to use these without the knowledge of their physicians, nurses may be the first health professional with whom clients have discussed this issue. Factors to assess include:

- CAM practices and products being used and their sources.
- Appropriateness of use of CAM practices and products.
- Side effects and risks associated with use of CAM.
- Conditions for which CAM currently is not used that could benefit by its use.

Through the assessment process nurses may identify the need to educate clients about the appropriateness of the CAM products and practices they are using. For example, a client with a pacemaker who uses magnets needs to be advised against continuing this practice; likewise, a client drinking ginseng tea at bedtime requires an explanation that his insomnia may be the result of the stimulant effects of the herb.

There may be situations in which nurses identify that specific conditions could benefit from the use of CAM therapies. As client advocates, nurses would bring this to the attention of the physician and other members of the health care team and make recommendations accordingly.

Nurses traditionally have been responsible for the coordination of client care. As CAM therapies are integrated into conventional care, nurses are the logical professional discipline to oversee the various parts and ensure that they are working in harmony for the client's benefit.

Nurses can learn to use many alternative healing measures to enhance nursing care. Among these are acupressure, aromatherapy, biofeedback, imagery, massage, and therapeutic touch. Nurses should seek whatever additional education and training required to gain competency in these therapies and ensure compliance with state licensing laws.

Integrating Complementary and Alternative Medicine Into Conventional Settings

Nursing leadership can be exercised in helping conventional clinical settings integrate CAM therapies. In fact, nursing's holistic orientation and traditional coordination responsibilities make nurses logical for this role. Let us look at the way in which one nurse accomplished this.

Becky Blake recently joined the nursing staff in a combined coronary care/step-down unit. It did not take her long to note the expert technical skill of her colleagues who could read monitors in a flash and respond to emergencies without missing a beat. The skill, efficiency, and organization of the nursing staff were evidenced by the lack of medication errors, infections, and pressure ulcers, coupled with the lowest length of stays of comparable hospital units in the area.

Yet there seemed to be something missing. Clients and their families often showed signs of anxiety and fear that were not addressed. Familiar faces reappeared as some clients were readmitted because they failed to alter lifestyle habits that contributed to their conditions. The same nursing staff who cared for people with hearts damaged by the effects of smoking, poor diet, and stress were guilty of the same practices themselves.

It came to a head for Nurse Blake one morning when she was at a bedside changing an intravenous bag and checking equipment. The client, a man in his 50s, pulled at her arm, looked Nurse Blake in the eyes, and tearfully said, "How do you think I'm going to do? I've been awake all night wondering if I'll be able to do my job, take care of my wife, see my grandkids grow up, do the things I like to do." For the first time, Nurse Blake saw beyond the body in the bed to a human being experiencing considerable emotional distress—distress that was hardly beneficial to his condition. We've managed to get this man's heart repaired, she thought, but we haven't begun to help him heal the emotional and spiritual pain that this illness created. This began a journey for Nurse Blake of discovering measures to help clients that went beyond the conventional treatments that were regularly prescribed.

Nurse Blake located a local network of holistic nurses and began attending their meetings. Through this group she learned of the difference between healing and curing and the importance of addressing the needs of body, mind, and spirit. She also heard nurses discussing their own need to be nurtured and committed to positive self-care practices. She met nurses who shared how they were using alternative healing practices and who led her to resources from which she could learn more.

Within the months that followed, Nurse Blake attended several workshops and learned how progressive relaxation, meditation, therapeutic touch, and aromatherapy could be used to benefit the clients on her unit. As her understanding of holism grew, she recognized that stress reduction and improved health habits of her co-workers were sorely needed.

After planting seeds through informal discussions and sharing of articles, Nurse Blake requested a formal meeting with the transdisciplinary team on the unit. In this meeting she described her areas of concern, which included the need to:

- Address clients' emotional and spiritual needs more effectively.
- Promote improved health habits of the staff.
- Develop practices that would reduce stress for clients, their families, and staff.

The staff concurred with these needs and expressed a desire to take actions to address them. Nurse Blake offered some suggestions:

- Coordinate with the staff development instructor to have classes offered on progressive relaxation, imagery, meditation, therapeutic touch, and stress reduction

- Form an ad hoc committee to develop guidelines, policies, and procedures on how these healing therapies could be safely and legally implemented.
- Begin to include healing therapies into the care plans.
- Arrange for the nutritionist to offer classes to staff on healthy eating.
- Add healthy snacks to the break room.
- Coordinate with the housekeeping and maintenance departments to introduce aromatherapy diffusers, plants, and piped-in music in the unit.
- Develop a system to remind staff to use stress reduction measures throughout their shift.
- Collaborate with the nutritionist, social worker, spiritual care counselor, and nursing clinical resources to provide group sessions for clients and their families on topics such as coping with illness, stress management, promoting healthy lifestyle habits.
- Request the quality improvement coordinator to monitor and evaluate the impact of these interventions.

It did not take long for the effects of these new approaches to be realized. Clients requested fewer sedatives and analgesics. Surveys of clients and families revealed higher levels of satisfaction. Staff sick days were reduced, and there seemed to be a greater sense of team spirit and cooperation. Soon staff in other parts of the hospital began requesting that similar interventions be implemented in their units.

Using Complementary and Alternative Medicine Competently

As increasing numbers of consumers and clinical settings are interested in or actually using CAM therapies, nurses are challenged to become knowledgeable about the uses, limitations, and precautions associated with these new practices and products. Maintaining a resource library and becoming familiar with websites to stay current are beneficial.

Nurses must become familiar with cultural factors that can influence acceptance and use of alternative healing practices. For instance, some individuals may object to therapeutic touch on the grounds that they associate it with occult practices, or they may have anxiety about meditation because they believe evil spirits could invade their minds. As comforting as a massage can be, some people who come from cultures that believe it is inappropriate for someone to touch someone of the opposite sex could become distressed with this measure. Knowledge and sensitivity to personal and cultural preferences are essential.

Legal Considerations

The use of CAM practices could present some legal issues for which nurses need to be concerned. As growing numbers of practitioners of healing therapies advocate for recognition and separate licensure, some of the healing therapies once considered part of nursing care may require separate licensure. Such is the case with massage. In some states nurses may not provide a massage unless they are licensed as massage therapists. Acupressure and biofeedback are among the other areas in which the nurse could be challenged if not licensed. Nurses need to clarify the therapies that fall within the realm of nursing practice and take a proactive role in ensuring that other disciplines do not attempt to limit them.

Another legal concern for nurses in the growing arena of CAM is the question of to whom the nurse is responsible when practicing CAM therapies. New, nonconventional practice settings are developing. For example, a nurse may be employed in a setting in which there is an acupuncturist, hypnotherapist, and homeopath. Among the questions that could arise are: *Who supervises the nurse? Can these therapists delegate responsibilities to the nurse? How does the nurse ensure that in such a practice setting diagnoses are not being made and treatments prescribed that are beyond the scope of the CAM practitioners?* Nurses need to begin to consider the implications of new practice models and develop clear practice guidelines that ensure a legally sound practice.

SUMMARY

An opportunity exists for nursing to demonstrate leadership in the integration of CAM with conventional care. Representing the largest number of health care professionals, nurses can have a significant impact on implementing CAM throughout the health care system. Nurses' historical holistic orientation to care enables them to ensure that the integration of CAM and conventional services is done in a manner that addresses the client's body, mind, and spirit. Without such coordinated efforts there is the risk that these new therapies will merely be additional ingredients of a fragmented system of care. Nurses have proven that they can coordinate and promote comprehensive care like no other discipline. Therefore nursing is the logical discipline to be the hub of the wheel of integrative services.

Critical Thinking Activities

1. Develop a care plan that integrates alternative healing therapies with conventional ones for a client who is experiencing pain.
2. Describe some potential constraints to integrating alternative healing measures into practice.
3. List risks and opportunities to nurses as they use alternative healing measures.
4. Describe alternative healing measures that nurses can use as part of their own self-care.

REFERENCES

Astin JA: Why patients use alternative medicine: results of a national study, *JAMA* 279(19):1548-1553, 1998.

Benson H, Beary JZ: The relaxation response, *Psychiatry* 37:37-46, 1974.

Chopra D: *Ageless body, timeless mind,* New York, 1993, Harmony Books.

Eisenberg DM et al: Trends in alternative medicine use in the United States, 1990-1997: results of a follow-up national survey, *JAMA* 280(18):1569-1575, 1998.

Eliopoulos C: *Integrating conventional and alternative therapies: holistic care for chronic conditions,* St Louis, 1999, Mosby.

Garfinkel MS et al: Yoga-based intervention for carpal tunnel syndrome. In Fontanarosa PB, editor: *Alternative medicine: an objective assessment,* Dover, Del, 2000, American Medical Association.

Herbal roulette, *Consumer Reports,* November, 1995, pp 698-705.

Horstman J: *The Arthritis Foundation's guide to alternative therapies,* Atlanta, 1999, Arthritis Foundation.

Kleiner SM: The true nature of herbs, *Phys Sports Med* 23:13-14, 1995.

Krieger D: *The therapeutic touch,* Englewood Cliffs, NJ, 1979, Prentice-Hall.

Krieger D: *Therapeutic touch inner workbook,* Santa Fe, NM, 1997, Bear & Co.

Larson DB, Sawyers JP, McCullough ME, editors: *Scientific research on spirituality and health: a report based on the Scientific Progress in Spirituality Conferences,* Rockville, Md, 1998, National Institute for Healthcare Research.

Nightingale F: *Notes on nursing,* London, 1860, Harrison.

Province MA: The effects of exercise on falls in elderly patients, *JAMA* 273(17):1341-1347, 1995.

Rogers M: *The theoretical basis for nursing,* Philadelphia, 1970, FA Davis.

Nursing Leadership and Management

Barbara Cherry, MSN, MBA, RN

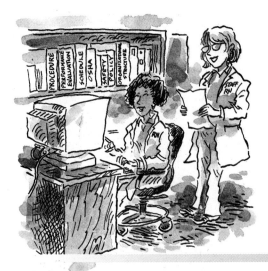

As a manager, the nurse will coordinate many aspects of care delivery.

Vignette

Nancy Brown, a new registered nurse (RN), has accepted a position in a busy outpatient dialysis unit. During nursing school Nancy worked in the facility as a patient care technician and is confident in her clinical skills because of this previous experience. The nurse manager of the dialysis unit has scheduled Nancy to attend the new-nurse orientation. Although Nancy thought to herself, "I know what the RNs do around here, I'd like to jump right in without attending orientation," she accepted the assignment.

The nurse manager began the orientation program with a discussion about the mission of the organization and the RN's responsibility to ensure that quality patient care is provided in a safe and cost-effective manner. As Nancy progressed through the orientation program, her confidence quickly faded. Nancy became overwhelmed as she listened to a description of her new responsibilities as an RN. The RN's duties involved much more than the expected physical assessment, identifying nursing diagnoses, and developing and implementing care plans. Some of Nancy's many new responsibilities as a staff RN were to:

- Supervise patient care technicians and manage the task assignments and use of supplies for a group of patients.
- Meet with the social worker, dietitian, nephrologist, nurse manager, and the patient and family to develop the patient's transdisciplinary care plan and then follow up to coordinate and implement the plan of care.

■ Serve on a task force whose goal is to develop and implement a new training and mentoring program for patient care technicians.

■ Perform chart audits to review patient education documentation, identify problems, develop recommendations, and report to the quality management committee.

As Nancy was trying to assimilate the information being presented, she almost failed to hear the nurse manager say that within 6 months of employment all staff RNs would be expected to begin orientation for the charge nurse position to provide back-up coverage. At the end of the orientation, Nancy had a new perspective about professional nursing practice—it seemed to be more about managing the delivery of patient care than actually giving the care!

Questions to consider while reading this chapter

1. What leadership and management skills will assist Nancy as she begins her new role as a staff RN responsible for supervising a group of patient care technicians, managing supply usage, and serving on a task force to implement a new training program?

2. Why is it important for the nursing staff to understand the mission and values of the organization in order to provide direct patient care?

3. What type of team building skills will help Nancy as she learns to work with the transdisciplinary team and coordinate the patient's plan of care with a diverse group of health professionals?

4. What resources are available to help Nancy learn and enhance her management and leadership skills?

Key Terms

Budget Financial plan for the allocation of the organization's resources (money) and a control document to ensure that resource utilization adheres to the plan.

External customers People in need of services from an organization who are not employed by the organization and include patients, families members, physicians, students, payers, and other facilities that are a source of patient referrals.

Health care organization Any business, company, institution, or facility (e.g., hospital, home health agency, ambulatory care clinic, health insurance company, nursing home) engaged in providing health care services or products.

Internal customers People who are employed by the organization to provide services to various groups and individuals across the organization (e.g., nurses and other patient care staff, administrators, social workers, dietitians, therapists, housekeeping staff, clerical support staff).

Leadership Guiding or influencing people to achieve desired outcomes; occurs any time a person attempts to influence the beliefs, opinions, or behaviors of an individual or group (Hersey and Blanchard, 1988).

Management Coordination of resources such as time, people, and supplies to achieve outcomes; involves problem-solving and decision-making processes.

Organizational chart Provides a visual picture of the organization and identifies lines of communication and authority.

Productivity The amount of outputs or work produced (i.e., home visits made) through the use of a specific amount of input or resources (i.e., nursing hours worked).

Resources Personnel, time, and supplies needed to accomplish the goals of the organization.

Learning Outcomes

After studying this chapter, the reader will be able to:

1. Relate leadership and management theory to nursing leadership and management activities.
2. Differentiate among the five functions of management and the essential activities related to each function.
3. Integrate principles of the customer service role in professional nursing practice.
4. Implement effective team-building skills as an essential component of nursing practice.
5. Implement the nursing process as a method of problem solving and planning.
6. Apply principles and strategies of change theory in the management role.
7. Integrate knowledge of human behavior and conceptual and technical skills into the role of the nurse leader and manager.

CHAPTER OVERVIEW

During nursing school students are often more concerned with learning and developing clinical knowledge and skills and less concerned with management and leadership skills. However, immediately after graduation the new nurse is placed in many situations that require leadership and management skills—managing a group of assigned patients, serving on a task force or committee, acting as team leader or charge nurse, or supervising unlicensed assistive personnel and licensed vocational/practical nurses. In addition to providing excellent clinical care, the challenges for RNs in the twenty-first century are to manage nursing units that are constantly admitting and discharging higher-acuity patients, motivating and coordinating a variety of diverse health professionals and nonprofessionals, and managing limited resources and shrinking budgets (Belcher, 2000).

Regardless of what position the nurse has or in which area the nurse is employed, the health care organization will expect the professional nurse to have leadership and management skills. Professional nurses in each employment setting are expected to:

- Make good clinical decisions based on quality, cost, legal, and ethical aspects of care.
- Make good business decisions based on the organization's goals.
- Coordinate patient care activities for the transdisciplinary team.
- Promote staff satisfaction, patient satisfaction, and overall unit productivity.
- Provide leadership to maintain compliance with governmental regulations and accreditation standards.

As the reader can easily visualize, leadership and management activities are a primary responsibility for the RN. In fact, it has been suggested that the activities of a professional nurse within the health care organization have more to do with managing the delivery of care rather than actually providing that care (Norman, 1997). This chapter presents key leadership and management concepts that will guide the professional nurse in meeting the employing organization's expectations.

Throughout this chapter the term *organization* is used to refer to the hospital, home health agency, postacute facility, long-term care facility, ambulatory clinic, managed care company, or any other area in which a nurse might be employed to practice professional nursing. Legal and ethical issues are a critical component of nursing management, although it is not within the scope of this chapter to discuss these issues. The reader is encouraged to review Chapter 8 regarding legal issues and Chapter 9 regarding ethical issues.

LEADERSHIP AND MANAGEMENT DEFINED AND DISTINGUISHED
Leadership Defined

Leadership occurs any time a person attempts to influence the beliefs, opinions, or behaviors of a person or group (Hersey and Blanchard, 1988). Leadership is a combination of intrinsic personality traits, learned leadership skills, and characteristics of the situation. The function of a leader is to guide people and groups to accomplish common goals. For example, an effective nurse leader is able to inspire others on the health care team to make patient education an important aspect of all care activities.

It is important to note that leaders may not have formal authority granted by the organization but are still able to influence others. "A job title alone does not make a person a leader. Only a person's behavior determines if he or she occupies a leadership position" (Marquis and Huston, 2000, p. 4). Leadership ability may be related to qualities such as unique personality characteristics, exceptional clinical expertise, or relationships with others in the organization.

Management Defined

Management refers to the activities involved in coordinating people, time, and supplies to achieve desired outcomes; it involves problem-solving and decision-making processes. Managers maintain control of the day-to-day operations of a defined area of responsibility to achieve established goals and objectives. Managers plan and organize what is to be done, who is to do it, and how it is to be done. A nurse manager will have:

- An appointed management position within the organization with responsibilities to perform administrative tasks such as planning staffing requirements, performing employee performance appraisals, controlling use of supplies and time, and meeting budget and productivity goals.
- A formal line of authority and accountability to ensure that safe and effective patient care is delivered in a manner that meets the organization's goals and standards.

Leadership vs. Management

Although leadership and management are intertwined concepts and it is difficult to discuss one without the other, these concepts are different. Leadership is the ability to guide or influence others, whereas management is the coordination of resources (time, people, supplies) to achieve outcomes. People are led, whereas activities and things are managed. Leaders are able to motivate and inspire others, whereas managers have assigned responsibility for accomplishing the goals of an organization. A good manager also should be a good leader, but this may not always be the case. A person with good management skills may not have leadership ability. Similarly, a person with leadership abilities may not have good management skills. Leadership and management skills are complementary; both can be learned and developed through experience, and improving skills in one area will enhance abilities in the other.

Power and Authority

Leadership and management require power and authority to motivate people to act in a certain way. Authority is the legitimate right to direct others and is given to a person by the organization through an authorized position such as nurse manager. For example, a nurse manager has the authority to direct staff nurses to work a specific schedule. Whereas authority is the formal right to direct others granted by the organization, power is the ability to motivate people to get things done with or without the formal right granted by the organization. Power originates from several sources as defined by Marriner-Tomey (2000):

1. *Reward power* comes from the ability to reward others for complying and may include such rewards as money, desired assignments, or the acknowledgment of accomplishments.

2. *Coercive power,* the opposite of reward power, is based on fear of punishment for failure to comply. Sources of coercive power include withheld pay increases, undesired assignments, verbal and written warnings, and termination.

3. *Legitimate power* is based on an official position in the organization. Through legitimate power, the manager has the right to influence staff members, and staff members have an obligation to accept that influence.

4. *Referent power* comes from the followers' identification with the leader. The admired leader is able to influence others because of the followers' desire to be like the leader.

5. *Expert power* is based on knowledge, skills, and information. For example, nurses who have expertise in areas such as physical assessment or technical skills or who keep up with current information on important topics will gain respect and compliance from others.

6. *Informal power* is based on personal characteristics. Informal power may result from personal relationships, connections with people in positions of power, being in the right place at the right time, or unique personal characteristics such as attractiveness, education, experience, drive, or decisiveness.

By understanding the authority of an assigned position and the sources of formal and informal power, the nurse manager will be better able to influence others to accomplish goals.

Formal and Informal Leadership

Both formal and informal leadership can exist in every organization. Formal leadership is practiced by the nurse who is appointed to an approved position (e.g., nurse manager, supervisor, charge nurse, coordinator) and given the authority to act by the organization. Informal leadership is exercised by the person who has no official or appointed authority to act but is able to persuade and influence others in the work group (Sullivan and Decker, 1997). The informal leader, who may or may not be a professional nurse, may have considerable power in the work group and can influence the group's attitude and significantly affect the efficiency and effectiveness of work flow, goal setting, and problem solving.

The nurse manager must learn to recognize and effectively work with informal leaders. Informal leadership may be positive if the informal leader's purpose is congruent with that of the nursing unit and organizational goals. For example, the informal leader of a patient care group may be highly supportive of a new nursing care delivery model being implemented on the unit, and, as a result, the other team members will be more willing to accept the change. However, an informal leader who is not supportive of the nursing unit's goals can create an uncomfortable work environment for the nurse manager and the entire team. Following are some strategies the nurse manager can use to work with informal leaders:

1. Identify the informal leaders in the work team and develop an understanding of their source of power.

2. Involve the informal leader, as well as other staff members, in decision-making and change-implementation processes.

3. Clearly communicate the goals and work expectations to all staff members.
4. Do not ignore an informal leader's attempt to undermine teamwork and change processes; counseling the person and setting clear expectations may be required.

LEADERSHIP AND MANAGEMENT THEORY

Understanding the development and progression of leadership theory is a necessary building block for developing leadership and management skills. Researchers began to study leadership in the early 1900s in an attempt to describe and understand the nature of leadership. Early leadership theory centered on describing the qualities or traits of leaders and has been commonly referred to as trait theory (Stogdill, 1974).

Leadership Trait Theory

Leadership trait theory sought to describe intrinsic traits of leaders and was based on the assumption that leaders were born with certain leadership characteristics. Traits found to be associated with leadership include intelligence, alertness, dependability, energy, drive, enthusiasm, ambition, decisiveness, self-confidence, a spirit of cooperation, and technical mastery (Stogdill, 1974). Although trait theories have been important in identifying qualities that distinguish today's leaders, these theories have neglected the interaction between other elements of the leadership situation. Trait theories also have failed to recognize the possibility that leadership traits can be learned and developed through experience. However, keeping in mind these traits associated with effective leadership, the new nurse can identify areas in which he or she should improve and develop.

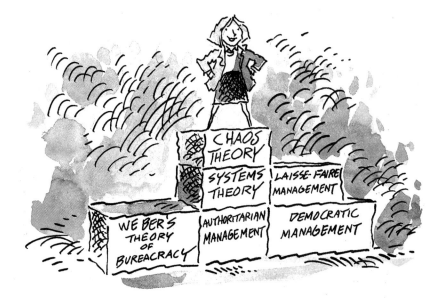

Leadership, management, and organizational theories provide the building blocks on which to build effective nursing management practices.

Interactional Leadership Theories

Researchers progressed from developing trait theory to studying the interaction between the leader and other variables of the leadership situation. Contemporary theories of leadership such as situational and behavioral theories have attempted to integrate the dynamics of the interaction between the leader, the worker, and elements of the leadership situation, arguing that effective leadership depends on several variables, including (Marquis and Huston, 2000):

1. Organizational culture.
2. Values of the leader.
3. Values of the followers.
4. Influence of the leader/manager.
5. Complexities of the situation.
6. Work to be accomplished.
7. Environment.

Situational leadership theory has explored the impact of the situation on the leadership role and suggests that leadership may vary in relation to the situation. The expectations, needs, attitudes, personalities, and developmental level of the leaders and followers will influence the style and effectiveness of leadership. Other aspects of a situation that influence the leadership role include the degree of interpersonal contact, time constraints, organizational structure, physical environment, and influence of the leader outside of the group. Situational theory suggests that a person may be a leader in one situation and a follower in another (Stogdill, 1974). By understanding the various elements that may influence the leadership situation, the nurse can become a more effective leader.

Transformational Leadership

In a contemporary concept of leadership, Burns (1978) identified and defined transformational leadership. Burns contends that there are two types of leaders: (1) the transactional leader, who is concerned with the day-to-day operations of the facility; and (2) the transformational leader, who is committed to organizational goals, has a vision, and is able to empower others with that vision. Box 16-1 compares characteristics of Burns' transformational and transactional leadership styles.

BOX 16-1   *Comparison of Transformational and Transactional Leaders*

Transformational leaders
- Identify and clearly communicate vision and direction.
- Empower the work group to accomplish goals and achieve the vision.
- Impart meaning and challenge to work.
- Are admired and emulated.
- Provide mentoring to individual staff members based on need.

Transactional leaders
- Focus on day-to-day operations and are comfortable with the status quo.
- Reward staff for desired work ("I'll do *x* in exchange for you doing *y*").
- Monitor work performance and correct as needed; *or*
- Wait until problems occur and then deal with the problem.

Studies have reported that, as nurse executives demonstrate more transformational leadership characteristics, they achieve higher levels of staff satisfaction and work group effectiveness. In one large national study of 396 randomly selected hospital nurse executives, Dunham-Taylor (2000) explored nurse executives' leadership characteristics and the relationship to staff satisfaction, work group effectiveness, and the nurse executive's effectiveness as rated by his or her superior. The study results demonstrated that staff satisfaction and work group effectiveness decreased as nurse executives were rated higher on transactional characteristics. The implication for nurse managers is that transformational leadership is very effective in increasing staff satisfaction and work effectiveness. The student is encouraged to read more about transformational leadership and to seek out transformational leaders as mentors.

Management Theory

Behavioral theories emerged to explain aspects of management and leadership based on behaviors of managers/leaders and followers. Three prevalent management behavior styles were identified by Lewin (1951) and White and Lippit (1960): authoritarian, democratic, and laissez-faire. Box 16-2 presents characteristics of these management styles. These three management styles vary in the amount of control exhibited by the manager and the amount of involvement that the staff has in decision making. At one extreme the autocratic manager makes all decisions with no staff input and uses the authority of the position to accomplish goals. At the opposite extreme is the laissez-faire manager, who provides little direction or

---

BOX 16-2   *Management Styles*

Autocratic/authoritative
- Determines policy and makes all the decisions
- Ignores subordinates' ideas or suggestions
- Dictates the work with much control
- Gives little feedback or recognition for work
- Makes fast decisions
- Successful with employees with little education or training

Democratic/participative
- Encourages staff participation in decision-making
- Involves staff in planning and developing
- Believes in the best in people
- Communicates effectively and provides regular feedback
- Builds responsibility in people
- Works well with competent, highly motivated people

Laissez-faire
- Does not provide guidance or direction
- Unable or unwilling to make decisions
- Does not provide feedback
- Initiates little change
- Rules by memos
- May work well with professional people

guidance and will forego decision making. Democratic management is also often referred to as participative management because of its basic premise of encouraging staff members to participate in decision making.

Depending on the situation, the nurse manager may need to use different types of management styles. This concept of situational leadership requires consideration of staff members' needs and experiences, the manager's abilities, and the goals and tasks to be accomplished. For example, in a life-threatening situation such as treating a patient in cardiac arrest, autocratic management might be appropriate. However, when structuring the weekend call schedule for a home health agency, a participative style of management would be more effective.

The health care system of the twenty-first century requires the use of a democratic or participative management style that will involve the staff in goal setting, problem solving, and decision making. Health care settings are driven to become increasingly cost-effective while continuing to improve quality, customer satisfaction, and positive patient outcomes. Staff directly involved in the challenges presented by patient care often can suggest the most workable, practical solutions. Problem solving and goal attainment are more likely to be successful when staff are involved in decisions affecting their daily work.

Research has shown that staff nurses' job satisfaction increases as the involvement in decision making and problem solving increases (Moss and Rowles, 1997). The new nurse manager should understand that his or her management style is what the staff perceives it to be, not what the manager has decided to practice. "What the staff perceives as the management style is the management style" (Moss and Rowles, 1997, p. 33). Managers have a responsibility to develop astute self-awareness about their intended leadership and management style and the style that the staff is perceiving. Although there is no one best leadership theory, nurses need to be aware of their own leadership behavior.

Organizational Theory

Just as leadership and management theories have evolved to provide a framework for understanding these two concepts, organizational theory has evolved to provide a framework for understanding complex organizations. A brief review of bureaucracy theory, systems theory, and chaos theory can provide the reader with insight into the value of using organizational theory to understand the management process within today's dynamic, complex health care organizations.

Weber's Theory of Bureaucracy. Max Weber, known as the father of organizational theory, began his work in the 1920s when he observed the growth of large organizations and predicted that this growth required a formal set of procedures. Weber, in his classic work on defining the characteristics of bureaucracy, argued that its great benefit was in its ability to apply general rules to specific cases, making the actions of management fair and predictable. The basis of Weber's concepts of bureaucracy revolves around explaining authority within organizations. He postulated that authority, thus the right to issue commands within an organization, is based on the impersonal rules and rights granted by virtue of the management position rather than related to the person who occupies that position. Weber's conceptualization of bureaucracy emphasized rules instead of individuals and competency instead of favoritism as important for effective organizations. Other characteristics of organizations identified by Weber include:

1. Managers are chosen because they have demonstrated knowledge, skill, and ability to fill the position.
2. The division of labor, authority, and responsibility is clearly defined.
3. Impersonal rules govern the actions of superiors over subordinates.

4. All personnel are chosen for their competence and are subject to strict rules that are applied impersonally and uniformly.
5. A system of procedures for dealing with work situations is in place.

Although the structure of bureaucracy described by Weber is still present in most organizations today, his work failed to recognize the complexity of human behavior within organizations and the constantly changing environment of today's organizations. As previously discussed, current leadership and management theory (participatory management, transformational leadership) recognizes the importance of supportive, respectful relationships between managers and employees, with employees being involved in decision making and problem solving.

Systems Theory. Systems theory views the organization as a set of interdependent parts that together form a whole (Thompson, 1967). The interdependent nature of the parts of the organization suggests that anything that affects the functioning of one aspect of the organization will affect the other parts of the organization. Open systems theory suggests that not only is the organization affected by internal changes among any of its parts, but also that external environmental forces will have a direct influence on the organization and vice versa—the internal forces will impact the external environment. In contrast to open systems theory, closed systems theory views the system as being totally independent of outside influences, which is an unrealistic view for health care organizations. To be successful, today's health care organizations must be able to continually adapt to both internal and external changes.

Consider the following example to help explain systems theory. The hospital in which Juan Hernandez, RN, works has reduced the number of RNs employed by the hospital and now requires that the remaining RNs work overtime "at the request of administration." The quality of patient care, patient safety, and the individual nurses' professional practice and personal health have been negatively affected by this change. Juan and his fellow RNs seek advice from their State Nurses Association (SNA) about their professional responsibility to work "mandatory overtime." The SNA is responding to the situation, which is occurring more frequently across the state and nation, by proposing legislation to mandate nurse/patient ratios and limit mandatory overtime. The SNA and state government may now require hospital administrators to respond to the need for increased staffing levels.

This example demonstrates open systems theory. As internal forces in one department (hospital administration) mandated changes that affected another area (RNs and patient care), internal forces (RNs) pushed for changes from the external environment (SNA and state government). The external environment may now force changes to the organization (hospital administration).

Systems theory has provided nurse managers with a framework to view nursing services as a subsystem of the larger health care organization and to realize the interrelatedness and interdependence of all the parts of the health care organization. Open systems theory suggests that shared responsibility among all groups is necessary to help patients gain and maintain health and wellness (McGuire, 1999). The nurse manager will be wise to consider open systems theory and the impact a change in one area will have in another area, both internal and external to the organization.

Chaos Theory. Chaos theory is a more recently developed organizational theory that attempts to account for the complexity and randomness in organizations. Despite the implications of the word "chaos," the theory actually suggests a degree of order by helping view complicated behaviors and situations as predictable. Nurse managers may wish for balanced and steady work environments, but in reality the they are dealing with, what seems at best, a chaotic system. Chaos theory says that variation is a normal part of managing health care systems. Examples of variation in health care are cultural diversity, constantly fluctuating patient census, and staffing shortages. Until nurse managers understand that these variations are a normal, predictable state in the organization, they may continue to experience discomfort and dissatisfaction with their role (McGuire, 1999).

MANAGEMENT FUNCTIONS

Classic theories of management suggest that the primary functions of managers are planning, organizing, and controlling (Stogdill, 1974). Leaders in nursing management have added two additional functions to this list and now recognize five major management functions as necessary for the management of nursing organizations: (1) planning, (2) organizing, (3) staffing, (4) directing, and (5) controlling (Marquis and Huston, 2000) (Fig. 16-1).

- Planning includes defining goals and objectives, developing policies and procedures; determining resource allocation; and developing evaluation methods.
- Organizing includes identifying the management structure to accomplish work, determining communication processes, and coordinating people, time and work.
- Staffing includes those activities required to have qualified people accomplish work such as recruiting, hiring, training, scheduling and ongoing staff development.

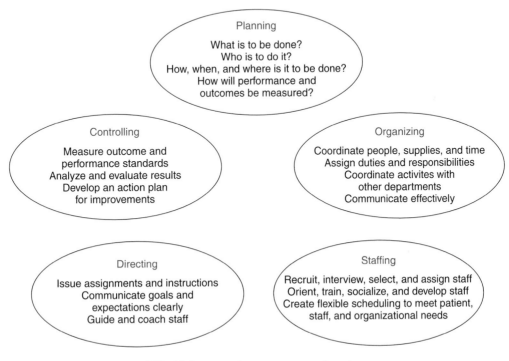

FIG. 16-1 Five major management functions.

- Directing encourages employees to accomplish goals and objectives and involves communicating, delegating, motivating, and managing conflict.
- Controlling analyzes results to evaluate accomplishments and includes evaluating employee performance, analyzing financial activities, and monitoring quality of care.

These management functions are interrelated; different phases of the process occur simultaneously, and the processes should be circular, with the manager always working toward improving the quality of health care, patient safety, and staff and customer satisfaction. Because understanding these five management functions is essential for success as a nurse manager, they will now be discussed in further detail.

Planning

Planning Questions

What is the right thing to do for the organization, its customers, and its employees?
What programs or services do customers need or want?
What financial and manpower resources are available?
What goals and objectives can be established to meet customer needs?
How can goals and objectives be communicated throughout the organization?

Planning is the first management function and has been defined as "deciding in advance what to do; who is to do it; and how, when, and where it is to be done" (Marquis and Huston, 1998, p. 49). All management functions are based on planning. Without effective planning, the management process will fail. Effective planning requires the nurse manager to understand the:

- Mission statement and philosophy of the organization.
- Organizational strategic plan.
- Goals and objectives for the entire organization.
- Operational plan for the individual unit or facility.

Mission and Philosophy. The mission statement, the foundation of planning for any organization, describes the purpose of the organization and the reason it exists. Most health care organizations exist to provide high-quality patient care, but emphasis may be on different concepts such as research, teaching, preventive care, spiritual care, or community service. The philosophy is the set of values and beliefs that guides the actions of the organization and thus serves as the basis of all planning. The philosophy statement should speak for the primary mission of the organization and reflect the values of the organization, any special approaches to care, and/or any particular beliefs regarding patients and/or employees (Marquis and Huston, 1998). New nurses should be aware of the mission and philosophy of the employing organization and understand the relationship between their own personal value system and that of the organization. Box 16-3 provides an example of an organization's mission and philosophy statement.

Strategic Planning. Strategic planning is long-range planning (extending 3 to 5 years into the future) and results from an in-depth analysis of (1) the business, community, and regulatory and political environment outside the organization (external assessment); (2) customer

BOX 16-3	*Sample Mission, Values, and Philosophy Statement*

The mission of Community Hospital is to provide high quality, cost-effective health services that patients and their families recommend, physicians prefer, employees, volunteers, and board members are proud of, health professional students learn and excel from, and the community values.

The philosophy and values of Community Hospital are:

- Commitment to professional and individual excellence with support for personal and professional growth within the organization.
- Continuous improvement by identifying the key needs of our customers, assessing how well we meet those needs, continuously improving our services, and measuring our progress.
- Ethical and fair treatment for ALL through a commitment to forming and maintaining relationships of fairness and trust with our patients, purchasers of our services, and our employees. Our business is conducted according to the highest ethical standards.
- Teamwork is consistently demonstrated as we work together to provide ever-improving customer service. People at all levels of the organization will participate in decision-making and process improvement.
- Compassion is our highest priority, we will always provide care and comfort to people in need, and our patients and families will receive respectful and dignified treatment from all of our people at all times.
- Innovation in service delivery is accomplished by investing in the development of new and better ways of deliver services.

needs; (3) technologic changes; and (4) strengths, problems, and weaknesses internal to the organization. The purposes of strategic planning are to:

- Provide direction for the organization.
- Identify strategies to respond to changes in customer needs, technology, health care legislation, the business environment, or the community.
- Dedicate resources to important services.
- Eliminate duplication, waste, and underused services.

The strategic plan is a written document that details organizational goals, allocates resources, assigns responsibilities, and determines time frames. Responsibility for development of the strategic plan rests with upper-level management, although there is increasing emphasis on including employees at all levels in strategic planning processes. Consider the following example.

Melanie Clements, an RN employed by the Quality Care Home Health Agency, noticed that the office had been receiving several calls per week for home nursing care for pediatric oncology patients. The agency did not provide services for pediatric patients. Melanie reported the situation to the administrator. Melanie soon was involved in gathering information about the number of home health agencies that offered pediatric oncology care, the standards of nursing care recommended for pediatric oncology patients, how many pediatric patients in the area might need such services, and what reimbursement was available for these services. Within the next few months, the administrator for Quality Care Home Health decided that, as part of the agency's strategic plan, a program for pediatric oncology services would be developed.

Goals and Objectives. Goals and objectives state the actions necessary to achieve the strategic plan and are central to the entire management process. Goals should be measurable, observable, and realistic. Objectives are more specific and detail how a goal will be accomplished with an established target date.

Goals and objectives serve as the manager's road map; without them it is difficult to know where one is going. Organization-wide goals will be established in the strategic planning process, and then unit goals that support the organization-wide goals should be developed. Every nurse manager should be able to clearly articulate the organization-wide goals, as well as the goals of the nursing unit for which he or she is responsible. In addition, goals and objectives must be communicated to everyone who is responsible for their attainment. Consider the following case example.

Judy Anderson, RN, recently has been appointed as nurse manager in a 150-bed, long-term care facility. The mission and philosophy of the organization is to "respect the dignity and worth of the individual and to provide care that will help restore the patient to the best possible state of physical, mental, and emotional health while maintaining his or her sense of spiritual and social well-being." Kenneth Cole, the administrator, has asked Judy to develop a set of goals that she views as priorities to accomplish in the next year. After gathering data about patient needs, costs, and staffing levels and meeting with the medical director, patient care staff members, and rehabilitation therapy, social services, dietary, and maintenance staff, Judy has developed the following goals: (1) increase the coordination of care activities between nursing, therapy, and social services to more effectively meet patient care needs for increased emotional well-being and socialization; (2) maintain a safe environment for patients and staff by implementing the patient safety program outlined in the safety manual; (3) improve the patient care staff's competencies in meeting the needs of the elderly patient. After reviewing Judy's goals, Kenneth agrees that they fit with the overall organizational plan and that the goals address needs identified in Judy's facility assessment activities. However, Kenneth has posed several questions. What is the specific plan for attaining goals? What costs are involved? How does the staff feel about these goals? How will results of the goals be measured?

Operational Planning. The nurse manager is most likely to be responsible for operational planning (i.e., short-range planning that encompasses the day-to-day activities of the organization). For example, short-range planning for a medical-surgical unit in a hospital might include maintaining the overall patient-to-staff ratio at 6:1, with 40% of the staff being RNs. As part of accomplishing organizational goals and objectives, the nurse manager involved in operational planning will be concerned with the:

- Number, type, and location of patients to be cared for.
- Qualifications and abilities of nursing and other health care staff.
- Type and amount of supplies and other physical resources available.
- Allocation of resources (staff, supplies, time) to meet budgetary requirements.

The nurse manager also must plan for a variety of other activities such as staff development, regulatory compliance, and quality improvement projects. The nurse manager should have a vision of how the day-to-day operational planning fits into the organizational plan as a whole.

Organizing

Organizing Questions

What lines of authority and levels of management are needed to accomplish goals?
How should communication and decision making occur?
What policies and procedures are needed to accomplish goals?
How can staff members' qualifications, functions, and responsibilities be defined?
How should work be assigned?

Organizing is the second management function. At the organizational level, organizing must occur to establish a formal structure that defines the lines of authority, communication, and decision making within an organization. The formal organizational structure helps define roles and responsibilities of each level of management. The organizational chart provides a visual picture of the organization and identifies lines of communication and authority. All nurses should be familiar with the organizational chart of their employing institution. Organizing also involves developing policies and procedures to help outline how work will be done and establishing position qualifications and job descriptions to define who will do the work.

At the unit level, the nurse manager has to determine how to best organize the work activities to meet organizational goals in an efficient and effective manner. Organizing involves:

- Using resources (people, supplies, time) wisely.
- Assigning duties and responsibilities appropriately.
- Coordinating activities with other departments.
- Effectively communicating with subordinates and superiors to ensure a smooth workflow.

Models for organizing the delivery of patient care are discussed in Chapter 19.

Staffing

Staffing Questions

What number and type of staff are needed to accomplish the necessary work?
How will appropriate staff members be recruited and hired?
How will staff members' work schedules be managed?
How will patient care and other task assignments be made?
How will ongoing staff development be managed?

Staffing is the third management function. The provision of health care is labor intensive, with a workforce composed of people with a variety of skill levels (i.e., professional nurses, physicians, pharmacists, social workers, therapists, dietitians, licensed vocational/practical nurses, technicians, and unlicensed assistive personnel). Hiring and managing staff to accomplish the work of the institution is an important function for all levels of managers. Staffing activities include:

- Recruiting, selecting, orienting, and developing personnel.
- Determining patient assignment systems.
- Scheduling staff to accomplish the goals of the organization.

Marquis and Huston (2000) have described the steps in the staffing function as follows:

1. Determine the number and type of staff needed based on organizational planning goals and budgetary requirements.
2. Recruit, interview, select, and assign personnel based on job description requirements and performance standards.
3. Use staff development resources to orient, train, socialize, and develop staff members.
4. Develop a staff-education program to assist personal and professional development and enhance knowledge and skill levels.
5. Implement creative and flexible scheduling based on patient care needs, employee needs, and organizational productivity requirements.

The staffing process most likely will prove to be one of the most time-consuming and challenging functions for the nurse manager. Recruiting and hiring staff is perhaps the nurse manager's most important job. Little can be accomplished without the right people to do the work.

Staff schedules are a key element to providing job satisfaction and keeping employees happy and productive, whereas patient assignment schedules are critical to ensure the provision of safe, effective patient care. In addition, the nurse manager has the important responsibility of assigning patients to staff members based on assessed patient needs, patient acuity levels, and the abilities and competencies of the staff members (Marrelli, 1997). Staffing and assignments are further discussed in Chapter 19.

While meeting staff and patient scheduling needs, the nurse manager also must meet organizational staffing and productivity goals. Productivity is the amount of work produced through the use of a specific amount of resources and is measured as outputs divided by inputs. For example, the number of nursing hours worked over a 24-hour period divided by the patient census is a standard productivity measurement used by many hospitals. Other examples of productivity measurements include number of home visits completed or number of procedures performed.

Directing

Directing Questions

How can managers clearly communicate to staff members what is expected?
How can staff members be motivated to work effectively and efficiently?
How can staff members be coached and guided to make a positive contribution to the work team?
How can delegation and assignments be used to accomplish work?

Directing is the fourth management function. After managers have planned what to do, organized how to do it, and staffed positions to do the work, they must direct personnel and activities to accomplish goals. Directing involves issuing assignments and instructions that allow workers to clearly understand what is expected, as well as guiding and coaching workers to contribute effectively and efficiently to achieve planned goals. Directing requires the nurse manager to:

- Establish a motivating climate and team spirit.
- Manage time efficiently.
- Manage conflict and facilitate collaboration.
- Demonstrate excellent communication skills.

Motivation.   Perhaps the most challenging aspect of directing is motivating staff. Motivation is the inner drive that compels a person to act in a certain way. The amount and quality of work accomplished by a person is a direct reflection of his or her motivation. A great deal of research has been undertaken to better understand human motivation. Most researchers will agree that motivation is complex and involves a combination of extrinsic or external rewards such as money, benefits, and working conditions and intrinsic or internal needs for recognition, self-esteem, and self-actualization (Marquis and Huston, 1998). Box 16-4 summarizes factors that influence nurses' job satisfaction, dissatisfaction, and motivation.

Positive Reinforcement.   Positive reinforcement is one of the most powerful and motivating, but often underused and overlooked, resources available to the nurse manager (Marquis and Huston, 2000). To be effective, positive reinforcement should (1) be specific, with praise given for a particular task done well or goal accomplished; (2) occur as close as possible to the time of the achievement; (3) be spontaneous and unpredictable (praise given routinely tends to lose its value); and (4) be given for a genuine accomplishment (Peters and Waterman,1982). "Managers can also create a motivating climate by being a positive and enthusiastic role model in the clinical setting. Managers who frequently project unhappiness to subordinates contribute greatly to low unit morale" (Marquis and Huston, 2000, p. 291).

BOX 16-4	*Factors Influencing Nurses' Job Satisfaction and Dissatisfaction*

Sources of satisfaction	**Sources of dissatisfaction**
Sense of achievement	Vague, inconsistent rules and regulations
Thanks and positive recognition	No thanks or recognition
Guidance, mentorship, and opportunities for professional development	No commitment by management to professional development
Open communication/being informed	Not being informed about changes
Challenging work and responsibility	Poor communication, unclear expectations
Advancement potential	Non-nursing duties
Pleasant work environment	No help from managers during crisis
Adequate staffing; help from managers during stressful times	Uncooperative physicians
Supportive managers who demonstrate respect and caring for each individual	Excessive workload negatively affecting quality
Ongoing feedback about performance	Inadequate feedback about performance
Agreeable working hours and flexibility in scheduling when necessary	Lack of involvement in decision making

Adapted from Marriner-Tomey A: *Nursing management and leadership,* St. Louis, 2000, Mosby; and McNeese-Smith D: The influence of manager behavior on nurses' job satisfaction, productivity and commitment, *J Nurs Admin* 27(9):47-55, 1997.

Several other skills are essential as nurse managers function in the directing role, including effective communication and conflict management skills (discussed in Chapter 17), delegation skills (discussed in Chapter 18), and team-building skills discussed later in this chapter. The nurse manager is challenged to create a climate that will generate worker satisfaction, motivate workers to accomplish goals, and encourage high productivity.

Controlling

Controlling Questions

What standards of performance should be established for the patient population cared for?
How can performance or nursing care outcomes be measured?
What process can be used to develop an action plan for improving performance?
What are some keys to good employee performance appraisals?

The purpose of controlling, the fifth management function, is to ensure that employees accomplish goals while maintaining a high quality of performance. Controlling involves:

- Establishing performance or outcome standards.
- Measuring and evaluating performance against established standards.
- Determining an action plan to improve performance.

Performance Standards. Controlling activities require the nurse manager to maintain a mindset that continually looks for ways to improve individual, team, and organizational performance. Performance standards describe a model of excellence for work activities and serve as the basis of comparison between actual and desired work performance. Examples of

BOX 16-5	*Tips for Successful Employee Feedback*

- Ask the employee if he or she will hear your feedback—it is helpful to ask if the person is open to your feedback
- Help employees not to take feedback personally—emphasize that feedback is to improve a process, not to blame for poor performance.
- Be specific and provide clear examples when possible; explain how your feedback can help improve a process or service.
- Focus on work-related outcomes and don't get personal.
- Allow time for a response.
- Thank the employee for listening.

Adapted from Grensing-Pophal L: Give-and-take feedback, *Nurs Manage* 31(2):27-28, 2000.

BOX 16-6	*Tips for Successful Employee Performance Appraisals*

- Each employee must understand the standard by which his or her work is being evaluated—at a minimum by receiving a copy of the appraisal form, and more effectively by being involved in developing the evaluation criteria.
- Conduct the appraisal during a time when there will be no interruptions for either party; select a comfortable seating arrangement that denotes collegiality such as side-by-side chairs.
- Avoid surprises—good leaders/managers will provide feedback and communicate with staff on a continual basis.
- Focus on the employee's performance and work-related outcomes, not on personal characteristics.
- Avoid vague generalities such as "your performance is fine" or "your attitude needs to improve"—give explicit examples; use positive examples liberally and negative examples sparingly (again, nothing should be a surprise!).
- Encourage input from the employee.
- Set goals together for continued growth and improvement; decide how goals will be accomplished and evaluated—then follow-up!
- Be sensitive and caring; demonstrate that you value the employee and his or her contribution to the organization.

Adapted from Marquis BL, Huston CJ: *Leadership roles and management functions in nursing, ed 3,* Philadelphia, 2000, JB Lippincott.

performance standards in an ambulatory outpatient clinic might include (1) that every patient is informed about all laboratory results within 48 hours, whether normal or abnormal; and (2) that all diabetic patients must remove their shoes and socks for a thorough foot examination each time they come into the clinic. Chapter 20 provides more discussion about performance standards and also presents an excellent process for measuring performance and planning for improvement. The nurse manager can draw on several resources for establishing performance standards, including:

1. Written organizational policies and procedures.
2. Standards for the practice of professional nursing developed by the American Nurses Association and published in *Standards of Clinical Nursing Practice* (ANA, 1998).
3. Standards for professional nursing specialty practices developed by the American Nurses Association such as the *Scope and Standards of Public Health Nursing Practice* (ANA, 1999) and *Standards and Scope of Gerontological Nursing Practice* (ANA, 1995).

4. Standards developed and published by specialty nursing organizations (e.g., American Association of Operating Room Nurses, 2001).

Employee Feedback. Other important controlling functions are continual employee feedback and employee performance appraisal activities. Employee performance appraisals must be ongoing, objective, and based on established performance standards. A manager should never wait until the "annual performance review" to discuss problems or deficiencies with a staff member. Consistent, day-to-day feedback and coaching about job performance clarifies expectations, improves the quality of work, and allows the manager to correct problems before they become serious. Ongoing documentation about an employee's job performance also is an essential management responsibility. The result of routine performance appraisals should be mutual goal setting designed to meet the employees' training, educational, and work-improvement needs. Box 16-5 presents some useful tips for providing employee feedback, and Box 16-6 presents some useful tips for successful employee performance evaluations.

The management functions of planning, organizing, staffing, directing, and controlling provide the nurse manager with a defined, practical set of skills to guide the implementation of management activities. The new nurse manager will be challenged to maintain the different stages of management that will occur in the span of just 1 day. In addition to managing different phases of the process occurring simultaneously, the nurse manager also will be functioning in many different management roles, each requiring the ongoing processes of planning, organizing, staffing, directing, and controlling.

ROLES OF THE NURSE MANAGER

Nurse managers will have to assume various roles as they function in leadership and management positions. Because a different set of roles and responsibilities will be required in almost any position in any health care setting, professional nurses should clearly understand the job description, roles and responsibilities, and policies and procedures related to the position in which they are employed or assigned. The following discussion presents information about the primary roles that a nurse will assume in any position. By understanding these roles, the nurse can (1) know what is expected to be effective, and (2) identify areas that require additional learning and improvement.

Customer Service Provider

Providing service or care to customers (patient or clients) is the primary reason any health care organization exists. The complex health care environment has created a competitive marketplace in which home health agencies, hospitals, ambulatory clinics, and even hospice agencies compete for patients. To survive and thrive in this competitive environment, the nurse must keep customer service first and foremost as the motivator of all plans and activities. Without customers, the organization will go out of business. "Client service is the key to future referrals and . . . revenues" (Taccetta-Chapnick and Rafferty, 1997, p. 45).

External and Internal Customers. Effective management requires that the health care organization and the nurse develop a comprehensive view of the term *customer.* Customers can be categorized as external or internal, depending on their relationship to the organization. External customers are not employed by the organization; they include patients and families, as well as physicians and other employees in facilities that serve as referral sources for new patients. For example, home health nurses should view hospital discharge planners as customers and find ways to meet their patients' discharge needs. Physicians will not refer patients to a particular hospital or clinic if they are not happy with the services provided by that facility.

Payers (insurance companies, managed care plans) are also being considered as primary external customers. For example, hospitals seek to contract with managed care plans to gain the plan's covered members as customers. Managed care companies seek to contract with hospitals that can demonstrate outstanding service that will please the plan's members. Thus the managed care company becomes the hospital's customer.

Internal customers are employed by the organization and may include patient care staff members, staff members of other departments (e.g., laboratory, dietary), faculty, administrators, social workers, dietitians, and therapists. For example, to facilitate effective and efficient work performance, nurse managers should view staff members as "customers" and determine how to meet their needs. Other departments—social services, laboratory, maintenance, housekeeping—are essential to manage an effective nursing unit, and the needs of these "customers" should be considered. If every department in the organization provided great service to both internal and external customers, just think how much more effective and efficient the entire organization would be!

Customer Service Standards. Certainly all customers have a need to be treated with kindness and respect, to have services provided in a timely and cost-effective manner, and to have effective communication about what is or will be occurring. Further service standards can be defined by listening to and observing customers and analyzing customer surveys, customer complaints, and unsolicited comments or letters. A sample customer service commitment for a health care organization is presented in Box 16-7. Meeting customer needs should be the focus in all planning, organizing, staffing, directing, and controlling activities, as well as in all meetings and communications with superiors and subordinates.

Team Builder

A team is a group of people organized to accomplish the necessary work of an organization. Teams have become important in the changing health care environment. Teams bring together a range of people with different knowledge, skills, and experiences to meet customer

---

BOX 16-7	*Sample Customer Service Commitment for a Healthcare Organization*

Community Clinics' Customer Service C sommitment
This is our customer service commitment. Translated, it stands for listening, caring, helping, and healing.
- Caring, friendly professional staff members
- Prompt and personal attention to requests
- Timely, convenient services with reasonable wait times
- Confidentiality and privacy respected and upheld
- Serious responses to concerns and complaints
- Ongoing efforts to improve our systems and processes

needs, accomplish tasks, and solve problems. Team members may include unit secretaries, nursing assistants, social workers, dietitians, therapists, physicians, licensed vocational/practical nurses, and RNs. A team should have clearly defined goals to accomplish work in the health care unit and should be empowered to make decisions within its realm of responsibility. Team building should create synergy. Synergy is the ability of a group of people working together to accomplish significantly more than each person working individually.

Bringing people together to work as a group does not necessarily make them a team. To create synergy, teams must have defined goals and objectives, a commitment to work together, good communication, and a willingness to cooperate. Wywialowski (1997) has suggested the following principles for promoting effective working relationships in teams:

1. Each member has a clear understanding of the team's overall purpose and goals, which gives meaning to the work.
2. Each member's contribution to meeting team goals is respected and valued.
3. The team receives relevant, timely, and constructive feedback about its success in meeting goals.
4. Team members are encouraged to seek help regularly, and that help is available from the manager.
5. Team members are encouraged to willingly help others.

Team members should be encouraged to communicate with each other to identify effective work division and solutions to problems so that synergy is accomplished. The nurse manager, as team builder, must serve as a role model to encourage and help develop team principles of respect, cooperation, commitment, and a willingness to accomplish shared goals. As a role model for team members, the nurse manager should:

- Show respect for all members of the team and value their input.
- Clearly define team goals. ("What do we want to accomplish?")
- Clearly define the decision-making authority within the realm of the team.
- Encourage the team members to develop a sense of stewardship (or ownership) for the success of the team.
- Exhibit a personal commitment to the team goals.
- Provide the resources necessary to accomplish goals (e.g., time for team meetings, information, supplies).
- Periodically review goal attainment with the team.

Resource Manager

Resources include the personnel, time, and supplies needed to accomplish the goals of the organization. Resources cost money and always will be in limited supply. Unfortunately, no health care organization can afford the luxury of an unlimited number of staff or supplies to accomplish the required work. With health care facilities' current focus on cost containment, it is essential that nurses develop an understanding of and expertise in resource management. It is the responsibility of the nurse manager to effectively manage resources to provide safe, effective patient care in an economic manner.

Budget. Planning resource management begins in the development of the budget, or fiscal planning. "A budget is a plan for the allocation of resources and a control for ensuring that results comply with the plans" (Marriner-Tomey, 2000, p. 198). Budgets are most often developed for a 1-year time period and are based on predicted amounts of services for the time period involved. For example, hospitals will predict patient census for the coming year and then allocate funds for nursing salaries based on this predicted census.

Historically nursing has had limited input into fiscal (or financial) planning and development of the organization's budget. Administrators with no nursing background and no understanding of nursing values, beliefs, and care requirements may have made decisions about resource allocation related to nursing. Participating in the budget process to determine resource allocation should be viewed as a fundamental responsibility of the nurse manager. Involving staff nurses in the budgeting process is also appropriate. Managers and staff members who participate in fiscal planning are more likely to be cost conscious and will have a better understanding of how their unit should function to meet the overall long- and short-term financial goals (Marquis and Huston, 2000).

The nurse manager will be concerned with three types of budgets: (1) the personnel budget, (2) the operating budget, and (3) the capital budget. In most organizations these budgets are outlined and explained in budgeting policies and procedures. Fiscal objectives and lines of authority and responsibility for budget and financial management should also be clearly stated. It is the responsibility of the nurse manager to learn about and understand these policies and procedures.

Personnel Budget. The personnel budget represents the funds allocated for employee salaries and benefits and is the largest expense for a health care organization. Factors that affect the personnel budget include salary rates, overtime, benefits, staff development and training, and employee turnover. In managing the personnel budget the nurse manager must be aware of the staffing mix, or the number of varied health care providers (experienced RNs, new graduates, licensed practical/vocational nurses, nursing assistants), required to competently meet patient needs and remain within budgetary guidelines (Marquis and Huston, 2000). Chapter 19 discusses staffing mixes in more detail.

One of the primary difficulties encountered in managing the personnel budget is accurately predicting future staffing needs. Because budgets are based on a predicted amount of services (i.e., patient census), variances between actual staffing levels and budget levels will occur if the facility experiences an unanticipated increase or decrease in patient services. At this point, the nurse manager might be required to complete a budget variance report to explain the difference between the budgeted and actual staffing levels.

Operating Budget. The operating budget represents the funds allocated for daily expenses required to operate the facility, including utilities, repairs, maintenance, and patient care supplies. After personnel costs, the operating budget is the second most important component of the organization's overall costs (Marquis and Houston, 2000). Maintaining an effective supply allocation system (how supplies are distributed and accounted for) and an inventory management system are key to helping the nurse manager control supply usage. The nurse manager who is able to effectively manage both personnel costs and supply costs will make a major contribution to the cost-containment goals of the organization.

Capital Budget. The capital expenditure budget represents funds allocated for construction projects and/or long-life equipment (e.g., cardiac monitor, defibrillator, computer hardware) that generally is more expensive than operating supplies. Because capital expenditures are associated with long-range planning and may be projected 1 to 3 years in advance, it is impor-

---

BOX 16-8	*Three Types of Budgets*

Personnel
Allocates funds for salaries, overtime, benefits, staff development and training, and employee turnover costs

Operating budget
Allocates funds for daily expenses such as utilities, repairs, maintenance, and patient care supplies

Capital budget
Allocates funds for construction projects and/or long-life equipment such as cardiac monitors, defibrillators, and computer hardware; capital budget items are generally more expensive than operating supplies

---

tant that the nurse manager be aware of the organization's capital expenditure plan to have input about future equipment needs for the unit or facility. The three types of budgets are summarized in Box 16-8.

Financial Reports. To be effective as a resource manager, the nurse should understand the organization's financial goals and how to track expenditures. Each organization should have a reporting mechanism in place to provide nurse managers with financial reports specific to their area of control. The variance report is a monthly or quarterly report that details budgeted expenses compared to actual costs for items such as the number of staff hours or cost of supplies per patient service provided. The variance report will provide the nurse manager with valuable information about the unit's financial performance and can be used to compare actual expenditures with predicted levels of service.

Other budget reports that the nurse manager might use include overtime, productivity, and supply usage reports. The more frequently the nurse manager analyzes financial reports, the more quickly he or she can make revisions to meet goals. Budget analysis requires the nurse manager to relate expenditures to actual patient care practices and to identify areas such as staffing levels or supply usage where adjustments might be necessary.

Each of the management activities of planning, organizing, staffing, directing, and controlling will come into play in the role of resource manager. The nurse manager needs to learn and develop skills in:

- Planning for the necessary resources to manage the unit.
- Organizing the resources to meet identified goals.
- Staffing appropriately as determined by patient needs and the budget plan.
- Directing to maintain resource allocations within budgetary guidelines.
- Controlling by analyzing financial reports and making adjustments where necessary.

This author would like to encourage all readers not to be unsettled by financial and budget reports and conversations. Instead, get involved! Don't be afraid to say, "I don't understand . . . please explain." Review budget and financial reports, ask questions, talk to seasoned nurse managers, talk to the organization's accountants and financial planners, and even consider taking an accounting or finance course at the local college. Understanding financial and budget management is one of the most useful and powerful tools you can have as a nurse manager.

Decision Maker and Problem Solver

Problem solving and decision making are essential skills for professional nursing practice. Not only are these skills required in clinical patient care, but they also are vital components of effective leadership and management. "Decision making is a purposeful and goal-directed effort using a systematic process to choose among options" (Yoder Wise, 1999, p. 91). Decision making is not always related to a problem situation; it is required throughout all aspects of the management functions of planning, organizing, staffing, directing, and controlling. Problem solving is focused on solving an immediate problem and includes a decision-making step.

The Nursing Process As a Guide for Decision Making and Problem Solving. The nursing process, familiar to nurses for addressing patient care needs, can be applied to all management activities requiring decision making and problem solving. The nursing process is a problem-solving process that includes assessment, analysis and diagnosis, planning, implementation, and evaluation and has proven to be effective to manage the complex decisions required in nursing practice (Howenstein et al., 1996). Table 16-1 summarizes the decision-making and problem-solving activities in each stage of the nursing process.

Assessment. During the assessment stage it is important for the nurse to separate the problem from the symptom by gathering information about the problem or situation. It often is appropriate to involve others who are familiar with the situation to provide a different viewpoint or information the manager lacks. For example, the nurse manager concerned about increasingly high absenteeism among the patient care staff may consider implementing a

TABLE 16-1	*The Nursing Process Applied to Problem Solving*			
ASSESSMENT	**ANALYSIS AND DIAGNOSIS**	**PLANNING**	**IMPLEMENTING**	**EVALUATION**
■ Gather information about the situation	■ Analyze results of information gathered	■ Identify as many solutions as possible	■ Communicate plans to everyone affected	■ Identify evaluation criteria in the planning stage
■ Identify the problem; separate the symptoms	■ Identify, clarify, and prioritize the actual problem(s)	■ Elicit participation from people or groups affected	■ Be sure plans, goals, and objectives are clearly identified	■ Identify who is responsible for evaluation, what will be measured, and when it will take place
■ Identify people and groups involved	■ Determine if intervention is appropriate	■ Review options and consider safety, efficiency, costs, quality, and legal issues	■ Maintain open, two-way communication with staff	■ Maintain open communication with all involved
■ Identify cultural and environmental factors		■ Consider positive and negative outcomes	■ Support and encourage compliance among all staff	■ Was the decision successful?
■ Encourage input from involved parties		■ Remain open-minded and flexible when considering options		■ What might have made it better?

strict policy to punish absentee staff members. In this situation the nurse manager may be addressing the symptom instead of the real issue. The following questions should be asked. What is causing the absenteeism? Are there problems on the unit that are creating an unhappy work environment? Are several staff members coincidentally having personal problems? Are absentee policies being unfairly administered? The nurse manager must correctly assess and diagnose the problem before planning can begin.

Analysis and Diagnosis. During the analysis stage decision makers use information gathered in the assessment phase to identify the specific problem to be solved. At this stage, the manager must also decide if the situation is important enough to require intervention and if it is within his or her authority to intervene. Managers should not attempt to intercede in every situation brought to their attention. Purposeful inaction is an intentional plan on the part of the manager and should not be confused with a "do-nothing approach" taken by a manager who chooses to do nothing when intervention is indicated. Purposeful inaction may be indicated when the problem or decision is beyond the manager's control or should be addressed by others. Often interpersonal conflicts are best resolved by the people involved in the conflict (Yoder Wise, 1999).

Planning. During the planning stage the goal is to identify as many options as possible and then objectively weigh the options as to possible risks and consequences and positive and negative outcomes; patient outcomes and staff effectiveness are key considerations. The decision maker should remain flexible, open-minded, and creative when reviewing options and avoid preconceived ideas or rigid thinking (Yoder Wise, 1999). "There is only one way to do this job," or "that's the way we have always done it" are examples of rigid thinking. At this stage of the process, it is also important to remember that decisions made with no input from those affected may be difficult to enforce. Cost, quality, and legal and ethical aspects of care also should be carefully considered.

Implementation. The implementation stage should include effective communication, delegation, and supervision. It is important for the manager to show positive support for the decision outcome and encourage compliance among all staff. Persons higher in the organizational structure may mandate some decisions, and, although not able to control those decisions, the nurse manager can influence a positive outcome.

Evaluation. The evaluation stage is necessary to ensure that the implemented plan effectively resolved the problem or decision. Considerable time and energy may be spent on identifying the problem, generating possible options, and selecting and implementing the best solution. However, time for follow-up evaluation must be allocated. It is important to establish early (during the planning stage) how and what evaluation and monitoring will take place, who will be responsible, and when it will be accomplished (Yoder Wise, 1999).

Staff input should be included in each stage of the decision-making, problem-solving process. In addition, the nurse manager might seek help from others who are more experienced and knowledgeable in specific areas. Even the most experienced nurse managers will not be able to effectively solve every problem, nor will any nurse manager have all the answers. The key to being a good manager is to understand and incorporate the decision-making, problem-solving process into all activities; know when and how to access resources; and learn and improve as successes and failures are experienced.

Change Agent

This text frequently has referred to the "changing" health care environment, and, true to the statement, change is an inevitable occurrence in health care organizations. Whether working with individuals, groups, or the entire organization, the professional nurse is certain to be involved in managing change. The nurse as the change agent is responsible for guiding people through the change process and needs to develop an understanding about the nature of change and effective change strategies.

People often feel threatened by change and may react with resistance and hostility. Change that is carefully planned and implemented slowly with all people continually informed and involved will be more successful in reaching the desired outcome (or change). "Regardless of the type of change, all major change brings feelings of achievement, loss, pride, and stress. What differentiates a successful change effort from an unsuccessful one is often the ability of a change agent—a person skilled in theory and implementation of planned changed—to deal appropriately with these very real emotions and to connect and balance all aspects of the organization that will be affected by that change" (Marquis and Huston, 2000, p. 71). Lewin (1951) has identified several rules that should be followed when change is necessary:

1. Change should be implemented only for good reason.
2. Change should always be planned and implemented gradually.
3. Change should never be unexpected or abrupt.
4. All people who may be affected by the change should be involved in planning for the change.

Change may be indicated for several reasons, including solving an identified problem, implementing a new program, improving work efficiencies, or adjusting to new mandates by regulatory agencies. For example, some states are implementing stricter "patient rights" regulations for long-term care facilities that will require changes to current patient care practices. Even though a strong reason for change may exist, it almost always will be met with some resistance. Resistance is demonstrated by refusing to cooperate with a course of action or showing active opposition to the change. The effective change agent will recognize that resistance is a natural response to change and will not waste time or energy attempting to eliminate it. Instead the effective change agent will identify and implement effective change strategies that will overcome resistance (Marquis and Huston, 2000).

Stages of Change. Effective change strategies can be developed through the three classic stages of change identified by Lewin (1951). These stages are:

1. Unfreezing stage—the change agent promotes problem identification and encourages awareness of the need for change. People must believe that improvement is possible before they are willing to consider change. The change agent's responsibilities during this stage include:
   a. Gathering information about the problem.
   b. Accurately assessing the problem.
   c. Deciding if change is necessary.
   d. Making others aware of the need for change.
2. Moving stage—the change agent clarifies the need to change, explores alternatives, defines goals and objectives, plans the change, and implements the change plan. The change agent's responsibilities during this stage include:
   a. Identifying areas of support and resistance.

    b. Setting goals and objectives.
    c. Including everyone affected in the planning.
    d. Developing an appropriate change plan with target dates.
    e. Implementing the change plan.
    f. Being available to help, support, and encourage others through the process.
    g. Evaluating the change and making modifications if necessary.
3. Refreezing stage—the change agent integrates the change into the organization so that it becomes recognized as the status quo. If the refreezing stage is not completed, people may drift into old behaviors. The change agent's responsibilities during this stage include:
    a. Requiring and enforcing compliance with the changed processes.
    b. Supporting and encouraging others until the change is no longer viewed as new but as part of the status quo.

In alignment with Lewin's three stages of change (unfreezing, moving, and refreezing), involvement of others and education and training are keys to successful change.

Involvement. The importance of involving all individuals, groups, or departments affected by the change cannot be overstated. Involvement will include clear, two-way communication throughout all phases of the change project and a concerted effort to garner information and feedback from all affected parties about the need for change. The effective change agent will take into consideration the needs of both external and internal customers and understand that a change in one area almost always will affect another group or department *(remember Systems Theory?)*. Consider the following case example.

As the number of procedures being performed in an outpatient surgery department continued to increase, Kevin Michaels, RN, nurse manager, recognized the need to extend the hours of the department to relieve the tight surgery schedule. When the staff began to complain about working through lunch and staying late some evenings, Kevin encouraged them to accept the need for a new department schedule. Kevin discussed the situation with the administrator and all nursing, technical, and clerical staff. He carefully assessed the department's scheduling needs, surveyed the physicians regarding their scheduling preferences, reviewed all options, and finally planned to add a half-day Saturday surgery schedule. Kevin carefully planned the new schedule with the staff and physicians and was pleased that the new plan seemed to be going smoothly. However, Jane, the housekeeping supervisor, who schedules heavy cleaning duties on Saturday mornings when the department was normally closed, was not informed or involved in the schedule change. Much to her dismay, Jane learned through a hallway conversation that she would have to quickly rearrange cleaning schedules and staff schedules to adjust to the new Saturday morning plan.

Peripheral departments (e.g., housekeeping, maintenance, security), crucial to safe, efficient operations, often are the forgotten piece in the planning activities. The nurse manager as the change agent is responsible for informing and involving all individuals and departments to ensure that change is implemented as smoothly as possible.

Education and Training. Education and training also are important components of effective change. People must have appropriate education and training to understand and comply with new policies, procedures, work processes, duties, or responsibilities. Early in the change process, the change agent must consider the training needs of all individuals, groups, and departments. Education and training can reduce fear of the unknown and allow the staff to feel prepared and comfortable with taking on new or different responsibilities.

Other Roles

In addition to the roles of customer service provider, team builder, resource manager, and change agent, nurses in leadership and management positions will find themselves functioning in many other roles. To perform effectively as a nurse manager, each of the management roles described in this chapter is equally important.

Clinical Consultant. Staff members will look to the nurse manager as a resource for clinical advice. For example, the nurse manager will frequently be called on to assess difficult or unusual patient cases and guide the staff nurse to make appropriate nursing judgments. In this role the nurse manager serves as a role model for excellence in nursing care and knowledge and provides ongoing staff training and education.

Staff Developer. The nurse manager should be ever mindful of the need for learning and training opportunities to enhance professional and personal growth for all employees for which he or she supervisors. Accessing resources and planning staff development activities that meet the needs of individual staff members, including RNs, licensed practical nurses/licensed vocational nurses, unlicensed assistive personnel, and clerical staff is a very important role for the nurse manager.

Mentor. As the nurse develops into an effective leader and manager, he or she should accept the responsibility to act as a mentor to new nurses, helping them develop effective leadership and management skills. Mentorship is key to developing our future nursing leaders and managers.

Corporate Supporter. The nurse manager, as a corporate supporter, has a responsibility to embrace the mission, goals, and objectives of the employing organization. In this role as corporate supporter, the nurse manager is a professional representative for the organization and is committed to supporting and accomplishing organizational goals.

CREATING A CARING ENVIRONMENT

Perhaps the most important responsibility for the nurse in any leadership or management role is to create an environment of caring—caring for staff members as well as for patients and families. Staff members who believe that their manager sincerely cares about them and the work they do are able to pass that feeling of caring on to their patients and other customers. Caring for the staff members can be demonstrated through (McNeese-Smith, 1997):

- Offering sincere positive recognition for both individuals and teams.
- Praising and giving thanks for a job well done.
- Spending time with staff members to reinforce positive work behaviors.
- Meeting the staff member's personal needs whenever possible, such as accommodating scheduling needs for family events and being flexible in times of illness.
- Providing guidance and support for professional and personal growth.
- Maintaining a positive, confident attitude and a pleasant work environment.

Staff members who believe that their work is valued and that they are respected and cared about as individuals are able to further contribute to a positive, caring environment in which to provide excellent patient care. Demonstrating respect and concern for every person at every level in the organization is an important leadership quality that the new nurse can use to develop a caring environment. "You show respect when you follow through on a staff concern or complaint. Other expressions of respect include active listening and taking an understanding approach to an employee's family needs" (Perra, 1999, p. 38).

Creating a caring environment in the highly technical, faced-paced, and often stressful health care facilities in which nurses work can be a significant challenge to the nurse manager. But it is a challenge that is at the heart of nursing if we are to promote the very best in patient care. "Failing to attend to caring practices will continue to fuel a technical cure approach to health care rather than attend to illness prevention, care of the chronically ill and health promotion. Sometimes care itself is the most significant outcome, as well as the most significant means to cure, healing and health" (Benner, 1999, p. 318).

LEADERSHIP AND MANAGEMENT SKILLS AND BEHAVIORS

Hersey and Blanchard (1988) have identified that effective leadership and management requires skills in three major areas:
- Technical skills—such as clinical expertise and nursing knowledge
- Human skills—the ability and judgment to work with people in an effective leadership role
- Conceptual skills—the ability to understand the complexities of the overall organization and where one's own area of management fits into the overall organization

At the staff nurse level of management, a considerable amount of technical skill and clinical expertise is needed because the nurse generally is involved in direct supervision of patient care and may be required to help train and mentor nurses and other health care providers. As one advances from lower to higher levels in the organization, more conceptual skills are needed. The common denominator at any level of management is the ability to work with people and provide effective leadership (Hersey and Blanchard, 1988).

Box 16-9 summarizes behaviors and practices that are essential to any nurse who strives to become an effective leader and manager. As the reader will note, human—or caring—skills encompass the largest part of the behaviors and practices identified.

SUMMARY

In every area of health care, the professional nurse is expected to provide leadership and management expertise to help manage complex and ever-changing health care organizations. The multifaceted set of theories, functions, roles, and skills presented in this chapter may at first seem overwhelming to the novice nurse. However, by learning and understanding the principles and concepts involved, the graduate nurse can become a successful nurse leader and manager.

Leadership, management, and organizational theories provide a framework on which to build effective nursing management practices. Although there is no one "best" leadership theory, professional nurses should maintain an awareness of their own behavior and how the key elements of the leadership situation influence outcomes.

The management functions of planning, organizing, staffing, directing, and controlling provide the nurse manager with a defined, practical set of skills to guide management activities. Professional nurses can apply these management functions to perform effectively in various management roles, including customer service provider, team builder, resource manager, change agent, clinical consultant, staff developer, mentor, and corporate supporter. The

BOX 16-9	*Effective Leading and Managing: Conceptual, Human, and Clinical Practices Required*

Conceptual practices

■ Make a commitment to support the mission, vision, and goals of the organization.

■ Accept the realities of the complex health care system—all health care organizations are under pressure to improve productivity, enhance quality, and cut costs, to "do more with less."

■ Understand the needs of external customers (patients, families, physicians, referring facilities) and internal customers (staff, administrators, executives, and other departments).

■ Incorporate legal, ethical, and nursing practice standards into all management functions and activities.

Caring practices

■ Maintain honesty and integrity in work and relationships—trust is an essential requirement for effective leadership. *"To trust a leader, it is not necessary to like him. Nor is it necessary to agree with him. Trust is the conviction that the leader means what he says. It is a belief in something very old-fashioned, called 'integrity'"* (Drucker, 1992).

■ Create a teaching and learning environment—earn a reputation for exceptional training and mentoring for everyone on the team.

■ Model the behavior desired—develop and exhibit a commitment to excellence.

■ Create an open, nonthreatening environment—share information, keep staff informed and encourage them to discuss issues.

■ Make an emotional investment—giving of yourself in a way that the staff understands your commitment to quality patient care. Care as much as one would like others to care.

■ Humanize the work environment—understand and respect both organizational and staff problems. Respect superiors. Coach, counsel, and correct subordinates in private; praise them in public.

■ Communicate effectively—develop good listening skills; listen more than you talk and clarify areas of potential misunderstanding.

■ Give frequent feedback—all staff should know when their performance is excellent or needs improvement.

■ Become a proactive problem solver—knowing how to solve problems is more important than knowing all the answers.

■ Get out of the office and into the patient care areas—listen to patients and staff.

■ Maintain a confident, positive outlook—identify areas in which you are weak and seek help to learn and grow.

Clinical practices

■ Keep your own clinical skills and knowledge current.

■ Train staff members adequately—be certain they are competent to perform their assigned responsibilities.

■ Know the organization's policies and procedures well—ensure that all staff members maintain compliance at all times.

■ Become results-oriented and outcomes-focused in all patient care activities—resource utilization (staff, time, supplies) is more effective when done with the end results in mind.

■ Act as a willing consultant for clinical problems—perform patient assessments, contribute to sound nursing judgments, and teach others.

professional nurse should use conceptual, caring, and technical skills in all leadership and management activities.

Developing effective leadership and management skills is an ongoing process that will continue throughout one's career as a professional nurse (see Box 16-10 for some nursing leadership and management resources). Nurses in management positions should routinely

| **BOX 16-10** | *Helpful Websites/Resources* |

Online resources
American Organization of Nurse Executives
www.aone.org/

American Nurses Association
www.nursingworld.org/

The purpose of the Best Practice Network is to promote information sharing in health care by nurses,
physicians, and other health care professionals. The Best Practice Network facilitates the exchange of
ideas, encourages collaboration in results-oriented problem solving, and enables health care
professionals to share best practices and other creative solutions that will positively impact patient care
and community well-being.
www.best4health.org/

The National Database of Nursing Quality Indicators (NDNQI) is a project of ANA's *Safety and Quality
Initiative,* which addresses the issues of patient safety and quality of care arising from changes in health
care delivery. NDNQI advances this initiative by developing an information resource that will be used to
quantify the specific role of nursing interventions in patient outcomes. Data are being collected from
hospitals across the United States for the NDNQI database.
www.mriresearch.org/health/ndnqi.html

Provides good advice and useful questions to be used when interviewing
www.vsearch.com/artic1.htm

Provides good information from the University of Missouri about behavioral interviewing, the latest interview
style that more and more companies are using in their hiring processes
http://web.missouri.edu/~cppcwww/behaviorlinterviewing.shtml

Journals
American Journal of Nursing
www.nursingworld.org/ajn/

Journal of Nursing Administration Quarterly

Nursing Management

Journal of Nursing Administration

Nursing and Health Care Perspectives

---

analyze personal strengths and weaknesses in each of these management roles and identify
areas in which learning and development are needed. Modeling effective nurse managers and
reading relevant professional journal articles and books are ways to increase leadership and
management knowledge and skills. Management and leadership roles are challenging and exciting and present a wonderful opportunity to grow professionally and personally.

Critical Thinking

1. Obtain a copy of the mission, values, philosophy, and goals of a nursing unit. How is the mission communicated to staff members? How are the goals accomplished? Identify and list behaviors that you observe on the unit that are not consistent with beliefs, values, and activities expressed in the document. If you were the nurse manager, how would you handle the behaviors that are inconsistent with the mission, values, philosophy, and goals of the nursing unit?

2. Identify experienced nurses who seem to be efficient at accomplishing their daily work. How do these nurses plan and organize their daily assignments? How do the experienced nurses interact with other members of the health care team? Identify and list several management skills that help the nurses accomplish their work more efficiently.

3. Think about a situation in the nursing unit in which an unsatisfactory management decision was made. Was the decision based on inaccurate or incomplete information or on an incorrectly identified problem? How could this situation have been avoided? What would you recommend to prevent a similar circumstance from occurring in the future?

4. Identifying and meeting customer (patients, clients, families) needs is an important management function. Identify and describe how an organization gathers and uses input from customers. What follow-up evaluation is done by the organization in response to positive and negative comments by customers?

REFERENCES

American Nurses Association: *Standards and scope of gerontological nursing practice,* Kansas City, Mo, 1995, ANA.

American Nurses Association: *Standards of clinical nursing practice,* ed 2, Kansas City, Mo, 1998, ANA.

American Nurses Association: *The scope and standards of public health nursing practice,* Kansas City, Mo, 1999, ANA.

Association of Operating Room Nurses: *Standards, recommended practices, and guidelines,* Denver, Co, 2001, AORN.

Belcher J: Improving managers' critical thinking skills: student-generated case studies, *J Nurs Admin* 30 (7/8):351-353, 2000.

Benner P: Nursing leadership for the new millennium: claiming the wisdom and worth of clinical practice, *Nurs Healthcare Perspect* 20(6):312-319, 1999.

Burns J: *Leadership.* New York, 1978, Harper & Row.

Drucker PF: *Managing for the future: the 1990s and beyond,* New York, 1992, Truman Talley Books/Dutton.

Dunham-Taylor J: Nurse executive transformational leadership found in participative Organizations, *J Nurs Admin* 30(5):241-250, 2000.

Hersey P, Blanchard K: *Management of organizational behavior: utilizing human resources,* ed 4, Englewood Cliffs, NJ, 1988, Prentice-Hall.

Howenstein MA et al: Factors associated with critical thinking among nurses, *J Cont Educ Nurs* 27(3):100-103, 1996.

Lewin K: *Field theory in social sciences,* New York, 1951, Harper & Row.

Marquis BL, Huston CJ: *Leadership roles and management functions in nursing,* ed 3, Philadelphia, 2000, JB Lippincott.

Marquis BL, Huston CJ: *Management decision making for nurses,* ed 3, Philadelphia, 1998, JB Lippincott.

Marriner-Tomey A: *Nursing management and leadership,* St Louis, 2000, Mosby.

Marrelli TM: *The nurse manager's survival guide,* St Louis, 1997, Mosby.

McGuire E: Chaos theory: learning a new science, *J Nurs Admin* 29(2):8-9, 1999.

McNeese-Smith D: The influence of manager behavior on nurses' job satisfaction, productivity and commitment, *J Nurs Admin* 27(9):47-55, 1997.

Moss R, Rowles C: Staff nurse job satisfaction and management style, *Nurs Manage* 28(1):32-34, 1997.

Norman L: Continuous improvement in nursing education, *Qual Connection* 6(20):4, 1997.

Perra BM: The leader in you, *Nurs Manage* 30(1):35-39, 1999.

Peters T, Waterman RH: *In search of excellence,* New York, 1982, Harper & Row.

Stogdill RM: *Handbook of leadership: a survey of theory and research,* New York, 1974, The Free Press.

Sullivan EJ, Decker PJ: *Effective leadership and management in nursing,* ed 4, Menlo Park, 1997, Addison Wesley Longman.

Taccetta-Chapnick M, Rafferty G: Promoting client satisfaction, *Nurs Manage* 28(1):45-48, 1997.

Thompson JD: *Organizations in action,* New York, 1967, McGraw-Hill.

White RK, Lippit R: *Autocracy and democracy: an experimental inquiry,* New York, 1960, Harper & Row.

Wywialowski EF: *Managing client care,* ed 2, St Louis, 1997, Mosby.

Yoder Wise P: *Leading and managing in nursing,* St Louis, 1999, Mosby.

SUGGESTED READINGS

Covey S: *The seven habits of highly effective people,* New York, 1990, Simon & Schuster.

Grensing-Pophal L: Give-and-take feedback, *Nurs Manage* 31(2):27-28, 2000.

McElhaney RM: Conflict management in nursing administration, *Nurs Manage* 27(3):49-50, 1996.

Scholtes PR, Joiner BL, Streibel BJ: *The team handbook,* Madison, Wisc, 1996, Joiner Associates.

Effective Communication

17

Anna Sallee, MSN, RN, CCRN

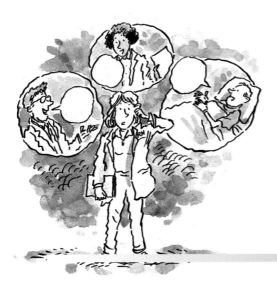

Effective communication
is a major component of successful
nursing practice.

Vignette

Lois Cox, RN, sighed. Things were not easy at home, this was her fourth 12-hour shift in a row, and now she was being told that the patient in 412 was just impossible. "Don't be surprised if you spend all day in there," Marilyn had said. "And, no matter what you do, it won't be right. Good luck; you'll need it."

Wearily, Lois started her morning assessments. Mr. Salcido in room 412 was grouchy and complained a lot. Lois could hardly complete a task before he expressed dissatisfaction or demanded something else. As Lois returned to the nurses' station to chart vital signs, she mentally reviewed her patient assignment and decided that she would save Mr. Salcido's morning care until last so that she could spend more time with him. The risk, of course, was that he would become impatient while waiting.

In addition to providing more time with Mr. Salcido, Lois resolved to use all of her communication skills. She would greet him cheerfully, respond with kindness and patience regardless of his demeanor, make pleasant conversation, and—above all—would listen for clues to explain his behavior. Maybe she could do something to make him happier.

Forty-five minutes later, Lois emerged from Mr. Salcido's room humbled and once again acutely aware of how easily a patient's deepest needs can go unrecognized. After rapport was finally established and Mr. Salcido decided he could trust Lois, he had confided to her that his wife had died in the same room 2 years earlier. He believed it was not masculine to cry or to express weakness with strangers. His anger was an expression of his unresolved grief over the death of his wife.

Questions to consider while reading this chapter
1. What communication techniques did Lois use to establish rapport with Mr. Salcido?
2. What nonverbal cues should Lois watch for as she begins initial care and communication with Mr. Salcido?
3. What strategies can Lois use to build trusting relationships with each of the patients she cares for?
4. How should Lois communicate her discovery about the source of Mr. Salcido's anger to the other staff members?

Key Terms

Blocking Obstructing communication through noncommittal answers, generalization, or other techniques that hamper continued interaction.

Communication components The sender, the receiver, the message.

Communication subcomponents Interpretation, filtration, feedback.

Feedback Response from the receiver, which can be verbal or nonverbal.

Filtration Unconscious exclusion of extraneous stimuli.

Interpretation Receiver's understanding of the meaning of the communication.

Negative communication techniques Behavior that blocks or impairs effective communication.

Nonverbal communication Unspoken cues (intentional or unintentional) from the communicant, such as body positioning, facial expression, or lack of attention.

Positive communication techniques Behavior that enhances effective communication.

Learning Outcomes

After studying this chapter, the reader will be able to:
1. Apply effective oral communication techniques in diverse situations.
2. Evaluate conflicting verbal and nonverbal communication cues.
3. Implement effective written communication skills.
4. Apply effective strategies for managing conflict.

CHAPTER OVERVIEW

Communication is one of the most basic human endeavors. At the moment of birth with the wail of new life, the infant begins a journey toward development of an effective way to interface with the world. Webster's New World Dictionary defines communication as, "**1.** the act of transmitting, **2.** a giving or exchanging of information, signals, or messages by talk, gestures, writing, etc . . . ."

There are many styles of transmitting information. Observation of a preverbal child for any time will yield creative, humorous, and usually fairly clear methods of disclosing desires and needs. The exchange of ideas and feelings is hardly limited to verbal communication. Although the spoken word is most commonly used for societal communication, a highly developed sign language exists for people who are unable to speak or hear. There are many types of nonverbal communication that often are as effective as, and in some instances more effective than, audible expression.

Effective communication is a major part of the nursing profession. Nurses interact with patients, families and significant others, nursing peers, student nurses, physicians, other members of the transdisciplinary team, and the public. Nurses communicate through a variety of media, including the spoken and written word, demonstration, role modeling, and, on occasion, public appearances. This chapter reviews the components of the communication process, communication styles, and principles of effective communication in professional nursing. In addition, communication issues related to cultural diversity, collaboration, dealing with conflict, effective delegation, and documentation are addressed.

HISTORY

Our nursing ancestors recognized the need for clear communication as a basic component of the profession. Their comments provide an interesting perspective on the development of nurse-patient and nurse-physician communication.

Florence Nightingale (1859) admonished persons attending the sick to be cautious in speaking about the patient as if he or she were not present or in tones too low for the patient to hear. *"I have often been surprised at the thoughtlessness . . . of friends or of doctors who will hold a long conversation just in the room or passage adjoining the room of the patient . . . who knows they are talking about him. . . . If it is a whispered conversation in the same room, then it is absolutely cruel."*

Later, in the chapter "Chattering Hopes and Advices," Nightingale inquires, *"Do, you who are about the sick or who visit the sick, try and give them pleasure, remember to tell them what will do so. . . . A sick person does so enjoy hearing good news. . . . A sick person also intensely enjoys hearing of any material good, any positive or practical success of the right."*

More than half a century later, Sue Parsons (1916) wrote regarding communication with the patient, *"Just by your expression you may assure him that he is among friends. If you cannot speak his language, you will attempt to get an interpreter to explain what the examinations mean, what the doctors are trying to do to help him, and to ask him if there is anything he wishes."* Regarding communication with physicians, Parsons advises the young nurse, *"When she becomes sufficiently experienced to detect a mistake, she will, of course, call his attention to it by asking if her understanding of the order is correct."*

Under the subtitle of "Discretion," Parsons (1916) warns, *"Nurses and doctors are sometimes thoughtless in conversation; they discuss a patient's condition before him, thinking he does not understand or care, and sometimes believing him too ill to notice what is said. This is a great mistake."* Regarding idle conversation that breaches patient confidentiality, Parsons observes, *"If a nurse, when meeting friends, finds herself invariably talking shop, gossiping about doctors, nurses, and patients, she must realize that she is on the road to unhappiness and cynicism."* In today's environment she would be on the road to litigation as well.

In the same era Katharine DeWitt (1917) penned, *"She [the nurse] must not only respect expressed preferences, but her imagination must be on the alert, ready to perceive, without the need of words, what is agreeable or disagreeable to her charge."* And, most profoundly, *"Every nurse should be a health missionary, telling how to keep well, how to avoid disease, how to aid in the great campaign for public health, good living and morality."*

COMPONENTS OF COMMUNICATION

Communication generally is thought to have three components—the sender, the receiver, and the message. As a dynamic process, communication is cyclic so that the receiver becomes the sender when responding. These roles then alternate as the communication process continues. Inherent in the process is a level of subcomponents, consisting of interpretation, filtration, and feedback. Fig. 17-1 is a visual representation of the basic communication process.

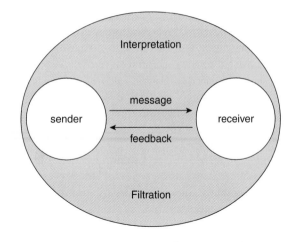

FIG. 17-1 Components of communication.

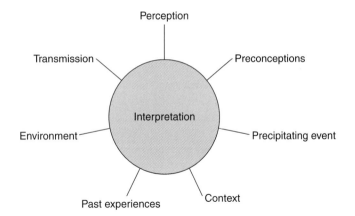

FIG. 17-2 Factors influencing interpretation of messages.

Interpretation

Interpretation of information can be influenced by such factors as context, environment, precipitating event, preconceived ideas, personal perceptions, style of transmission, and past experiences. Because of the interaction of these factors, the sender's message may mean to the receiver something that was entirely unplanned or unexpected by the sender (Fig. 17-2).

Context and Environment. Context refers to the entire situation relevant to the communication, such as the environment, the background, and the particular circumstances that lead to the discussion. Environment can denote physical surroundings and happenings and the emotional conditions involved in the communication.

Precipitating Event. Precipitating event refers specifically to the event or situation that prompted the communication. Precipitating event refers to a specific single event, whereas context describes the whole ambiance of the situation, with the inclusion of multiple circumstances that have led to the precipitating event.

Preconceived Ideas. Preconceived ideas are conceptions, opinions, or thoughts that the receiver has developed before the encounter. Such ideas can dramatically affect the receiver's acceptance and understanding of the message.

Style of Transmission. Style of transmission involves many aspects of the manner of conveyance of the message. Transmission styles include aspects such as open or closed statements or questions, body language, method of organizing the message, degree of attention to the topic or to the receiver, vocabulary chosen (professional jargon vs. language a layperson could easily understand), and intonation.

Past Experiences. Each person comes to any type of communication, whether it is friendly conversation, informational lecture, staff meeting, performance evaluation, or any other possible scenario, with baggage in terms of past experiences. Because past experiences will be a variety of positive, neutral, and negative events, the influence that the experiences can and will have on communication may be positive, neutral, or negative. The importance of recognizing that any reaction from the receiver may be biased by previous experiences cannot be overstated. A perfect example is presented in the vignette when Mr. Salcido was hospitalized in the same room in which his wife died 2 years earlier. An astute sender will begin to investigate such a possibility if the receiver reacts in an unexpected or inappropriate manner to information that was not expected to produce such a response, which may range from nonresponse to overly vehement response.

Personal Perceptions. Personal perceptions can have a profound effect on the quality of communication. Perception is awareness through the excitation of all the senses. Perception can be described as all that the person knows about a situation or circumstance based on what each of the senses—taste, smell, sight, sound, touch, and intuition—discover and interpret.

Consider the processes of interpretation that occur in the following example. Donna was an industrious young wife who managed a job, children, and housekeeping. She rarely became sick, but, when an illness did occur, she felt considerable dismay at the response she received from her husband, Dave. When she most needed him to provide assistance and care, he seemed to grow irritable and pull away, leaving her with less physical and emotional support than when she was well.

On one such occasion tempers flared, and an argument ensued. Suddenly Dave burst out, "You're just like Mom. Sick all the time." Donna and Dave were shocked at the remark. Donna was not sick all the time. Dave's mother was sick all the time. Once the real issue, that of Dave's frustration with his mother's frequent illnesses, had been identified, Donna and Dave were able to work through the reality of the situation, and the problem was resolved.

Filtration

The most concise delivery of information is subject to some amount of filtration. Compare the process to washing vegetables in a colander. A large amount of water is poured over the pro-

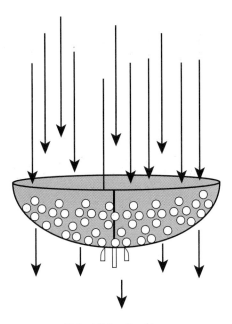

FIG. 17-3 Filtration.

duce. Some of the water comes quickly through the colander holes, some water drips through more slowly; and some water hangs on the contents or settles in the solid portions of the colander and never filters through. If people were not able to filter out a part of the stimuli that bombard them daily, the clutter would be unmanageable! At the same time, however, it is possible to filter out some part of intended communication that is essential to facilitate understanding (Fig. 17-3).

Feedback

Feedback, simply put, is the response from the receiver. However, as with all communication, feedback is a dynamic process. As the receiver interprets and responds to the original message, the sender begins the same process of feedback to the receiver. Because of this circular property, the process frequently is referred to as the "feedback loop" (van Servellen, 1997). As with the original message, feedback is not confined to verbal responses alone. Both communicants constantly assess nonverbal communication as well. Feedback is formed based on all the components of interpretation and filtration.

VERBAL VS. NONVERBAL COMMUNICATION
Verbal Communication

Verbal communication refers to the spoken word. Many factors influence the meaning of oral speech. An abundance of words can have several meanings. For example, consider the phrase, "He flew the plane." Suppose more information is provided. "The cropduster flew the plane." "The Air Force pilot flew the plane." "The Coast Guard Search and Rescue pilot flew the plane." The visual image of the plane changes with each statement from a small fixed-wing plane capable of dusting crops, to a jet, to an aquatic plane with pontoons for landing on water. To carry the interpretation a step farther, it is likely that the impression of the intensity or style of flying also will change.

Another clue to the meaning of oral communication is the tone or inflection with which the words are spoken. Suzette Haden Elgin (1993, p. 186) refers to the "... tune the words are set to." More of Elgin's work is available at www.sfwa.org/members/elgin/. The key to the true meaning of a statement may be contained in the emphasis placed on a specific word. Consider how differently the following phrase could be perceived based on the inflection or the emphasis on the wording:

- You are going **to bed.**
- **You** are going to bed.
- You **are going** to bed.

With an emphasis on bed, the first phrase most likely will be perceived as an inquiry. The second phrase might imply that you are going to bed, but no one else is. The last phrase, an imperative, gives the impression of increased emotion such as anger or frustration.

Nonverbal Communication

Nonverbal communication involves many factors that either confirm or deny the spoken word. Facial expression, the presence or absence of eye contact, posture, and body movement all project a direct message. Indirect messages that are nonverbal might include dressing style, lifestyle, or material possessions. Never presume that external trappings and physical presentation do not influence the quality of communication. Preconceived ideas and expectations interpret input from all such sources, often on an almost subconscious level.

No one can miss the message regarding "body language" sung by the sea witch in the film *The Little Mermaid* (Ashman and Menken, 1988), which says that Ariel can win the Prince without her voice because of the power of body language. Body language can speak volumes—sometimes in support of the verbal message, but other times in direct opposition to the spoken words.

Imagine being greeted by a door-to-door salesman with a proverbial silver tongue. He makes all the right statements about the lovely home and darling children but holds out a limp hand to shake and draws back when one of the children reaches toward him. Which message seems more likely to be true—the verbal or the nonverbal?

The inability to make eye contact can be construed to mean that the speaker is shy, scared, or not telling the truth. The judgment of which condition is the correct one then is based on all the factors that feed into the receiver's interpretation—perception, preconceptions, precipitating event, context, past experiences, environment, and transmission. Faced with the many opportunities for incorrect interpretation, is it any wonder that misunderstandings occur?

An important concept to remember is that, when the verbal and nonverbal messages do not agree, the receiver is more likely to believe the nonverbal message. Jan Hargrave (2001) tells us that our bodies give "hidden messages" all the time. We can't get away from what our bodies say; they don't lie!

An understanding of the importance prescribed to body language and other nonverbal clues to the intent of the message explains the advantage of face-to-face communication whenever possible. Although a telephone conversation supplies verbal messages, intonation, and feedback, other signals are missing such as facial expression, body position, and environmental clues. The perils inherent in written communication are discussed later in this chapter.

LOGICAL FALLACIES

Many times we find ourselves influenced by what appear to be justifiable arguments of others. Sometimes these arguments are not based on sound logic. Recognition of faulty logic will promote effective communication and save a lot of confusion or even conflict. The following are some logical fallacies that are frequently encountered. For more information on logical fallacies, you can visit the following sites: www.nizkor.org/features/fallacies/ or www.datanation.com/fallacies/index.htm.

Ad Hominem Abusive

Ad hominem abusive is an argument that attacks the person instead of the issue. The speaker hopes to discredit the other person by calling attention to some irrelevant fact about that person. Perhaps a nurse has just had a disagreement with a physician about laboratory results that were not properly reported. The nurse makes the following comment to colleagues: "She thinks she's so smart just because she's a doctor." What does that have to do with the disagreement? Nothing. It is an unwarranted attack on the doctor. Does it accomplish the purpose? Very likely the group will be influenced by the disparaging comment. They may even become angry at the physician who had legitimate cause to be upset about not receiving laboratory results. Ultimately the issue of unreported laboratory values is lost in the attack against the doctor.

Appeal to Common Practice

Appeal to common practice occurs when the argument is made that something is okay because most people do it. This logic is likely to be faulty in two ways: (1) do "most" people really do it? (2) does common practice really make an action okay? It's easy to imagine a situation in which using an explanation that you did something because you'd seen someone else do it that way, rather than checking the organization policy and procedure manual, could lead to significant professional and legal problems.

Appeal to Emotion

Appeal to emotion is an attempt to manipulate other people's emotions to avoid the real issue. For example, consider Deb, RN, who has made a medication error. She has been called into the nurse manager's office to discuss the incident and receives a written warning. She comes out tearful. It is obvious to her colleagues that she has been reprimanded. She begins to discuss the problem and makes the following statements: "I am the first person in my family to even go to college. I'm a single parent and I've worked so hard to get where I am. Our manager doesn't care anything about that. She just wants to pass out written warnings to cover herself. She doesn't care about us as individuals." After a bit of this type of talk, the entire staff is probably becoming angry with the nurse manager—who may feel very badly about having had to give the written warning because she *does* care about her staff. However, Deb has successfully deflected the attention away from the real issue, the medication error that was legitimately addressed, and appealed to the emotions of her colleagues.

Appeal to Tradition

Appeal to tradition is the argument that doing things a certain way is best because they've always been done that way. This argument is often expressed as, "that's just how it's done here."

Another version would be, "Oh, we tried that once, and it didn't work, so we went back to the old way." Change always brings some uncertainty, but choosing to continue a practice just because "that's the way we've always done it" is not very sound reasoning. Health care is a very dynamic arena. The old ways of doing things seldom work out to be the best in this time of rapid change.

Confusing Cause and Effect

Confusing cause and effect occurs when we assume that one event must cause another just because we often see the two events occur together. Amber and Chyane are nurses in labor and delivery. One night shift, two mothers delivered babies with significant "birthmarks." It happened to be a night with a full moon. Amber states, "Clearly, babies born on a night during the full moon are more likely to have birthmarks." She makes the assumption that since the moon was full and two babies were born with birthmarks, some cause-and-effect relationship must exist.

Hasty Generalization

Hasty generalization involves coming to a conclusion based on a very small number of examples. A hasty generalization occurs whenever an assumption is made that a small group represents the whole population. Two nurses are discussing a co-worker who seems a bit disorganized and always leaves a mess. One of the nurses makes the following statement, "Well, what do you expect from a blonde? You know how ditzy Capri was, and she was a blonde, too." The hasty generalization here is that, because the nurse knew two blondes who were disorganized and messy, all blondes must be disorganized and messy.

Red Herring

Red herring is the introduction of an irrelevant topic to divert attention away from the real issue. Two nurses, Brian and Nikoah, are having an argument regarding Brian's failure to complete his assigned tasks. Brian states, "It's not my work that you're really mad about. It's that I'm a guy. You just don't like male nurses." Nikoah then begins to defend herself, denying any prejudice against male nurses. The focus of the argument has been turned from the real issue, Brian's failure to complete his assigned tasks, to a situation in which Nikoah is on the defensive about her opinion of male nurses.

Slippery Slope

Slippery slope is the belief that an event will inevitably follow another without any real support for that belief. In fact, this type of logic often leads from a fairly harmless situation to an assumption akin to the notion that the sky is falling. Kathy and Janet are talking in the nurses' lounge over lunch. Kathy is upset over the recent announcement that the unit is going to convert to computerized bedside charting. Kathy states, "It was bad enough having to chart all we do. Now we have to learn to use computers and make all kinds of entries. We'll probably have just as much paperwork. We'll end up spending even less time with the patients. The next thing you know, nurses will be sitting at a computer terminal, and someone else will be taking care of patients. Then they'll decide they don't really need nurses at all!" Kathy's logic takes her from a simple unit change to the end of nursing as we know it! Yet we often hear that kind of "escalating disaster" logic when change is introduced.

Straw Man

Straw man occurs when the actual issue is ignored and replaced with a distorted or exaggerated version. Cindy and Toi, both labor and delivery nurses, are discussing one of the local politician's stand on abortion. Toi states, "Dave Stroud said in an interview that he is very strongly opposed to late-term abortions." Cindy becomes angered immediately and says, "Oh, so he doesn't believe in abortion. He thinks a woman doesn't have a right to choose, to say what happens to her own body. I figured him for that kind of a person." In actuality, the interview said nothing about the politician's opinion on abortion earlier in a pregnancy. Cindy's faulty logic has effectively represented Mr. Stroud as insensitive to women, with nothing to support that position. She has not only exaggerated his stated opinion but distorted it to imply an attitude that was never addressed in the statement.

Understanding these logical fallacies should help the nurse recognize the difference between legitimate and faulty reasoning. A clear understanding and use of sound logic will help health care providers present issues and resolve problems effectively.

POSITIVE COMMUNICATION TECHNIQUES
Trust

Trust between the nurse and the patient is essential to effective communication and often must be cultivated. Factors that enhance the development of trust include openness on the part of the nurse, honesty, integrity, and dependability. These can be achieved by:

- Communicating clearly in language that laypersons can understand.
- Keeping promises.
- Protecting confidentiality.
- Avoiding negative communication techniques such as blocking and false reassurance.
- Being available to the patient.

The need for trust is not limited to the nurse-patient relationship, but rather it pervades all associations. Care is more effective when the nursing team and the transdisciplinary team share the essential element of trust.

"I Messages"

The use of "I messages" is a fundamental component in acceptable communication. Consider the following exchange.

Laura: "You make me so mad, Donald."
Donald: "I don't mean to make you mad."
Laura: "Well, you do. You never think about how I feel. You know I hate it when you leave a patient's room as cluttered as 103."
Donald: "You don't have the vaguest idea what went on here last night! That's what I hate about you—always so quick to judge. You are so critical. You must think that you're perfect!"

When a comment starts with "you," most commonly the receiver's defenses will promptly go on alert. The use of "you" in such a context sounds—and most probably is meant to be—accusatory. Notice how the emotions quickly escalate to anger. Notice that, although initially the receiver tries to sound conciliatory, he soon begins to respond in like form. Instead of using accusatory and defensive language, the sender should place emphasis on his or her feelings, rather than on the receiver as the cause of the feelings.

"Donald, I feel so upset when I find a cluttered room like 103 at the beginning of my shift. I feel as if I'm behind when I start." The difference is obvious. When "I messages" are used, they become less likely to sound accusatory. By using such an opening, the sender allows the receiver to respond to the true message rather than start to mount a defense. It allows for more effective communication because the receiver is more likely to offer an explanation such as the following.

"I'm really sorry about room 103, Laura. I guess the wheel that doesn't squeak doesn't get oiled, as they say. Our shift started last night with a patient coding right after he arrived from the Emergency Department. There was no family here. It took forever to find them and then to support them through the shock. About the time things settled down, the patient in room 110 coded. It was quite a night."

In this instance the "I message" enhances communication by giving Donald the opportunity to address the real concern. In addition, if Laura is truly astute, she has a wonderful opportunity to support her colleague by voicing appreciation for the working circumstances of his shift. Most people respond gratefully to recognition and commiseration. The exchange could build collegiality between the two co-workers and perhaps between the two shifts.

Eye Contact

As mentioned previously, avoiding eye contact can be interpreted a number of different ways. A person who does not make eye contact may be thought to be shy, scared, insecure, preoccupied, unprepared, dishonest—the list could go on and on. None of these qualities is likely to be appreciated in a primary caregiver. By making direct eye contact, the nurse gives undivided attention to the patient, and the patient is likely to feel valued and understood by the nurse. Eye contact in essence says, "I am wholly available to you. What you are saying is important to me."

Eye contact is equally important in communication with co-workers and other members of the transdisciplinary team. This quality is lost in telephone conversations or written communications.

Keep in mind that the use of direct eye contact is a Western value. In some cultures avoidance of eye contact is more appropriate social behavior. By careful observation, the nurse quickly will recognize whether direct eye contact is interpreted as inappropriate or disrespectful. Nurses must make every effort to be sensitive to the cultural values of the client and their co-workers to enhance effective communication.

Promise Keeping

Little else can destroy the fragile trust developing in any interpersonal relationship as quickly as making and then breaking promises. Inherent in the concept of promise keeping are the qualities of honesty and integrity. Once a commitment is made, every effort must be expended to fulfill the expectation. Sometimes the request is impossible to satisfy. If this happens, the nurse must explain the situation or circumstances. The fact that the patient understands that the nurse has made an effort to meet his or her needs or desires often is more important than whether the goal is accomplished. If the nurse responds, "I'll check on that," and then finds the request impossible to fulfill but never returns with an explanation, the lack of dependability perceived by the patient (or colleague) will surely drive a wedge into the relationship.

Empathy

Empathy is the ability to mentally place oneself in another person's situation to better understand the person and to share the emotions or feelings of the person. Empathy is not feeling sorry for another. Empathy is understanding the experiences of the other person. Development of empathy builds the nurse's ability to help the patient through a true understanding of the patient's feelings and needs. Empathy is integral to the therapeutic relationship. The nurse is able to perceive and address the needs of the patient without emotional involvement to the point of becoming inappropriately immersed in the situation.

Open Communication Style

Certain styles of phrasing questions and statements lend themselves to obtaining more information. For example, suppose Chris asks Mr. Barrow, "Do you know where you are?" and Mr. Barrow responds, "Yes." Can Chris assume that Mr. Barrow knows he is in the hospital? Not necessarily. Chris may be surprised to hear a completely unexpected response if he rephrases the inquiry.

> "Mr. Barrow, tell me where you are."
> "Why I'm in the honeymoon berth of the Titanic, of course. Have you seen my lovely bride?"

Using open-ended questions or statements that require more information than "yes" or "no" can augment gathering enough facts to build a more complete picture of the circumstances. Questions or statements that are phrased to require only one- or two-word responses may miss the mark entirely.

Clarification

Both communicants have a responsibility to clarify anything not understood. The sender should ask for feedback to be certain the receiver is correctly interpreting what is being said. The receiver should stop the sender anytime the message becomes unclear and should provide feedback regularly so that misinterpretation can be identified quickly. Such phrases as, "What I hear you saying is . . ." or "I understand you to mean . . ." help to communicate to the sender what is being perceived. Other techniques of clarification include using easily understood language, giving examples, drawing a picture, making a list, and finding ways to stimulate all the senses to enhance the ability to understand.

Body Language

Body positioning and movement send loud messages to others. The nurse can imply openness that facilitates effective communication by awareness of body position and movement. In addition to eye contact, effective communication is enriched through an open stance, such as holding one's arms at the side or out toward the patient, rather than crossed, or leaning toward the patient as if to hear more clearly rather than away from the patient.

Touch

Most people have a fairly well-defined personal space. It is important for the nurse to be sensitive to each patient's personal preference and cultural differences in terms of touch. However, for many people a gentle touch can scale mountains in terms of demonstrating genuine interest and concern. A pat on the back, a hand held, a back rub are all behaviors that indicate availability and accessibility on the part of the nurse.

NEGATIVE COMMUNICATION TECHNIQUES

Several negative communication techniques have been alluded to in the previous discussion. Closed communication styles such as asking yes-no questions or making inquiries or statements that require single-word answers potentially limits the response of the person and may prevent the discovery of pertinent facts. Closed body language also can hinder effective communication. Crossed arms, hands on the hips, avoidance of eye contact, and turning or moving away from the person all impose a sense of distance in the relationship.

Blocking

Another technique that is detrimental to good communication and the development of a trusting relationship is blocking. Blocking occurs when the nurse responds with noncommittal or generalized answers. For example:

"Nurse, I've never had surgery before. I'm afraid I might not ever wake up." Mr. Clayton is twisting the bedsheet as he speaks.

"Oh, Mr. Clayton, many people feel that way. It'll be okay." Amanda Butler, RN, smiles brightly, pats his hand, picks up the dirty linen bag, and bounces out of the room.

Does Mr. Clayton feel reassured? Not likely. Will he be inclined to broach the subject with Amanda again? Probably not. Amanda has incorporated some important aspects of communication into her response—cheerfulness and touch—but she has not truly communicated. She has effectively blocked Mr. Clayton's attempt to get the reassurance he wanted from her. He may be too intimidated to ask anyone else, assuming that his fear is invalid.

By generalizing in this way, Amanda has trivialized Mr. Clayton's concerns. He is not "many people." He needs to be validated as a person experiencing a legitimate feeling. Amanda can validate his fear and put it into perspective at the same time with a different approach.

Nurse: *What makes you think you might not wake up, Mr. Clayton?*
Patient: *Well, my wife's cousin's husband had surgery about 25 years ago, and he never woke up.*
Nurse: *What kind of surgery did he have?*
Patient: *Uh, it was some kind of heart surgery, and he had another heart attack on the table and died right there.*
Nurse: *It sounds like his condition was critical going into surgery.*
Patient: *Yes, ma'am. He'd been sick for a long time.*
Nurse: *It's not uncommon to feel afraid of being put to sleep, especially if you have never had surgery before. There are rare cases in which complications do occur during surgery. That's why we put the disclosures on the consent form, so that you will know just what the risks are. Thankfully most surgeries are without such drastic problems. Although your gallbladder certainly has made you uncomfortable, you are otherwise in good health. The tests that were done before surgery, like the chest radiograph and the laboratory work, show that you are healthy and should do well with the anesthesia. That drastically decreases the chance for complications in your case. I would be glad to answer any other questions you have or to ask the anesthetist to come and talk with you some more.*

Amanda has validated Mr. Clayton's feeling as legitimate, provided an explanation with reasonable reassurances, and offered to explore the issue with him further, or to have someone else talk with him.

Some things are difficult to talk about with another person. The dying patient may want to talk about how he or she feels, ask questions, or perform a life review. A nurse who is uncomfortable with such topics may consciously or unconsciously block communication through generalizations or closed responses. Avoiding the blocking technique requires a good understanding of oneself. If unable to provide the open communication the patient obviously needs, the nurse should access other personnel who are more comfortable in the situation. This might be another nurse, a social worker, a physician, a member of the clergy, a family member, or a friend of the patient.

False Assurances

False assurances are similar to and have about the same effect as blocking. When someone is trying to get real answers or express serious concerns, an answer such as "Don't worry," or "It'll be okay" sends several unintended messages. Such an answer can be interpreted by the patient as placating or showing a lack of concern or a lack of knowledge. The patient might even conclude that the nurse is being neglectful through trivialization of an issue that is important to him or her. At the very least, the nurse has neither recognized the need the patient has expressed nor provided validation.

Conflicting Messages

Conflicting messages also have been alluded to in the previous discussion. If a person professes pleasure at seeing someone but draws back when that person extends a hand of greeting, the nonverbal message speaks more loudly than the words spoken. If a nurse enters a room and goes through the routine greeting by rote (even with a smiling face and a bouncing step), a patient can quickly perceive this and consider the nurse less approachable.

The nurse's statement that the patient's condition is important to the nurse followed by failing to answer the call bell in a timely manner or by forgetting to bring items promised to the patient sends a double message. Such behavior can leave the patient confused, frustrated, or angry. Carrying through with a commitment, no matter how unimportant it may seem, is a premier method of saying to the patient, "You are important to me."

LISTENING

Neal Samuels, RN, decided to make an unplanned stop at the clinic one evening after hours, arriving without his magnetized name badge that would let him in select doors. As he pushed the intercom button outside the door to contact security, he formulated a concise message to explain his predicament. He could see the security guard through the tinted window. A clear voice sounded through the speaker, "Police Department. Can I help you?"

Neal responded, "Yes, my name is Neal Samuels. I am on the School of Nursing faculty. While I was out shopping, I realized I needed to stop by my office, and I don't have my badge with me to open the door. Would you let me in?"

"Do you work here?" the officer asked.

"Yes, I work in the School of Nursing."

"Then use your badge to get in."

"I don't have it with me," Ned repeated.

"What did you say your name was?" the officer responded.

And so it went.

Listening certainly is as important an element in clear and effective communication as any other component. Many distracters contribute to poor listening habits. Framing an answer while the other person is still talking interferes with receiving the entire message. Environmental disturbances can provide major disruption. A crying baby, a call light buzzing, or multiple concurrent conversations in a busy nurses' station are a few of the interruptions that jumble the simplest of instructions. Preexisting concerns or worries can block absorption of conversation because of the preoccupation. Attempts to continue work in progress leads to inattention. Ineffective engagement or peculiar mannerisms on the part of the speaker can be distracting. A person who does not make eye contact, shuffles through papers while talking, or overuses hand movements actually can deter communication.

A number of techniques can be used by the receiver to facilitate the ability to listen.

- Give undivided attention to the sender by moving to a quieter area and stopping the speaker to clarify any points not understood.
- Provide feedback in terms of perceived meaning of the message rephrased in the receiver's own words.
- Give attention to positioning to face the sender and make eye contact.
- Note nonverbal messages such as body language and respond to them.

Mindful listening will dramatically improve the likelihood of receiving the correct message. However, equally important is the fact that attentive listening implies a respect for the speaker and communicates a regard for what the speaker has to offer. The nonverbal message that keen listening delivers is, "I value you, and what you have to say is important to me."

WRITTEN COMMUNICATION

Rhonda stared at the sign in amusement. Concurrent seminar sessions had been planned in a large room equipped with sliding soundproof panels that could be rolled along a track to effectively divide the large room into two smaller conference rooms. However, the sections had not been moved into place to create the dividing wall—the panels remained in two rows on short tracks against a structural wall. For the past 20 minutes, Rhonda had watched several of the attendees struggle to move the dividers along the track.

The group quickly realized that the sections would need to be moved in an alternating fashion from first one side row and then the other row. When the last piece should have slid into place, it became obvious that the panels should have been pulled out in reverse order. All the panels had to be replaced in storage position. The process then was redone starting with the opposite panel row.

When the last section finally was pulled into place, the audience burst into a round of applause. Simultaneously, the following sign, written in large black print on white paper and posted at eye level, came into view (Fig. 17-4).

The message certainly is clear. Did the sign accomplish its intended mission? Not by a long stretch! Undoubtedly the placard was effective when the dividing wall was in use because it could be clearly seen. However, when the panels were stored, the sign was completely covered. Even the most carefully worded and designed message can go astray if not properly directed to the intended audience.

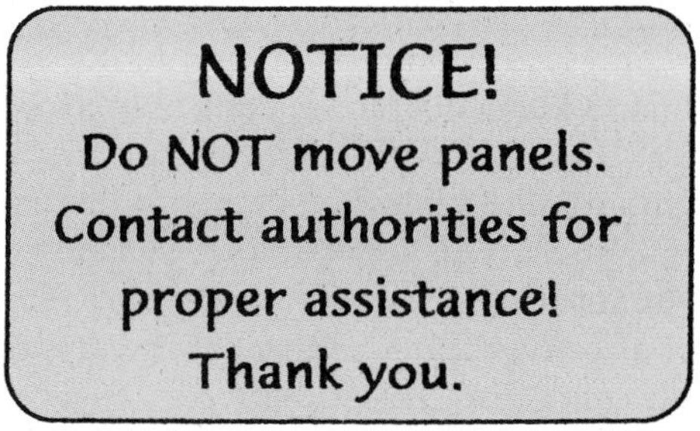

NOTICE!
Do NOT move panels.
Contact authorities for
proper assistance!
Thank you.

FIG. 17-4

The professional nurse must interface with many forms of written communication on a daily basis. Nursing documentation includes a variety of reports—the nurse's notes in patient charts, memos, kardexes, incident reports, discharge teaching forms, and written shift reports, to name a few. Many of the forms that nurses use for documentation are part of the legal record and require careful consideration. Unclear instructions or reports either written or read by the nurse can lead to misunderstandings, errors, and the potential for litigation. Most profoundly, misinformation potentially can lead to patient harm or injury. Therefore special attention must be paid to communicating effectively in writing.

Accuracy

Absolute accuracy is paramount in recording legal documentation. For the nurse, this most specifically applies to the nursing notes or any other entry in the patient's chart. Every effort should be made to report concisely, descriptively, and truthfully. To write "Patient walked today" is not adequate. A more concise and descriptive entry reads, "Patient walked to the nurses' station and back three times this shift, a total distance of 96 yards." (Many hospitals have distance measures marked in the hallway for this purpose.)

Cody Johnson, RN, entered a patient's room and found her agitated and speaking loudly into the phone as she twisted her hair with her free hand. She was crying and periodically pounded the bedside table with her fist. Later the patient told Cody that she had been talking with her mother. Would it be appropriate for Cody to chart, "Patient became very angry with her mother while talking on the phone." No! The nurse must be diligent not to include personal judgments or quantify the patient's emotional state in such terms.

More accurately, Cody could chart, "Patient found crying while talking on the phone in a loud tone to her mother. Patient was twisting her hair and hitting bedside table with her fist." The information is descriptive and states exactly what Cody observed factually without any judgmental conclusions. If, however, the patient had said, "My mother makes me so mad," Cody could have charted the statement as a direct quote (enclosed in quotation marks).

Attention to Detail

In addition to absolute accuracy, written documents should be descriptive. As mentioned in the previous section, information should be quantified whenever possible. How many feet did the patient walk? How many times was the patient out of bed? How many milliliters of fluid did the patient drink? Precisely what did the patient say?

Words can be used to depict a verbal picture of a wound, rash, bruise, or any type of injury or situation. Illustrative terms can create a mental image for the person reading the notes, memo, or other communication. Descriptive categories can include measurement, color, position, location, drainage, or condition when speaking of a physical condition; or time, setting, people present, issues or goals discussed, or direct quotes when speaking of a meeting, conference, evaluation, or other interchange.

Consider the differences between the following written communications.

"1000 Dressing change completed. Site healthy."
"1000 Dressing change completed. Edges of 4-inch surgical wound approximated, no drainage noted. Skin pink without any redness or edema."

BOX 17-1	*Incomplete Memo*

Anecdotal report
Memo
To: Bonnie Thompson, RN, BSN, Nurse Manager
From: Jessica Lindsay, RN, BSN, Charge Nurse
Date: August 18
Subject: Lucas Alfred, RN

I have had lots of complaints about Lucas Alfred's treatment of students. I do not think he should be assigned as a preceptor anymore and do not plan to do so from now on.

The second entry allows the reader to "see" the wound mentally and follow the progress of healing even when unable to be present at the time of the dressing change. A good rule when describing any kind of break in skin integrity—whether from a stabbing, a surgical wound, an intravenous line, and so on—is to describe color, drainage, and presence or absence of edema.

Consider the memo written in Box 17-1. What does this memo really tell the nurse manager? Not much—only that there is some kind of perceived problem between Lucas and the students. The nurse manager does not know based on the information provided if the problem is "real," if it is based on a bias of Jessica's or a student bias, if it has occurred more than once, if an interpersonal communication problem or misunderstanding exists, or if obvious mistreatment of a student or students has occurred.

Now consider the memo written in Box 17-2. Carefully constructing a factual memo of this length is more time-consuming initially, but it will save a lot of frustration in the long run. The nurse manager now has a clear picture of what has occurred and knows that an ongoing problem exists. Most appropriately, Jessica will speak to Bonnie about the problem, even if only briefly, when she delivers the memo. However, a written account of the incident must be submitted and should be composed promptly while the facts are freshly remembered. In addition, written communication often is the first source of contact because the nurse manager is not likely to be immediately available on all shifts.

The skill of writing concisely yet descriptively must be developed. Over some time, nurses build a repertoire of phrases and illustrative terminology that are useful and effective. Often, when a nurse is stumped as to how to express a situation, she or he will ask a colleague, "How would you write . . . ?" Accessing the experience and expertise of nursing peers is productive in terms of problem solving while also demonstrating respect for the colleague.

Thoroughness

The memo example in the previous section also illustrates the need for thoroughness. In addition to being descriptive in terms of the incident, Jessica reported her interview with other

---

BOX 17-2   *Descriptive, Thorough Memo*

Anecdotal report
Memo
To: Bonnie Thompson, RN, BSN, Nurse Manager
From: Jessica Lindsay, RN, BSN, Charge Nurse
Date: August 18
Subject: Student Precepting

Today (Monday, August 18) at 0710 I observed what appeared to be an animated conversation between Lucas Alfred, RN, and John Roberts, SN, a student nurse from North Hills University. As I moved toward them, I heard Lucas say loudly, "Well, you better stay with me because I am not going to come looking for you all day. I know how lazy students are." I asked Lucas, "Is there a problem?" He replied, "Oh, no problem. I just hate having students, that's all. They're more trouble than they're worth." I asked Lucas, "Would you prefer that I reassign the student?" He shrugged his shoulders and walked away. I suggested to the student that I assign him to another nurse for the day. He responded, "I'd really appreciate that. Mr. Alfred has let me know since I arrived that he didn't want to work with me."

Because this group of students has been on the unit 2 days a week for the past 3 weeks, I spoke to the other students who had worked with Lucas and asked them how things had gone. The other three students who have worked with him reported similar experiences.

I would like to arrange a time to meet with you and Lucas to address this problem.

---

nursing students. By doing so, Jessica has been thorough in describing and reporting the extent of the problem she has discovered. Providing such complete information helps to avoid communication breakdown. Anticipating and answering relevant questions before they are asked exemplifies thoroughness and clarifies communication.

Conciseness

Written communication must be concise. The message must state the necessary information as clearly and as briefly as possible. Consider the memo written in Box 17-3.

Whew! Extraneous details tend to confuse more than clarify. An inherent dilemma often develops as the nurse attempts to determine how to be descriptive and concise at the same time. One must determine what facts are pertinent to enable the reader to understand the true message. When in doubt and when appropriate, the writer can ask another party to read the message and provide feedback to the writer as to what the reader believes the message means. However, the right to confidentiality and privacy of the people involved must be observed. This basic principle applies to patients, families, students, members of the health care team—to all persons. Consequently, the nurse must be as judicious in handling written material in a confidential matter as with any other form of communication.

BOX 17-3	*Anecdotal Note*

Subject: Student precepting

Today at about 0730 (it may have been earlier because I don't remember whether the breakfast trays had been served or not), I observed what appeared to be an animated conversation between Lucas Alfred, RN, and John Roberts, SN, a student nurse from North Hills University. I thought they might be arguing, but I couldn't tell for sure, so I decided to go over and see what the conversation was about. It really seemed like Lucas was angry because he was talking loudly and not smiling, and neither was the student smiling, and I heard Lucas say, "Well, you better stay with me because I am not going to come looking for you all day. I know how lazy students are." Well, I could just imagine how that made the student feel, so I asked, "Is there a problem?" even though it was pretty obvious that something was wrong. Lucas said, "Oh, no problem. I just hate having students, that's all. They're more trouble than they're worth." I asked Lucas, "Would you prefer that I reassign the student?" He shrugged his shoulders and walked away. Well, I don't know for sure about the student, but I really thought that was rude. I suggested to the student that I assign him to another nurse for the day. He responded, "I'd really appreciate that. He has let me know since I arrived that he didn't want to work with me." Well, I know how that would make me feel—to be a student and be treated that way.

The same group of students has been on the unit 2 days a week for the past 3 weeks (maybe a month, I'm not sure, and some of them may have been here on make-up days, too), so I talked to other students who had worked with Lucas and asked them how things had been going. They said he'd acted the same way to them. We need to talk to him.

ELECTRONIC COMMUNICATION

More and more communication is computer-based using e-mail, chat rooms, attachments, and other electronic modes. The computer-based written record can be somewhat more transient than other written documents. For example, e-mails are often read and then deleted. However, remember that communication via the computer can be saved and is often retrievable even after deletion. As with any form of written communication, computer-based interaction loses nonverbal cues. Therefore it is important for the sender to elicit feedback and/or for the receiver to ask for clarification if the meaning of the communication is not clear.

COMMUNICATION STYLES

Development of truly effective communication necessitates understanding various communication styles. In addition to the concepts discussed up to this point, characteristics exist that might impede efficacious exchange of information. Issues such as gender differences, cultural diversity, assertiveness vs. aggressiveness, and dissimilarities in the professional approach of the various health care disciplines all contribute to disparate understandings and interpretations.

Communication and Gender Differences

A significant clarification must be made regarding communication between men and women. Although research and many years of observations and writings have produced information about gender differences resulting from socialization, these are generalizations and should be viewed from that perspective. Attributes described do not necessarily apply to all persons or all

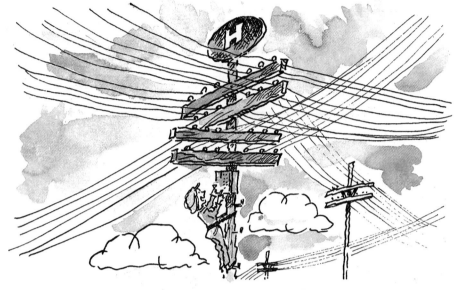

Nurses have the big job of keeping the wires from getting crossed.

of the time. Nevertheless, a plethora of observations indicate that men and women solve problems, make decisions, and communicate from different perspectives based on socialization that begins shortly after birth (Cummings, 1995; Elgin, 1993; Heim, 1995). Typically boys are taught to be tough and competitive; girls are taught to be nice and avoid conflict. Dr. Pat Heim (1995, p. 8) suggests, "Playing team sports boys learn to compete, be aggressive, play to win, strategize, take risks, mask emotions, and focus on the goal line." Regarding girls' play, Dr. Heim comments, "Relationships are central in girls' culture and therefore they learn to negotiate differences, seek win-win solutions, and focus on what is fair for all instead of winning."

Clearly, learning to approach life on such different terms—with different rules—can lead to frustration, sometimes a sense of total defeat in the communication arena! For the most part women work toward compromise, even when it means relinquishing some of the original goal. Preserving relationships is usually of paramount importance to women. The role of peacemaker and nurturer has been a traditional expectation of women throughout the ages.

Generally men work toward winning. Traditional role expectations of men have included provider and protector. Men learn early in life how to focus on goals and move aggressively toward accomplishment. Team sports teach men that relationships are not destroyed in the "battle" (Heim, 1995). Consequently, men have been socialized to behave assertively when such performance is needed in pursuit of the goal and then move on without loss of friendships. Women have been socialized that assertive behavior will endanger relationships and that conflict should be avoided to preserve friendships.

On the other hand, men tend to communicate with a purpose to achieve an identified goal. If conflict occurs during the process, it is simply dealt with as part of the routine. Men are more likely to give concise responses and make prompt, straightforward decisions. Women most often seek to communicate with sensitivity (i.e., how the information is being received and what adjustments need to be made in the presentation, and perhaps the proposed solution, to avoid outright conflict). Decision making involves discussion as part of the problem-solving process.

Men typically use communication as a tool to deliver information, whereas women value the process of communication itself as an important part of the relationship. Therefore, in an effort to improve communication, men might try spending more time in discussion, and women might try to phrase comments more succinctly. Consider the following conversation.

Nurse: *Dr. Vernon, I'm calling to talk to you about Mrs. Guevara. She says she's having more pain and feels a little dizzy. I've given her her pain medicine as soon as I can each time. She says she's a little nauseated. Her husband's in the room, and he says she feels worse too. She did not sleep much last night and has not been able to nap today . . .*

Doctor: *I have patients to see! Just give me the facts.*

Nurse: *Okay, she's had her medication every 4 to 5 hours this shift. I don't know if she needs a higher dose or just needs the medication more frequently, or maybe we should try a different medicine.*

Doctor: *What are her vitals? Does she have any drug allergies?"*

Nurse: *Just a second, and I'll get the chart.*

Doctor: *Confound it, when you get your act together, call me back!*

Dr. Vernon slams down the phone.

Consider the many communication styles and concepts illustrated by the previous conversation. Preparedness, conciseness, contributing environmental conditions (patients waiting), and even courtesy are issues that could be more competently addressed. The fact that the conversation is occurring by telephone instead of in person also is a factor, responsible for the lack of eye contact and the lost potential for additional information through other body language. Telephone conversations are a fact of life in health care. Careful planning and preparation of what will be said will facilitate effective information exchange. In the professional setting especially, men are more prone to favor brief, concise information exchange. In the professional setting women still tend to prefer verbal problem solving as the situation is discussed. Knowledge of the gender differences in communication style could have altered the nurse's telephone call in the following manner.

"Dr. Vernon, this is Holly Michaels, RN, from Fairmont General calling about Mrs. Guevara in room 496. She has been receiving her pain medication exactly every 4 hours and continues to complain of incisional pain. She currently is complaining of slight dizziness and nausea, although she has had no emesis. Her blood pressure is 135/86; pulse, 112; and respirations, 24, which are higher than they have been running. Her temperature is 98.8° F. She has no drug allergies. How would you like to change her orders?" Holly has prepared the information the physician will need and communicates it in an orderly fashion.

The issue of gender differences deserves special consideration in health care. Most nurses are women, whereas male physicians significantly outnumber female physicians (Heim, 1995). The current gender mix in medical schools is approaching 50-50 (Heim, 1995), although a number of years will pass before that balance permeates the population of practicing physicians. Unfortunately the general public continues to view nurses and physicians somewhat stereotypically—the female nurse as the helper of the male physician. Consequently, the health care arena is almost "set up" to experience increased problems associated with differing communication styles between genders. Dealing with resultant conflict is discussed later in the chapter.

Cultural Diversity

Although Chapter 11 is devoted to cultural and social issues, it is important to highlight cultural issues specific to communication. Sensitivity to cultural differences is an integral part of the nurse's responsibility. Many cultural beliefs are tightly interwoven with strong religious convictions. Societies throughout the world depend as strongly or even more strongly on a variety of alternative healing sources as they do on medical science. Some people rarely have an opportunity to interface with medical science as it is known in the "developed" countries.

The obvious difficulty is a potential language barrier. Even if the person speaks English as a second language, the preponderance of slang terms and colloquialisms can confound a literal translation. In addition, the stress associated with illness and possibly hospitalization only adds to the potential for misunderstanding and frustration. Fortunately most communities have interpreters willing to translate in the health care setting. The variety of language interpreters (including sign language for the deaf) available even in smaller communities is surprising.

Although many persons of various cultural backgrounds willingly access the health care system, they concurrently adhere to the beliefs and traditions of many generations of their ancestors. Health customs often involve a faith healer and the use of alternative treatments such as herbal remedies, rituals, and blessings. Attributing healing powers to material objects such as stones, statues, or blessed water (whether in containers or rivers) is not uncommon.

Latasha Williams, RN, an intensive care unit nurse with many years of experience, recently relocated to the southwestern United States. On entering the room of a septic patient, she observed a family member slowly moving an egg above the prone body of the patient. Latasha was shocked at the peculiar behavior, hardly knowing how to respond. Because other family members encircled the bed in what appeared to be an almost prayerful stance, Latasha quickly backed out of the room and went to the nurses' desk.

Sitting down with a stunned expression, she said to a colleague, "Manuel, you will never believe what I saw in your patient's room when I went in to check the monitor alarm." Latasha proceeded to describe the scene.

Manuel Garcia, RN, chuckled and responded, "Latasha, the family is removing the patient's fever. The egg will absorb the fever and help make the patient well."

"You have got to be kidding," snapped Latasha. "What kind of hocus-pocus is that?"

"It is part of faith healing." Manuel looked irritated.

"Surely you do not believe in such a thing. Why don't you stop them and teach them what will really help the patient? We're supposed to teach patients and their families real health care." Latasha was incredulous.

"How can we judge what part faith plays in healing? I have taught the patient and family about sepsis and explained every procedure and treatment. They have expressed an understanding of what we are doing and how it is helping. Their use of the egg to remove fever is not disrupting patient care. They're not even touching the patient! Don't you think that in this case nontraditional healing practices and medical science can combine for the best treatment of the patient and the family?"

Latasha's reaction to a behavior unknown to her is neither surprising nor unusual. Her commitment to patient teaching to promote understanding of the medical beliefs she embraces as a nurse is exactly as it should be. However, Manuel's approach to tolerance of cultural healing beliefs while delivering competent, scientific nursing care is vastly more sensitive. The balance between alternative healing and medical science sometimes is precarious. Maintaining equilibrium with quality patient care at the center requires knowledge and perceptivity.

Many forms of communication do not carry the same meanings in various cultures. In some instances direct eye contact is to be avoided if possible. Touch, also considered a positive communication technique in Western culture, may be perceived as a serious invasion of privacy. Some gestures considered innocuous in one culture may represent vulgarity in another. Some cultures strictly adhere to paternalism; unless the male head of the family agrees to a procedure or treatment, the family member will refuse under any circumstance. Although a sense of modesty is shared by many people, some cultures experience a greater feeling of violation at having to expose certain body parts than do others. The consumption of certain foods, the use of blood or blood products—the possibilities of culturally diverse practices are endless. The prudent nurse will become familiar with the specific cultural practices in the region of her or his employment.

Assertiveness vs. Aggressiveness

There is a clear distinction between the terms *assertive* and *aggressive*. Aggressiveness implies an inclination to start quarrels or fights, whereas assertiveness connotes a style of positive declaration, a persistent demonstration of confidence. The difference becomes obvious—aggression conveys dominance, assertion conveys confidence and competence. The line between the two behaviors can easily become blurred if one or both parties direct or receive controversial comments personally. A review of the vignette involving Donald and Laura ("I Messages") provides an example of how easily a conversation can be perceived as a personal attack and escalate into aggressive behavior.

All of the positive communication techniques and styles that have been discussed must be used to produce assertive rather than aggressive communication. To speak assertively, the person must be sure of the facts, have carefully considered the options, and exude confidence while making the observation, request, or point. Aggressive behavior often leads to conflict and seldom to resolution or effective communication.

The Transdisciplinary Team

The transdisciplinary team is composed of a variety of disciplines approaching health care from the unique perspective of the theories and therapies of the individual profession. Consider the variety represented by nurses, physicians, dietitians, respiratory therapists, pharmacists, physical therapists, psychologists, and social workers. Then add to the mosaic the sublevel of specialists: cardiologists, endocrinologists, oncologists, orthopedists, recreational therapists, occupational therapists, licensed vocational (or practical) nurses, registered nurses, nurse anesthetists, nurse practitioners, nurse scientists, and unlicensed assistive personnel. Registered nurses with varied educational backgrounds (diploma, associate degree, bachelor or master of science in nursing) and licensed vocational nurses sometimes can be found in the same unit with similar assignments. Now add managers, administrators, clerical staff, accountants, and housekeeping, to name a few. Also consider cultural differences among health care professionals and workers. Is it any wonder that communication disasters occur?

All of the positive communication techniques have to be used to clearly understand another's perception. Listening is an essential tool for determination of the intended message as seen from the unique perspective of the other discipline. Frequent clarification and a sense of "safety" are paramount as people explore the meanings that each person attributes to the situation and the discipline-specific suggested solutions. Realization that the fundamental basis of all health care professionals and of ancillary staff is to provide quality patient care should keep all interactions focused on a common goal.

Confidentiality and Privacy

No discussion of communication would be complete without reference to the proverbial "grapevine," which, despite consistent efforts to the contrary, appears to be alive and well. Breach of confidentiality and the patient's right to privacy through careless gossip has ethical and legal ramifications. Thoughtless conversation in the elevator, the dining room, the parking lot, or any other public place has created heartache for the client and the health care provider.

Other sites where communication about confidential or personal patient issues needs to be controlled include the nurses' station, any desks or tables along the halls commonly used for charting, and the utility rooms. Such locations are not often viewed as "public" places, but many people pass by these areas and overhear information they should not, especially during change-of-shift reports. Unfortunately there is a great curiosity among people regarding illness and health care issues, and some people may linger in these areas to glean information. In some circumstances diagnoses carry major social implications that can easily lead to prejudicial treatment in terms of employment, insurance coverage, and social standing. The nurse is bound by the ethics of the profession and the laws of the United States to protect the patient and the patient's family from improper disclosure of personal information.

To carry the concept a step further, the nurse is limited in the type of information that is appropriate to access. In the age of informatics, more information is available, literally at the fingertips.

For example, accessing the record of an acquaintance simply to know "what's going on" with the patient is an absolute infraction of ethical and legal standards. The professional nurse is obligated to know only information that will facilitate quality physical, spiritual, and emotional care to his or her assigned patients. Satisfying curiosity beyond the legitimate requirements of providing care, engaging in gossip, or otherwise compromising the patient's confidentiality is a grievous breach of nursing standards.

Delegation

Although an entire chapter is dedicated to delegation (Chapter 18), the importance of effective communication in the delegation process cannot be overemphasized. Hansten and Washburn (1992) suggest that communication is frequently the primary stumbling block to the successful completion of a delegated task.

Work satisfaction from the point of view of the delegatee is negatively affected by ambiguity and lack of courtesy (Hansten and Washburn, 1992). The delegation of duties requires a thorough explanation of exactly what is expected in terms of what is to be done, as well as any other information not likely to be known to the delegatee. Such information might include the location of supplies needed, time frame for completion of the work, how to document properly (if applicable), and who is available to answer questions or provide assistance if needed. Solicitation of verbal feedback for assurance of understanding can avoid complications that may result from delegation.

The use of everyday courtesies such as "please," "thank you," and "you're welcome" helps establish rapport in a situation that sometimes lends itself to the development of

| BOX 17-4 | *Professional Response to Verbal Conflict* |

1. When a conversation is obviously escalating, try to move to a more private location.
2. Speak in a normal tone of voice.
3. Use "I messages."
4. Maintain eye contact (keeping cultural differences in mind). This may be difficult, but it conveys to the other party that you are confident and competent.
5. Maintain an open body stance with your hands at your side or open toward the person (but not invading the other person's space). Do not cross your arms, tap your toe, wag your finger, or perform any body language that is commonly associated with anger.
6. Do not physically back away unless you perceive you actually are in physical danger. By standing your ground, your carriage will convey the message of assurance.
7. Offer explanations, but do not make excuses.
8. If you say you will take care of something, report something, or change something, do it. Then seek out the person to whom you made the commitment and report your action and the result. Little else will go as far as demonstrating that you are dependable and want to work toward a solution.

interpersonal friction. Establishing an interaction as a win-win situation and demonstrating intent to be available enforces a sense of collegiality and team work.

DEALING WITH VERBAL CONFLICT

The many styles of communication, varying beliefs and traditions, and even a level of "turf protection" can lead to misunderstandings. The stress inherent in the care of the sick, injured, and dying only adds to the likelihood that disagreements will occur. Box 17-4 presents some basic principles that can augment professional response to verbal conflict.

For the most part, verbal conflict is the result of poor communication, distraction, or varying perspectives. However, some persons use verbal abuse as a tool. Whether the behavior is meant to draw attention, express anger, build a sense of power, or accomplish any other equally inappropriate objectives often is immaterial. Problems can be solved without demeaning another human or creating an unpleasant scene. The principles listed are remarkably effective in cases of verbal abuse. Considered together, the principles demonstrate a person of confidence, assurance, and competence who will not react to inappropriate behavior in like form but also will not withdraw from the issues. As always, the focus should be kept on the delivery of quality patient care.

PROFESSIONAL NURSING IMAGE

The discipline of nursing is recognized as a profession because of the standards of advanced education, licensure, intellectual challenge, and commitment to the greater good of humankind. The professional nurse will touch many lives during a career of caregiving, teaching, and leading. Through capable role modeling for patients, families and significant others, nurse colleagues, other health care professionals, and students, the professional nurse can facilitate positive health practices in unlimited numbers of people—just as the ripple of a stone thrown into a stream creates an ever-widening circle. The nurse who astutely uses positive communication techniques, provides a safe environment for a patient to ask questions and learn, and focuses energy toward the resolution of conflict has the opportunity to bring the best of nursing to the most of humanity. Through clear, open, sensitive communication, nurses portray the consummate professional image.

SUMMARY

The first attempts at communication begin shortly after birth and continue throughout life. Effective communication is an essential part of competent professional nursing care. Historically nurses recognized communication to be integral in the duties of the caregiver. Communication has three basic components: the sender, the receiver, and the message. Subcomponents consist of interpretation, filtration, and feedback. Interpretation of messages involves such factors as context, environment, precipitating event, preconceived ideas, personal perceptions, style of transmission, and past experiences.

Communication can be verbal and nonverbal. If the verbal and nonverbal messages do not match, most people will believe the nonverbal message; they will be correct in that belief most of the time. Positive communication techniques include the development of trust; use of "I messages," eye contact, empathy, open communication style, clarification, open body language, and touch; and commitment to keeping promises. Listening is an essential element in efficacious communication. Negative communication techniques include closed communication style, closed body language, blocking, false assurances, and conflicting messages.

There are many differences in communication styles. Such variances include gender differences, cultural diversity, assertiveness vs. aggressiveness, and dissimilarities in the professional approach of various health care disciplines. Other concepts pertinent to communication within the health care arena include written communication techniques, the patient's right to confidentiality and privacy, delegation, and the skill of dealing with verbal conflict.

As a professional, the nurse must be committed to quality patient care. An essential component of quality care is the ability to communicate clearly and to listen well. The strong public image of the nurse is that of nurturer, caregiver, teacher, and leader. The development of effective communication skills can only enhance each nurse's professional image while building strong relationships with patients and colleagues.

Critical Thinking Activities

1. You have been assigned to care for Rhonda, a young wife and mother who was admitted through the Emergency Department last night with significant abdominal pain. As you inquire about her symptoms, she repeatedly glances at her husband, Tommy, before she answers. Although she denies any pain at this time, you observe that she guards her stomach, has a "clinched" jawline, and does not make eye contact with you. Her skin is warm and slightly diaphoretic. As you assess and question Rhonda, Tommy often interrupts with comments such as, "She's just fine. It was only a big stomachache, and it's gone this morning, isn't it, dear?" You suspect that Rhonda is experiencing pain but is reluctant to increase her husband's obvious concern. How will you address the nonverbal cues? How will you evaluate the conflicting cues? What strategies will you use to enhance communication with this couple?

2. Dr. Blademan, whom you recently paged to report an abnormal laboratory result, approaches you shouting angrily, "Why did you page me with that report? You know I make rounds in the evenings, and I would have been here soon." You attempt to explain that the client was symptomatic, that the abnormal laboratory result was high enough to be labeled critical value, and that you believed

prompt reporting was in the best interest of the client. You also are thinking about the fact that "in the evening" could be anytime from 6:00 PM to 11:00 PM for this particular physician. Nothing you say in defense of your decision appeases the physician, who has digressed to general statements about the lack of consideration that nurses give doctors. What do you perceive to be the true message here? How will you respond to the physician's comments? What techniques can you use to prevent the situation from escalating? If the situation continues to escalate, what would be your next course of action?

3. You are talking with Mr. Phillips about his new diagnosis of diabetes mellitus. You state, "Mr. Phillips, I noticed that the diabetic educator was in to talk with you this morning. What did you talk about?" His response is, "Oh, she told me about the special diet . . . you know . . . no sugar and that stuff. But I'm going to tell you now that I drink sodas, and nobody is going to take those away from me!" You comment, "Have you tried diet sodas?" to which he responds, "Are you kidding? That stuff tastes like crankcase oil! I'm not using any of that sweetener stuff!" The conversation continues along the same lines, indicating a lack of commitment to healthy self-regulation on his part. What will you do? It appears that Mr. Phillips is resistant to the restrictions of his new diagnosis. What additional resources can you use to help interpret his health beliefs? What techniques will you use to clarify the issues he must address?

REFERENCES

Ashman H, Menken A: *The little mermaid,* Burbank, Calif, 1988, Walt Disney Pictures.

Cummings SH: Attila the Hun versus Attila the hen: gender socialization of the American nurse, *Nurs Admin Q* 19(2):19-29, 1995.

DeWitt K: *Private duty nursing,* Philadelphia, 1917, JB Lippincott.

Elgin SH: *Genderspeak: men, women, and the gentle art of verbal self-defense,* New York, 1993, John Wiley & Sons.

Elgin SH: www.sfwa.org/members/elgin/

Hansten R, Washburn M: What do you say when you delegate work to others? *Am J Nurs* 92(7):48-50, 1992.

Hargrave J: *Nonverbal communication,* 2001, www.janhargrave.com/index.html

Heim P: Getting beyond "she said, he said," *Nurs Admin Q* 19(2):6-18, 1995.

Nightingale F: *Notes on nursing: what it is, and what it is not,* London, 1859, Harrison.

Parsons SE: *Nursing problems and obligations,* Boston, 1916, Whitcomb & Barrows.

van Servellen G: *Communication skills for the healthcare professional: concepts and techniques,* Gaithersburg, MD, 1997, Aspen Publishers.

Effective Delegation and Supervision

18

Barbara Cherry, MSN, MBA, RN, and Margaret Elizabeth Strong, MSN, RN, CAN

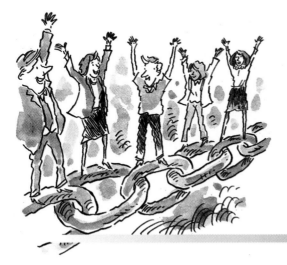

Delegaton: linking together for better patient care.

Vignette

Glenda Miller, a registered nurse (RN), works on a medical-surgical floor of a small hospital. She has just received report from the 11 PM to 7 AM shift and is about to make assignments for the 7 AM to 3 PM shift. The philosophy of the unit is that the RN coordinates all patient care. Today on this 12-bed unit there are eight patients and four empty beds. The nursing staff consists of you as the RN, one licensed practical nurse (LPN), 1 nursing assistant, and one unit secretary. The following members of the transdisciplinary health care team are available to help with patient care needs: one respiratory therapist, one physical therapist, one occupational therapist, one speech therapist, one medical social worker, one nutritional support nurse and one chaplain. The patients are medically complex, many tasks are required to complete their care, and they need a great deal of emotional support. The patients are described to you as follows:

502: Mr. A is ventilator dependent with an infection that requires IV antibiotics every 12 hours. He needs to be OOB in a chair BID. He has a stage I sacral decubitus and a PEG tube with bolus feedings. He is very hard of hearing, tries to speak, and becomes very frustrated and uncooperative.

503: Mrs. B is on day 2 of 40 days of antibiotics for osteomyelitis. She is dehydrated with a central line in her right subclavian and on TPN. She needs to be OOB and AMB in the room. She receives a respiratory treatment every 4 hours and needs assistance with AM care. Her daughter is at her bedside and very upset that mother may need to go to a nursing home.

411

504: Mr. C is to be discharged to a rehabilitation hospital today. His chart needs to be copied. The family is at his bedside and extremely anxious.

507: Mr. D has TPN infusing into his left subclavian and is on multiple antibiotics. He has vancomycin-resistant enterococcus in his urine and a stasis ulcer on his left leg that requires pulsavac every day.

508: Mr. E is a ventilator-dependent patient who will start weaning this AM. He is on continuous tube feedings and IV antibiotics and needs to be assessed for a PICC line. He is to ambulate in the hall twice a day per doctor's orders. He also needs to have a pharyngeal speech evaluation scheduled.

509: Mrs. F is 3 days' post-CVA and is unable to move her right extremities. She has an IV infusing via her left arm. Her blood pressure is 170/100. She needs total care with personal hygiene and feeding. The doctor just ordered ROM exercises every day. Her husband is at her bedside crying continuously and asking, "What am I going to do now?".

510: Mr. G has been off the ventilator for the past 24 hours and is doing very well. He continues on q4h respiratory treatments. His TPN is being decreased, and his PEG feedings are increasing. He has accuchecks ordered every 4 hours, a Foley to straight drainage, and IV antibiotics every 12 hours. He needs to be out of bed, ambulating in the hall with assistance. If he stays off the ventilator, he will be discharged in 5 days. The family needs to find a nursing home for him; however, the family has not visited Mr. G since his admission 18 days ago.

511: Mr. H is a new admission that will be coming from ICU sometime during your shift.

In addition to the tasks mentioned, routine activities of taking vital signs, giving scheduled medications, updating care plans, and answering call lights must be assigned. When reviewing the tasks to be accomplished, Glenda must consider several issues in order to make safe and effective delegation and supervision decisions.

Questions to consider while reading this chapter
1. Which of the above tasks must the RN perform as required by your state's Nursing Practice Act?
2. What are the training, skills, and competencies of the licensed vocational nurse (LVN) and nursing assistant?
3. How can other members of the transdisciplinary health care team be used to most effectively meet the patients' needs?

Key Terms

Accountability In the context of delegation, accountability means bearing responsibility for both the action and inaction of the nurse and those to whom he or she delegates tasks (Fisher, 1999).

Assignment The downward or lateral transfer of both the responsibility and accountability of an activity from one individual to another. The transfer must be made to an individual of appropriate skill, knowledge, and judgment; and the assigned activity must be within the individual's scope of practice (ANA, 1997).

Delegation Transferring to a competent individual the authority to perform a selected nursing task in a selected situation; the nurse retains accountability for the delegated task (National Council of State Boards of Nursing, 1995).

Supervision The active process of directing, guiding, and influencing the outcome of an individual's performance of an activity or task (ANA, 1997).

Unlicensed assistive personnel An unlicensed individual who is trained to function in an assistive role to the RN by performing patient care activities as delegated by the nurse (ANA, 1997).

Competency Determination of an individual's capability to perform up to defined expectations (Joint Commission on Accreditation of Healthcare Organizations, 2000).

Learning Outcomes

After studying this chapter, the reader will be able to:

1. Evaluate the impact of changes in the current health care system on nursing staffing patterns and responsibilities.
2. Apply principles of delegation and supervision to specific examples of professional nursing practice.
3. Incorporate principles of delegation and supervision in professional nursing practice to ensure safe and legal patient care.

CHAPTER OVERVIEW

The delivery of patient care is a fundamental goal of every health care organization. To accomplish this goal in a cost-effective manner, teams of diverse professionals and assistants are used to deliver care. Because the RN is most often responsible for coordinating care provided by the various team members, he or she must clearly understand and be able to effectively use the management processes of delegation and supervision to ensure high-quality, safe patient care. This chapter highlights current issues that are influencing staffing patterns and delegation and supervision processes. The chapter also discusses the RN's role and responsibility in delegating to and supervising unlicensed assistive personnel (UAP), LPNs, and LVNs and will provide useful guidelines for establishing a safe and effective delegation and supervision practice.

DELEGATION AND SUPERVISION IN THE HEALTH CARE SYSTEM

Several factors affecting the health care industry have influenced staffing patterns and the provision of patient care. First, the balanced budget act of 1997 has led to decreased funding of health care organizations, which has led to expanded cost-cutting measures and continued reorganizing and restructuring of health care systems. Second, managed care and the prospective payment system continue to drive health care organizations to provide care in the most cost-efficient manner possible. Third, the current nursing shortage has affected staffing patterns and will continue to do so for the next decade.

To continue to care for patients in an efficient and cost-effective manner, the employment of UAP such as nursing assistants, nursing technicians, patient care technicians, and medical office assistants has increased. In 1996 a survey of RNs in the United States was conducted by the *American Journal of Nursing* to examine nursing practice in the U.S. health care system. Following are some highlights of the responses from the 7560 RNs who responded to the survey (Shindul-Rothschild, Berry, and Long-Middleton, 1996).

- 60.2% reported a decrease in the number of RNs providing direct patient care within the preceding year.
- 65.5% reported increased patient loads.
- 35.8% reported spending more time supervising UAP.
- 41.9% reported hiring UAP to provide direct care previously provided by RNs.
- 87% reported that the use of UAP has not improved the quality of patient care in their organizations.

As the use of UAP increases, the RN is forced to delegate more and more tasks to a person who does not have clearly defined parameters for education, training, job content, responsibilities, and role limitations. Therefore it is up to the RN to know the law and regulation that governs his or her practice. The quality of health care may be adversely affected by nonclinical hospital administrators who fail to recognize the assessment and decision-making activities performed by the RN.

There is also a growing concern that the roles and responsibilities of care providers, including RNs, LPN/LVNs, and UAP are significantly overlapping. In some practice settings LPNs/LVNs are functioning as managers and supervisors and are performing more complex and invasive procedures. In some states UAP are trained to perform complex procedures such as venipunctures and catheter insertions. This trend has prompted many nurses, nursing organizations, and state boards of nursing to reexamine the scope of nursing practice and the nurses' delegation and supervision responsibilities.

Despite these concerns related to the use of caregivers who are not RNs, the use of UAPs and LPNs/LVNs is an economic necessity in today's health care system. The National Council of State Boards of Nursing (1995) states, "there is a need and a place for competent, appropriately supervised, unlicensed assistive personnel in the delivery of affordable, quality health care. However, it must be remembered that unlicensed assistive personnel are equipped to assist—not replace—the nurse" (p. 2).

As the number of RNs continues to decrease, it is imperative that the nurse learns new ways of managing care and delegating tasks. This requires nurses to understand the importance of our nursing presence with the patient, value what we know, and delegate effectively (Boucher, 1998). Benner (1984) defines nursing presence as focusing on the patient's responses to interventions, not on the skills used during interventions.

In the twenty-first century the reality exists that RNs are becoming increasingly responsible for delegation and supervision. Therefore it is imperative that RNs have confidence with delegation skills and understand the legal responsibility that they assume when delegating to and supervising licensed personnel and UAPs. RNs should know what aspects of nursing and health care to delegate and what level of supervision is required to ensure that the patient receives safe, competent, and effective care.

WHAT IS DELEGATION?

Delegation, as defined by the American Nurses Association (ANA) (1997), is "the transfer of responsibility for the performance of an activity from one individual to another while retaining accountability for the outcome" (p. 4). Although RNs can transfer the responsibility and authority for the performance of an activity, they remain accountable for the overall nursing care.

Delegation is a two-way process in which the RN requests that a qualified staff member (UAP, LPN/LVN) perform a specific task. When a task is delegated, the delegator shares with the delegatee the ultimate responsibility and authority for the accomplishment and outcome of the task. However, the RN delegator remains accountable for the nursing care outcomes. When delegating, the RN delegator is accountable for:

- The act of delegation.
- Supervising the performance of the delegated task.
- Assessment and follow-up evaluation.
- Any intervention or corrective actions that may be required to ensure safe and effective care.

The delegatee (LPN/LVN, UAP) is accountable for:

- His or her own actions.
- Accepting delegation within the parameters of his or her training and education.

- Communicating the appropriate information to the delegator.
- Completing the task.

Delegation is a management strategy that, when used effectively, can ensure the accomplishment of cost-effective health care services.

WHAT SHOULD AND SHOULD NOT BE DELEGATED?

Unfortunately there is no easy answer to what can and cannot be delegated. The answer will vary, depending on the (1) Nursing Practice Acts and other applicable state laws, (2) patient needs, (3) job descriptions and competencies of the UAP and LPN/LVNs, (4) policies and procedures of the health care organization, (5) clinical situation, and (6) professional standards of nursing practice. To establish a safe, effective delegation practice, the RN will have to seek guidance and integrate information from each of these areas as discussed in the following paragraphs (Fig. 18-1).

State Nursing Practice Acts

Each state's Nursing Practice Act provides the legal authority for nursing practice, including delegation (Hutcherson, Sheets, and Williamson, 1998). However, each state's Nursing Practice Act expresses delegation criteria differently, and the criteria often are not clearly spelled out in the act or they may be presented in various parts of the act. It is absolutely essential that every RN be familiar with his or her state Nursing Practice Act and know the delegation criteria contained within the act. Johnson (1996) has identified 10 essential elements related to delegation criteria in nursing practice acts as follows.

1. Definition of delegation
2. Items that cannot be delegated

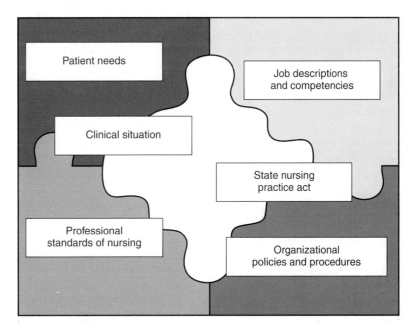

FIG. 18-1 Solving the delegation puzzle.

BOX 18-1	*Policies Common to Many State Nursing Practice Acts*

- Only nursing tasks can be delegated, not nursing practice.
- The RN must perform the patient assessment to determine what can be delegated.
- The LPN/LVN and UAP do not practice professional nursing.
- The RN can delegate only what is within the scope of nursing practice.
- The LPN/LVN works under the direction and supervision of the RN.
- The RN delegates based on the knowledge and skill of the person selected to perform the tasks.
- The RN determines the competency of the person to whom he or she delegates.
- The RN cannot delegate an activity that requires the RN's professional skill and knowledge.
- The RN is accountable and responsible for the delegated task.
- The RN must evaluate patient outcomes resulting from the delegated activity.
- Health care facilities can develop specific delegation protocols, provided they meet the state board delegation guidelines.
- Delegation requires critical thinking by the RN.

From Johnson SH: Teaching nursing delegation: analyzing nurse practice acts, *J Cont Educ Nurs* 27(2):52-58, 1996.

3. Items that cannot be routinely delegated
4. Guidelines for the RN about what can be delegated
5. Description of professional nursing practice
6. Description of LPN/LVN and unlicensed nursing assistant roles
7. Degree of supervision required
8. Guidelines for decreasing the risk of delegation
9. Warnings about inappropriate delegation
10. Restricted use of the word "nurse" to licensed nurse

Although not every state's Nursing Practice Act contains all 10 elements, the RN can use this list to assist in understanding delegation criteria in his or her own Nursing Practice Act and to apply the information to enhance delegation activities. Box 18-1 presents policies common to many nursing practice acts.

If the Nursing Practice Act does not provide clear direction regarding delegation, the state board of nursing may be able to offer guidance. The board of nursing may have developed definitions, rulings, advisory opinions, or interpretations of the law to provide guidance regarding delegation activities. Many state boards of nursing may also have practical tools available such as delegation decision trees or delegation checklists. Fig. 18-2 is a delegation decision tree recommended by the National Council of State Boards of Nursing and provides an excellent framework for making delegation decisions.

Most states also have a practice act to govern practice by LPN/LVNs. Because the practice of LPN/LVNs varies significantly from state to state, RNs should know the LPN/LVN practice act in the state in which they practice and understand the LPN/LVN's legal scope of practice. State law generally does not define practice by UAP, although such practice should be governed by the health care organization's standards.

Patient Needs

When deciding to delegate, the RN must remember that tasks can be delegated, nursing practice cannot. The functions of assessment, evaluation, and nursing judgment cannot be

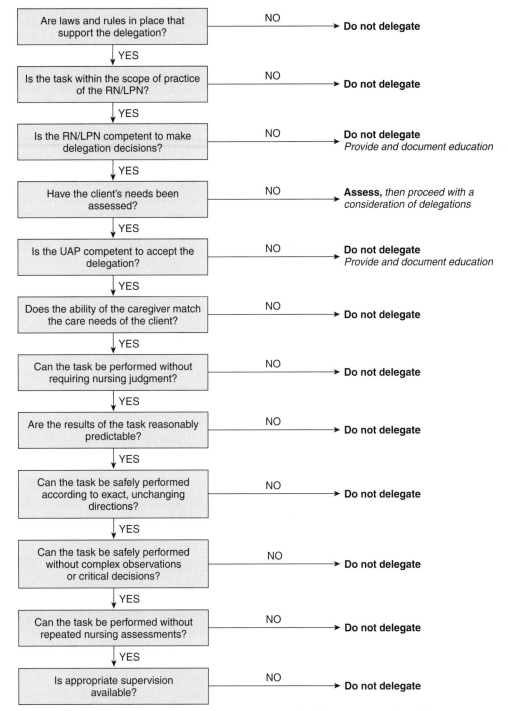

Note: Authority to delegate varies, so licensed nurses must check the statutes and regulations of the jurisdiction. RNs may need to delegate to the LPN the authority to delegate to the UAP.

FIG. 18-2 Delegation decision-making tree. (Used with permission from the National Council of State Boards of Nursing, 1997.)

delegated. Generally the more stable the patient, the more likely delegation is to be safe. However, it also is important to remember that many tasks that can be delegated may also carry with them a nursing responsibility. Taking vital signs on a physiologically stable, postcardiovascular accident patient could be delegated to UAP, but the task presents an opportunity for the RN to assess the patient's cognitive functioning. In the vignette presented previously, Glenda cannot delegate any care on the newly admitted patient until the nursing assessment is complete and the plan of care is developed.

Job Descriptions and Competencies

The RN who is delegating also has the responsibility of knowing the background, skill level, training received, and job requirements of each person to whom tasks are delegated. The job description provides important information about what a staff member is allowed to do and delineates the specific tasks, duties, and responsibilities required of the person as a condition of employment. Job descriptions generally comply with state laws and the health care organization's standards of care. However, in all cases, legal requirements related to delegation supersede any organizational requirement or policy. The RN should be aware of what type of education and training the person received to function as described in the job description. The RN should also know what kind of orientation is provided to new employees and be part of the orientation process. In the vignette presented previously, the LPN's job description most likely will include duties such as "perform dressing changes" and "administer oral medications," but Glenda also should know the LPN's knowledge and skill level for the patient population being cared for.

Documented competencies confirm that the person has demonstrated specific knowledge and skills. For example, a UAP may have documented competency in performing Foley catheter care for adult patients. Various regulatory and accrediting agencies such as the Joint Commission on Accreditation of Healthcare Organizations require written documentation of staff competencies. It is important for the RN to be aware of the documented competencies for all staff members whom he or she supervises.

Organizational Policies and Procedures

When delegating, the RN should comply with the specific skill requirements designated in the organization's written policies and procedures, which usually describe the supervision required for a specific task and how problems or incidents should be reported and documented. Again, it is important for the nurse to remember that the legal requirements related to delegation supersede any organizational requirement or policy. The RN should also know the organization's general standards of care, such as infection control, and ensure that the delegatee has the necessary knowledge and skills to comply with the standards. In the previous vignette Glenda should be aware of the hospital's policy regarding the orientation process. All the clinical staff members should have received training about the unit's infection control, emergency, and safety procedures.

Clinical Situation

Each delegation opportunity presents the RN with a variety of considerations, including the delegatee's current workload and the complexity of the task in relationship to the patient. Does the staff member realistically have time to accomplish the task? Is the staff member familiar with characteristics of the patient population (i.e., pediatrics or geriatrics) and with the task to be performed? Other considerations include the availability of resources such as supplies and equipment and the appropriate level of supervision.

Professional Standards of Nursing Practice

Professional standards of nursing practice as established by professional nursing organizations exist to guide the RN in providing patient care. "A standard is a model of established practice which has general recognition and acceptance among registered professional nurses and is commonly accepted as correct. Standards of practice are agreed-on levels of competence as determined by the ANA and specialty nursing organizations" (ANA, 1996). To practice safe delegation, the RN should be familiar with the standards of practice outlined in the ANA's Standards of Clinical Nursing Practice (1991) and with the standards for any specialty area in which the RN practices. (Refer to Appendix A for a list of most of the specialty nursing organizations in the United States.)

The ANA has addressed delegation directly in its position statement *Registered Nurse Utilization of Unlicensed Assistive Personnel* (1997). As an accepted standard of care, the RN should use professional judgment to determine activities that are appropriate to delegate based on the concept of providing safe and effective patient care and protecting the public. In delegation the RN will consider the following:

- Assessment of the patient condition
- Capabilities of the nursing and assistive staff
- Complexity of the task to be delegated
- Amount of clinical oversight (supervision) the RN will be able to provide
- Staff workload

The RN cannot delegate activities that include the core of the nursing process and require specialized knowledge, judgment, and/or skill (ANA, 1996).

The ANA (1997) has also delineated activities that can be delegated by the nurse. The RN may delegate direct or indirect patient care activities. Direct-care activities assist the patient to meet basic human needs and include activities related to feeding, drinking, positioning, ambulating, grooming, toileting, dressing, and socializing. They may involve the collecting, reporting, and documenting of data related to these activities. The patient-related data are reported to the RN, who uses the information to make clinical judgments about patient care. Indirect care activities that may be delegated focus on maintaining a clean, safe, efficient environment in which to practice nursing. Indirect care activities, which only incidentally involve patient contact, include activities involved in housekeeping, transporting, record keeping, stocking, and maintaining supplies. *Activities that the nurse may not delegate include:*

- Initial nursing assessment and any subsequent assessment that requires professional nursing knowledge, judgment, and skill.
- Determination of nursing diagnoses, establishment of nursing care goals, development of the nursing plan of care, and evaluation of the patient's progress with the nursing plan of care.
- Any nursing intervention that requires professional knowledge, judgment, and skill (ANA, 1996).

Box 18-2 presents a list of questions to assist the nurse in making delegation decisions.

BOX 18-2	*Questions to Guide Delegation Decision Making*

A. State Nursing Practice Act
1. Is the task within the RN's scope of practice?
2. Does the Nursing Practice Act address delegation of the task?
3. Does the task to be delegated require the exercising of nursing judgment?
4. Is the RN delegator willing to accept accountability for the performance of the delegated task?

B. Job description and competencies
1. Does the RN delegator understand the nature of the task and have the knowledge, skills, and competency required to perform the task?
2. Does the delegatee have the appropriate education, training, skills, and experience to perform the task?
3. Is there documented or demonstrated evidence that the delegatee is competent to perform the task?
4. Does the delegatee perform the task on a routine basis?
5. Is the delegatee familiar with the patient population?

C. Organizational policies and procedures
1. What skill level and level of supervision are required for the task as stated in the procedure manual?
2. What is the policy or procedure for documenting tasks and reporting results, observations, problems, or unusual incidents?
3. Does the delegatee have the necessary knowledge and skills to comply with general standards of care such as infection control?

D. Clinical situation and task
1. Is adequate supervision by the delegator available?
2. Are adequate resources available, including supplies and equipment, to the delegatee?
3. What is the delegatee's current workload? Does the person realistically have time to perform the task?
4. How complex is the task? Does it frequently reoccur in the daily care of patients? Does it follow a standard and unchanging procedure?

E. Patient needs
1. Has the nursing assessment and plan of care been completed by the RN?
2. What is the patient's clinical, physiologic, emotional, cognitive, and spiritual status?
3. Is the patient's condition considered stable?
4. What is the potential for change in the patient's condition as a result of the delegated task?
5. Can the patient's safety be maintained with delegated care?

F. Professional Standards of Nursing Practice
1. What specific standards of nursing practice apply to the specific situation?
2. Does the delegated task include health counseling, teaching, or other activities that require specialized nursing knowledge, skill, or judgment?

DEVELOPING SAFE DELEGATION PRACTICES

For the RN to make safe, effective delegation decisions and develop a sound delegation practice, he or she must have a strong foundation of knowledge related to the legal criteria and standards of practice governing delegation decisions. The RN also must know the patient, the staff members to whom he or she is delegating, and the tasks to be performed. In addition, the RN must provide for effective outcomes by clearly communicating expectations, supporting and appropriately supervising the delegatee, evaluating the outcomes, and reassessing the patient after the delegated task is completed. Following is a brief discussion about these essential requirements for safe and effective delegation.

Establish a Foundation of Knowledge As a Basis for Decisions

Know the criteria regarding delegation specified in the Nursing Practice Act for the state in which the RN is practicing. Knowledge of the delegator's (RN) and the delegatee's (LPN/LVN, UAP) scope of practice, documented competencies, and job description should guide the RN in the delegation process. Know and comply with the specific skill requirements designated in the organization's written policies and procedures and standards of care. Know the professional standards for nursing practice as recommended by the ANA and by the related specialty nursing organizations, including specific recommendations on delegation. Clearly, any task that requires health counseling, teaching, or other activities that require specialized nursing knowledge, skill, judgment, or the application of the nursing process cannot be delegated.

Know the Patient

A nursing assessment must be completed before delegation—know the level of care required by the patient, considering the clinical, physiologic, emotional, cognitive, and spiritual status. Is the patient's condition considered stable? Generally the more stable the patient, the more likely delegation is to be safe. What is the potential for change in the patient's condition as a result of the delegated task? If there is moderate-to-high risk that the task will result in a change in the patient's condition, delegation should not be considered. Can the patient's safety be maintained with delegated care? The answer to this question must be a firm "Yes" for delegation to be considered.

Know the Staff Member

Before the task is delegated, the delegatee must have the skills and knowledge necessary to perform it, as evidenced by the person's job description, training program, and documented competencies. Experience and past job performance should also be a consideration. Is the staff member knowledgeable and trained to perform the task? Does the staff member perform the task on a routine basis? Select the right person for the right task. It is very helpful for the RN to be involved in training programs and development of job descriptions for UAPs and LPN/LVNs.

Know the Task(s) To Be Delegated

The RN delegator must be competent and skilled in performing any task he or she is considering delegating, and the task must be in the RN's scope of practice. Routine, standardized tasks that are performed according to a standard and unchanging procedure and have predictable outcomes are the safest to delegate. These routine tasks are most likely to have been documented in the staff member's competencies and may require fewer directions and less supervision. Complex tasks or activities that are high risk for patient complications or unpredictable outcomes should be examined closely before delegation is considered.

Explain the Task and Expected Outcomes

The RN should explain the delegated task, what must be done, and the expected outcomes. If necessary, outline the task in writing. Failure to effectively communicate what is expected may result in unsatisfactory performance, errors, and possible harm to the patient. Directions should be provided in a clear, concise manner. Demonstration and return demonstration by the delegatee or inservice education may be required. The delegated task is acceptable only when the staff member understands the task and is adequately prepared to carry it out.

Expect Responsible Action From the Delegatee

When the staff member accepts and understands the task, he or she should then be allowed to perform the task. The staff member becomes responsible for his or her own actions and is obligated to complete the task as mutually agreed. The RN should provide appropriate supervision but should not intervene in task performance unless assistance is requested or an unsafe situation is recognized. Interfering with the delegatee's task will negate his or her responsibility and obligation. The RN should expect responsible actions, give authority, and retain accountability.

Assess and Supervise Job Performance

Supervising job performance provides a mechanism for feedback and control. Job performance is assessed by making frequent rounds, observing, and communicating (ask about progress and determine if there are any questions or concerns). Determine the appropriate level of supervision. The RN should be available to the delegatee if there are any questions or unexpected problems. Supervise in a positive and supportive manner to reassure the staff member that his or her work is important and appreciated. Intervene immediately if the task is not being performed in a safe and appropriate manner. Poor performance must be documented and reported to the nurse manager. Never ignore poor performance! When a mistake is made, use it as a learning opportunity for the staff member involved.

Provide for the Achievement of Outcomes and Effective Performance

Ongoing communication and support are vital to the achievement of positive outcomes and effective performance. The necessary resources (e.g., equipment, forms, supplies, personnel, and time) to perform the tasks should be available to the delegatee.

Evaluate and Follow-Up

Once the task is complete, evaluate the staff member's performance and reassess the patient to ensure that the expected outcomes were achieved. Follow up with any interventions that may be required based on the patient's care outcomes or the delegatee's job performance. Review and document the skills that were learned. Appropriate evaluation and follow-up will ensure a positive outcome for both patient and staff member. Box 18-3 presents some important steps to remember after the decision to delegate has been made.

High-Risk Delegation

The RN often expresses concern about legal liability—"putting my license on the line"—when delegating to UAPs and LPN/LVNs. How does the RN know if he or she might be at risk when delegating tasks to the UAP or LPN/LVN? The RN may be at risk if the (ANA, 1996):

- Delegated task can only be performed by the RN according to law, organizational policies and procedures, or professional standards of nursing practice.
- Delegated task could involve substantial risk or harm to a patient.
- RN knowingly delegates a task to a person who has not had the appropriate training or orientation.
- RN fails to adequately supervise the delegated activity and does not evaluate the delegated action by reassessing the patient.

RNs can avoid being placed into an unsafe, risky delegation situation by adhering to the safe delegation practices recommended in this chapter.

BOX 18-3	*From Deciding-to-Delegate to Delegating: Steps to Remember*

A. Communicate effectively.
  1. The delegatee accepts the delegation and accountability for carrying out the task correctly.
  2. The RN delegator provides clear directions to the delegatee: What specific task is to be performed, for whom is the task to be done, when is the task to be done, how is the task to be performed, what data are to be collected, and any patient specific instructions.
  3. The RN delegator clearly communicates expected outcomes and timelines for reporting results.
B. Provide appropriate supervision.
  1. Monitor performance to ensure compliance with established standards of practice, policies, and procedures.
  2. Obtain and provide feedback.
  3. Intervene if necessary.
  4. Ensure proper documentation.
C. Evaluate and reassess.
  1. Reassess the patient.
  2. Evaluate the performance of the task and the delegatee's experience.
  3. Reassess and adjust the overall plan of care as needed.

Delegation and the Nursing Process

Understanding safe delegation practices may seem overwhelming for the novice nurse, although the components of the delegation process become familiar when compared with the nursing process. After assessing the patient and planning the care, the RN identifies tasks that someone else can perform. Implementing the plan of care includes assigning and supervising task performance. Finally, evaluating the delegatee's performance, planned outcomes, and patient response completes the process.

Another method to simplify the delegation process has been recommended by the National Council of State Boards of Nursing (1995) and is referred to as the "Five Rights of Delegation":

1. *The right task:* delegated tasks must conform to the established guidelines.
2. *The right circumstances:* delegate tasks that do not require independent nursing judgment.
3. *The right person:* one who is qualified and competent.
4. *The right direction and communication:* clear explanation about the task and expected outcomes, and when the delegatee should report back to the RN.
5. *The right supervision and evaluation:* invite feedback to assess how the process is working and how to improve the process. Also evaluate the patient's outcomes and results of the tasks.

Box 18-4 provides a list of online resources related to delegation and supervision.

SUPERVISION

Supervision is defined by the ANA (1997) as "the active process of directing, guiding and influencing the outcome of an individual's performance of an activity" (p. 20). Supervision may be categorized as on-site, in which the nurse is physically present or immediately available while the activity is being performed, or off-site, in which the nurse has the ability to provide

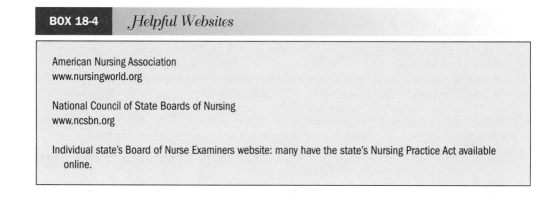

direction through various means of written, verbal, and electronic communication (ANA, 1997). On-site supervision generally occurs in the acute care or ambulatory care settings where the RN is immediately available. Off-site supervision may occur in home health practice, community settings, and long-term care facilities.

As a result of the rapidly increasing use of telecommunication technologies, the distinction between on-site and off-site supervision has become unclear. Some operational guidelines of supervision are (ANA, 1996):

1. Who is in control of the activity? If the nurse is responsible, he or she should incorporate measures to determine if an activity or task has been completed to meet the expectations.
2. How should controls be instituted? Controls must be in place that allow the person delegating an activity or task to stop the task when inappropriately done, review the measures taken, and take back control of the task.

The necessary frequency of periodic instruction dictates the level of supervision required. Hansten and Washburn (1998) have identified three levels of supervision based on the task delegated and the education, experience, competency, and working relationship of the people involved.

1. *Unsupervised:* One RN is working with another RN in a collegial relationship, and neither RN is in the position of supervising the other. Each RN is responsible and accountable for his or her own practice. However, the RN in a supervisory or management position (e.g., team leader, charge nurse, nurse manager) as defined by the health care organization will be in a position to supervise other RNs.
2. *Initial direction/periodic inspection:* The RN is supervising a licensed or unlicensed caregiver, knows the person's training and competencies, and has developed a working relationship with the staff member. For example, the RN has been working with the nursing assistant for 6 months and is comfortable in giving initial directions to ambulate two new postoperative patients and following up with the assistant once during the shift.
3. *Continuous supervision:* The RN has determined that the delegatee will need frequent to continual support and assistance. This level of supervision is required when the working relationship is new, the task is complex, or the delegatee is inexperienced or has not demonstrated an acceptable level of competence.

It is absolutely essential that the RN understands and provides the appropriate level of supervision whenever tasks are delegated.

ASSIGNING VS. DELEGATING

Assigning tasks is not the same as delegating tasks. Assignment as defined by ANA (1997, p. 4) is "the downward or lateral transfer of both the responsibility *and accountability* of an activity from one individual to another." An assignment designates those activities that a staff member is responsible for performing as a condition of employment and is consistent with the staff member's job position and description, legal scope of practice, and training and educational background. The staff member—RN, LPN/LVN, or UAP—assumes responsibility and is accountable for completing the assignment.

Assignment Considerations

Assigning groups of patients to various care providers, including UAP and LPN/ LVNs, is not appropriate. For example, UAP cannot be assigned to a patient or group of patients but rather should be assigned to an RN. Typical assignments for UAP would include passing trays, assisting with transfers, transporting patients, and stocking supplies. The LPN/LVN may be assigned specific patients for whom to perform care, but the RN remains responsible for all nursing practice activities, including patient assessment, care planning, and patient teaching.

The RN is also responsible for assignments made to personnel in the clinical setting. Several factors should be considered when making assignments.

1. *Patient's physiologic status and complexity of care:* Are vital signs unstable? Is the patient's condition changing rapidly? Does the patient have multisystem involvement? Does the patient need extensive health education? Does the patient need extensive emotional support? What technology is involved in the care (e.g., cardiac monitor, intravenous pump, and patient-controlled analgesic pump)? Patients with more unstable physiologic status or complex care requirements need a higher level of skilled care.
2. *Infection control:* To what extent are isolation procedures required? Which patients could be adversely affected as a result of cross-contamination? For example, a new patient is admitted with a history of night sweats and chronic cough. The results of a sputum culture are pending. Another patient on the unit was admitted with complications resulting from chemotherapy. The same caregiver should not be assigned to a potentially infectious patient and an immunosuppressed patient.
3. *Degree of supervision:* What level of supervision, direct or indirect, is required based on the staff member's education, experience, skill level, and competence? Is the appropriate supervision available? The "on-call" RN who works an occasional weekend may require more supervision than the LPN who has worked in the unit full time and has demonstrated competence within his or her scope of practice.

Note that the most experienced skilled staff members should not be exclusively assigned to the most complex, difficult cases. Assignments should be used as a staff development tool. Assigning a less experienced nurse to a more complex patient, but increasing the level of supervision, increases that nurse's skill level and competence while maintaining safe, effective patient care.

Working With Transdisciplinary Health Care Team Members

Other health professionals who are members of the transdisciplinary health care team, including respiratory therapists, physical therapists, occupational therapists, speech therapists,

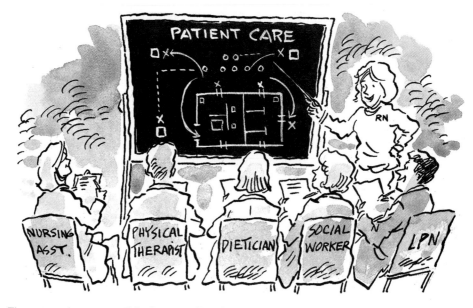

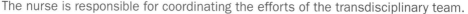

The nurse is responsible for coordinating the efforts of the transdisciplinary team.

nutritionists, medical social workers, and chaplains, will be very valuable in helping meet patient care needs. In the vignette Glenda will need to coordinate the efforts of each of the transdisciplinary team members available to her unit to accomplish the many and varied tasks needed by the patients for whom she is responsible and accountable.

The RN must be knowledgeable about the scope of practice and training background of the transdisciplinary team members in order to ensure the very best care for patients. The RN also needs to understand how the work is delegated or assigned to the transdisciplinary team members and where they fit in the organizational structure of the unit. In some organizations some or all of the transdisciplinary team members report to the RN, and it is the RN who is responsible for assigning and delegating patient care tasks to the team members. In other organizations the transdisciplinary team members report to supervisors in their individual disciplines and work in a collaborative manner with the RN to provide patient care based on their individual legal scope of practice, knowledge, and experience.

In the vignette the transdisciplinary team members do not report directly to Glenda but to a supervisor in their respective disciplines. However, each of the team members is available and willing to work collaboratively with Glenda to meet the needs of the patients on the unit. For example, the respiratory therapist monitors all patients on ventilators and assists in the weaning process. The medical social worker provides valuable assistance to identify family support and assists with nursing home placement for Mr. G. The speech therapist can work on communication techniques with Mr. A, the ventilator-dependent patient who becomes very frustrated when he tries to speak. Chapter 24 provides the reader with an overview of various transdisciplinary team members and their related skills and education level.

BUILDING DELEGATION AND SUPERVISION SKILLS

Effective delegation is an underlying quality for the success of working with others efficiently and cost-effectively. Delegating can be very difficult, especially for the novice nurse. Some of the struggles the nurse has are the fear of being disliked, losing control, taking risks, making mistakes, lack of confidence, and lack of knowledge of the delegation process itself. Because delegation and supervision involve interactions between two people, the RN needs to develop strong interpersonal skills and a supportive work environment to guarantee an effective delegation situation. Following are management skills RNs need to develop to become proficient at delegation and supervision.

Communicate Effectively

Clear communication is the key to successful delegation. The first step toward effective communication is for the RN to know exactly what needs to be done and what outcomes are expected. What is the specific task to be done? For whom is the task to be done? When is the task to be done? How is the task to be performed? What is the expected outcome? What feedback is expected? Why does the task need to be done in a certain way?

Maintaining self-control and confidence is an important communication skill. New RNs often have expressed concern about delegating to more seasoned LPN/LVNs or UAP. "I have been working here for 12 years, and I do not need you telling me what to do" might be a typical response directed to the new RN. The RN's correct response is to maintain composure and confidence and remain positive. "I appreciate your experience and knowledge, but I need you to . . . (describe the task clearly)."

It also is important to listen carefully to the delegatee's response. Did the delegatee appear to listen and understand the directions? Did he or she appear to be hesitant to accept the task? Angry? Uninterested? Frustrated? If a delegation action elicits a negative response from the delegatee, ask for feedback using open-ended, nonthreatening statements. "You seem unsure about performing this task." Always provide an opportunity for the delegatee to ask questions. The positive communication techniques discussed in Chapter 17 provide additional information for the reader to enhance delegation skills.

Create an Environment of Trust and Cooperation

Staff members will report problems more quickly if they know that the reaction from the supervisor will be nonthreatening and nonjudgmental. When mistakes occur, the person should not be blamed or criticized, but rather the supervisor should look for root causes such as inadequate training or too heavy a workload. Encourage staff members to report and discuss problems as a method of improving patient care and maintaining a helpful, supportive attitude. Just as the RN establishes trust and rapport with patients, he or she should strive for the same type of supportive relationships with the staff members.

Create an Environment of Teaching and Learning

Inadequate training is a common cause for poor performance in the work setting. RNs should identify the learning needs of the staff members with whom they work and either directly or indirectly provide educational programs aimed at building skills and competencies. Parkman (1996) has identified the following areas in which UAP need training and skill development:

- Basic care procedures, including vital signs, transfer and body mechanics, infection control procedures, basic emergency procedures, privacy and confidentiality, and documenting care activities
- Communication skills, including greeting patients and families, handling complaints, resolving conflicts, and reporting to the supervisor
- Decision-making skills, including prioritizing tasks and deciding when and what to report
- Critical thinking skills, including recognizing abnormal vital signs, identifying risks to patient safety, and reporting appropriately to the RN

By creating an environment that encourages teaching and learning, the RN will enhance the quality of care in the nursing unit. The RN should be willing to teach and demonstrate how to perform a task rather than merely tell how it should be done. The RN should strive to earn a reputation for exceptional training and mentoring, involving everyone on the health care team, including LPNs/LVNs and UAP, in educational and staff development activities.

Promote Patient Satisfaction

Patients need and want to know who their caregivers are and what qualifications they have. In this day when a variety of nursing apparel is acceptable in the clinical setting, it often is difficult to tell the RN from the housekeeper. The RN is responsible for describing the health care team to the patient. For example, "Hello, my name is Marjorie Will. I am a registered nurse, and I will be responsible for your care until 11 PM tonight. Mary James, a nursing assistant, is working with me and will be in to take your vital signs and help with your meal tray. Also John Howle, the physical therapist, will be in to work with you on your knee exercises. Please call me if you have any questions."

Provide Feedback and Follow-Up Evaluation

The delegation process is not complete until the RN reassesses the patient and adjusts the plan of care as indicated. The RN also should provide honest feedback to the delegatee about his or her performance. An easy, although often overlooked, delegation skill is to praise good performance. More difficult for the RN, and frequently ignored, is the duty to address poor job performance.

The RN should tell the staff member about mistakes in a supportive manner—in private—with a focus on "learning from mistakes." However, if the LPN/LVN or UAP performs in an inappropriate, unsafe, or incompetent manner, the RN must intervene immediately and stop the unsafe activity, document the facts of the performance, and report to the nurse manager or supervisor. In addition, the RN should request additional training or other appropriate action for the staff member to ensure that patient safety is protected. The RN has a professional responsibility to intervene appropriately when poor performance is observed.

SUMMARY

Effective delegation and supervision are essential skills for the professional nurse in any practice role or setting, especially with the increased use of UAP to provide health care services.

Although there is no definitive list of what can and cannot be delegated, the RN is guided to safe, effective delegation and supervision through an assessment of (1) the clinical situation; (2) patient needs; (3) the job descriptions and competencies of the assistive and vocational/practical nursing personnel; (4) the health care organization's policies and procedures; (5) nursing practice acts and other regulations and applicable state laws; and (6) professional standards of nursing practice. This chapter presents information to assist the RN with delegation decisions and also discusses effective delegation and supervision skills, including communicating effectively, creating an environment of trust and cooperation, creating an environment of teaching and learning, promoting customer or patient satisfaction, and providing feedback and follow-up evaluation. These activities and skills provide the tools the RN needs to develop a safe and legal delegation practice.

Critical Thinking Activities

1. Review the tasks to be accomplished that are described in the vignette. Analyze the factors that the RN should consider when deciding which tasks can and cannot be delegated. Develop a plan for delegating these activities and explain the rationale for each delegation decision.
2. Analyze the delegation criteria contained in your state's Nursing Practice Act. Explain how delegation practices in a selected clinical site are influenced by the delegation criteria in the Nursing Practice Act.
3. Request to view copies of job descriptions for RNs and LVNs/LPNs and for UAP at a selected clinical site. Compare and contrast the responsibilities and duties described in each job description and analyze how delegation decisions would be influenced by information contained in the job descriptions.
4. Compare and contrast the levels of supervision you have received as a student. How have these supervision levels changed as you progressed from a beginning to a senior nursing student?

REFERENCES

American Nurses Association: *Standards of clinical nursing practice,* Kansas City, Mo, 1991, ANA.

American Nurses Association: *Registered professional nurses & unlicensed assistive personnel,* ed 2, Washington, DC, 1996, ANA.

American Nurses Association: Position statement: registered nurse utilization of unlicensed assistive personnel, *NursingWorld,* 1997, www.nursingworld.org/readroom/position/uap/uapuse.htm.

Benner PE: *From novice to expert: excellence and power in clinical nursing,* Menlo Park, Calif, 1984, Addison-Wesley.

Boucher M: Delegation alert! *Am J Nurs* 98(2):26-33, 1998.

Fisher M: Do your nurses delegate effectively? *Nurs Manage* 99(5):23-25, 1999.

Hansten RI, Washburn MJ: *Clinical delegation skills: a handbook for professional practice,* ed 2, Gaithersburg, Md, 1998, Aspen Publishers.

Hutcherson C, Sheets V, Williamson S: What five regulatory trends mean to you, *Nursing* 98(5):54-57, 1998.

Johnson SH: Teaching nursing delegation: analyzing nurse practice acts, *J Contin Educ Nurs* 27(2):52-58, 1996.

Joint Commission on Accreditation of Healthcare Organizations: *Hospital accreditation standards,* Oakbrook Terrace, Ill, 2000, JCAHCO.

National Council of State Boards of Nursing: *Delegation: concepts and decision-making process,* Chicago, 1995, Author, www.ncsbn.org/files/publications/positions/delegati.asp.

Parkman CA: Delegation: are you doing it right? *Am J Nurs* 96(9):46-48, 1996.

Shindul-Rothschild JB, Berry B, Long-Middleton E: Where have all the nurses gone? Final results of our patient care survey, *Am J Nurs* 96(11):25-39, 1996.

SUGGESTED READINGS

Canavan K: Combating dangerous delegation, *Am J Nurs* 97(5):57-58, 1997.

Fisher M: Do you have delegation savvy, *Nursing* 2000(9):58-59, 2000.

Parsons L: Building RN confidence for delegation decision-making skills in practice, *J Nurse Staff Dev* 15(6):263-269, 1999.

VanCura B, Gunchick D: Five key components for effectively working with unlicensed assistive personnel, *Medsurg Nurs* 6(5):270-274, 1997.

Staffing and Nursing Care Delivery Models

Barbara Cherry, MSN, MBA, RN

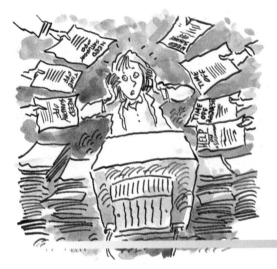

Staffing and assigning work is probably the most important and challenging role of the nurse manager.

Vignette

As a student nurse John Knox noticed that during rotations through the different clinical areas the registered nurses (RNs) had various types of responsibilities and duties. On the medical-surgical units, the RN supervised a group of licensed vocational nurses (LVNs) and nursing assistants who provided direct patient care and the RN spent her time doing patient assessments, care planning, and education. In the critical care unit the RN provided all the care required by the patient with little help from any other caregivers. In the obstetric unit two RNs worked as a team to provide care to laboring mothers. In the outpatient health clinic each RN was assigned to perform specific tasks (e.g., one nurse assigned to do all diabetic teaching and one nurse assigned to screen the results of all laboratory work performed). John had many questions about why care delivery was very different in the different clinical sites where he worked as a student.

Questions to consider while reading this chapter
1. Why is the RN's work assignment very different in different units—obstetrics, critical care, medical-surgical, and the outpatient clinic?
2. How do nurse managers on nursing units decide how assignments will be made?
3. Who has responsibility and authority for making patient care assignments?

Key Terms

Clinical pathways Also called critical paths, practice protocols, or care maps; delineate a predetermined, written plan of care and specify the desired outcomes and transdisciplinary intervention required within a specified time period for a particular health problem (Birdsall and Sperry, 1997).

Multiskilled worker Unlicensed caregiver trained to perform multiple tasks such as phlebotomy, vital signs, housekeeping, and assisting patients with hygiene and ambulation.

Nursing care delivery models Also called care delivery systems or patient care delivery models; detail the way work assignments, responsibility, and authority are structured to accomplish patient care; models depict which health care worker is going to perform what tasks, who is responsible, and who has the authority to make decisions.

Patient classification systems Method used to group or categorize patients according to specific criteria and care requirements and thus help quantify the amount and level of nursing care needed.

Staff mix Combination of categories of workers employed to provide patient care (e.g., RNs, LVNs/licensed practical nurses [LPNs], nursing assistants, multiskilled workers, or unlicensed assistive personnel [UAP]).

Staffing Ensuring that an adequate number and mix of health care team members (e.g., RNs, LVNs/LPNs, unlicensed assistive personnel, clerical support) are available to provide safe, quality patient care; usually a primary responsibility of the nurse manager.

Unlicensed assistive personnel An unlicensed individual who is trained to function in an assistive role to the RN by performing patient care activities as delegated by the nurse (ANA, 1997).

Learning Outcomes

After studying this chapter, the reader will be able to:

1. Outline key issues surrounding staffing for a health care organization.
2. Evaluate lines of responsibility and accountability associated with various types of nursing care delivery models.
3. Analyze the advantages and disadvantages of nursing care delivery models in relation to patient care in various settings.
4. Integrate essential components of the critical pathway model into patient care planning.
5. Differentiate among several nursing care delivery models by evaluating their defining characteristics.
6. Explain the purpose and components of nursing case management.

CHAPTER OVERVIEW

Of all the nurse manager's varied and complex roles, staffing and assigning work is probably the most challenging and certainly the most important to the delivery of safe, quality patient care. Staffing ensures that an appropriate number and level of staff members are available to provide care; assigning is the method used to divide work tasks among the various staff members. This chapter presents a brief introduction to staffing and its surrounding issues such as acuity levels and staff satisfaction. A description of various nursing care delivery models, which detail how work assignments are structured, follows. Case management as a nursing care delivery model and the use of clinical pathways are also presented. The chapter attempts to answer the following questions related to staffing and nursing care delivery models:

1. How does staffing affect patient care, staff satisfaction, and the organization's bottom line?
2. What staff mix (e.g., combination of RNs, LVNs or LPNs, UAP, technicians) is required to provide quality patient care?

3. Who is responsible for making work assignments?
4. What factors should be considered when making patient care and other work assignments?
5. Is the work assigned by task or by patient?
6. How is communication about patient issues managed?
7. What factors are considered when choosing a nursing care delivery model?
8. What is case management and how is it used to provide patient care?

STAFFING

Staffing can be defined as the activities required to ensure that an adequate number and mix of health care team members (e.g., RNs, LVNs/LPNs, UAP, clerical support) are available to meet patient needs and provide safe, quality care. Several considerations surround staffing; they can be categorized in three general areas: (1) patient needs, (2) staff satisfaction, and (3) organizational needs.

Staffing and Patient Needs

The primary considerations for staffing a specific nursing unit are the number of patients, the level of intensity of care required by those patients, and the level of preparation and experience of the staff members providing the care (ANA, 1999). Knowing only the number of patients that require care is an ineffective way to plan staffing because of the wide range of care requirements needed by individual patients. To account for the diverse care needs and quantify the intensity of care required by a group of patients, various patient classification systems have been used.

Patient Classification Systems. Patient classification systems group or categorize patients according to specific criteria and care needs and thus help quantify the amount and level of care needed. This may be referred to as the "acuity level." The higher the acuity level, the more intense the patient's nursing care needs. For example, patients may be grouped in such categories as "uncomplicated postpartum" or "ventilator dependent." As the reader can easily visualize, these two groups of patients would require very different levels and amounts of care and therefore would be categorized at different acuity levels. Imagine the many different kinds of patients treated by a health care facility and you can begin to picture the complexity of patient classification systems.

Because of this complexity and the differences in patient populations across different health care facilities, patient classification systems vary from organization to organization. However, the American Nurses Association (ANA) has recommended in its publication, *Principles for Nurse Staffing* (ANA, 1999), that the following physical and psychosocial factors be considered when determining the intensity of care required for any group of patients:

- Age and functional ability
- Communication skills
- Cultural and linguistic diversities
- Severity and urgency of the admitting condition
- Scheduled procedures
- Ability to meet health care requisites
- Availability of social supports
- Other specific needs identified by the patient and by the RN

Understanding the intensity of care required by individual patients and groups of patients based on these factors is the first step in developing effective patient classifications systems and planning for appropriate staffing levels. The second step is knowing the level of preparation, skill, and experience of the staff members who are available to provide patient care.

Level of Staff Preparation and Experience. It is of critical importance that the staff members available to provide patient care have the educational preparation, skill, and experience necessary to meet patient care needs. Clinical competencies required to care for the population being served should be well defined. The nurse manager who is responsible for making staffing decisions must be aware of each individual staff member's competencies, experience, skill, and training. Clinical support from experienced RNs should be readily available to support and advance the skills of those RNs and other staff members with less experience. If the nurse manager does not believe that adequate numbers of appropriately skilled and experienced staff members are available to provide safe patient care, he or she should immediately address those concerns with the executive level managers.

Staffing and Staff Satisfaction

Nurses who are satisfied with their work generally provide higher-quality, more cost-effective care. "It has been shown that the quality of work life has an impact on the quality of care delivered" (ANA, 1999, p. 5). Marquis and Houston (2000, p. 264) report that staff scheduling "factors significantly in promoting job dissatisfaction or job satisfaction and subsequent nurse retention." However, because of the requirements for 24 hours/day, 365 days/year staffing needs in many health care facilities, meshing staffing needs with each nurse's personal needs is often very difficult. Various creative staffing options are available to meet the varied needs of staff members, including:

- 10-hour shifts/4 days per week.
- 12-hour shifts/3 days per week.
- Premium pay or part-time staff for weekend work.
- Job sharing, flextime, and/or staff self-scheduling.
- Use of supplemental, or agency staffing.

Each of these options has various advantages and disadvantages. For example, long shifts over consecutive days can result in clinical errors when nurses become fatigued. The excessive use of part-time or supplemental nurses can result in poor continuity of care (Marquis and Houston, 2000). Self-scheduling is becoming a popular staffing technique in which the responsibility for staffing the unit is delegated to the employees on the unit who work collectively to design the schedule based on preestablished staffing criteria and some guidance from the manager. No one scheduling system has proven to be best overall for staff satisfaction. However, when staffing, methods that gain staff input and enhance staff autonomy seem to be the key to staff satisfaction (Davidhizar, Dowd, and Brownson, 1998).

Staffing and Organizational Needs

The three basic organizational needs that are significantly affected by staffing are (1) financial resources, (2) licensing regulations and Joint Commission on Accreditation of Healthcare Organizations (JCAHO) standards, and (3) customer satisfaction. Productivity, the ratio of the amount of outputs produced (i.e., home visits) to the use of a specific amount of input (nursing hours worked), is the measure of staffing efficiency. Productivity will have a direct effect on the organization's bottom line. Staff salaries are by far the largest expense for a health care organization. Thus the efficient management of staffing is critical to ensure the organization's financial solvency. The nurse manager is accountable for appropriately managing staffing to stay within budgetary guidelines for:

- Numbers of staff working at any given time to provide care to a given number of patients.
- Staff mix, the combination of types of workers present to provide patient care (e.g., RNs, LVNs/LPNs, nursing assistants, multiskilled workers, or UAP).

Because RNs are the most expensive of the staff members listed here, most health care organizations have established goals for the ratio of RNs to other types of care providers. For example, a medical-surgical unit may be budgeted for a 30% RN staff, with the remainder of the staff members being LVNs/LPNs or UAP.

Health care facility licensing agencies such as a state's Department of Health and accreditation agencies such as JCAHO address minimum staffing levels. However, these agencies do not impose mandatory staffing ratios. For example, licensing regulations for long-term care facilities stipulate minimum RN coverage for the unit but do not mandate specific nurse-to-patient ratios. However, these agencies do look for evidence that patients are adequately cared for, which can only occur with adequate staffing. They also require documentation of staff training and competency to care for the organization's specific patient population.

Perhaps most critical to an organization's success in a competitive health care environment is customer satisfaction. The key to customer satisfaction is the customer's personal interaction with the organization's employees. "Interactions with patients and their families . . . have remarkably strong effects on clinical outcomes, functional status and even physiologic measures of health" (Kenagy, Berwick, and Shore, 1999, p. 663). Appropriate staffing within budget constraints with well-trained, competent, professional staff members who are committed to providing safe, high-quality care is the nurse manager's number one challenge.

This section has provided the reader with a very brief introduction to staffing issues such as scheduling options, patient classification systems, and productivity and staff mix. These issues related to staffing in a health care organization are much more complex than may appear from this introduction. The reader, especially the person interested in entering nursing management, is encouraged to learn more about staffing and these related issues. Box 19-1 presents some online resources to begin learning more about staffing.

| **BOX 19-1** | *Helpful Staffing Websites* |

ANA's *Principles for Nurse Staffing*
http://www.nursingworld.org/readroom/stffprnc.htm

Nursing-Sensitive Quality Indicators for Acute Care Settings and ANA's Safety and Quality Initiative
http://www.nursingworld.org/readroom/fssafe99.htm

ANA's Nationwide State Legislative Agenda on Nurse Staffing
http://www.nursingworld.org/gova/state/2001/agstaff.htm

Analysis of ANA's Staffing Survey
http://www.nursingworld.org/staffing/

NURSING CARE DELIVERY MODELS

Nursing care delivery models, also called care delivery systems or patient care delivery models, detail the way task assignments, responsibility, and authority are structured to accomplish patient care. The nursing care delivery model describes which health care worker is going to perform what tasks, who is responsible, and who has the authority to make decisions. The basic premise of nursing care delivery models is that the number and type of caregivers are closely matched to patient care needs to provide quality care in the most cost-effective manner possible.

The four classic nursing care delivery models used during the past five decades are (1) total patient care, (2) functional nursing, (3) team nursing, and (4) primary nursing. However, variations of these four classic models have been adopted more recently in an effort to continually improve both the quality and cost-effectiveness of patient care. These more recent innovations include modular nursing, partnership model (or co-primary nursing), patient-centered or patient-focused care, and case management. This section describes these models and discusses advantages and disadvantages of each model. Although no care delivery model is perfect, some methods may be more conducive to specific health care settings, such as home health care, ambulatory care, or hospital care.

Total Patient Care

The oldest method of organizing patient care is total patient care, sometimes referred to as case nursing. In total patient care nurses are responsible for planning, organizing, and performing all care, including personal hygiene, medications, treatments, emotional support, and education required for their assigned group of patients during the assigned shift. A diagram of the total patient care model is shown in Fig. 19-1.

Total patient care was used in the 1800s when most nursing care was provided in the home. As the popularity of public health nursing increased in the early 1900s, nurses practiced total patient care, and as nursing care moved into the hospital setting, this method continued to be the primary means of organizing patient care. Today nursing students typically perform total patient care for their assigned patients.

Advantages of the Total Patient Care Model
1. The patient receives holistic, unfragmented care by only one nurse per shift.
2. At shift change the RN who has provided care and the RN assuming care can easily communicate about the patient's condition and collaborate about the plan of care to ensure continuity because so few caregivers are involved.

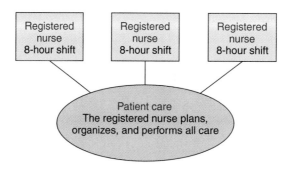

FIG. 19-1 The total patient care (case method) delivery model.

3. The nurse maintains a high degree of practice autonomy.
4. Lines of responsibility and accountability are clear.

Disadvantages of the Total Patient Care Model

1. The number of RNs required to provide total patient care to a group of patients is very costly for the health care facility.
2. The RN performs many tasks that could be performed by a caregiver with less training and at a lower cost.
3. The nursing shortage will affect RN availability, making total patient care difficult to accomplish.

Today the total patient care method is commonly used in the hospital's critical care areas such as intensive care units and postanesthesia care units, where continuous assessment and a high degree of clinical expertise are required. This method is less widely used in other patient care settings as health care organizations move to more efficient, transdisciplinary team approaches to patient care. However, variations of the total patient care method exist, and it is possible to identify similarities to this method when reviewing other methods of nursing care delivery.

Functional Nursing

The functional nursing model evolved during World War II when the demand for nurses both for the war effort and at home, greatly increased. Because of the shortage of nurses, ancillary personnel, UAP, and LVNs and LPNs were used to provide care to patients. It was found that, after training, relatively unskilled workers became proficient at performing routine, simple tasks such as taking blood pressures, giving baths, and administering medications. The nursing shortage persisted even after the war ended, and hospitals continued to use a variety of workers with different levels of skill and education to provide patient care. This practice continues today (Marquis and Huston, 2000).

In the functional nursing method of patient care delivery, staff members are assigned to complete certain tasks for a group of patients rather than care for specific patients. For example, the RN performs all assessments and administers all intravenous medications; the LVN/LPN gives all oral medications; and the assistant performs hygiene tasks and takes vital signs. A charge nurse makes the assignments and coordinates the care. A diagram of the functional nursing model is shown in Fig. 19-2.

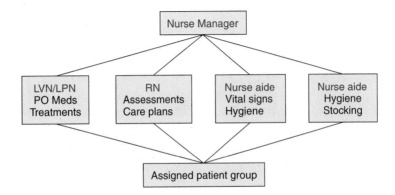

FIG. 19-2 The functional nursing care delivery model.

Advantages of the Functional Nursing Model

1. Patient care is provided in an economic and efficient manner because more less-skilled, lower-cost workers are used who focus on task completion.
2. A minimum number of RNs is required to supervise and to perform strictly nursing duties.
3. Tasks are completed quickly, and there is little confusion about job responsibilities.

Disadvantages of the Functional Nursing Model

1. Care may be fragmented, and the possibility of overlooking priority patient needs exists because of the number of different workers focused on performing specific patient care tasks.
2. The patient may feel confused because of the many different care providers he or she sees in 1 day.
3. Caregivers may feel unchallenged and unmotivated when performing repetitive functions.

   Although the functional model is considered efficient and economical, the patient is treated by many caregivers who are not able to give personalized care because they are focused on performing a task—not on meeting patient needs. This model may not fit well in the new health care system, which focuses on customer service. However, functional nursing care delivery is still appropriate in some care settings and often is used in the operating room.

Team Nursing

The concept of team nursing evolved in the 1950s in an effort to improve patient satisfaction and solve the problems associated with functional nursing. The goal of team nursing was to reduce fragmented care and provide a more personalized approach to patient care. In team nursing the RN functions as a team leader and coordinates a small group (no more than four or five) of ancillary personnel to provide care to a small group of patients. "As coordinator of the team, the registered nurse is responsible for knowing the condition and needs of all the patients assigned to the team, and for planning the care of each patient" (Marquis and Huston, 2000, p. 192). The team leader also is responsible for encouraging a cooperative environment and maintaining clear communication between all team members. The team leader's duties include planning care, assigning duties, directing and assisting team members, giving direct patient care, teaching, and coordinating patient activities. A diagram of the team nursing model is shown in Fig. 19-3.

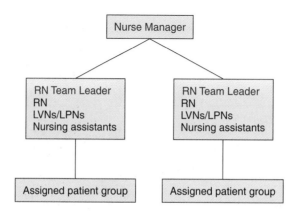

FIG. 19-3 Team nursing model.

Advantages of the Team Nursing Model *(Marquis and Huston, 2000)*

1. High-quality, comprehensive care can be provided with a relatively high proportion of ancillary staff.
2. Each member of the team is able to participate in decision making and problem solving.
3. Each team member is able to contribute his or her own special expertise or skills in caring for the patient.

Disadvantages of the Team Nursing Model

1. Continuity of care may suffer if the daily team assignments vary and the patient is confronted with many different caregivers.
2. The team leader may not have the leadership skills required to effectively direct the team and create a "team spirit."
3. Insufficient time for care planning and communication leads to unclear goals. Therefore responsibilities and care may become fragmented.

   Team nursing is an effective, efficient method of patient care delivery and has been used in most inpatient and outpatient health care settings. However, for team nursing to succeed, the team leader must have strong clinical skills, good communication skills, delegation ability, decision-making ability, and the ability to create a cooperative working environment. In an attempt to overcome some of its disadvantages, the team nursing design has been modified many times since its original inception, and variations of the model are evident in other methods of nursing care delivery, such as modular nursing.

Modular Nursing

Modular nursing is a modification of team nursing and focuses on the patient's geographic location for staff assignments. The patient unit is divided into modules or districts, and the same team of caregivers is assigned consistently to the same geographic location. Each location, or module, has an RN assigned as the team leader, and the other team members may include LVNs/LPNs and UAP (Yoder Wise, 1999).

The concept of modular nursing calls for a smaller group of staff providing care for a smaller group of patients. The goal is to increase the involvement of the RN in planning and coordinating care. Communication is more efficient among a smaller group of team members (Marquis and Huston, 2000). To maximize efficiency, each designated module should contain all the supplies needed by the staff to perform patient care. A diagram of the modular nursing model is shown in Fig. 19-4.

Advantages of the Modular Nursing Model *(Yoder Wise, 1999)*

1. Continuity of care is improved when staff members are consistently assigned to the same module.
2. The RN as team leader is able to be more involved in planning and coordinating care.
3. Geographic closeness and more efficient communication saves staff time.

Disadvantages of the Modular Nursing Model *(Yoder Wise, 1999)*

1. Costs may be increased to stock each module with the necessary patient care supplies (medication cart, linens, and dressings).
2. Long corridors, common in many hospitals, are not conducive to modular nursing.

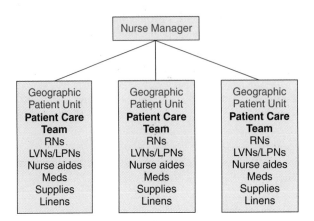

FIG. 19-4 Modular nursing model.

Just as in the team-nursing concept, the team leader in the modular model is accountable for all patient care and is responsible for providing leadership for the team members and creating a cooperative work environment.

Primary Nursing

The primary nursing model evolved in the 1970s in an effort to improve autonomy and quality care in professional nursing practice. In primary nursing the RN, or "primary" nurse, assumes 24-hour responsibility for planning, directing, and evaluating the patient's care from admission through discharge. This model differs significantly from the total patient care model in that the "primary nurse" assumes 24-hour responsibility for directing the patient's plan of care. While on duty, the primary nurse may provide total patient care or he or she may delegate some patient care tasks to LPN/LVNs or UAP. When the primary nurse is off duty, care is provided by an associate nurse who follows the care plan established by the primary nurse. The primary nurse, who has 24-hour responsibility, is notified if any problems or complications develop and directs alterations in the plan of care. A fundamental responsibility for the nurse in the primary nursing model is to maintain clear communication among all members of the health care team, including the patient, family, physician, associate nurses, and any other members of the health care team. A diagram of the primary nursing model is shown in Fig. 19-5.

Advantages of the Primary Nursing Model

1. Direct patient care provided by a few nurses allows for high-quality, holistic patient care (Marquis and Huston, 2000).
2. The patient is able to establish a rapport with the primary nurse, and patient satisfaction is increased (Yoder Wise, 1999).
3. Job satisfaction is high because nurses are able to practice with a high degree of autonomy and feel challenged and rewarded (Marquis and Huston, 2000).

Disadvantages of the Primary Nursing Model *(Marquis and Huston, 2000)*

1. Implementation may be difficult because the primary nurse is required to practice with a high degree of responsibility and autonomy.

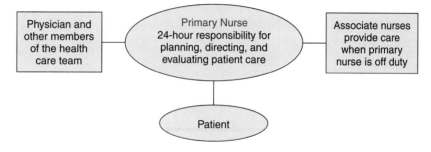

FIG. 19-5 Primary nursing model.

2. An inadequately prepared primary nurse may not be able to make the necessary clinical decisions or communicate effectively with the health care team.
3. The RN may not be willing to accept the 24-hour responsibility required in primary nursing.
4. The number of nurses required for this method of care may not be cost-effective and may be difficult to recruit and train, especially with the current nursing shortage.

The primary care nursing model lends itself well to home health nursing, hospice nursing, and long-term care settings in which the patient requires nursing care for an extended time period. Primary nursing may be more difficult to provide in acute care settings where stays are short and the nurse may see the patient for only 1 or 2 days. Because the concept of primary nursing is sound, some organizations have modified this nursing care model and implemented partnership models that use a wider staff mix.

Partnership Model

The partnership model, sometimes referred to as co-primary nursing, is a modification of primary nursing and was designed to make more efficient use of the RN. In the partnership model the RN is partnered with an LVN/LPN or UAP, and the pair work together consistently to care for an assigned group of patients.

Advantages of the Partnership Model
1. The model is more cost-effective than the true primary care nursing system because fewer RNs are needed.
2. The RN can encourage the training and growth of his or her partner.
3. The RN can perform the nursing duties while the partner can perform the nonnurisng tasks.

Disadvantages of the Partnership Model
1. The RN may have difficulty delegating to the partner.
2. Consistent partnerships are difficult to maintain based on varied staff schedules.

Patient-Centered Care

Patient-centered care, sometimes referred to as patient-focused care, is a more recent development in nursing care delivery models and is a result of work redesign in health care organizations in an effort to become more patient-oriented rather than hospital- or department-oriented. This patient-centered care model is a concept in which cross-functional teams of professionals and assistive personnel from nursing and other departments work together as a unit-based team to provide care to a given group of patients.

Patient-centered care "involves all departments that deal with the patient, including the nursing department, and is truly multidisciplinary in approach" (Marrelli, 1997, p. 111). Patient care functions such as diet teaching, phlebotomy, housekeeping, transportation, and respiratory treatments, which at one time had no relationship to the nursing department, now are centralized in a patient care unit under the direction of a nurse manager. The ancillary workers who once performed only one function such as phlebotomy now are cross-trained to increase their level of productivity.

A typical patient-centered team may include, in addition to a nurse manager and RNs, patient support assistants, health unit coordinators, and multiskilled workers often called patient care technicians. Patient care technicians support RNs and are trained to perform multiple duties, including bedside care, phlebotomy, oxygen therapy, and computer order entry. The patient support assistants perform various tasks in the unit, including housekeeping, stocking supplies, transporting patients, and assisting with patient care duties. The health unit coordinator performs nonclinical aspects of patient care, including medical record keeping, admitting and discharge, financial counseling, and clerical tasks (Reisdorfer, 1996). The job roles and titles used in the patient-centered model vary among health care facilities as they determine how patient care needs are best met. A diagram of a typical patient-centered care model is shown in Fig. 19-6.

Advantages of the Patient-Centered Care Model

1. The workers who come in contact with the patient are unit-based, are able to spend more time in direct care than in transit between patient-care areas, and are supervised by an RN who is familiar with the patient's plan of care (Kerfoot, 2000).
2. The RN is accountable for a wider range of services to the patient and thus is able to ensure more consistent patient care.
3. The model is more cost-effective for the health care organization.

Disadvantages of the Patient-Centered Care Model *(Douglass, 1996)*

1. Major change is required not only in the structure of the health care organization, but also for the nurse manager and the team members.

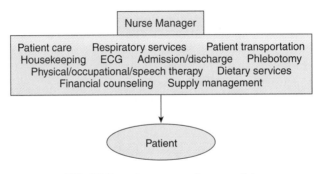

FIG. 19-6 Patient-centered care model.

2. Departments other than nursing must be willing to accept nursing leadership, and the nurse manager must be willing to accept the responsibility to understand and manage other types of workers.
3. Because many different types of workers and disciplines are involved as a team, new and different issues arise involving team conflict, problem resolution, and standards of care.

The patient-centered model is a variation of the team-nursing model and may be used in a variety of inpatient and outpatient settings. Just as in team nursing, the RN coordinator of the cross-functional team is responsible for planning patient care, encouraging a cooperative environment, and maintaining clear communication between all team members. However, the patient-centered model may vary considerably from facility to facility, depending on the patient's needs and the facility's resources.

CASE MANAGEMENT
Evolution of Case Management

Case management is a model of care delivery in which an RN case manager coordinates the patient's care throughout the course of an illness. The concept of case management was first introduced in the 1970s by insurance companies as a method to monitor and control expensive health insurance claims, usually created by a catastrophic accident or illness (More and Mandell, 1997). Today, virtually every major health insurance company has a case management program to direct and manage the use of health care services for their clients. Case management by payer organizations (e.g., health insurance companies, health maintenance organizations [HMOs]) is known as external case management.

By the mid-1980s hospitals had recognized the need for a case management model to manage the treatment plan and length of stay of hospitalized patients (More and Mandell, 1997). When the Medicare prospective payment program was implemented in 1983, hospitals were reimbursed a set payment based on the patient's diagnosis, or diagnosis-related group (DRG), regardless of how long the patient was hospitalized or what treatment was provided. To keep costs lower than the diagnosis-related payment, the hospitals had to efficiently manage the treatment provided to a patient and reduce the patient's length of stay. Thus internal case management, or case management "within the walls" of the health care facility, was created to maintain quality care while streamlining costs. Several studies have since demonstrated the value of case management in both improving patient health outcomes and reducing costs (Galvin and Baudendistel, 1998; Huggins and Lehman, 1997; Gonzalez-Calvo et al., 1997).

Definition of Case Management

The ANA has defined nursing case management as "a dynamic and systematic collaborative approach to providing and coordinating health care services to a defined population. It is a participative process to identify and facilitate options and services for meeting individuals' health needs, while decreasing fragmentation and duplication of care and enhancing quality, cost-effective clinical outcomes. The framework for nursing care management includes five components: assessment, planning, implementation, evaluation, and interaction" (ANCC, 2001, p. 1).

Nursing case management is clinically and business oriented and is based on achieving specified patient outcomes. Patient outcomes should be achieved within a specified time frame while using available resources as efficiently as possible to decrease costs. Preestablished patient outcomes may be designated in critical pathways, which are discussed in the following section of this chapter.

Other disciplines, most notably social work, have been involved in developing case management programs and have identified themselves as case managers. Social workers have demonstrated their effectiveness in coordinating care needs and resource utilization in the outpatient setting, but the inpatient programs require a clinical practitioner (Birdsall and Sperry, 1997). It is common to see the term *case manager* used for many types of caregivers in many different health care settings. However, when clinical knowledge and experience is required, the RN is most effective in the case management role.

The ANA recommends that the case manager be a baccalaureate-prepared RN and preferably have a master's degree and advanced clinical and managerial skills. "Professional nurses are uniquely prepared to be case managers by virtue of their broad-based education in the life, social, and nursing sciences; their experiences in arranging and providing patient education and referrals; their awareness of the vital link between health and environment; and their orientation toward holistic health and its promotion" (ANCC, 2001, p. 2). Variations of case management models now are found in almost all health care organizations, including home health agencies, rehabilitation and long-term care facilities, hospitals, and ambulatory care organizations. A nursing case management model is shown in Fig. 19-7.

Components of Case Management

Assessment. The first role of the case manager is to collect and analyze comprehensive information about the client, his or her significant others, and available health care resources such as health insurance coverage. The comprehensive assessment includes collecting and analyzing information in the following areas: physiologic status, psychologic status, cognitive and functional abilities, sociocultural and lifestyle, spiritual beliefs, and financial resources. The nurse case manager may also find, appraise, and use research findings as the basis for clinical treatment decisions to ensure evidence-based practice. During the assessment phase the nurse case manager interacts with the client, his or her significant others, physicians and other

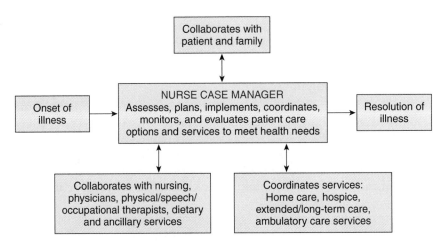

FIG. 19-7 Case management model.

health care providers, and representatives from the health insurance company to gather detailed information.

Planning. The plan of care is developed based on a comprehensive analysis of information obtained in the assessment phase and delineates desired, realistic patient goals and outcomes. The care plan, which should be client-centered, evidence-based, and transdisciplinary, is developed in collaboration with the client, family members and/or significant others, health care team members, employers, and payers. A primary responsibility of the nurse case manager is to ensure that all parties have had a part in developing the plan of care and are in agreement with the final established plan.

Implementation. During this stage the nurse care manager becomes involved in actual implementation of the plan of care. The nurse case manager's responsibilities might include performing care or, more usual, delegating care activities and facilitating and coordinating various aspects of the plan of care. Communication and documentation about progress toward desired outcomes are of primary importance to the nurse manager, as is ensuring that interventions are consistent with the established plan of care and are implemented in a safe, timely, and cost-effective manner.

The internal case manager assumes an important responsibility for understanding and monitoring the patient's payment source (e.g., private insurance, Medicare, or Medicaid). Not only will case managers confirm payment rates for the facility and initiate treatment preauthorization when required, they also will keep the patient and family members informed about available insurance benefits and how much out-of-pocket expense the patient may expect. For example, the discharge plan for a patient might include home health care. However, if the patient does not have health insurance coverage for home health services and if the patient is not able to pay for the home health services, a different plan of care will have to be developed.

Evaluation. The evaluation process is important to monitor the client's progress toward accomplishing established goals and outcomes, as well as evaluating the components of the case management process. Evaluation can be accomplished through (1) direct observation; (2) interviews, surveys, and/or verbal feedback from the client, significant others, and members of the health care team; (3) documentation review and/or chart audits; and (4) cost-benefit analysis of the client's treatment plan. "Nurse case managers continually evaluate each individual's health plan and challenge and attempt to overcome those obstacles that affect outcomes. Such obstacles may require the nurse case manager to reassess and revise the plan of care" (ANCC, 2001, p. 4)

Interaction. Ongoing interaction and collaboration with all members of the health care team, the client, the family and significant others, and the payer representatives is a key responsibility of the nurse case manager and is inherent in all phases of the nursing case management process. To effectively interact and collaborate with all parties involved in the client's care, the nurse case manager needs good communication skills and the ability to motivate a diverse group of individuals to cooperate and collaborate to meet client needs.

Case Management Example. The nurse case manager "manages" a "caseload" of patients from preadmission, or onset of illness, to discharge, or resolution of illness. Although case managers generally do not perform direct care duties, they assume a planning and evaluative role and collaborate with the transdisciplinary health care team to ensure that goals are met, quality is maintained, and progress toward discharge is made. The goal of case management, whether internal or external, is to focus attention on the quality, outcomes, and cost of care throughout the patient's episode of illness and to assist the patient to move through the continuum of care. For example, the nurse case manager coordinates arrangements to move the patient from acute care—to rehabilitation—to home health—to independent living as determined by patient needs. Following is an example to demonstrate the functions of the case manager.

Mr. Smith, a 58-year-old man, was diagnosed with lung cancer 1 year ago. He has been in Medical Center Hospital with multiple complications for more than 3 weeks. Debra Welch, RN, the internal case manager assigned to Mr. Smith's case, is working with the patient, family, physician, other members of the health care team, and the insurance company to determine a timely, cost-effective discharge plan. Debra has performed a comprehensive health assessment and understands the patient's condition and the available support systems. The physician, patient, family, and health care team agree that Mr. Smith's prognosis is grave and the treatment plan should be for palliative care only. Pain management is most important at this stage of the disease. Mr. Smith has a strong desire to go home, and his wife and adult daughter are willing to share the responsibility for home care. Debra also has identified the family's need for emotional support to deal effectively with the terminal illness.

After contacting Mr. Smith's insurance company, Debra learns that the company does not provide home health benefits, but the patient could be transferred to a subacute facility for continued care. Knowing Mr. Smith's strong desire to go home and the support systems in place, Debra identifies all the costs for home care (hospital bed, bedside commode, oxygen, wheelchair, and hospice support with pain management) and reports the comparative costs of home care vs. subacute care to the insurance company. By demonstrating that home care is slightly less expensive than inpatient, subacute care, Debra is able to negotiate successfully a payment for home care from Mr. Smith's insurance company.

As case manager, Debra's next responsibilities are to coordinate Mr. Smith's discharge and to arrange for home services needed, including hospice care and medical equipment. The home plan of care is developed by the health care team and approved by the physician. Debra communicates the plan of care to the home care providers to ensure nonfragmented care. As a result of case management, Mr. Smith and his family are able to go home with continued support and a smooth transition of care.

Box 19-2 presents a review of the components of the nursing case management process and related activities.

Case Management and Other Nursing Care Delivery Models

Nursing case management in a health care facility is a supplemental form of nursing care delivery and does not take the place of the nursing care delivery model in place to provide direct patient care. For example, if a hospital's medical-surgical unit uses a team nursing approach to patient care, a system of case management also might be in place to assist with coordinating the patient's total care through discharge. Case management is not needed for every patient in a health care facility and generally is reserved for the chronically ill, seriously ill or injured, and long-term, high-cost cases.

Case Management As a Nursing Specialty

Certification. The American Nurses' Credentialing Center (ANCC) offers certification in nursing case management and has established two categories of requirements for the certification examination. If an individual currently holds a core nursing specialty certification such

| **BOX 19-2** | *Components of Nursing Case Management and the Related Activities* |

Assessment

- Review the client's history and current status
- Perform comprehensive health assessment
- Identify available resources and support system (e.g., individual, family, financial, health insurance, community)
- Identify barriers to accessing necessary treatment (e.g., lack of health insurance coverage; no family support)
- Identify health promotion and disease prevention opportunities
- Identify adherence patterns, educational needs, and ability to learn
- Determine potential for overuse or underuse of resources
- Find, appraise, and use research findings as the basis for treatment decisions (evidence-based practice)

Planning

- Prioritize needs and set realistic, measurable goals and outcomes
- Identify realistic treatment options
- Coordinate various providers involved in the plan of care (e.g., physician, physical therapist, dietitian)
- Determine appropriate levels of care and realistic treatment settings (e.g., home, long-term care, rehabilitation facility)
- Identify and address gaps in care
- Ensure continuity of care
- Negotiate and manage financial aspects of care

Implementation

- Ensure implementation of the care plan in a safe, timely and cost-effective manner
- Coordinate services and referrals to providers or agencies
- Ensure compliance with federal, state, and local regulations and standards
- Use appropriate community resources
- Document progress toward achieving goals and outcomes
- Accept accountability for implementation of the care plan

Evaluation

- Measure clinical goals, functional improvement, satisfaction with services and cost-benefit of treatment plan
- Is/was the plan of care realistic, collaborative, and mutually beneficial to all involved?
- Are/were the established time frames realistic?
- Are/were the best possible and most cost-effective treatments used?
- Are/were individual educational opportunities maximized?

Interaction

- Interact on a daily basis with diverse groups of people: client, family members, and significant others; health care team members; payer representatives; representatives from other health care agencies and community organizations
- Motivate diverse groups to cooperate, collaborate, and work in the best interest of the client
- Use good communication, negotiation, facilitation, and documentation skills

BOX 19-3	*Helpful Case Management Resources*

Online Resources

Case Management Society of America website
http://www.cmsa.org

Case management resource guide with searchable listings of over 110,000 health care facilities and companies from the following categories: home care, rehabilitation, subacute care, nursing facilities, assisted living facilities. hospice, long-term acute hospitals, psychiatric and addiction treatment facilities
http://www.cmrg.com/guide.htm

Case management resource guide with links to disease management resources for the following diseases: acquired immune deficiency syndrome/human immunodeficiency virus, asthma, bone stimulation/healing therapies, bone marrow transplant, burn care, cancer/oncology, cardiovascular disease, diabetes, end-stage renal disease
http://www.cmrg.com/guide.htm

American Nurses Credentialing Center, a division of the ANA has information on case management and certification as a nurse case manager
http://www.nursingworld.org/ancc/

Journals

Nursing Case Management

Lippincott's Case Management: Managing the Process of Patient Care

Books

Cohen E, Cesta T: *Nursing case management: from essentials to advanced practice*, St Louis, 2001, Mosby.

Powell SK: *CMSA Core Curriculum for Case Management*, Philadelphia, 2001, JB Lippincott.

as the Critical Care Registered Nurse (CCRN) from the American Association of Critical Care Nurses, then the following requirements must be met to take the case management certification examination (ANCC, 2001):

- Hold an active RN license in the United States or its territories
- Hold a baccalaureate or higher degree in nursing (transcript showing conferral of degree must be submitted)
- Have functioned within the scope of an RN case manager a minimum of 2000 hours within the past 2 years
- Show proof of a current, core nursing specialty certification

Candidates without a nursing core specialty certification must complete an additional 50 questions related to the ANA's *Standards of Clinical Nursing Practice*. These candidates receive two separate scores, one for the nursing care management component and one for the core clinical practice components. The candidate must pass both examinations to become certified in case management (ANCC, 2001).

Case Management Professional Organization. The Case Management Society of America (CMSA), the largest professional organization of case managers, is an international not-for-profit membership society of case managers, nurses, and allied health care professionals. CMSA was founded in 1990 and is dedicated to the support and development of the profession of case management through educational forums, networking opportunities, and legislative involvement. CMSA developed the nationally recognized *Standards of Practice for Case Management* and offers its members, which number over 7500, opportunities to network and obtain continuing education in the fields of case management, nursing, social work, disease management, and rehabilitation (CMSA, 1997).

Box 19-3 offers online resources for case management.

CLINICAL PATHWAYS

Clinical pathways, also called critical paths, practice protocols, clinical practice guidelines, patient care protocols, or care maps, delineate a predetermined written plan of care for a particular health problem (Birdsall and Sperry, 1997). Clinical pathways specify the desired outcomes and transdisciplinary intervention required within a specified time period for a specified diagnosis or health problem. Clinical pathways were developed in response to the need to identify quality, cost-effective care plans to reduce the patient's length of stay in the hospital. The JCAHO now stipulates that health care facilities use clinical pathways to meet accreditation standards (JCAHO, 2000). Clinical pathways dictate the type and amount of care given and therefore have financial implications for the health care facility (Marrelli, 1997).

In essence, the "pathway" can be viewed as a road map the patient and health care team should follow to guide the patient's care management and recovery. As the patient progresses along the path, specified goals should be accomplished. If a patient's progress deviates or leaves the planned path, a variance has occurred. A positive variance means that the patient has progressed ahead of schedule, and a negative variance means that the identified goals are not accomplished as planned. The RN generally identifies that a variance has occurred and mobilizes the transdisciplinary team members to create an action plan to address the problem or issue.

Clinical Pathway Terminology

- *Patient outcomes* are the end result of intervention by the health care team.
- *Transdisciplinary intervention* is the collaborative effort by all disciplines (e.g., nursing, physician, dietitian, physical therapy, occupational therapy, pharmacy), along with the patient and the family, to help the patient reach the desired health outcomes.
- *Variance* is any event that may alter the patient's progress through the clinical pathway.
- *Trigger* alerts the caregiver that an unexpected event has occurred and identifies potential and actual variations in the patient's response to the planned intervention (Birdsall and Sperry, 1997).

Clinical Pathway Components

Components of a clinical pathway include (1) consultations, (2) laboratory and diagnostic tests, (3) treatments and medications, (4) safety and self-care activities, (5) nutrition, and (6) discharge planning (Yoder Wise, 1999). Many clinical pathways also address triggers (potential negative variances from the path) in addition to patient and family education needs. Clinical paths are written to address common medical diagnoses such as heart failure and pneumonia, nursing care needs such as immobility, and medical complications such as weaning from mechanical ventilation (Birdsall and Sperry, 1997).

Clinical Pathway Goals

Health care organizations develop clinical pathways to meet the specific needs of their patients and health care providers. The goals for developing and using clinical pathways are:

- Identify client and family needs.
- Determine realistic patient outcomes and the time frames required to achieve those outcomes.
- Reduce length of stay and inappropriate use of resources.
- Clarify the appropriate care setting, providers, and timeliness of intervention.

Development of Clinical Pathways

Clinical pathways should be based on accepted standards of practice. The ANA and specialty nursing organizations publish standards of practice for professional nursing. For example, the American Nephrology Nursing Association publishes standards of practice for nursing care of the patient with end-stage renal disease. Medical specialty boards also recommend standards of practice and actually have developed clinical practice guidelines for a variety of conditions. The American Academy of Pediatrics recommends several practice guidelines, including one on "Managing Otitis Media with Effusion in Young Children." This guideline can be found online at www.aap.org/policy/otitis.htm.

The Agency for Healthcare Research and Quality (AHRQ), (formerly know as the Agency for Health Care Policy and Research), in conjunction with medical specialty associations, professional societies, and various other health care organizations, has developed a series of 19 clinical practice guidelines. The reader is strongly encouraged to view current clinical practice guidelines at www.ahcpr.gov/clinic/cpgonline.htm. Additional information about clinical practice guidelines is also available through the National Guideline Clearinghouse at www.guideline.gov.

Clinical pathways most often are developed for the health care organization's most common or costly diagnoses. For example, a general hospital may develop pathways for the treatment of congestive heart failure from admission in the Emergency Department—to care in the coronary care—to care on the general floor—to discharge home. It is important that the clinical pathway be individualized to meet unique patient needs.

A team supported by management, with representatives from various disciplines, including nursing, medicine, therapy, pharmacy, and dietary, develops clinical pathways for the organization. As a starting point, samples of clinical pathways can be found in the literature. In addition, professional medical associations and the AHRQ are excellent sources for currently recommended clinical guidelines. Although these resources provide a place to start, pathways developed by the health care organization's own team result in an individualized plan of care supported by all team members and avoid a "cookbook" approach to care. An excellent, easy-to-follow process for guideline development and implementation can be found in the JCAHO Accreditation Manual (2000). The success of clinical pathway development and implementation depends on input and support from all disciplines, including physicians, involved in using the pathway and caring for the patient.

CHOOSING A NURSING CARE DELIVERY MODEL

The nursing care delivery models presented in this chapter can be integrated into a variety of health care settings, including acute care, long-term care, ambulatory care, home care, and hospice. The organizational structure, patient needs, and staff availability influence which delivery system will be used.

Acute care settings may use different types of care delivery models for various patient care units. Emergency Departments often use functional approaches to care because emphasis is on efficient assessment and immediate treatment. Team nursing frequently is used in medical-surgical units, whereas total patient care is common in critical care units. As identified in this chapter's vignette, acute care hospitals demand that the RN understand and be able to function in the diverse patterns of care that are in place throughout the organization.

In long-term care settings such as nursing homes, skilled nursing facilities, and rehabilitation settings, patients remain in the care settings for extended time periods. Therefore the care delivery models may be structured differently than in the acute setting. Because of its economy and efficiency, functional nursing may be used for daily care tasks, whereas a form of primary care nursing is used for assessment and care planning. The RN is assigned to function as the primary nurse for a group of patients. The primary nursing care duties include assessment, planning, and monitoring care over an extended period of time.

The variety of ambulatory care settings continues to grow as health care moves out of the more expensive inpatient settings to the less costly outpatient settings. Outpatient surgery centers, minor emergency clinics, outpatient cancer centers, outpatient dialysis units, outpatient birthing centers, health clinics, and physicians' offices are examples of ambulatory care settings. The nursing care delivery model in ambulatory settings varies widely, depending on the type of patients being treated. For example, in outpatient dialysis units a combination of functional and primary care nursing usually works well. Patient care technicians are assigned to perform specific patient care functions such as dialysis machine set-up, whereas the RN is assigned primary nurse responsibilities for a group of patients to ensure effective assessment, care planning, and care coordination with the transdisciplinary team.

Home health agencies often use a variation of the total patient care model. Although in home care the RN does not provide 24-hour care, he or she is responsible for the patient's needs for a 24-hour period and will coordinate care provided by others, including the home health aide and therapists involved in the patient's care. In the home health setting the RN may function in the role of case manager for his or her assigned patients.

In every care setting the nurse manager must carefully evaluate the nursing care delivery model to ensure safe, efficient, and effective patient care. When evaluating nursing care delivery models, the following questions should be asked (Marquis and Huston, 2000; Marrelli, 1997):

- Are patient outcomes being achieved in a timely, cost-effective manner?
- Are patients and families satisfied with care?
- Are physicians and other health team members satisfied with the care?
- Does the system allow for implementation of the nursing process?
- Does the system facilitate communication among all members of the health care team?

SUMMARY

Managers of health care organizations are concerned that patient care is delivered in the most efficient and cost-effective method possible and that staffing is appropriate to ensure safe, high-quality care and contribute to staff satisfaction. Because staffing is the highest cost area for a health care organization, managers always will focus on ways to structure the delivery of care to maximize the use of staff time and minimize the use of high-cost staff such as RNs. For this reason, nursing care delivery models have undergone tremendous changes throughout the past decade and will continue to evolve as organizations look for ways to reduce costs and improve quality, customer satisfaction, and staff satisfaction. Regardless of changes that may occur, the RN will retain responsibility to evaluate nursing care delivery models to ensure that patient care is delivered safely and efficiently, that caregivers are competent and legally qualified to perform the duties they have been assigned, and that quality care and staff satisfaction are maintained.

Critical Thinking Activities

1. Describe the nursing care delivery models you have observed in the clinical setting. List the advantages and disadvantages of each one, and note the delivery models you liked best and why.
2. Review a critical pathway from a selected clinical setting. How is patient care based on the critical pathway implemented in the facility? How is the patient's progress through the critical pathway communicated to the entire health care team and documented in the chart? What action does the nurse take if the patient "falls off" the pathway?
3. Your nurse manager has asked you to serve on a committee to review the nursing care delivery system currently in place on the nursing unit and to make recommendations to improve the current system. What factors should you consider when evaluating the current system and reviewing new systems?

REFERENCES

American Nurses Association: Position statement: registered nurse utilization of unlicensed assistive personnel, *NursingWorld,* 1997, http://www.nursingworld.org/readroom/position/uap/uapuse.htm.

American Nurses Association: *Principles for nurse staffing,* 1999, http://www.nursingworld.org/readroom/stffprnc.htm.

American Nurses Credentialing Center: *Modular certification: basic eligibility requirements, 2001,* http://www.nursingworld.org/ancc/certify/cert/catalogs/2000/bcc/modspec.htm.

Birdsall C, Sperry SP: *Clinical paths in medical-surgical practice,* St Louis, 1997, Mosby.

Case Management Society of America: 1997, www.cmsa.org.

Davidhizar R, Dowd SB, Brownson K: An equitable nursing assignment structure, *Nurs Manage* 29(4):33-35, 1998.

Douglass LM: *The effective nurse,* ed 5, St Louis, 1996, Mosby.

Galvin LG, Baudendistel D: Case management: a team approach, *Nursing Manage* 29(1):28-31, 1998.

Gonzalez-Calvo J et al: Nursing case management and its role in perinatal risk reduction: development, implementation, and evaluation of a culturally competent model for African American women, *Public Health Nurs* 14(4):190-206, 1997.

Huggins D, Lehman K: Reducing costs through case management, *Nurs Manage* 28(12):34-37, 1997.

Kenagy JW, Berwick DM, Shore MF: Service quality in health care, *JAMA* 281(7):661-665, 1999.

Joint Commission on Accreditation of Healthcare Organizations: *2000-2001 Comprehensive accreditation manual for ambulatory care,* Oakbrook Terrace, Ill, 2000, JCAHO.

Kerfoot K: The health care organization and patterns of nursing care delivery. In Zerwekh J, Claborn JC: *Nursing today: transition and trends,* ed 3, Philadelphia, 2000, WB Saunders.

Marrelli TM: *The nurse manager's survival guide,* ed 2, St Louis, 1997, Mosby.

Marquis BL, Huston CJ: *Leadership roles and management functions in nursing,* ed 3, Philadelphia, 2000, JB Lippincott.

More PK, Mandell S: *Nursing case management,* New York, 1997, McGraw-Hill.

Reisdorfer JT: Building a patient-focused care unit, *Nurs Manage* 27(10):38-44, 1996.

Yoder Wise P: *Leading and managing in nursing,* St Louis, 1999, Mosby.

Nursing's Role in Improving the Quality of Health Care

Kathleen M. Werner, MS, BSN, RN

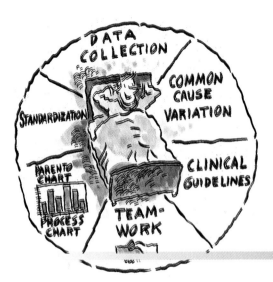

The focus of all quality management activities must be what customers need and want.

Vignette

It was a typical day on 4 East, a busy medical-surgical unit in General Hospital. Patients were being admitted, discharged, and transported to surgery at a brisk pace. For Maureen Harper, RN, the day was like most others, until one of her patients was to be discharged. All of the necessary paperwork was documented, the patient's belongings were packed, and all discharge instructions were completed. But Maureen's patient could not be discharged until the pharmacy delivered the newly prescribed medication that was to be taken at home. This was not the first time a patient had to wait for a prescription, and for Maureen it was becoming a repeated pattern in the normal course of discharge preparations. The patient eventually received the medication after an hour's wait and was sent home, but Maureen began to ponder the impact of this repeating set of circumstances.

Maureen calculated the additional cost that resulted from this patient's wait. It was an extra hour of hospital care, an extra hour of nursing care, and because this occurred during lunch time, it also meant that an extra meal needed to be served to the patient while he waited. Each of these costs was small in its own right, but Maureen began to think of the implications of these costs as they multiplied across dozens of patients throughout the many different nursing units at General Hospital. More important, Maureen was beginning to see the impact that this waiting had on patients' perceptions of the hospital. Family members often arrived early in the morning to take patients home, only to find they had to wait. Likewise, patients were not pleased when told they would need to wait. An entire positive hospital stay could be tainted with the experience of having to wait for discharge medication. Would that perception stay with them as they spoke to other friends and family about their hospitalization? Maureen began to feel more pressed to do something about the situation.

The next week, Maureen approached her nurse manager and expressed her concern with the discharge situation. Maureen's manager thanked her for the feedback and expressed similar interest in resolving this problem. Pharmacy staff members already had been in preliminary conversations with Maureen's manager about the discharge medication process and were willing to work collaboratively with the nursing staff to find a solution to this problem. Maureen eagerly volunteered to participate in a work group that was charged with understanding the common causes of delays in filling discharge medication prescriptions and implementing key changes to eliminate the delay. The team met regularly for several weeks and gained a clear understanding of what was contributing to the medication delay. This was accomplished through creation of a detailed "picture" of what typically happened in filling discharge medication prescriptions and working on constructive ways to prevent breakdowns in this process. The project involved data collection to validate the sources of the breakdowns; what surfaced were surprises for staff members in each of the major departments involved, who always thought that "someone else" was to blame for the problems. In reality, the interaction of multiple departments leads to delays. Over time, with constant monitoring of the turnaround time between the writing of the discharge medication order and delivery of drugs back to the units, progress was demonstrated. Maureen now knows that the proper steps are in place to guarantee an efficient way for medication orders to be tracked and filled. When her patients are ready for discharge, so are their medications, and Maureen feels like she is a vested part of this success!

Questions to consider while reading this chapter

1. What key principles of quality improvement are demonstrated in the vignette?
2. What quality improvement tools did Maureen and the team most likely use to identify the causes for delays in filling discharge medications?
3. What resources are available to help Maureen and others in her organization learn more about improving the quality of health care?

Key Terms

Cause-and-effect diagram Tool that is used for identifying and organizing possible causes of a problem in a structured format. It is sometimes called a "fishbone" diagram because it looks like the skeleton of a fish.

Clinical indicators Measurable items that reflect the quality of care provided and demonstrate the degree to which desired clinical outcomes are accomplished; clinical indicators help to identify the goals of quality improvement.

Customer Individual or group who relies on an organization to provide a product or service to meet some need or expectation. It is these customer needs and expectations that determine quality.

Flowchart Picture of the sequence of steps in a process. Different steps or actions are represented by boxes or other symbols. A top-down flowchart shows the sequence of steps in a job or process. It can have different levels of detail. A deployment flowchart shows the detailed steps in a process and the people or departments that are involved in each step.

JCAHO Joint Commission on the Accreditation of Healthcare Organizations; a national agency that conducts surveys of inpatient and ambulatory facilities and certifies their compliance with established quality standards.

IOM National Academy of Sciences Institute of Medicine; a nonprofit organization with a mission of advancing and disseminating scientific knowledge to improve human health. The Institute provides objective, timely, authoritative information and advice concerning health and science policy to government, the corporate sector, the professions, and the public.

ISMP Institute for Safe Medication Practices; a nonprofit organization that is well known as an education resource for the prevention of medication errors.

NCQA National Committee for Quality Assurance; an accreditation body that has become the primary group that accredits health maintenance organizations.

Pareto Chart A graphic tool that helps break a big problem down into its parts and then identifies which parts are the most important.

Process Series of linked steps necessary to accomplish work. A process turns inputs, such as information or raw materials, into outputs, like products, services, and reports. Clinical processes are a series of linked steps necessary for the provision of patient care. It is through the improvement of processes that an organization improves its work and the way it sustains itself.

Process variation Variation results from the lack of perfect uniformity in the performance of any process. Understanding variation helps one to know the real limits to quality and productivity inherent in the system and to understand the capability of the system. Understanding variation points to the direction that improvement efforts must take.

Quality management Philosophic framework for managing organizations that recognizes that quality is determined by customer needs and expectations. Attention is paid to how the work is done, with an emphasis on involving the people who best understand the detail of the work processes with which they are involved. Health care quality management (QM) is specifically related to the quality of health care services provided.

Root cause analysis Defined by the JCAHO (2000) as a process for identifying the basic or causal factors that underlie variation in performance, including the occurrence or possible occurrence of a sentinel event. A root cause analysis focuses primarily on systems and processes, not individual performance. It progresses from special causes in clinical processes to common causes in organizational processes and identifies potential improvements in processes or systems that would tend to decrease the likelihood of such events in the future, or determines, after analysis, that no such improvement opportunities exist.

Sentinel event Defined by the JCAHO (2000) as an unexpected occurrence involving patient death or serious physical or psychologic injury or the risk thereof. Serious injury specifically includes loss of limb or function. The phrase "or the risk thereof" includes any process variation for which a recurrence would carry a significant chance of a serious adverse outcome. Such events are called "sentinel" because they signal the need for immediate investigation and response.

Standardization Approach to process improvement that involves developing and adhering to best known methods and repeating key tasks in the same way, time and time again, until a better way is found, thereby creating exceptional service with maximum efficiency.

Time plot Graph of data in time order that helps identify any changes that occur over time. Another name for a time plot is a run chart. A time plot that has a centerline and statistical control limits added is known as a control chart. Control limits help detect specific types of change in a process.

Learning Outcomes

After studying this chapter, the reader will be able to:

1. Apply principles of QM to the role of the professional nurse.
2. Critique key evolutionary facts that led to the development of QM in health care.
3. Analyze the role of health care regulatory agencies and how they have embodied the principles of QM.
4. Analyze the basis for the increasing emphasis on medical errors.
5. Discuss the role process improvement can play in ensuring patient safety.
6. Discuss the tools and skills necessary for QM activities in relation to the professional nurse.

CHAPTER OVERVIEW

Although Maureen Harper's story depicted in the vignette seems credible and would be a logical way for any organization to begin addressing customer concerns, far too often that has not been the case. Hospitals and health care organizations have been slow to recognize the necessity of a true customer perspective and to emphasize quality in a proactive manner. Donald Berwick (1990) wrote, "The paradox is infuriating. In some ways, it is the best of times for American health care . . . . But in equally striking ways, it is the worst of times for American health care, at least since it entered the scientific era of twentieth-century practice. Almost no one is happy with the health care system. It costs too much; it excludes too many; it fails too often; and it knows too little about its own effectiveness" (Berwick, Godfrey, and Roessner, 1990, p. xv). Although Dr. Berwick made this statement over 10 years ago, it is still timely because unfortunately we have documented little progress in addressing the quality issues that continue to plague the U.S. health care system.

In an alarming 1999 report by the National Academy of Science's Institute of Medicine (IOM), authors extrapolated and summarized data from two major studies and concluded that up to 98,000 patients are killed each year from medical errors, confirming that poor quality of health care is a major problem in the United States (Kohn, Corrigan, and Donaldson, 1999). Contributing factors cited in the report included:

- Overuse of expensive invasive technology.
- Underuse of inexpensive care services.
- Error-prone implementation of care that could potentially harm patients and waste money.

The intention of this chapter is not to solve the nation's health care crisis, but rather to address the following questions.

- What is quality in health care?
- Who determines the degree to which quality is evident in our health care system?
- What do the potential answers to the first two questions mean in relationship to professional nursing accountability?

The responses to these questions, particularly in relation to nursing's commitment to become involved with QM and to participate in its implementation, provide the elements of hope in determining and implementing sustainable, positive improvements in the design and delivery of health care in the United States.

QUALITY MANAGEMENT PRINCIPLES

There are many buzzwords meant to describe activities associated with QM. The most prevalent are total quality management (TQM), continuous quality improvement (CQI), continuous process improvement, statistical process control, and performance improvement. The terms themselves are not as important as the principles they embody: that of assessment and improvement of work processes while focusing on what customers want and need. In the example of Maureen and her patient waiting for discharge medication, the work process would be that of filling discharge prescription medication orders. The customer in this situation would be Maureen's patient, who wants to receive the medication quickly so that he can go home as soon as possible. Essentially the cornerstones of QM include the following.

1. Recognition and understanding by all who serve a customer that it is the customer who defines quality. In health care, primary customers are patients, and they are the ones who determine what quality is, not those who are in the position of providing the care and service. Historically caregivers frequently have assumed the role of determining "what is best for the patient."

2. Organizational support for all employees to develop quality knowledge and skills and to begin thinking of their work as a series of processes that can be more deeply understood and improved through data measurements. As employees within an organization work to improve their work processes, they begin to understand the interrelationship and impact of process work across departments, such that ultimately the final product or service offered to the customer can be vastly improved. This chapter's vignette demonstrated this concept through Maureen's participation on a work team on which pharmacy and nursing both studied their contribution to the discharge medication process and found ways to better meet the patients' expectations of timeliness.

3. Belief in the people who are working to serve the customer. By recognizing the insight and knowledge held by those who are closest to the work and allowing them to be involved with the study and improvement of their own work, the potential for dramatic improvements can be realized.

Brian Joiner (1994) refers to these cornerstones of QM graphically in what he terms the "Joiner Triangle," labeling each point respectively as "quality," "scientific approach," and "all one team." He compares this model to a three-legged stool; all legs are necessary for the stool to stand. Remove any leg, and the stool falls. Maureen's example is one that demonstrates these three principles of QM.

1. Maureen began to consider the patient as the one who would define the quality of his hospital stay. She recognized that the perceived quality of the entire hospital stay could suffer if the timeliness of delivering discharge medications could not be improved.

2. Maureen was supported organizationally by her manager, who provided the opportunity for Maureen to collaborate with other key department employees to better understand the current series of processes that were in place for medication delivery. This group's work led to a clearer understanding of the interrelationship of the processes across multiple departments, which together impacted the overall timeliness of medication delivery and enabled the group to make the necessary improvements to achieve the desired result.

3. There was faith in the people who were working on the medication delivery team. These people were recognized as those who had the best understanding of how the medication delivery "work" was happening and where the system was breaking down.

Quality

To better appreciate the importance of these three QM cornerstones, Joiner (1994) elaborates on what quality means to customers, noting that customers pay attention to all personal interactions that they may have with an organization and do not just focus on the characteristics of the product or service they receive. The products or services provided to the customer are not made up just of a physical item or a one-time experience that the customer encounters but rather of all the services that go with it. Organizations actually provide a "bundle" of products and services to customers to satisfy some need. If the service and product or outcome together are perceived as a good value, a loyal customer following will be established. In the case of Maureen and her patient, this is clearly represented by Maureen's concern that the patient's entire hospital stay could be remembered negatively because of the delay in receiving the medications before discharge.

Scientific Approach

The scientific approach, the second leg of Joiner's three-legged stool of QM, emphasizes that, to develop process thinking and manage organizations as systems, decisions must be based on sound, valid data, and the people managing the processes must have a clear understanding of the nature of variation in these processes. Processes that demonstrate common cause variation are those that are stable, predictable, and statistically in control.

Processes that demonstrate both common cause and special cause variation are those that are unstable, unpredictable, and not in statistical control. The actions that would be taken in implementing improvements under each scenario would be significantly different. For example, to respond to common cause variation with a special cause focus could grossly upset an otherwise stable process and would be considered tampering, otherwise known as overreaction to variation. Tampering or overreaction holds the potential for being a major source of increased cost and waste.

To use Maureen's example again, team members collected data over time regarding the length of time it took from the writing of the discharge medication order to delivery of the drugs back to the clinical unit. Overall the time interval showed variability because of numerous factors associated with this process, one example being the total volume of orders written on any given day. The team recognized the total volume of orders written as common cause variation and realized that, to minimize the degree of this variation, the overall process would need to be studied to determine the best ways to change the medication delivery system, regardless of the total order volume.

The team was aware of a significant time delay in medication delivery during the week of the computer system conversion. This variation was special cause, one of extreme impact but related to a clearly identified single source. If the team had modified the overall medication delivery process based solely on the special cause factor, the computer conversion, the underlying problem most likely would not have been improved for the long term.

"All One Team"

The "all one team" concept, the third leg of Joiner's three-legged QM stool, embodies the principles of believing in people; treating everyone in the workplace with dignity, trust, and respect; and working toward win-win situations for all customers, employees, shareholders, suppliers, and perhaps even the broader community as a whole. The team referred to here is not an individual team, a project team, or even a cross-functional team. Joiner (1994) uses the term team to mean an organizational environment in which everyone from the front lines, or the direct care provider level in health care, to the executive level understands and acts like they are all on the same team, working together to continually enhance customer satisfaction. For people to work this way, they must believe it is in their best interest to cooperate; they need to be more concerned with how the system as a whole operates rather than optimizing their own contributing area. In other words, all team members must rely more on cooperation and less on competition.

QUALITY MANAGEMENT IN HEALTH CARE AND THE ROLE OF REGULATORY AGENCIES

TQM in the United States did not begin to grow until well after World War II following Dr. W. Edwards Deming's work with the Japanese in their postwar reconstruction efforts (Neave, 1990). The Western business world was slow to embrace Dr. Deming's philosophy, but by the time of his death, it was evident that quality efforts in U.S. industry were more than a passing fad. As QM moved from manufacturing to service industries, penetration into the health care environment began.

From Quality Assurance to Quality Management

Initially hospitals were some of the first health-related organizations to seriously explore the potential value in adopting a total quality mindset in the 1980s and wrestled with more traditional models of quality assurance vs. those of quality improvement. Health care leaders began to recognize that quality improvement was not necessarily a replacement for existing quality assurance activities but rather an approach that broadened perspectives on quality, and therefore they introduced tools that helped facilitate the improvement process previously lacking in quality assurance (Box 20-1).

Another way to think about this shift from quality assurance to QM is that health care quality was historically gauged through "inspection"-type methods, frequently relying on retrospective reviews of patient incidences or adverse responses and outcomes. For example, an adverse patient response to a medication would have been reviewed through quality assurance auditing. This kind of inspection process is important in understanding the circumstances surrounding the event, but using this information to impact the broader level of quality of care was challenged by the quality improvement perspective on variation, suggesting

---

BOX 20-1   *Quality Assurance vs. Quality Improvement*

Quality assurance	Quality improvement
Inspection-oriented (detection)	Planning-oriented (prevention)
Reaction	Proactive
Correction of special causes	Correction of common causes
Responsibility of few people	Responsibility of all involved with the work
Narrow focus	Cross-functional
Leadership may not be vested	Leadership actively leading
Problem solving by authority	Problem solving by employees at all levels

From Koch MW, Fairly TM: *Integrated quality management: the key to improving nursing care quality,* St. Louis, 1993, Mosby.

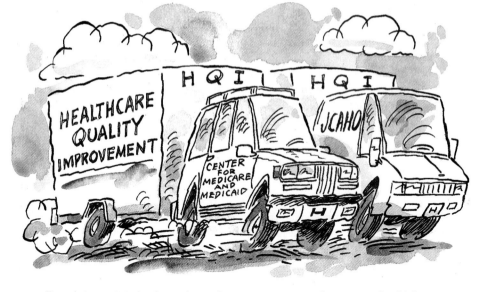

Regulatory standards and requirements are very important in driving the quality management movement in health care.

that these incidences may be special cause in nature. Although special causes need to be addressed, the historical approach was focused on specific incidents rather than more widely sweeping improvements that could address the more common causes of declining quality care delivery and lead to preventing problems and improving care.

Regulatory Agencies

Equally important in driving this movement from quality assurance to QM was the incorporation of quality principles into health care regulatory standards and requirements (Bliersbach, 1992). Almost all regulatory and voluntary accrediting agencies now require QM in some form. The Centers for Medicare and Medicaid Services (CMS) (formerly the Health Care Financing Administration [HCFA]), which administers the U.S. Medicare program, has "Conditions of Participation" for its quality foundation, and many state licensing authorities also have QM standards.

Voluntary accrediting organizations such as the Commission on Accreditation of Rehabilitation Facilities and the Accreditation Council of Developmental Disabilities promote QM requirements primarily for community-based providers serving various populations. The National Committee for Quality Assurance (NCQA) is becoming the primary voluntary accreditation body for managed care organizations, including outpatient clinic and medical practice group settings. The committee's emphasis revolves around performance measures of patient outcomes and results of practice patterns. The NCQA has grown significantly during the 1990s and now surveys at least half of the U.S. health maintenance organizations (HMOs).

Joint Commission on Accreditation of Healthcare Organizations. The Joint Commission on Accreditation of Healthcare Organizations (JCAHO) was one of the first regulatory agencies to embrace quality improvement principles in hospital-based settings. The JCAHO introduced its "Agenda for Change" in 1987, moving away from standards that reflected structures and processes of health care that established a capability to provide quality care to those that now required evidence of actual performance. Four general approaches demonstrated the Joint Commission's move: (1) changes in the accreditation survey process itself, (2) establishment of indicator development task forces, (3) implementation of research projects, and (4) development and revisions of standards.

By 1992 the JCAHO's *Accreditation Manual for Healthcare Organizations* included seven standards that addressed the role of hospital leadership and were included in what formerly was known as the "Quality Assessment" chapter. The chapter was changed to "Quality Assessment and Improvement," with language changed or added to include the following:

- Expanding the scope of monitoring activities beyond strictly clinical processes to include management and support services
- Emphasizing CQI vs. problem solving
- Using other sources of feedback, such as from patients themselves, to identify and trigger evaluation and improvement of care
- Organizing improvement activities around interdepartment, interdisciplinary patient care processes vs. department-specific indicators
- Emphasizing the process of care vs. the performance of individuals

The current JCAHO Accreditation Manual reflects even more clearly this emphasis, with yet another change in the quality chapter now titled, "Improving Organization Performance." The chapter overview states clearly, "The goal of the improving organization performance function is to ensure that the organization designs processes well and systematically monitors, analyzes, and improves its performance to improve patient outcomes. Value in health care is the appropriate balance between good outcomes, excellent care and services, and costs" (JCAHO, 2000). Other evidence of the JCAHO's quality focus is found in chapters that were once organized by hospital department and their respective functions and now are written around direct care and supporting processes, which may be cross-functional. For example, the current standards addressing core and critical competencies relevant to personnel are organized within the manual across multiple departments collectively; the older manuals isolated performance expectations by an individual department area.

It cannot be emphasized enough that professional nurses are key in enabling an organization to successfully meet the established regulatory standards. Nurses have the unique position of supporting the overall management of patient care throughout the length of stay in the facility, working collaboratively with other health care professionals to initiate changes, and monitoring ongoing effectiveness of the care provided.

CLINICAL INDICATORS AND PROCESS IMPROVEMENT TOOLS AND SKILLS

The basic foundation of the monitoring and evaluation process required by QM principles within the JCAHO regulatory context resides in the use of clinical indicators, measurable items that reflect the quality of care. Development of such indicators involves choosing aspects of care that can show the degree to which clinical care is or is not carried out as it should be. Indicators focus on clinical actions and outcomes vs. structures or supporting process procedures, which are separate from clinical decision making. Take an example of an intravenous solution stock cart: replacing the correct solutions as they are used would be a

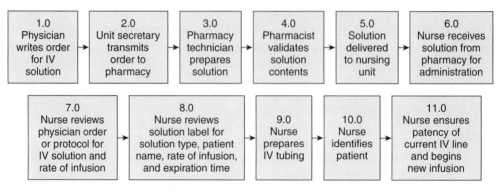

FIG. 20-1 Top-down flowchart of process for administering intravenous solutions.

supporting process as opposed to administering the correct solution at the correct rate as prescribed, which is appropriate clinical care. Both items are measurable, but only the latter is truly a clinical indicator. Indicators are not meant to define quality but rather to point the way to assessment of areas in which issues of quality may be present.

How do process improvement skills and tools fit with clinical indicator work? Clinical indicators help to identify the goals of quality improvement, whereas process improvement skills and tools support the quantitative understanding of key work processes. There are many process improvement models that incorporate these principles, but each of them has the following in common:

1. Analyzing and clearly understanding the process
2. Selecting the key aspects of the process to improve
3. Establishing "trial" targets to guide the improvement measures
4. Collecting and plotting data
5. Interpreting results
6. Implementing improvement actions and evaluating effectiveness

Various tools such as flowcharts, Pareto charts, cause-and-effect diagrams, and run charts may be used to accomplish each of these six steps (Joiner Associates, 1995), and it will become increasingly necessary for professional nurses to understand and apply these tools.

Flowcharts

The analysis of a work process usually is initiated through construction of some sort of flowchart or flow diagram. These are indispensable tools in mapping out what actually occurs during the process vs. what is intended (Fig. 20-1). There are several different types of flowcharts, each of which is valuable in its own way. A top-down flowchart simply lists the main steps and substeps of a process in a linear fashion. A deployment flowchart maps out the steps of a process under headings designating people or departments who actually carry out the step. This type is especially helpful when dealing with processes that cross multiple caregivers or areas and when there is a need for common understanding of what the process is doing as a whole (Fig. 20-2). As illustrated in Fig. 20-2, both a top-down and deployment flowchart can be used to view the process of administering the correct intravenous solution at the correct rate.

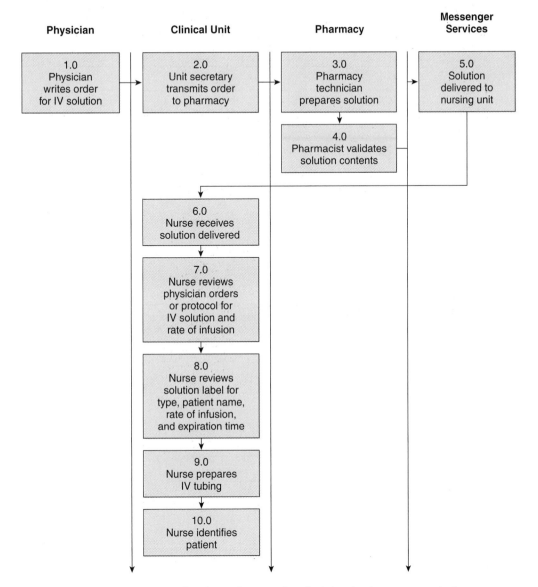

FIG. 20-2 Deployment flowchart of process for administering intravenous solutions.

Pareto Chart

In selecting key aspects to focus on within the process, a Pareto chart may be an appropriate tool. By collecting data on presumed or known problems in a given process, areas of focus or concentration can be achieved. This tool itself is a type of bar chart, with the height of bars reflecting the frequency with which events occur or the impact events have on a process problem. The bars are arranged in descending order, so the most commonly occurring problems are

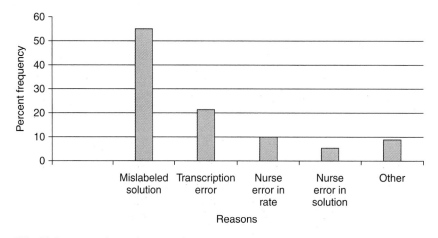

FIG. 20-3 Pareto chart of reasons for incorrect intravenous solution administration.

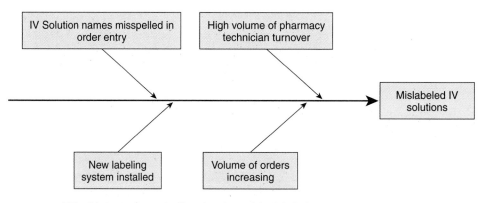

FIG. 20-4 Cause-and-effect diagram of mislabeled intravenous solutions.

readily visible. Fig. 20-3 is based on the Pareto principle, which proposes that 80% of process or system problems are generated from only 20% of the possible causal factors. Therefore by focusing on the significant few causes, a much broader impact can be achieved in improvement efforts (Fig. 20-3).

Cause-and-Effect Diagrams

Cause-and-effect diagrams are other worthy tools that can help determine the potential causes of a problem. These diagrams essentially are lists of potential causes, arranged by categories to show their potential impact on a problem. The categories usually are broad, with subsequent levels of detail pursued under each as the "might cause" question is asked of each subsequent level of detail. This diagram sometimes is referred to as a "fishbone" diagram because it resembles a fish skeleton when complete. Cause-and-effect diagrams (Fig. 20-4) are useful when the major problem areas have been localized using the Pareto chart.

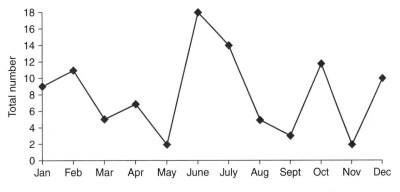

FIG. 20-5 Run chart of number of mislabeled intravenous solutions.

Run Charts

Measuring data over time to evaluate patterns in process variation typically is suited for tools such as run charts and control charts. Run charts also are known as "time plots" and are graphs of data points as they occur over time. Valuable information can be obtained regarding process variation by studying the trends in the run chart. A control chart is a slightly more sophisticated tool in helping distinguish between common and special cause variation. A control chart is nothing more than a run chart with statistical control limits added (Fig. 20-5).

Through use of these tools, results can be analyzed with interpretations subsequently guiding appropriate improvement actions. Once improvements are initiated, ongoing monitoring follows to evaluate the effectiveness of the changes implemented.

UNDERSTANDING, IMPROVING, AND STANDARDIZING CARE PROCESSES

Standardization processes, otherwise referred to as "best known methods" or "best practices," when effectively managed, have shown themselves to be the foundation for improvements in all areas of business today, but especially in the clinical care setting. There is a typical resistance to standardizing practices, especially when they involve providing patient care and services, but the realistic impact of care without standardization must be considered in the following context as described by Joiner (1994, p. 191):

- "Management has never effectively emphasized the use of documented standards.
- Few employees have experienced the benefits of effective standardization; many have been subject to rigid implementation of arbitrary rules.
- Virtually no one sees the need for standards.
- Most employees receive little training on how to do their jobs. Instead, the majority are left to learn by watching a more experienced employee.
- Most employees have developed their own unique versions of any general procedures they witnessed or were taught. They think, 'my way is the best way.'
- Changes to procedures happen haphazardly; individuals constantly change details to counteract problems that arise or in hopes of discovering a better method. Tampering is rampant."

Each of Joiner's points could easily be applied to caregiver situations. At first glance it would be assumed that all care practices are based on scientific evidence and research, and although many are, others exist simply because that was how the practitioner originally was educated. Those practices that are research-based, even though they represent "best known methods," may still not be widely practiced and therefore result in lack of standardization.

During the past few years a number of methods have been used in health care settings for the purpose of supporting standardization of care processes. Clinical guidelines, critical pathways, and case management are standardization methods that are more prevalent and familiar. Although these terms sometimes are used interchangeably, the following is offered as a context in which to understand their potential differences.

Clinical Guidelines or Critical Pathways

A clinical guideline or critical pathway typically defines the optimal sequencing and timing of interventions by physicians, nurses, and other staff for a particular diagnosis or procedure. These guidelines typically are developed through collaborative efforts of the transdisciplinary team that includes physicians, nurses, pharmacists, and others to improve the quality and value of the patient care provided. Among the most obvious benefits of using clinical guidelines are (1) reduction in variation of the care provided, (2) facilitation and achievement of expected clinical outcomes, (3) reduction in care delays and ultimately lengths of stay in the inpatient setting, and (4) improvements in cost-effectiveness of the care delivered while maintaining or increasing the satisfaction of patients and their families regarding care received.

One model (Owen, 1996) suggests that the effectiveness of clinical guidelines should be monitored through review of data in three major areas:

1. Patient health outcomes—the actual results of the treatment and care provided in terms of health status
2. Patient satisfaction outcomes—the perceptions that patients have of the care and treatment they received
3. Financial outcomes—the overall charges the patient or payer bears for all aspects of care. All are important and must be appropriately managed to achieve the desired overall outcomes

Clinical Protocols or Algorithms

Other tools and methods may be used to standardize clinical practice. Examples are clinical protocols or algorithms, which are different from clinical guidelines because they represent more of a decision path that a practitioner might take during a particular episode or need. For example, common algorithms exist for treatment of hypertension, provision of both basic and advanced life support, and general diagnostic screening (Fig. 20-6).

Case Management

Case management embraces somewhat different elements of professional caregiving. Traditionally case management has been provided by professional registered nurses and physicians, although there are appropriate settings in which psychologists or social workers may assume the role. The original intent of case management was to match the most appropriate services to the care needs evident for patients in an efficient manner. This potentially could result in reduced costs and lengths of stay, particularly in inpatient settings. Case management is discussed further in Chapter 19.

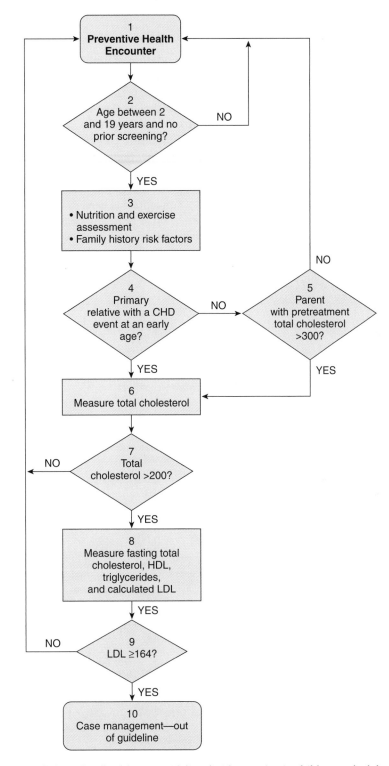

FIG. 20-6 Clinical algorithm/health care guideline: lipid screening in children and adolescents. (From Institute for Clinical Systems Integration, *1996 Health care guidelines,* vol 1, Bloomington, Minn, 1996, ICSI, p 141.)

BREAKTHROUGH THINKING

Just as standardization is critical to the foundation of health care improvement, so is the notion of breakthrough thinking. The premise behind breakthrough thinking and its resulting action is threefold: (1) substantial knowledge exists about how to achieve better performance than currently prevails; (2) strong examples already exist of organizations that have applied that knowledge and "broken through" to substantial results; and (3) the stakes are high and relevant to the most crucial strategic needs of health care (Berwick, 1997).

The Institute for Healthcare Improvement (IHI), a voluntary organization formed to assist leaders in all health care settings actively involved in improving quality, has established and teaches a results methodology that begins with what they term "change concepts" (Berwick, 1997). A list of change concepts has been developed by a planning group of national experts in several topic areas such as reducing cesarean deliveries, reducing patient delays and waiting times, and reducing adverse drug events and medical errors. Organizations use these change concepts to develop specific changes that they test, refine, and implement. For example, hospital systems have tested, refined, and implemented

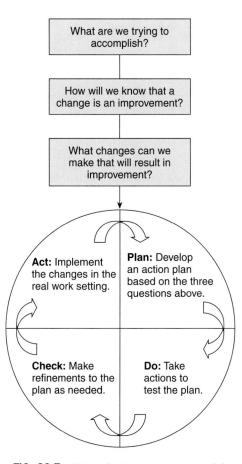

FIG. 20-7 IHI quality improvement model.

changes that have effectively reduced cesarean section rates while maintaining maternal and infant outcomes.

The model that IHI proposes for improvement essentially is made of two parts (Berwick, 1997). Part one asks three fundamental questions:

1. What are we trying to accomplish?
2. How will we know that a change is an improvement?
3. What changes can we make that will result in improvement?

Part two uses a sequence of steps, starting with developing an action plan based on these three questions, taking actions to test the action plan, making refinements as needed, and last implementing the resulting changes in real work settings. This also is known as a "plan-do-check-act" cycle, or "PDCA" (Fig. 20-7). Organizations are supported in determining measurements that provide guidance for further action. Donald Berwick, MD, President and CEO of IHI, states, "Much is known about how to improve health care, but too little of that knowledge is used."

PROCESS IMPROVEMENT AND PATIENT SAFETY

Nowhere is the need for quality improvement more evident than in the area of health care errors. As discussed previously in the chapter, the IOM report, *To Err Is Human: Building a Safer Health System* (Kohn, Corrigan, and Donaldson, 1999), placed the issue of medical mistakes and patient safety on the pages of many national newspapers, on the agendas of health care governing boards, and at the forefront of federal government legislation. The report, which concluded that up to 98,000 patients die each year as a result of medical errors, went on to promote the following recommendations:

1. A national center for patient safety should be developed.
2. A nationwide mandatory, state-based error-reporting system should be established.
3. Systems should be implemented that do not blame individuals but rather look at processes.
4. Safety performance standards for health organizations should be established.
5. Proven medication safety systems and practices should be implemented.

Other credible sources for patient safety improvements mirrored the IOM report. The Risk Management Foundation of the Harvard Medical Institutions (2000) summarized the following themes based on reviews of numerous patient care cases reported within its respective organizations:

1. It is critical to look beyond individual performance to the systems that underlie events, including human, team, organizational, and cultural factors.
2. Active and latent failures in care systems must be identified and addressed and are the basis for effective error reduction efforts.
3. By analyzing details about the process of work and the reasons people sometimes fail, significant flaws in care that effect patients, families, and providers are discovered.
4. By constantly adapting to demanding, complex, and fragmented systems, the clinician's struggle to reach the elusive goal of providing safe care is heroic.
5. Because barriers to communication and teamwork are significant, improvements must be focused in this area to protect patients and providers from the inevitability of error.
6. Health care providers whose mistakes cause or contribute to patient injury are the "second victims" and are often blamed, instead of being viewed as part of the larger system of care.
7. Increasing patient involvement is fundamental to building safer care systems.

To more clearly understand which systems should be of priority concern and what actions should be taken for safety improvements, comprehensive and comparable data must be tracked and made available to all health care organizations. The Institute for Safe Medication Practices (ISMP) is a nonprofit organization that is well known as an education resource for the prevention of medication errors. The ISMP provides independent, multidisciplinary, expert review of errors reported through the U.S. Pharmacopeia—ISMP Medication Errors Reporting Program (MERP). Through MERP, health care professionals across the nation voluntarily and confidentially report medication errors and hazardous conditions that could lead to errors. The reporting process is simple and easily accessible by clinicians. All resulting information and error prevention strategies are shared with the Federal Food and Drug Administration (FDA).

The ISMP has also developed a self-assessment tool for hospitals, which is designed to "heighten awareness of distinguishing characteristics of a safe hospital medication system and create a baseline of hospital efforts to enhance the safety of medication and evaluate these efforts over time" (*Medication Safety Self Assessment,* 2000, p. 1).

Role of Regulatory Agencies and Patient Safety

The leaders of regulatory agencies (i.e., the Centers for Medicare and Medicaid Services [CMS]) and accrediting agencies (i.e., JCAHO) are trying to develop new accountability models, emphasizing their consulting role and, when possible, collaborating with the organizations and individuals they oversee. Because these regulators and accreditors remain ultimately responsible to the public they serve, they implement their functions under extreme scrutiny by the media. Accreditors and regulators are continually developing ways to migrate through these tensions while trying to forge successful partnerships with health care organizations and other provider groups.

As one response to the increasing emphasis on patient safety, JCAHO established its Sentinel Event Standard. This standard requires organizations to carry out designated steps in order to fully understand the factors and systems associated with adverse patient events, given that certain defining characteristics have been confirmed. The steps revolve around a "root cause analysis," which is a direct application of the quality improvement principles and methods defined earlier in this chapter. The intention behind the root cause analysis is to understand the systems at fault within the organization so that improvements can be determined and implemented to prevent any future occurrences. The JCAHO allows organizations a degree of latitude in determining the policy for disclosure of these events to the commission. The commission does validate that organizations have policies and systems in place to address sentinel events. (O'Leary, 2000).

The Professional Nurse and Patient Safety

Many experts argue that the answers for improved patient safety cannot lie within regulatory agencies alone. The answers reside in every care provider pulling together to review critical circumstances and learning from key events. Basic improvement principles can help direct possible solutions within an organization by pinpointing warning flags through data analysis, applying tools and methods to address the concerns, and continually evaluating the resulting patient outcomes. For nurses, the challenge starts with making patient safety improvement and reducing errors not just an organizational priority, but a personal one as well. This means buying into a state of mind that recognizes the complexity and high risk nature of modern health care and subscribing to implementing standardized "best practices" and eliminating "never do" events. Specific steps that can be taken by nurses include:

- Educating patients and family members about their medications.
- Implementing mechanisms with primary care providers to ensure follow up.
- Prominently displaying critical, patient-specific information on every record.
- Questioning accessibility to high-hazard drugs such as potassium chloride and epinephrine if limitations have not already been instituted.
- Insisting on the use of protocols for highly toxic drugs or those with a narrow therapeutic range.
- Acknowledging errors and reporting them immediately in error tracking systems.
- Seeking restorative or remedial care immediately when warranted.
- Participating in improvement strategies including root cause analyses.
- Apologizing to those impacted when appropriate.

There are lessons for all nurses from one of the original patient safety and quality improvement mentors, Florence Nightingale. Ms. Nightingale used data to support her efforts to reduce the incidence and spread of infections in the patient wards she was accountable for during the Crimean War. What resulted from Ms. Nightingale's work was a broader shift in the culture of health care at that time. Culture is defined as a system of shared beliefs, values, customs, behaviors, and material objects that members of a society use to cope with their world and with each other that is passed on from generation to generation through learning. Culture may be viewed as almost any form of behavior that is 'learned' rather than instinctive or inherited (Bates and Fratkin, 1999). What can result from the current emphasis on patient safety is a shift in the health care culture of today. "Building health care systems that do no harm" will increasingly be the shared value and goal of all those involved in patient care delivery.

ROLE OF PROFESSIONAL NURSING IN PROCESS IMPROVEMENT

There has been a dramatic shift in the role of nursing over the past 3 years, with the health care industry's pronounced emphasis on managed care, downsizing of acute care organizations, and expansion of home care services (Norman, 1997). It has been suggested that the key functions of nursing within the health care team have less to do with being providers of primary care and more to do with the management of the delivery of that care (Norman, 1997). As a result, there is a stronger focus on delegation and management of other care providers, processes, and the overall continuity of care.

Nurses must be knowledgeable about the broad picture of patient care and assume accountability that it occurs in the proper time period. Nurses also are intimately involved in resource allocation and utilization and are being taught in basic education programs about the cost and efficiency of patient care. Historically these concepts were learned "on the job." Nursing education is also shifting to emphasize principles of managed care and health care delivery systems within the curriculum. Educational experiences are being geared toward clinical interactions with transdisciplinary teams. These efforts are being received well by other disciplines who are also moving in the same direction (Norman, 1997).

The traditional approach to education in health care was to educate each discipline separately (Pyatt, 1997). Changes are being implemented based on the awareness of the need for partnerships, collaboration, and measurement of performance. The model of the future will be team learning, in which physicians, nurses, and other health care professionals will convene as teams to design improved care, measure performance, and improve outcomes.

BOX 20-2	*Organizations Dedicated to Quality Improvement*

The Institute for Healthcare Improvement (IHI)
www.ihi.org
IHI was established in 1991 as an independent not-for-profit organization working to accelerate improvement in health care systems in the United States, Canada, and Europe by fostering collaboration rather than competition among health care organizations. IHI provides bridges connecting people and organizations that are committed to real health care reform and who believe they can accomplish more by working together than they can separately.

"We envision a system of care in which those who give care can boast about their work and those who receive care can feel total trust and confidence in the care they are receiving." Donald M. Berwick, M.D., MPP President and CEO, Institute for Healthcare Improvement

The Agency for Healthcare Research and Quality (AHRQ)
www.ahcpr.gov
AHRQ supports research to provide evidence-based information on health care outcomes, quality, cost, use, and access. Information from AHRQ's research helps people make more informed decisions and improve the quality of health care services. AHRQ is funded by the federal government and was formerly known as the Agency for Health Care Policy and Research.

National Association for Healthcare Quality (NAHQ)
www.nahq.org
The NAHQ is dedicated to improving the quality of health care and to supporting the development of professionals in health care quality by providing educational and development opportunities for professionals at all management levels and within all health care settings. NAHQ is the nation's leading organization for health care quality professionals and comprises more than 6000 individual members and 100 institutional members.

Joint Commission on Accreditation of Healthcare Organizations (JCAHO)
www.jcaho.org
The JCAHO is an independent not-for-profit organization whose mission is to continuously improve the safety and quality of care provided to the public through the provision of health care accreditation and related services that support performance improvement in health care organizations. JCAHO is the nation's predominant standards-setting and accrediting body in health care and evaluates and accredits nearly 19,000 health care organizations and programs in the United States.

Furthermore, these same providers will partner more with patients, payers, and industry representatives to manage health care (Pyatt, 1997).

Paul Batalden, MD (1997), of the Dartmouth Medical School, sums it up nicely by writing that the problem surfacing in health care today is that improvement of care has relied on organization- and issue-based strategies, which are no longer adequate. Batalden describes organization-based strategies that arise when an entire organization decides to focus its work around improvement and designs strategic plans to support the accomplishment of the improvements. The difficulty with this strategy is that organizations themselves are changing so rapidly that they are not stable enough to last through a cycle of deploying a systematic approach to improvement.

| BOX 20-2 | *Organizations Dedicated to Quality Improvement—cont'd* |

The Institute for Safe Medication Practices (ISMP)
www.ismp.org
The ISMP is a not-for-profit organization that works closely with health care practitioners and institutions, regulatory agencies, professional organizations, and the pharmaceutic industry to provide education about adverse drug events and their prevention. ISMP is dedicated to the safe use of medications through improvements in drug distribution, naming, packaging, labeling, and delivery system design. The Institute provides an independent review of medication errors that have been voluntarily submitted by practitioners to a national medication errors reporting program (MERP) operated by the United States Pharmacopeia in the United States. All information derived from the MERP is shared with the U.S. Food and Drug Administration and pharmaceutic companies whose products are mentioned in reports.

American Society for Quality (ASQ)
www.asq.org
The ASQ is dedicated to the ongoing development, advancement, and promotion of quality concepts, principles, and techniques and offers products, services, and information to help people in all walks of life grapple with perplexing issues such as total QM, benchmarking, and productivity. ASQ has more than 120,000 individual and 1,100 organizational members.

Picker Institute
www.picker.org
The Picker Institute offers a variety of products and services for health care providers and organizations looking to develop practical approaches for improving care through the eyes of the patient.

Partnership for Patient Safety (p4ps)
www.p4ps.com
p4ps is a collaborative network of people and organizations dedicated to reducing the harm caused by health care errors. With the existing network, p4ps is developing a responsive portfolio of services and products that will enable creation of a continuously safer health care system.

Issue-based strategies focus on pressing health care needs and the actions necessary to convert learning strategies into real-time changes, as done with the IHI breakthrough approach. These strategies, although extremely valuable, are likened to playing catch-up, which is a costly way to approach improvements on an ongoing basis. The challenge is to prepare health care professionals so that they enter into practice having the knowledge and skills to make quality improvement part of their regular work. Quality improvement should not be considered a separate function within care provider roles but rather an ongoing part of the professional role for all health care professionals. Box 20-2 presents a list of on-line resources to help the professional nurse seek more information about how to improve the quality of care for all patients.

SUMMARY

For today's graduating nurses, the challenge is to find whatever means are available to refine the knowledge and skills fundamentally necessary to enter into partnership with all others in the ongoing improvement of health care. This will be every nurse's accountability in what will be lifelong professional development; the solutions and strategies are not to be left to an amorphous organizational hierarchy, but rather within each practitioner to pursue collectively.

Critical Thinking Activities

1. Interview a nurse manager in a clinical setting. What type of QM program is in place in the facility? How are staff members involved in the QM program? How are patient care needs addressed through the QM program? How does the QM process in the selected clinical site relate to the principles presented in this chapter?

2. Think about a situation in the clinical setting that may cause the patient frustration and possibly interfere with nursing care. What areas in the clinical setting does the situation impact (e.g., patient and family perception of care, nursing time, supply costs)? Describe the processes involved in the situation from beginning to end.

3. You have been appointed to serve on a committee to identify causes for nursing staff not receiving laboratory results in a timely manner. What tool or tools would you suggest to help create a picture of the processes involved in obtaining laboratory results?

4. In assessing your patient's medication schedule, ordered therapies, and current infusion pump settings, you realize that the continuous heparin solution he is receiving has been administered incorrectly, resulting in a dosage twice what would be prescribed according to the existing protocol. It appears that this occurred within the preceding shift. What actions would you take?

REFERENCES

Batalden P: Continuous improvement in health professions education, *Qual Connection* 6(2):1, 1997.

Bates D, Fratkin E: *Cultural anthropology,* ed 2, Toronto, 1999, Prentice Hall Canada.

Berwick D: The breakthrough series, *Qual Connection* 6(2):11, 1997.

Berwick D, Godfrey AB, Roessner J: *Curing health care,* San Francisco, 1990, Jossey-Bass.

Bliersbach CM: *Guide to QM,* Skokie, Ill, 1992, The National Association for Healthcare Quality.

Joiner BL: *Fourth generation management,* New York, 1994, McGraw-Hill.

Joiner Associates: *Plain & simple: introduction to the tools,* Madison, Wisc, 1995, Joiner Associates.

Joint Commission on Accreditation of Healthcare Organizations (JCAHO): *Comprehensive accreditation manual for hospitals: the official handbook,* Oakbrook Terrace, Ill, 2000, JCAHO.

Kohn L, Corrigan J, Donaldson M, editors: *To err is human: building a safer health system,* Washington, DC, 1999, National Academy Press.

Medication Safety Self-Assessment, Huntingdon Valley, Pa, 2000, Institute for Safe Medicine Practices, www.ismp.org.

Neave HR: *The Deming dimension,* Knoxville, Tenn, 1990, SPC Press.

Norman L: Continuous improvement in nursing education, *Qual Connection* 6(2):4, 1997.

O'Leary D: Accreditation's role in reducing medical errors, *West J Med* 6(172):357, 2000.

Owen L: *CMGs: clinical management guidelines,* unpublished manuscript, Madison, Wisc, 1996, Meriter Hospital.

Pyatt R: Improvement in health care continuing education, *Qual Connection* 6(2):7, 1997.

Risk Management Foundation of the Harvard Medical Institutions: *Case study: key themes,* unpublished paper, Cambridge, Mass, 2000, RMF.

Nursing Research

Jill J. Webb, PhD, RN, CS

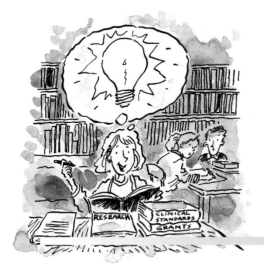

Nursing research provides
the foundation for evidence-based
nursing practice.

Vignette

"I didn't understand why I had to take a research class when all I want to do is be a staff nurse in a critical care unit. I thought I would never need to know anything about research. However, now that I've taken the course, I have an entirely different way of addressing clinical questions. I have an appreciation for research journals, and I see how important it is to read nursing research reports. I have discovered by reading widely and critically that research reports contain many implications that will apply to my practice in the critical care unit. Now I understand that, by keeping up with the latest research in my practice area, I will provide better care to patients."

Questions to consider while reading this chapter
1. How can faculty encourage students to read research journals?
2. How does research affect nursing practice?
3. How can nurses motivate colleagues to base their practice on research?

Key Terms

Clinical nurse specialist An advanced practice nurse who provides direct care to clients and participates in health education and research.

Clinical nurse researcher An advanced practice nurse who is doctorally prepared and directs and participates in clinical research.

475

Control group Subjects in an experiment who do not receive the experimental treatment and whose performance provides a baseline against which the effects of the treatment can be measured. When a true experimental design is not used, this group is usually called a comparison group.

Data collection The process of acquiring existing information or developing new information.

Ethnography A qualitative research method for the purpose of investigating cultures that involves data collection, description, and analysis of data to develop a theory of cultural behavior.

Evidence-based practice The process of systematically finding, appraising, and using research findings as the basis for clinical practice.

Experimental design A design that includes randomization, a control group, and manipulation between or among variables to examine probability and causality among selected variables for the purpose of predicting and controlling phenomena.

Generalizability The inference that findings can be generalized from the sample to the entire population.

Grant Proposal developed to seek research funding from private or public agencies.

Grounded theory A qualitative research design used to collect and analyze data with the aim of developing theories grounded in real world observations. This method is used to study a social process.

Meta-analysis Quantitative merging of findings from several studies to determine what is known about a phenomenon.

Methodologic design A research design used to develop the validity and reliability of instruments that measure research concepts and variables.

Naturalistic paradigm A holistic view of nature and the direction of science that guides qualitative research.

Needs assessment A study in which the researcher collects data for estimating the needs of a group, usually for resource allocation.

Phenomenology A qualitative research design that uses inductive descriptive methodology to describe the lived experiences of study participants.

Pilot study A smaller version of a proposed study conducted to develop or refine methodology such as treatment, instruments, or data collection process to be used in a larger study.

Qualitative research A systematic, subjective approach used to describe life experiences and give them meaning.

Quantitative research A formal, objective, systematic process used to describe and test relationships, and examine cause-and-effect interactions among variables.

Quasi-experimental research A type of quantitative research study design that lacks one of the components (randomization, control group, manipulation of one or more variables) of an experimental design.

Randomization The assignment of subjects to treatment conditions in a random manner (determined by chance alone).

Secondary analysis A research design in which data previously collected in another study are analyzed.

State-of-the-science summary A merging of findings from several studies concerning the same topic. Examples include meta-analysis with a quantitative approach and integrative review with a descriptive approach.

Survey A nonexperimental research design that focuses on obtaining information regarding the status quo of some situation, often through direct questioning of participants.

Triangulation The use of a variety of methods to collect data on the same concept.

Learning Outcomes

After studying this chapter, the reader will be able to:

1. Summarize major points in the evolution of nursing research in relation to contemporary nursing.
2. Evaluate the influence of nursing research on current nursing and health care practices.
3. Differentiate among nursing research methods.
4. Evaluate the quality of research studies using established criteria.
5. Participate in the research process.
6. Use research findings to improve nursing practice.

CHAPTER OVERVIEW

This chapter provides basic knowledge regarding the research process and the ultimate importance of evidence-based nursing practice. The intent is to inspire an appreciation for nursing research and to show how it can improve nursing practice and how results can be translated into health policy. Nursing research is defined as a systematic approach used to examine phenomena important to nursing and nurses. A summary of major points in the evolution of nursing research in relation to contemporary nursing is presented. A description of private and public organizations that fund research is given, and their research priorities are listed. Major research designs are briefly described, and examples of each are given. Nurses of all educational levels are encouraged to participate in and promote nursing research at varying degrees. The process of locating research is reviewed. Students are introduced to the research process and guided through the process of critically appraising published research. Ethical issues related to research are examined, and historical examples of unethical research are given. The functions of the Institutional Review Board (IRB) and the use of informed consent in protecting the rights of human subjects are emphasized.

DEFINITION OF NURSING RESEARCH

Research is a process of systematic inquiry or study to build knowledge in a discipline. The purpose of research is to "validate and refine existing knowledge and develop new knowledge" (Burns and Grove, 1999, p. 3). The results of research process provide a foundation on which practice decisions and behaviors are laid. Research results can create a strong scientific base for nursing practice (Mateo and Kirchoff, 1999), and application of results demonstrates professional accountability to insurers and health care consumers (Fain, 1999). In recent decades the nursing discipline has begun to pay much greater attention to the necessity of participating in research.

Nursing research is a systematic approach used to examine phenomena important to nursing and nurses. Because nursing is a practice profession, it is important that clinical practice be based on scientific knowledge. Evidence generated by nursing research provides support for the quality and cost-effectiveness of nursing interventions. Thus recipients of health care and particularly nursing care reap benefits when nurses attend to research evidence and introduce change based on that evidence into nursing practice. The introduction of evidence-based change into the direct provision of nursing care may occur at the individual level of a particular nurse or at varied organizational or social levels.

In addition to nursing research aimed at impacting the direct provision of nursing and health care to recipients of nursing care, nursing research also is needed to generate knowledge in areas that affect nursing care processes indirectly. Research within the realms of nursing education, nursing administration, health services, characteristics of nurses, and nursing roles provides evidence for effectively changing these supporting areas of nursing knowledge (Burns and Grove, 1999). Today the importance of nursing research to the discipline is recognized. But much nursing history underlies the current state of acceptance.

EVOLUTION OF NURSING RESEARCH

Nursing research began with the work of Florence Nightingale during the Crimean War. After Florence Nightingale's work, the pattern that nursing research followed was closely related to the problems confronting nurses. For example, nursing education was the focus of most research studies between 1900 and 1940. As more nurses received their education in a university setting, studies regarding student characteristics and satisfactions were conducted. As more nurses pursued a college education, staffing patterns in hospitals changed because students were not as readily available as when more students were enrolled in hospital-affiliated diploma programs. During this period researchers became interested in studying nurses. Questions such as, "What type person enters nursing?" and "How are nurses perceived by other groups?" guided research investigations. Areas such as teaching, administration, and curriculum were studies that dominated nursing research until the 1970s. By the 1970s more doctoral-prepared nurses were conducting research, and there was a shift to studies that focused on the improvement of patient care.

The 1980s brought nursing research to a new stage of development. There were many more qualified nurse researchers than ever before, widespread availability of computers for collection and analysis of data, and a realization that research is a vital part of professional nursing (Polit, Beck, and Hungler, 2001). Nurse researchers began conducting studies based on the naturalistic paradigm. These studies were qualitative rather than quantitative. In addition, instead of many small, unrelated research studies being conducted, teams of researchers, often transdisciplinary, began conducting programs of research to build bodies of knowledge related to specific topics such as urinary incontinence, decubitus ulcers, pain, and quality of life. The 1990s brought increasing concern about health care reform, and research studies that focus on important health care delivery issues such as cost, quality, and access are being conducted.

Research findings are being used increasingly as the basis for clinical decisions. Evidence-based practice can be defined as the process of systematically finding, appraising, and using research findings as a basis for making decisions about patient care. The technology age, information, and the flow of information worldwide have transformed the decision-making processes of practitioners. No longer do nurses compare outcomes of patient care with other units in the same hospital. Nurses and other health care professionals are more likely to look for solutions, choices, and outcomes for patients that represent the best available knowledge internationally (Hamer and Collinson, 1999). To implement clinical practice based on evidence such as legitimate research findings, nurses must ask the question, "Is this treatment effective?" The next step would be to break that question down into something that is answerable. The revised question might contain information about the disease and the patient such as the specific diagnosis and the patient's age. Evidence might be found in published research journals or in presentations at research conferences (Dawes et al., 1999) (Box 21-1).

BOX 21-1	*Helpful Websites*

National Guidelines Clearing House—resource for evidence-based clinical practice guidelines:
www.guidelines.gov/

US National Institute for Health Consensus Statements:
odp.od.nih.gov/consensus

Centre for Evidence-based Nursing, based at University of York—United Kingdom:
www.york.ac.uk/depts/hstd/centres/evidence/ev-intro.htm

RESEARCH PRIORITIES

Why set priorities for research in the nursing discipline? Can't nurses do research in areas that match personal areas of interest? The answer to the second question is, "yes, certainly!" But nursing exists to provide high quality nursing care to individuals in need of health-promoting, health-sustaining, and health-restoring strategies. The main outcome of research activity for a nurse is to eventually put the knowledge gained to work in health care delivery. Research priorities, often set by groups that fund research, encourage nurse researchers to invest effort and money into those areas of research likely to generate the most benefit to recipients of care. Of course, the funding opportunities offered by such groups don't hurt the research enterprise either. Research costs money! Thus nurses engaged in research often match personal interest with funding opportunities that are available during the planning phase for a proposed investigation. Two major sources of funding for nursing research are the National Institute for Nursing Research (NINR) and the Agency for Healthcare Research and Quality (AHRQ) (formerly known as the Agency for Healthcare Policy and Research [AHCPR], reauthorized as AHRQ by Congress in 1999). Both of these organizations are funded by federal congressional appropriations. Private foundations and nursing organizations also provide funding for nursing research.

The National Institute for Nursing Research

As part of the National Institutes of Health (NIH), the NINR supports research on the biologic and behavioral aspects of critical health problems that confront the nation. The NINR seeks to:
1. Understand and ease the symptoms of acute and chronic illness.
2. Prevent or delay the onset of disease or disability or slow its progression.
3. Find effective approaches to achieving and sustaining good health.
4. Improve clinical settings in which care is provided (NINR Mission Statement, 2001). With major emphases on at-risk, underserved populations and on quality cost-effective health care, the NINR promotes and supports research in universities, research centers, and at the NINR research campus in Bethesda, Md. Objectives of the NINR address the following six broad science areas:
   a. Chronic conditions—arthritis, diabetes, urinary incontinence, long-term care, and caregiving

b. Health promotion and risk behaviors—women's health, adolescence, menopause, environmental health, exercise, nutrition, and smoking cessation

c. Cardiopulmonary health—prevention and care of persons with cardiac or respiratory conditions, including research in critical care, trauma, wound healing, and organ transplantation

d. Neurofunction and sensory conditions—pain management, sleep disorders, and symptom management in persons with cognitive impairment and chronic neurologic conditions

e. Immune and neoplastic diseases—symptoms primarily associated with cancer and acquired immune deficiency syndrome, such as fatigue, nausea and vomiting, and cachexia, as well as risk-factor prevention research

f. Reproductive and infant health—prevention of premature labor, reduction of health-risk factors during pregnancy, delivery of prenatal care, care of neonates, infant growth and development, and fertility issues

These areas are not considered to be prescriptive in nature. NINR accepts funding proposals from investigators with unique interests, as well as those specifically detailed in NINR priority research lists.

Annually the NINR conducts a roundtable discussion with multiple nursing organizations to obtain the feedback of the disciplines regarding the need for continued or new research emphases. In addition, NINR listens to discussions at regional nursing research meetings across the nation to get a grassroots look at ongoing nursing research initiatives (personal communication, Daniel O'Neil, NINR, January 24, 2001). Information obtained is used in setting future research agendas and making decisions about funding of proposals submitted by researchers. NINR provides a website detailing current announcements regarding research priorities (www.nih.gov/ninr/roep.html).

The Agency for Healthcare Research and Quality

As an agency of the Department of Health and Human Services, AHRQ aims to improve the outcomes and quality of health care, reduce its costs, address patient safety and medical errors, and broaden access to effective services (AHRQ, 2000). The AHRQ broadly defines its function as the provision of evidence-based information to health care decision makers to improve the quality of health care in the nation. Since the inception of the agency in 1989, strategic goals have centered on supporting improvements in health outcomes, strengthening measurement of health care quality indicators, and fostering access to and cost-effectiveness of health care. The 1999 reauthorizing legislation expanded the role of the agency by directing the AHRQ to:

- Improve the quality of health care through scientific inquiry, dissemination of findings, and facilitation of public access to information.
- Promote patient safety and reduce medical errors through scientific inquiry, building partnerships with health care providers, and establishment of Centers for Education and Research on Therapeutics (CERTs).
- Advance the use of information technology for coordinating patient care and conducting quality and outcomes research.
- Establish an Office on Priority Populations to ensure that the needs of low-income groups, minorities, women, children, the elderly, and individuals with special health care needs are addressed by the agency's research efforts.

The research-related activities of the AHRQ are quite varied. In a process similar to that used by the NIH, investigators are invited to submit research proposals for possible funding through grant announcements. A listing of current areas of the agency's research interests can be found at www.ahrq.gov/fund/grantix.

The AHRQ actively promotes evidence-based practice, partially through the establishment of 12 evidence-based practice centers (EPCs) in the United States and Canada. EPCs conduct research on assigned clinical care topics and generate reports on the effectiveness of health care methodologies. Health care providers may then use the evidence in developing site-specific guidelines that direct clinical practice. AHRQ also actively maintains the National Guideline Clearinghouse (www.guidelines.gov), an Internet site that makes available to health care professionals a wide array of clinical practice guidelines that may be considered in health care decision making. Although most AHRQ activities are intended to support health care professionals and institutions, the agency supports health care recipients by designing some information specifically for dissemination to the lay public. In addition, AHRQ supports the design and development of databases for use in outcomes research (AHRQ, 2000).

Private Foundations

Federal funding is available through the NIH and the AHRQ. However, because obtaining money for research is becoming increasingly competitive, voluntary foundations and private and community-based organizations should be investigated as possible funding sources. Many foundations and corporate direct-giving programs are interested in funding health care projects and research. Computer databases and guides to funding are available in local libraries.

Private foundations such as the Robert Wood Johnson Foundation (2001, a, b) or the WK Kellogg Foundation (2001) are sources that offer program funding for health-related research. Investigators should be encouraged to pursue funding for small projects through local sources or private foundations until a track record is established in research design and implementation. After several years of experience in the research arena, investigators are more likely to be successful in securing funding through federal sources such as the NIH.

Nursing Organizations

Nursing organizations such as Sigma Theta Tau International (STTI), the American Nurses Association (ANA), and the Oncology Nurses Society (ONS) are a few of the nursing organizations that fund research studies.

STTI makes research grant awards to increase scientific knowledge related to nursing practice. STTI supports creative interdisciplinary research and places importance on identifying "best practices" and benchmark innovations. Awards are made at the international and local chapter levels.

The ANA awards small grants through the American Nurses Foundation. Specialty nursing organizations offer grants to support research related to their specialty. For example, the ONS awards grants that focus on issues related to oncology.

To summarize, multiple potential sources of funding are available for research projects. The individual or group wishing to conduct research will need to carefully develop a proposal, search for a possible funding source, and submit the proposal. Libraries and the Internet provide ample information about the many foundations and organizations interested in funding research endeavors. Most research institutions establish offices that help in the search and procurement of funding. Thus researchers are supported in their work of knowledge building.

| BOX 21-2 | *Components of the Research Process* |

Research is a process that takes place in a series of steps:
1. Formulating the research question or problem
2. Defining the purpose of the study
3. Reviewing related literature
4. Formulating hypotheses and defining variables
5. Selecting the research design
6. Selecting the population, sample, and setting
7. Conducting a pilot study
8. Collecting the data
9. Analyzing the data
10. Communicating conclusions

COMPONENTS OF THE RESEARCH PROCESS

The research process involves conceptualizing a research study, planning and implementing that study, and communicating the findings. The process involves a logical flow as each step builds on the previous steps. These steps should be included in published research reports so that the reader has a basis for understanding and critiquing the study (Box 21-2).

STUDY DESIGNS

Study designs are plans that tell a researcher how data are to be collected, from whom data are to be collected, and how data will be analyzed to answer specific research questions. Research studies are classified into two basic methods: quantitative and qualitative. Quantitative research is a formal, objective, systematic process in which numeric data are used. Qualitative research is a systematic approach used to describe and promote understanding of human experiences such as pain. Human experiences related to health (such as pain) are of primary importance to nursing (Marcus and Liehr, 1998); thus qualitative research design provides a dimension of understanding to nursing science that adds to traditional quantitative methodology. The most common designs used in health care research are case study, survey, needs assessment, experimental, quasiexperimental, methodologic, meta-analysis, and secondary analysis. A brief overview of these study designs is given. If terminology is unfamiliar, refer to the key terms at the beginning of the chapter.

Nonexperimental Designs

Case Study. Case study designs are used to present an in-depth analysis of a single subject, group, institution, or other social unit. The purpose is to gain insight and provide background information for more controlled broader studies, develop explanations of human processes, and provide rich descriptive anecdotes (Wilson and Hutchinson, 1996). Practitioners or researchers may publish results from a unique case. An example of a unique case would be that of an obstetric client who had an allergic reaction to latex material that is common in surgical gloves. Disadvantages of the case study include the fact that the cost of studying one case, or even two, can approach the same cost of studying a larger sample and yet lack the ability to generalize the results.

Survey. Survey research designs are popular in nursing research studies that are designed to obtain information regarding the prevalence, distribution, and interrelationships of variables within a population. Surveys are a good design to use when collecting demographic information, social characteristics, behavioral patterns, and information bases. Surveys might be used by ambulatory clinics to assess demographic information of the population geographically near the clinic to better know what services potential clients in the area might need.

Advantages of surveys include the ability to collect large amounts of information with little expenditure of time and money; they are easy to replicate and can use standardized scales and questionnaires. Disadvantages include low rate of return, the possibility that prestructured questions are confusing or irrelevant, and the tendency for data to be superficial because cause-and-effect relationships about study variables are not included (Polit, Beck, and Hungler, 2001).

Needs Assessment. Needs assessments are used to determine what is most beneficial to a specific aggregate group. This design can be used by organizations to determine needs of their employees or by agencies to determine the needs of their consumers (Talbot, 1995). For example, employers may conduct a needs assessment to determine the employees' needs for on-site exercise facilities. An advantage of this type of design is that it is possible to make changes that reflect the perceived need. Disadvantages include the limitation of people providing input and the potential that it will not be politically correct to institute the change that is desired (Talbot, 1995).

Experimental Designs

Experimental. Experimental studies are quantitative studies that include the manipulation of one or more independent variables, random assignment to either a control or treatment group, and observation of the outcome or effect that is presumably a result of the independent variable. Rigor and control of extraneous variables allow researchers to establish cause-and-effect relationships, testing causal relationships (Polit, Beck, and Hungler, 2001). Experimental designs include pretest–posttest control group design, posttest-only design, Solomon four group design, factorial design, randomized block design, and clinical trials. The randomized clinical trial is the premier study design used to evaluate the effectiveness of medical interventions. It is a prospective design in which subjects are randomly assigned to treatment and control groups and effects are measured in terms of statistical significance of the extent that differences in outcomes are the result of interventions (Abdellah and Levine, 1994).

Disadvantages of the experimental design are that it is not always suitable for real world conditions, it is not always ethical or feasible to manipulate some variable if the standard of care of some clients would be compromised, random selection often is not a possibility, and many of the phenomena of concern to nursing are multidimensional and therefore not appropriately studied in such a reductionistic way (Polit, Beck, and Hungler, 2001).

Quasi-experimental. Quasi-experimental design includes one-group posttest-only design, static group comparison, one-group pretest-only design, nonequivalent control group designs, and interrupted time series designs. This study design is one that is lacking one of the required components of the experimental design. When randomization, a control group, or the manipulation of one or more variables is not possible, this is a useful design. A researcher may design a study to examine the efficacy of different bereavement interventions. Participants could be assigned to one of two or three interventions. A control group might not be appropriate for this study because it would not be ethical to withhold bereavement intervention from a group of participants. Therefore this study would be quasiexperimental on the basis of lacking a control group.

Methodologic. Methodologic research focuses on the development of data collection instruments such as surveys or questionnaires. The goal is to improve the reliability and validity of instruments. This work is time-consuming and tedious but necessary for the implementation of research studies. However, when quality instruments are developed, they can be used in multiple studies. An example of a methodologic study would be the development of a measure of pain, such as a visual analog scale.

Meta-analysis. Meta-analysis is an advanced process whereby research on a specific topic is reviewed and findings of multiple studies are statistically analyzed and expressed quantitatively. Meta-analysis synthesizes quantitative data from different studies, thus enlarging the power of the results and allowing more confident generalizations than a single study. The larger the sample of studies, the greater the confidence in the results (Abdellah and Levine, 1994). An example of this design could be an examination of the literature and a meta-analysis of findings related to pediatric preparation for hospitalization. The researcher would decide to include published studies exclusively or also nonpublished studies during specific years of publication. The researcher also might limit the review to studies of specific design, such as experimental and quasiexperimental. Other factors would include age of the sample and time frame of the experience of the children with hospitalization. By using this research method, studies can be compared, conclusions drawn about the topic of study such as the most effective preparation methods, and findings can be incorporated into practice.

A limitation of meta-analysis is that the findings are only as good as the studies that are included in the review. In addition, using completed studies as primary data may present a problem because studies that were conducted several years ago may not be relevant to current practice.

Secondary Analysis. Secondary data can be valuable for many types of studies. Meta-analysis is a prime example of a research design that uses secondary data. Many computerized record systems such as Medicare and Medicaid patient systems contain large data sets that can be used for research studies. There are literally hundreds of federal, public, and private databases in the health care field that can be accessed for the implementation of outcomes research (Abdellah and Levine, 1994). A researcher might examine the effectiveness of a newly developed statewide managed care program by examining hospital and outpatient records to determine use of nursing personnel and services. Advantages of secondary data analysis include saving time and expense related to data collection (Talbot, 1995). Disadvantages include missing data and the fact that the data may not be exactly what the researcher would like.

Although the trend in nursing research has been toward large, complex studies, there is a need for small, simple studies that can be conducted by a single researcher with modest resources. Many issues could be addressed without the involvement of large samples and complex methodology (Abdellah and Levine, 1994). Esoteric and overly complicated methodology cannot substitute for well-designed and creatively conducted research on important topics (Abdellah and Levine, 1994).

Quantitative and qualitative research are two distinctly different approaches to conducting research. The researcher chooses the method based on the research question and the current level of knowledge about the phenomena and the problem to be studied (Talbot, 1995).

Qualitative Designs

Qualitative research is a method of research designed for discovery rather than verification. It is used to explore little-known or ambiguous phenomena. The researcher is looking to explain a phenomena or process rather than to verify a cause and effect. Qualitative methods can be important to the complex study of humans. Concepts that are important to health care professionals often are difficult to reduce in a quantitative way. Interviewing is the main technique used in qualitative methods to explore the meaning of certain experiences to individuals. This method is time-consuming and costly and uses small samples; therefore generalizations cannot be made from findings. However, when exploring issues such as caregiver strain or hardiness, it might be more appropriate to interview participants to get their perspective than to send out a standard questionnaire that might not encompass everything the researcher would discover from personally interviewing the participant. The main types of qualitative research designs include phenomenology, ethnography, and grounded theory.

Phenomenology. Phenomenology is a valuable approach for studying intangible experiences such as grief, hope, and risk-taking. Phenomenology is designed to provide understanding of the participants' "lived experience." For example, the researcher might conduct interviews with women who have had breast cancer to discover their experience of living with breast cancer.

Ethnography. Ethnography is a method used to study phenomena from a cultural perspective. Ethnographers spend time in the cultural setting with the research participants to observe and better understand their experience. For example, a researcher might seek to discover the experience of terminally ill children. To gain insight into their experience with parents, other terminally ill children, and medical staff, the researcher might spend time observing them in a pediatric cancer facility. Observation and interview would be the main techniques used for data collection.

Grounded Theory. Grounded theory is designed to explore a social process. It is a method used to explore a process that people use to deal with problematic areas of their lives, such as coping with a terminal illness or adjusting to bereavement. Personal interviews conducted in the homes of participants would likely be the main form of data collection.

Although there is a need for qualitative research studies in health care research, qualitative methods are time-consuming and costly. One-on-one interviews take time; and the interviews must be recorded, typed, transcribed, and analyzed. Data analysis is conducted by the researcher who reviews each transcribed interview line by line to group common conceptual meanings. Concepts are combined to describe the experience for the particular group being studied. Qualitative studies usually have small samples, and results are not generalizable to the whole population. The researcher cannot assert that findings from a small unique sample would be the same in a large heterogeneous population. However, findings should be transferable. The researcher should give a thorough description of the sample and setting so that findings could be expected to occur in similar individuals in a similar setting. In addition, triangulation studies might provide the strength needed to recommend change based on qualitative research findings.

Triangulation

Triangulation is the use of various research methods or different data collection techniques in the same study. Triangulation commonly refers to the use of qualitative and quantitative methods in the same study. This method can be useful when data from multiple sources and methods are needed to provide a relatively complete understanding of the subject matter.

Pilot Studies

Pilot studies are small-scale studies often referred to as feasibility studies. The purpose of the pilot study is to identify the strengths and limitations of a planned larger-scale study. Pilot work is preliminary research that can be used to assess the design, methodology, and feasibility of a study and typically includes participants who are similar to those who will be used in the larger research study. By performing each step of the procedures to be used in a planned larger-scale study, the researcher can evaluate the effectiveness of the proposed data collection methods. Information can be gained that will aid the improvement of the study, as well as help assess the feasibility of the study (Polit, Beck, and Hungler, 2001).

Before the initiation of a 3-year longitudinal study designed to examine the effectiveness of a small, structured, nurse-led support group on grief reconciliation and health of bereaved older adults whose spouses had hospice care, a smaller-scale pilot study was conducted (Jacob, 1997). Procedures for recruitment of participants were refined during the pilot study. Relationships were established with five different hospice programs, and bereavement coordinators were educated regarding the aims and value of the study. The pilot study involved the facilitation of four groups of bereaved adults, whereas the larger-scale study involved nine groups. Four groups were sufficient to test the methods of facilitation and the clinical model of grief support that was used. A pretest and posttest design was used so that the instruments could be tested, even though the larger-scale study included a pretest and posttests at 6 weeks, 6 months, and 12 months. The methods for collecting, coding, and analyzing the data also were refined during the pilot study. Based on the outcomes of the pilot study, changes were made that facilitated the effectiveness of the 3-year study. It was cost-effective to conduct the smaller scale study before the large study because the most efficient methods were determined in advance.

Pilot studies can serve to determine the feasibility of using interventions and to discover preliminary trends in outcomes for a particular agency, personnel, and clients. Most funding agencies favor research that is based on pilot work, although a pilot study may not be warranted if the researcher has used the same techniques, instruments, and participants in the same or similar setting.

RESEARCH UTILIZATION

Currently there is extensive concern that nurses have failed to realize the potential for using research findings as a basis for making decisions and developing nursing interventions. The case study illustrates the process of research utilization and demonstrates how useful it is to nurses in everyday practice.

Mary, a clinical nurse researcher in a medical center, asks the staff nurses on a pediatric oncology unit to identify patient care problems that need to be investigated. The nurses identify pain control as a major problem for the children admitted to the unit. In talking with the nurses on the unit, Mary discovers that the nurses routinely use physiologic measures such as heart rate and blood pressure as indicators of pain. Occasionally the nurses rely on parents' reports, but rarely do they consult the child. Mary conducts a review of the literature to determine proven ways to assess pain in children. In the *Western Journal of Nursing Research,* Mary discovers a meta-analysis of pediatric pain assessment techniques. Findings from this study indicate that self-report tools are appropriate for most children 4 years and older and provide the most accurate measure of children's pain. Mary discovers a pediatric pain interview tool in the literature that she thinks would be practical and feasible for use on the unit. She then writes a utilization memo to the nurse manager citing the problem (inadequate pain control), the research findings documented in the literature, and a suggestion for change in practice (use of the self-report pain assessment) on the pediatric oncology unit. Next Mary organizes a meeting with the nurses to discuss conducting a pilot study on the unit for the purpose of comparing the effectiveness of the pediatric pain assessment interview tool and their usual procedures for assessing pain in the pediatric oncology patients. Findings from this study are incorporated into practice by documenting the preferred method of pain assessment in the unit's protocol. The change instituted by the pediatric oncology unit is cited in the medical center's accreditation report as an example of how the medical center is meeting standards of care in pain management.

Barriers related to research use include quality of research findings, the characteristics of nurses who need to use the findings in practice, and the characteristics of organizations in which the research should be used (Burns and Grove, 1999). Barriers related to the quality of the research findings include:

■ Studies are not focused on clinical problems.

■ Studies are not replicated.

■ Findings are not stated in terms that are understood by most practicing nurses.

There is evidence that nurses are not always aware of research results and do not effectively incorporate these results into their practice (Polit, Beck, and Hungler, 2001). Major barriers related to nurses include:

■ Nurses do not value research.

■ Nurses are unaware or unwilling to read research reports.

■ Nurses lack the ability to access research findings.

■ Nurses do not know how to apply research findings in practice.

Opinions among nurses that research is not relevant to current practice and views that theory and practice are not related are common. However, even when nurses have an appreciation for research and want to incorporate findings into their practice, they are unsure of what process to use and where to find quality studies on a specific topic or practice issue. In the wake of the increasingly greater amounts of research evidence, the nursing discipline and other health care professions are in need of more detailed guidance in using research and other types of evidence. Uncertainty of how to go about the process of using research evidence in practice has spawned recent attention to this issue. Much literature has been written to inform health care professionals about the myriad of issues to be considered when seeking to make an evidence-based change in practice. Whole texts are now available that explain the process of evidence-based practice (Brown, 1999; Dawes et al., 1999; Hamer and Collinson, 1999), and various models have been proposed that more carefully detail the process of incorporating research findings into practice (Brown, 1999; Mackay, 1998; Stetler, 1994).

Brown offers a model for achieving research-based practice that incorporates three pathways:

1. Appraisal of the findings of a single study
2. Appraisal of collective evidence from two or more studies
3. Appraisal of a state-of-the-science summary

A pathway begins with the shaping of a clinical question. Next several reports of relevant studies are obtained and evaluated. Once the research findings from the initial set of articles are understood, it is often necessary to narrow or broaden the clinical question and obtain additional reports. Narrowing may be necessary if a very large set of reports is available, or broadening may be necessary if few articles are found. On occasion a single study may be all that is available on a given topic. More often, several studies are available. If research on a topic has been particularly rich, it may be possible to locate a state-of-the-science summary. Brown suggests that appraisal of the evidence should be specific to the breadth of the research evidence and to the particular design(s) of the study(s) reviewed. Careful evaluation may or may not lead one to make a change in practice. If change is implemented, there is an ethical responsibility to evaluate the quality of patient outcomes derived from the change (Brown, 1999).

Rather than being a simple process of implementing the practice suggestions found at the end of a research report, use of research requires careful and complex analysis, wise implementation, and patient outcome assessment. On the way to becoming a seasoned user of research evidence, the novice nurse should avail himself or herself of expert guidance from clinical nurse researchers, clinical nurse specialists, and other experienced health care professionals.

Health professionals should be familiar with two major projects on research utilization that were implemented to address the problem of nurses failing to review and use research findings. These formal projects were the Western Interstate Commission for Higher Education (WICHE) regional nursing research development project and the Conduct and Utilization of Research in Nursing (CURN) project. These projects were federally funded for the purpose of designing and implementing strategies to promote research use in practice.

Western Interstate Commission for Higher Education Project

The WICHE project was a 6-year project funded by the U.S. Public Health Service's Division of Nursing and directed by Krueger and others in the mid 1970s (Krueger, 1978: Krueger, Nelson, and Wolanin, 1978). Members for the WICHE project were recruited from various clinical settings and educational institutions to participate in a workshop that focused on improving their skills in critiquing research. Participants selected research-based interventions that they were willing to implement in practice and developed detailed plans for using selected research findings in practice. Participants in the WICHE project also functioned as change agents in clinical agencies when the research was used in practice. One of the major findings of the WICHE project was that there were few well-designed clinical studies with clearly identified implications for nursing care (Burns and Grove, 1999).

Conduct and Utilization of Research in Nursing Project

The CURN project was a 5-year (1975 to 1980) project funded by the Division of Nursing and directed by Horsley (Horsley, Crane, and Bingle, 1978; Horsley et al., 1983). The major goal of the CURN project was to increase the use of research findings in nursing practice by disseminating research findings. Facilitating organizational changes necessary for implementation of findings and encouraging collaborative research (Polit, Beck, and Hungler, 2001) also were integral to this project. For this project, research utilization was considered an organizational process rather than a process that should be implemented by an individual nurse. From this perspective clinical agencies needed to make a commitment to implement research findings and then develop policies and procedures to guide the implementation process. An outcome of the CURN project was the development of clinical protocols to direct the use of selected research findings in practice. The research utilization process included the following steps:

- Synthesizing multiple studies on a selected topic
- Organizing the research knowledge into a clinical protocol for practice
- Transforming the protocol into nursing actions
- Evaluating the protocol to determine if it produced the desired outcome (Burns and Grove, 1999)

During the CURN project clinical studies were examined for scientific merit, clinical relevance, feasibility for changing practice in an agency, and cost-benefit ratio. Protocols in the following 10 areas were developed by participants in the CURN project:

1. Structured preoperative teaching
2. Reducing diarrhea in patients fed by tube
3. Sensory preparation to promote recovery
4. Preventing decubitus ulcers
5. Intravenous cannula change
6. Closed urinary drainage systems
7. Distress reduction through sensory preparation
8. Mutual goal setting in patient care
9. Clean intermittent catheterization and pain
10. Deliberate nursing interventions

Protocols were implemented in clinical trials and evaluated for effectiveness. Based on the evaluation, decisions were made by individual agencies to reject, adopt, or modify the intervention. These protocols still are available for use in practice (CURN Project, 1981, 1982).

Clinical Practice Guidelines

In 1992 the federal government again demonstrated support for research utilization activities when the AHCPR within the Department of Health and Human Services (DHHS) convened panels of experts to summarize research and develop clinical practice guidelines. These panels summarized research findings and developed practice guidelines in the following three areas:

1. Acute pain care management in infants, children, and adolescents
2. Prediction and prevention of pressure ulcers in adults
3. Identification and treatment of urinary incontinence in adults

Under the reauthorization of 1999, the AHRQ (formerly AHCPR) continues to support research utilization through its oversight of the National Guideline Clearinghouse. Although AHRQ is no longer mandated to directly develop practice guidelines, the agency continues to make guidelines available to health care professionals and to the public.

Strategies To Promote Research

Strategies for Administrators. Burns and Grove (1999) predict that in the future accrediting agencies will require health care agencies to have protocols that are documented with research. Therefore procedure manuals, standards of care, and nursing care plans will need to reflect current nursing research. Progressive nurse executives are fostering a positive environment for conducting research and implementing findings into practice. To challenge traditional practice, an attitude of openness and intellectual curiosity must exist (Polit, Beck, and Hungler, 2001). Administrators should use the following strategies suggested by Polit, Beck, and Hungler (2001):

- Foster a climate of intellectual curiosity by making staff aware that their experiences and problems are important.
- Offer support in the way of encouraging individual staff members.
- Establish research utilization committees.
- Establish journal clubs.
- Serve as a role model for staff nurses.
- Offer financial and resource support for research utilization.
- Include research utilization as a criterion in performance evaluation.

Individual nurses must be empowered to be self-directed and encouraged to initiate innovative care based on research findings from sound, well-designed studies. It is important to determine the overall cost-benefit of implementing findings from research into practice, as well as their effectiveness, before incorporating new techniques.

Strategies for Practicing Nurses. Strategies suggested by Polit, Beck, and Hungler (2001) for practicing nurses to promote research utilization are:

- Read widely and critically.
- Attend professional conferences.
- Expect evidence that a procedure is effective.
- Seek environments that support research utilization.
- Become involved in a journal club.
- Collaborate with nurse researchers.
- Participate in institutional research utilization projects.
- Pursue appropriate personal utilization projects.

All nurses should participate in nursing research at some level, depending on the level of educational preparation (Fig. 21-1). The researcher role expands with advanced educational preparation, although nurses at all levels of preparation should at least be consumers of research (Burns and Grove, 1999).

Nurse Researcher Roles

Two nursing roles are specifically focused on research: the clinical nurse specialist (CNS) and the clinical nurse researcher (CNR).

Clinical Nurse Specialist. The CNS is a master's degree–prepared nurse who is an expert clinician with additional responsibility for education and research. A CNS is in an ideal position to link research to practice by assessing the agency's readiness for research utilization; working with staff to identify clinical problems; and helping staff find, implement, and evaluate findings that are relevant to current practice (Pepler, 1995). All CNSs are educated in the research process and can conduct their own investigations and collaborate with doctoral prepared nurses.

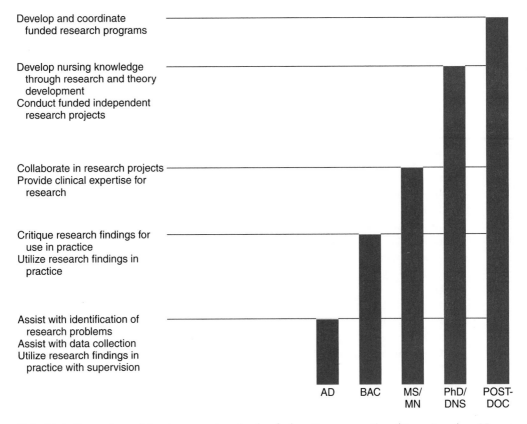

FIG. 21-1 Research participation at various levels of education preparation. (From American Nurses Association: *Education for participation in nursing research,* Kansas City, Mo, 1989, ANA.)

Clinical Nurse Researcher. The CNR should be a doctoral-prepared nurse with clinical and research experience. A CNR can either focus on the conduct or facilitation of research and should possess knowledge of statistics, grantsmanship, evaluation research, and administration. Interpersonal skills such as patience, flexibility, and approachability are imperative (Pepler, 1995). A CNR employed by a hospital or home health agency must develop relationships with staff nurses to identify the research questions that staff nurses see as most significant in the particular setting. The CNR would be responsible for designing studies and assisting staff nurses with understanding the implications of the study. In addition, the CNR would provide guidance to the staff regarding their role in the research process. This role could involve patient recruitment for studies or actual data collection. The CNR also would be responsible for disseminating findings of the research not only to staff nurses, but also to administrators of the agency so that findings would be incorporated into practice. The CNR also may need to communicate results to legislators if the results potentially affect health policy. An example of findings that could affect health policy is the findings related to the efficacy of hospice bereavement intervention. Currently legislation mandates that hospice programs provide bereavement services, although there is no reimbursement for bereavement by Medicare. When hospice Medicare legislation was enacted in 1986, there were no well-designed studies documenting the effectiveness of bereavement programs. Therefore bereavement was not included in the funding to hospice programs provided by Medicare. If bereavement intervention studies are conducted and bereavement is found to have a positive effect on morbidity, mortality, and health care costs, legislation could be changed to include reimbursement for bereavement services.

If agencies do not have a CNR, they should be encouraged to develop relationships with researchers in university settings or other agencies. Professors in academic settings are expected to conduct research and often are interested in collaborating with health care agencies that might serve as a site. These agencies often have the patient population that can serve as a study sample. For example, a university professor interested in home health care issues might collaborate with an agency to examine the efficacy of various health care delivery models for patients with congestive heart failure. In a managed care environment it would be essential for the agency to offer care that is the most effective and efficient. Therefore this collaborative relationship would have benefits for the researcher and the health care agency.

Researchers have an obligation to take steps to ensure use of findings. Polit, Beck, and Hungler (2001) suggest the following steps:

- Conduct high-quality research.
- Replicate studies.
- Collaborate with practitioners.
- Disseminate findings aggressively.
- Communicate clearly, eliminating jargon.
- Provide nursing implications as a standard section of research reports and articles.

Locating Published Research

Many health care practitioners may routinely read clinical practice journals but are unfamiliar with research journals. Other than reading the occasional research report that may be disseminated through a practice journal, busy clinicians may not spend time browsing the library for research. Computerized databases have aided the process of locating research relevant to current practice. The Cumulative Index to Nursing and Allied Health Literature (CINAHL) print index or database indexes 1284 journal titles (March 2001) categorized as follows: 423 nursing; 299 allied health; 56 consumer health; 57 computer/information science; 428 biomedicine; and 113 alternative/complementary therapies, education, health services, and administration (www.cinahl.com/prodsvcs/cinahldb). MEDLINE (Medical Literature Analysis, and Retrieval System Online) is the most comprehensive online resource for national and international medical literature. MEDLINE includes about 11 million articles from approximately 4300 life science and biomedical journals in 30 languages (www.nlm-nih.gov/pubs/factsheets/medline)(U.S. National Library of Medicine, 2000). Computerized literature databases may simply list article information, include short summaries of the article contents, or provide full-text information.

Traditionally, printed journal articles have been available on the shelves of libraries in paper or microfiche format. If not available locally, users request the library to procure the articles from another library (interlibrary loan). Increasingly in the last few years, university and public libraries have been able to increase collections by purchasing electronic databases of full-text online articles. Although it greatly reduces the time required to access certain articles, this feature is also expensive for libraries to obtain. In addition, there is a temptation to novice users to limit searches to only those articles that are available as full-text. This is a serious mistake that any student or researcher should avoid. Literature searches should be conducted with the intent of procuring all or most of the current articles appropriate to the topic of interest, regardless of the ease of obtaining sources. A truly comprehensive reading of the literature may include all articles of current and historical relevance to the topic. Therefore a relatively comprehensive literature search must anticipate by many weeks the time when the searcher needs the articles in hand.

Even though nurses may have access to computerized databases to assist with a literature search, they often are unaware of the journals that are devoted entirely to the publication of research studies. Box 21-3 contains a list of research journals and other health-related journals that publish research.

Another important publication is the *Annual Review of Nursing Research.* As of 2000 the book was in its eighteenth volume. The purpose of this annual publication is to conduct systematic reviews of nursing literature, to provide guidance to graduate students and faculty in specific fields for research, and to provide critical evaluations for health policy makers (Abdellah and Levine, 1994). These volumes are an excellent resource for those involved in the development and use of research. For example, if a nurse wanted to study quality of life in renal transplant patients, a good starting point in the literature review stage would be to read the review of "Quality of Life" studies published in the *Annual Review of Nursing Research.* This review would give a summary of all the studies focusing on quality of life that have been published. Important information would include study designs, variables considered, instruments, important findings from each of the reviewed studies, and gaps that exist in the body of research that has already been conducted. Reviews usually include suggestions for further study on the particular topic reviewed.

Critical Appraisal of Nursing Research

Nurses of all levels of educational preparation should read research journal articles critically. A journal article is a summary of a research study. Research reports are published in research

---

BOX 21-3 *Nursing and Health-Related Research Journals*

Advances in Nursing Science	Qualitative Health Research
Applied Nursing Research	Research in Nursing and Health
Clinical Nursing Research	Scholarly Inquiry in Nursing Practice
Clinical Effectiveness in Nursing	Western Journal of Nursing Research
International Journal of Nursing Studies	American Journal of Public Health
Journal of Nursing Scholarship	Hastings Report
Journal of Advanced Nursing	Health Affairs
Journal of Health Economics	Healthcare Management Review
Journal of Transcultural Nursing	Health Services Research
Nursing Clinics of North America	Heart and Lung
Nursing Economics	Hospice Journal
Nursing Policy Forum	Journal of the American Medical Association
Nursing Research	New England Journal of Medicine
Nursing Science Quarterly	Oncology Nursing Forum
Online Journal of Knowledge Synthesis for Nursing	Social Science and Medicine
www.stti.iupui.edu/library/ojksn	

or specialty clinical journals. These articles are accepted on a competitive basis and are peer-reviewed. Researchers who are doing work in the particular field of study are asked to review the article and recommend whether the journal should publish the article. The review is called a blind review because the reviewers are unaware of who wrote the article. Therefore readers generally can assume that experts have scrutinized it for merit and relevance to nursing. If the article is reporting the results of a study that has been funded by a grant, this is acknowledged in the credits of the article. This is added verification for the reader that the study has gone through review and probably is valid. However, readers cannot assume that findings are valid; therefore articles must be critically appraised. Critical appraisal of the validity of research findings through detailed analysis of study design and measurement strategies is another layer of evaluation that must be incorporated into appraisal of research evidence for possible use in practice. The abstract section of the article gives an overview of the study, and the discussion section offers suggestions for nursing practice based on the findings of the research study. These two sections often are the easiest for the novice to interpret. If sections on methods or statistics are confusing, the reader should consult a CNR to help interpret results.

ETHICAL ISSUES RELATED TO RESEARCH
Institutional Review

In institutional review a committee called an institutional review board (IRB) or Human Subjects Committee examines research proposals to make sure that the ethical rights of those individuals participating in the research study are protected. Persons participating in research must be assured that their right to privacy, confidentiality, fair treatment, and freedom from harm is protected. They must sign an informed consent that explains the study and assures them of their rights, including their right to refuse to participate or to withdraw from the study. Institutions that receive federal funding or conduct drug or medical device research regulated by the Food and Drug Administration (FDA) are required by federal regulations to establish an IRB. Studies that are funded federally have to meet strict guidelines to ensure the protection of the human rights of subjects such as self-determination, privacy, anonymity and confidentiality, fair treatment, and protection from discomfort and harm. The IRB is responsible for reviewing the study procedures and process of informed consent to ensure the protection of subjects. The informed consent must include essential study information and statements about potential risks and benefits, protection of anonymity and confidentiality and voluntary participation, compensation, alternative treatment, and the investigator's name and telephone number (Talbot, 1995).

Historical Examples of Unethical Research

In addition to the institutional review process, a number of codes and regulations have been implemented to ensure ethical conduct in research. The two historical documents are the Nuremberg Code and the Declaration of Helsinki, which were developed in response to unethical acts such as the Nazi experiments. These experiments occurred in the 1930s and 1940s and included experiments with untested drugs, sterilization, and euthanasia on prisoners of war. These experiments were unethical not only because they caused harm to the subjects, but the subjects were not given the opportunity to refuse participation (Polit, Beck, and Hungler, 2001).

Another famous incident of unethical research that has prompted the need to oversee the conduct of research is the famous Tuskegee syphilis study. This study, which was initiated by the U.S. Public Health Service, continued for 40 years. The study was conducted to determine the natural course of syphilis in African-American men. Many participants were not adequately informed about the purpose and procedures of the study. The subjects were examined periodically but did not receive treatment for syphilis, even when penicillin was determined to be effective. The study was not stopped until 1972, when public outrage was sparked by published reports of the study (Talbot, 1995).

As late as the 1960s another famous study that violated human rights took place. The Jewish Chronic Disease Hospital in New York was the setting for a study to determine patients' rejection of liver cancer cells. Twenty-two patients were injected with liver cancer cells without being informed that they were taking part in the research. In addition, the physician directing the study did not have institutional approval for a study that had the potential to cause the subjects harm or even death (Polit, Beck, and Hungler, 2001).

In institutions where IRB approval is not required for nonfederally funded programs, the researcher should seek external advice regarding ethical considerations. When an IRB is an option, researchers should seek its approval because IRB approval demonstrates scientific rigor to the audience when the research is disseminated either through presentation or publication.

SUMMARY

Educators must prepare health care professionals to have an appreciation of research and to participate in research design implementation and evaluation at the level of their preparation. Practicing nurses of various educational levels must actively seek, develop, and adopt evidence-based practice protocols while encouraging affiliated institutions to support this effort. Health care administrators must facilitate an environment that fosters intellectual curiosity and supports research efforts. Collaborative arrangements between health care agencies and universities must be developed for such activities as student projects, continuing education, development of clinical practice guidelines, and research endeavors. Consumers must be educated about the value of health care research, and policy makers must be informed of pertinent findings so that results can be translated into health policy.

Critical Thinking Activities

1. Identify a research study in the literature and evaluate the findings for application to your practice in a particular clinical setting.
2. As a critical care nurse, you learn that there have been several research studies about open visitation in the critical care area. How would you find this information and use it in your practice?
3. As a home health nurse, you learn that there have been several studies on long-term caregiving and caregiver burden. What strategies could you use to facilitate staff involvement in reviewing and critiquing the literature related to this problem?
4. As a hospice nurse, you learn that there have been reports demonstrating the effectiveness of two different alternative methods of pain control: relaxation techniques and music therapy. How would you compare the effectiveness of these two methods in controlling the pain of hospice patients?

REFERENCES

Abdellah F, Levine E: *Preparing nursing research for the 21st century,* New York, 1994, Springer.

Agency for Healthcare Research and Quality: *AHQR profile: quality research for quality health care,* AHRQ Publication No. 00P005, Rockville, Md, 2000, Department of Health and Human Services, AHRQ, www.ahrq.gov/about/profile.

Brown S: *Knowledge for health care practice: a guide to using research evidence,* Philadelphia, 1999, WB Saunders.

Burns N, Grove S: *Understanding nursing research,* ed 2 , Philadelphia, 1999, WB Saunders.

Cumulative Index to Nursing and Allied Health Literature, The CINAHL Database, 2001, www.cinahl.com/prodsvcs/cinahldb

CURN PROJECT: *Using research to improve nursing practice,* Series of Clinical Protocols: Clean intermittent catheterization (1982), Closed urinary drainage patient care, (1982), Pain: deliberative nursing interventions (1982), Preventing decubitus ulcers (1982), Reducing diarrhea in tube-fed patients (1981), Structured preoperative teaching (1981), New York, 1981, 1982, Grune and Stratton.

Dawes M et al: *Evidence-based practice: a primer for health care professionals,* Edinburgh, 1999, Churchill Livingstone.

Fain JA: *Reading, understanding, and applying nursing research,* Philadelphia, 1999, FA Davis.

Hamer S, Collinson G: *Achieving evidence-based practice: a handbook for practitioners,* Edinburgh, 1999, Ballière Tindall.

Horsley JA, Crane J, Bingle JD: Research utilization as an organizational process, *J Nurs Admin* 8(7):4-6, 1978.

Horsley JA et al: *Using research to improve nursing practice: a guide,* CURN project, New York, 1983, Grune and Stratton.

Jacob S: Outcomes of pilot work with bereaved older adults. Presented at Annual Midsouth Conference for Research in Nursing and Health Care, April 8, 1997.

Krueger J: Utilization of nursing research: the planning process, *J Nurs Admin* 8(1):6-9, 1978.

Krueger JC, Nelson AH, Wolanin MO: *Nursing research: development, collaboration, and utilization,* Germantown, Md, 1978, Aspen.

Mackay, M: Research utilization and the CNS: confronting the issues, *Clin Nurse Spec* 12:233-237, 1998.

Marcus MT, Liehr PR Qualitative approaches to research. In LoBiondo-Wood G, Habe J, editors: *Nursing research: methods, critical appraisal and utilization,* ed 4, St Louis, 1998, Mosby.

Mateo M, Kirchoff K: *Using and conducting nursing research in the clinical setting,* Philadelphia, 1999, WB Saunders.

National Institute of Nursing Research: *About NINR,* 2001, www.nih.gov/ninr/a_mission.

Pepler C: Using research to improve nursing practice. In Talbot L, editor: *Principles and practice in nursing research,* St Louis, 1995, Mosby.

Polit D, Beck C, Hungler B: *Essentials of nursing research: methods, appraisal and utilization,* ed 5, Philadelphia, 2001, JB Lippincott.

Robert Wood Johnson Foundation: *About RWJW,* 2001a, www.rwjf.org/app/rw_about_rwjf/rw_abo_main_set.

Robert Wood Johnson Foundation: *Grantmaking priorities,* 2001b, www.rwjf.org/app/rw_applying_for_a_grant/rw_app_main_set.

Stetler CB: Refinement of the Stetler/Marram model for the application of research findings to practice, *Nurs Outlook* 42:15-25, 1994.

Talbot L: *Principles and practice of nursing research,* St Louis, 1995, Mosby.

US National Library of Medicine, Fact Sheet Medline, 2000, www.nlmnih.gov/pubs/factsheets/medline.

Wilson H, Hutchinson S: *Consumer's guide to nursing research,* Albany, 1996, Delmar Publishers.

WK Kellogg Foundation: *Who we are,* 2001, www.wkkf.org/WhoWeAre.

Making the Transition From Student to Professional Nurse

Tommie L. Norris, DNS, RN

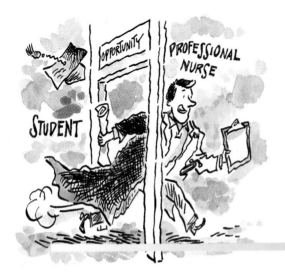

Moving from student to professional can be frightening: plan your strategies.

Vignette

Moving from student to professional can be both exciting and frightening: plan your strategies. "Every nurse has experienced the transition from student to professional nurse. Why can't we learn from our experiences and help our future nurses have a positive first impression of nursing?"

Questions to consider while reading this chapter

1. What could educators incorporate into the curriculum to decrease the "reality shock" of transition from student to professional nurse?
2. What could employers of novice nurses do during the orientation phase to help the nurse learn the "ropes of their organization," which may differ somewhat from the learning environment?
3. What strategies should novice nurses use to gain self-esteem and prove themselves capable of having the required skills, but still needing help with specific tasks and skills which come with experience?
4. Should professional nurses form official task teams to look at the role of mentoring as one means of transitioning novice nurses into the profession?

Key Terms

Biculturalism The merging of school values with those of the workplace.

Mentoring A mutual interactive method of learning in which a knowledgeable nurse inspires and encourages a novice nurse.

Novice nurse A nurse who is entering the professional workplace for the first time; usually occurs from the point of graduation until competencies required by the profession are achieved.

Preceptor An experienced professional nurse who serves as a mentor and assists with socialization of the novice nurse.

Reality shock A condition that exists when a person prepares for a profession, enters the profession, and finds that he or she is not prepared.

Role modeling Observing experienced nurses, often in leadership positions, to internalize desired qualities during rule transition (Strader, 1995).

Socialization The nurturing, acceptance, and integration of a person into the profession of nursing; the identification of a person with the profession of nursing.

Transition Moving from one role, setting, or level of competency in nursing to another; change.

Learning Outcomes

After studying this chapter, the reader will be able to:

1. Compare and contrast the phases of reality shock.
2. Differentiate between the novice nurse and the expert professional nurse.
3. Design strategies to ease the transition from novice to professional nurse.
4. Make the transition from novice to professional nurse.

CHAPTER OVERVIEW

According to Webster, transition is defined as the "passage from one state, place, stage, or subject to another: change." As nurses prepare to enter the profession from student to registered nurse (RN), they move not only from one role to another, but also from the school or university setting to the workplace. Transition is a complicated process during which many changes may be happening at once. The novice nurse tries to juggle all these changes while continuing his or her life outside of nursing (e.g., as mother, father, husband, wife, daughter, or active church leader).

To help students gain an understanding of the issues involved in the transition from the student role to that of the professional nurse, this chapter discusses the various stages of reality shock. Strategies that may alleviate this shock and ease the transition are also suggested.

REAL LIFE SCENARIO

The first impression the novice nurse has of his or her chosen profession is valuable and sets the stage for entry into nursing. This first impression occurs during the transition phase from student to professional. Consider the following scenario.

Rachel Stevens had wanted to be a nurse for as long as she could remember. As a child she donned a pretend laboratory jacket and set to work providing care to teddy bears and dolls. She softly spoke to her pretend patients, explaining that she was a nurse and would make everything better. After graduation from high school, Rachel entered nursing school and visualized her dream coming true. She was a high achiever and received comments from her instructors such as "shows evidence of applying the nursing process to the clinical environment," "psychomotor skills improving," and "becoming more autonomous." Her patients complimented her nursing abilities and caring attitude. Finally Rachel graduated from nursing school, passed the national licensure examination, and accepted her first position as an RN. She proudly entered the hospital and felt confident that she would be a caring nurse and assist patients to achieve their highest level of health.

The hospital provided a 2-month orientation period. The first week consisted of classes to explain benefits, safety education, standard precaution protocols, and computer classes. Rachel loved her new job! The next step in her employment was orientation to the medical-surgical unit where she would be working. The nurse manager welcomed her to the unit and introduced her to the staff. Because all the seasoned nurses wanted to transfer to the day shift, Rachel was hired to work the evening shift, which had a lower nurse-patient ratio than the day shift. Rachel proudly sat through the shift report, jotting down reminders that were stressed by the previous shift, such as the patient in room 200 needs a blood glucose test drawn at 6:00 PM, and the patient in room 215 is to receive a unit of blood. Rachel's assignment consisted of six patients. The charge nurse encouraged Rachel to ask if she had any questions. The nursing assistants hurried to complete their tasks. Rachel reread her assignment and entered the first room. "Hello, my name is Rachel Stevens, and I'll be your nurse tonight." She assessed her patients and reviewed their medication sheets. No medications were due until 6:00 PM, so she began researching those medications with which she was not familiar. At 5:30 PM, the charge nurse informed Rachel that the only other nurse on the floor would be going for dinner, and that Rachel should respond to her patients during her absence. Rachel was a little nervous about the responsibility, but positively acknowledged the assignment.

Moments later, Rachel was paged to respond to a newly admitted patient who was assigned to the nurse on break. As soon as she entered the room, the patient complained of nausea and began vomiting. Rachel assessed and comforted the patient and reviewed the medication record for orders related to antiemetics. The physician had not ordered medication for nausea, so Rachel quickly telephoned his office to report the patient's condition. She received an order to insert a nasogastric tube and place to suction. Rachel was anxious; she had only inserted one such tube with her instructor's assistance. She gathered supplies and reentered the patient's room. She measured for correct placement and was just positioning the patient when she received a page that the blood had arrived for the other patient and the laboratory assistant could not obtain a blood culture ordered on yet another of Rachel's patients.

After numerous unsuccessful attempts to insert the nasogastric tube, Rachel became more anxious and requested assistance from the charge nurse. The charge nurse replied, "I'm admitting a new patient and can't help you. Don't you know how to insert the nasogastric tube?" Rachel explained that she had made numerous attempts, and the patient was continuing to vomit. Rachel returned to the patient's room and attempted again to insert the tube. The nurse originally assigned to the patient returned to the floor; however, neither the secretary nor the charge nurse informed her of the new admission with orders, so she proceeded to care for her other patients. Finally Rachel again requested help, and the charge nurse inserted the tube to the relief of Rachel and the patient. Now the medications were late, she had forgotten to check the patient's blood sugar, and she had not completed the charts. "Where are my notes?" Oh well, she would just have to remember. Finally at 10 o'clock, 1 hour before the shift ended, Rachel sat down to chart. She took out scrap paper and began writing her notes, but what time did she start the blood? She became more and more anxious. The clock continued to advance to 11 o'clock, and Rachel was still charting. "You need to give the shift report to the on-coming shift," said the charge nurse. Rachel complied and 15 minutes later returned to her charting. At one o'clock in the morning, Rachel left the unit feeling depressed and incompetent.

REALITY SHOCK

Nursing students are in college for several years and "learn the ropes" of that role, becoming an expert student (Tingle, 2000). When the expert student moves into the novice nurse role, uncertainty takes over, and the support of both classmates and the nursing instructors are gone. This time marks the end of one era as a student and the beginning of a new era in a nursing career.

Novice nurses often suffer reality shock as described by Kramer (1974), which is the result of inconsistencies between the academic world and the world of work. Reality shock occurs in novice nurses when they become aware of the inconsistency between the actual world of nursing and that of nursing school. As the novice nurse enters the new profession, reality shock begins. The excitement of passing the licensure examination quickly fades in the struggle to move from the student to the staff nurse role. Reality shock leads to stress, which can cause exacerbation of symptoms that affect health and loss of time at work (Brown, 2000). There are four phases of reality shock: honeymoon, shock or rejection, recovery, and resolution (Kramer, 1974).

Honeymoon Phase

During the honeymoon phase, everything is just as the new graduate imagined. The new nurse is in orientation with former school friends or other new graduates who often share similarities. Many novice nurses in this phase are heard making the following comments: "Just think, now I'll get paid for making all those beds." "I'm so glad I chose nursing; I will be a part of changing the future of health care."

Shock (Rejection) Phase

Then orientation is over, and the novice nurse begins work on his or her assigned unit. This nurse receives daily assignments and begins the tasks.

"But wait! I've only observed other nurses hanging blood. Where is my instructor?"

Now the shock or rejection phase comes into play. The nurse comes into contact with conflicting viewpoints and different ways of performing skills, and lacks the security of having an expert available to explain uncertain or gray areas. The security of saying, "I am just the student nurse," is no longer valid. During this phase the novice nurse may be frightened or react by forming a hard cold shell around himself or herself. Vague feelings of discomfort are experienced, and the inexperienced nurse wonders if the other nurses care about the patients. After going home in the afternoon, the new nurse may experience feelings of rejection and a sense of lack of accomplishment. The novice nurse may reject the new environment and have a preoccupation with the past when he or she was in school. A need to contact former instructors, call schoolmates, or visit the nursing school may occur. Others may reject their school values and adopt the values of the organization. Therefore they may experience less conflict (Kramer, 1974).

During this phase, Kramer (1974) suggests that novice nurses must ask themselves two important questions:

1. What must I do to become the kind of nurse I want to be?
2. What must I do so that my nursing contributes to humankind and society?

Dealing with the shock phase is approached in many different ways. Some common approaches for dealing with it are reviewed and then each nurse must decide which method best allows the questions to be answered. Other suggestions for dealing with each stage of reality shock can be found at http://www.jps.net/yvonnea/WWW.NewGradProgram.htm.

Native. Many nurses choose to "go native" (Kramer, 1974). They decide they cannot fight the experienced nurses or the administration; thus they adopt the ways of least resistance. These nurses may mimic other nurses on the unit and take short cuts, such as administering medications without knowing their action and side effects and the associated nursing responsibilities.

Runaways. Others choose to "run away." They find the real world too difficult. These new nurses may choose another occupation or return to graduate school to prepare for a career in nursing education to teach others their "values in nursing."

Rutters. Some adopt the attitude that, "I'll just do what I have to do to get by," or "I'm just working until I can buy some new furniture." These nurses are termed *rutters*. They consider nursing just a job.

Burned Out. These nurses bottle up conflict until they become burned out. Kramer (1974) describes the appearance of these nurses as having the look of being chronically constipated. In this situation, patients may feel compelled to nurse their nurse. Inexperienced nurses may become burned out because they assume too many responsibilities in a short period of time (Domrose, 2000). Some common symptoms of burnout include extreme fatigue, headaches, difficulty sleeping, mood swings, anxiety, poor work quality, depression, and anger (Larsen, 2000). The more intelligent, hard-working nurses are the most prone for burnout, but, if you exhibit these symptoms remember they can be reduced. Go to the website and click on *beating burnout, how to deal with it* to find out ways to overcome burnout.

Loners. These nurses create their own reality. They adopt the attitude of "just do the job and keep quiet." These nurses may prefer night shifts, during which they often are "left alone."

New Nurse on the Block. These nurses change jobs frequently. They go from the hospital setting to community health to the doctor's office. They always are new in their setting and therefore adopt the attitude, "teach me what you want; I'm new here."

Change Agent. These nurses are termed bicultural troublemakers by Kramer (1974). They are the nurses who care enough to work within the system to elicit change. They frequently visit the nurse manager or head nurse to suggest change or a better way. They keep the welfare of the patient at the forefront.

Recovery Phase

The return of humor usually is the first sign of the recovery phase. The novice nurse begins to understand the new culture to a certain degree. There is less tension and anxiety, and healing begins. The nurse in this phase may comment, "I'll hang that blood, and I'll bet I can infuse it before 8 hours this time."

Resolution Phase

The resolution phase is the result of the shock phase and the novice nurse's ability to adjust to the new environment. If the nurse is able to positively work through the rejection phase, he or she grows more fully as a person and a professional nurse during the resolution phase. Work expectations are more easily met, and the nurse will have developed the ability to elicit change.

Most novice nurses experience each phase of reality shock (honeymoon, shock or rejection, recovery, and resolution); however, the degree of shock is individualized. For example, the

| BOX 22-1 | *Reality Shock Inventory* |

Respond to the following statements with the appropriate number.

1—strongly agree	4—slightly disagree
2—agree	5—disagree
3—slightly agree	6—strongly disagree

____ I think often about what I really want from life.

____ Nursing school and/or my work has brought stresses for which I was unprepared.

____ I would like the opportunity to start anew, knowing what I know now.

____ I drink more than I should.

____ I often feel that I still belong in the place where I grew up.

____ Much of the time my mind is not as clear as it used to be.

____ I am experiencing what would be called a crisis in my personal or work setting.

____ I can't see myself as a nurse.

____ I must remain loyal to commitments, even if they have not proven as rewarding as I had expected.

____ I wish I were different in many ways.

____ The way I present myself to the world is not the way I really am.

____ I often feel agitated or restless.

____ I have become more aware of my inadequacies and faults.

____ I often think about students or friends who have dropped out of school or work.

____ I am still finding new challenges and interest in my work.

____ My own personal future seems promising.

____ There's no sense of regret concerning my major life decision of becoming a nurse.

____ My views on nursing are as positive as they ever were.

____ I have a strong sense of my own worth.

____ My sex life is as satisfactory as it has ever been.

Scoring

To compute your score, reverse the number you assigned to statements 1, 3, 9, 10, 11, and 19. For example, 1 would become a 6, 2 would become a 5, 3 would become a 4, 4 would become a 3, 5 would become a 2, and 6 would become a 1. Total the numbers. The higher the score, the better your attitude. The range is 20-120.

From Zerwekh J, Claborn JC: *Nursing today: transition and trends,* ed 2, Philadelphia, 2000, WB Saunders.

new graduates who complete their clinical rotation during school in the same institution as they choose to begin their career may suffer reality shock to a much lesser degree because they already may be familiar with the environment, staff, and overall personality of the nursing unit. However, many students choose another institution for various reasons, such as better hours, better pay, or less travel time to work. Nurses who choose to work in an institution different from the one in which they worked as student nurses may experience a higher degree of shock. This does not imply that all nurses should work in the institution where they received their clinical educational experience. The staff in the institution where novice nurses were educated may continue to see them as only "student nurses," and this presents another barrier for novice nurses to overcome.

Zerwekh and Claborn (2000) suggest completing a reality shock inventory to make nurses more aware of how they feel about themselves and the situation at present. The higher the score, the better the attitude. It might be helpful to take the test at different times throughout one's career or when trying to decide if a career change would be advantageous (Box 22-1).

CAUSES OF REALITY SHOCK

Many nurses are familiar with the term culture shock. Culture shock occurs when people are immersed into a culture different from their own with norms that are unfamiliar and uncomfortable. This is exactly what happens in reality shock. Colleges stress patient-centered nursing, whereas the workforce stresses management of tasks, which may lead to feelings of failure due to the inability to provide holistic care (Charnley, 1999). First consider how students were taught to think in nursing school. When they prepared a care plan that took all night to complete, how were they to view the patient? Nursing schools teach holistic, or rather, "wholistic" nursing. Students were taught to look at the patient as a whole and even incorporate the family and significant other into the care plan. However, in the real world nurses may function with a partial-person approach. Different members of the health care team divide the patient care into parts.

Partial-Task vs. Whole-Task System

This type of health care in which different members of the health care team divide the patient care into parts is termed the partial-task system and only requires partial knowledge (Kramer, 1974). For instance, one nurse may be assigned to administer all medications, one may be assigned to dressing changes, the nursing assistant aids with personal hygiene and grooming, the physical therapist provides range-of-motion exercises, and the respiratory therapist teaches pulmonary hygiene techniques. There are many other nursing care delivery models in which the role of the RN varies considerably. The partial-task system just described is also congruent with the model known as "functional nursing," which places a high emphasis on completion of tasks. It is an efficient method when working with large numbers of clients, but the nurse cannot provide holistic care (Huber, 2000). With functional nursing and the partial-task system, the nurse is seen as only part of the care picture, but the RN is the central organizer and responsible for follow-through on all care given by other members. This type of system is popular because fewer professional staff members are required, and it is frequently used on the evening and night shifts when staffing is considerably less. This type of partial-task system encourages loyalty to the organization because it forces the nurse to focus on task completion and productivity. The nurse ensures that all tasks are carried out but is not the sole provider of care. A simple check mark often assesses quality, with initials being placed by completed tasks (Box 22-2).

Most novice nurses are more comfortable with the whole-task system because it is more consistent with what they were taught in school. The whole-task system requires complete knowledge and encourages loyalty to the profession. The nurse provides total patient care, which incorporates physical, emotional, spiritual, and cultural components. The model of nursing care consistent with the whole-task system is "Primary Nursing," in which the nurse is responsible for all the needs of the patient (Huber, 2000). This model provides increased satisfaction for the caregiver, as well as the nurse. However, because of the need to use an increasing number of lower-salaried employees and the shortage of RNs, few institutions use this model.

Evaluation Methods

Another inconsistency between the school and work environment is the means of evaluation (Kramer, 1974). The school environment evaluates care from the correct step aspect, whereas the evaluation phase in the work environment is based on whether components of care were completed according to established policies and procedures. Were all the steps carried out in a logical, correct, and efficient way? This is exemplified in the following scenario.

A graduate nurse was involved in a resuscitation effort. After the incident she exclaimed, "I remembered to keep the time recorded and even had all the equipment needed on hand. I did everything right." But what about the patient? This nurse may have enacted all the steps correctly but not have completed the components of care according to policies and procedures.

Think back to your first few weeks in school. Can you remember the hours of practice you spent in learning how to correctly make a patient's bed? Remember the stress you felt when the instructor observed you making your first patient bed? How much error did the instructor allow? Probably not much. This is not to say that you should become lax in your tol-

BOX 22-2	*Whole-Task and Partial-Task Check List*

Whole task-check list (completed by same nurse)			**Partial-task check list** (completed by different members of the health care team)		
Initials		Task	Initials		Task
TN	√	Nursing history	SJ	√	Nursing history
TN	√	Nursing assessment	TN	√	Nursing assessment
TN	√	Patient education	BC	√	Patient education
TN	√	Medication teaching	CS	√	Medication teaching
TN	√	Bed made	CS	√	Bed made
TN	√	Intake and output recorded	SJ	√	Intake and output recorded
TN	√	Dressing changed	SJ	√	Dressing changed
TN	√	IV fluids hung	CS	√	IV fluids hung
TN	√	Patient turned	BC	√	Patient turned

erance for error. For example, it is never acceptable to have errors in the five rights of medication administration. You must and will develop your own system and quality check for performing nursing care. Nursing texts often list supplies followed by a flow diagram for procedures in which each step is listed. Let's go back to the resuscitation scenario: even basic and advanced life support courses focus on algorithms that direct, step by step, the care of the patient. *Always remember that patient safety comes first.*

The transition from student to professional nurse is difficult, and changes in the health care environment have only added to the strain. Nursing as a profession is thought to be based on how novice nurses are socialized (Boyle and Taunton, 1996).Often new nurses are greeted with open hostility rather than open arms (Meissner, 1999). Nursing administrators may not support the novices' need to learn and may expect them to perform at the same level as experienced nurses. Unfortunately the novice nurse may become bewildered and discouraged.

FROM NOVICE TO EXPERT

Benner (1984) described the following five stages through which novice nurses proceed to become clinically competent:

- Stage 1: The nurse has few experiences with clinical expectations, and skills are learned by rote; this stage usually occurs while completing the nursing educational requirements.
- Stage 2: Exemplifies advanced beginners who are able to perform adequately and make some judgment calls based on experience; most novice nurses enter the workforce during this stage.
- Stage 3: Includes competent nurses who are able to foresee long-range goals and are mastering skills.
- Stage 4: Includes proficient nurses who view whole situations rather than parts and are able to develop a solution.
- Stage 5: Includes expert nurses with whom intuition and decision making are instantaneous.

During these five stages of transition from novice to expert, nurses will most likely to experience stress. Charnley (1999) identified four categories that lead to stress in novice nurses: (1) reality of practice: novice nurses think that they are supposed to have all the answers, are overwhelmed by the volume of work, and feel guilty because they cannot spend time with patients; (2) unfamiliar with the structure of the organization: valuable time is spent looking for supplies; (3) lack of professional relationships, lack of understanding roles of health care providers, and being dependent on other staff may cause anxiety; and (4) lack of clinical judgment: decreased confidence in skills and decision-making abilities leads to apprehension.

SPECIAL NEEDS OF NOVICE NURSES

The following skills have been identified as needing further refinement in novice nurses. Discussion about each of these areas follows.

- Interpersonal skills/communication skills (Brown, 2000; Tingle, 1999)
- Clinical skills (Charnley, 1999; Gries, 2000)
- Organizational skills (Charnley, 1999; Tingle, 1999)
- Delegation skills (Huber, 2000; Tingle, 1999)
- Priority setting skills (Gries, 2000; Huber, 2000)

Interpersonal Skills

Most physicians, administrators, and head nurses expect the novice nurse to immediately develop interpersonal skills that they take for granted. These feelings probably are rooted in the past when nurses in training spent most of their time on units caring for patients and received little theoretic information or content in the classroom setting. They had time to get to know the members of the health care team and felt comfortable interacting with them. It is difficult for many people, including novice nurses, to be comfortable with interpersonal skills at work when they feel incompetent and inadequate as a member of the transdisciplinary health care team. They are often uncomfortable making rounds, clarifying orders, and participating in transdisciplinary team conferences. However, effective communication is critical. For example, the novice nurse receives the following order from the patient's physician: give Tylenol as needed for pain. The unit secretary transcribes the order and hands the chart to the new nurse, stating, "You will need to clarify this order: I can't take the new order." Feelings of fear and uncertainty invade the novice nurse as he or she practices what to say to the physician.

"Can you clarify the Tylenol order on your patient?" Or possibly, "How much Tylenol did you want your patient to have" or maybe "Hey stupid, can't you write your orders using the five rights?"

Well, perhaps the conversation would go as follows.

"Dr. Jones, this is the student nurse, I mean the nurse taking care of your patient. I don't understand your order, I mean, can you clarify how much Tylenol you want me to take, I mean how much Tylenol do you want the patient to have?" The inexperienced nurse hangs up feeling ineffective, and the physician questions the nursing care the patient is being given.

Before asking the physician to clarify the order, it *is* a good idea to practice what will be said and even write it down so as not to forget. Then, when face-to-face with the person, state the facts simply and allow time to consider the correct answer. A smile during the exchange in conversation might provide the receiver with a little more patience. Gaps in communication may also occur between the experienced staff and the novice nurse because staff are so familiar with the routines that they may leave out information, causing the novice to not be able to complete the task. Novice nurses must listen, ask the appropriate person, and avoid distractions when communicating (Tingle, 1999).

Clinical Skills

The novice nurse has a basic knowledge of how to perform nursing skills. However, doubt in his or her own ability to perform skills without instructor supervision becomes a reality. In other words, the knowledge is there, but the experience is not (Charnley, 1999). Practice increases the effectiveness, efficiency, and correctness of performing skills. However, until the nurse has experience, there are actions the novice nurse can take. For example, it is wise to be familiar with the procedure manual on the unit. Also, during the orientation phase the novice nurse should ask to observe or assist an experienced nurse with procedures for which there is a lower comfort level or a lesser degree of experience. It is important to remember that no skill is "basic" and step-by-step instructions such as those found in procedure manuals are helpful (Gries, 2000). Remember that everyone had to learn these skills. No one was born with a Foley catheter in one hand and the set of directions engraved in memory.

Organizational Skills

The novice nurse may lack organizational skills. This lack of proficiency may be exaggerated by feelings of being "overwhelmed" by the new environment. Typically student nurses are responsible for a limited number of patients, and, although they must answer for their care, they typically are not responsible for as many patients as they will be assigned as new nurses. Someone is usually with students to offer suggestions on how to organize their time. The instructor might question: "Now what do you plan to do, and what supplies will you need to accomplish the task?" New nurses might consider asking these same questions. If unsure, the procedure book not only lists the steps to follow but also the supplies that will be needed. List specific time-limited tasks. Avoid scheduling time so tightly that a slight delay causes chaos. Charnley (1999) describes the novice nurse as lacking general organizational and prioritizing skills. Chapter 23 offers valuable tips on getting organized, setting priorities, and managing time.

Delegation Skills

Most students have limited exposure to delegation. Uncertainty or feeling uncomfortable with delegation may be a result of the characteristics of the personnel to whom one is delegating. Consider the licensed practical nurse, the nursing assistant, or other nonlicensed staff. Often these personnel are older and more experienced; therefore the new nurse might feel intimidated. Novice nurses should familiarize themselves with policies concerning which tasks that can be performed by which category or level of health care provider. The question, "who can perform this task other than myself," should be considered. Due to the broad span of responsibility for most nursing jobs, it is impossible for one person to complete all the work alone (Huber, 2000). Delegation relies on trust and leadership skills, both of which may be deficient in the novice nurse. Chapter 18 presents a comprehensive overview of delegation.

There are also times when the novice nurse should decline to accept a delegated responsibility because he or she may not be competent, to perform the task even though it is within his or her scope of practice. Remember, patient safety is the priority! Show your willingness to learn and ask someone to demonstrate the task. Tingle (1999, p. 3) suggests simply stating, "I haven't done this; who can talk me through it?" or "I don't know how to do that, but I am willing to help with it."

Priority-Setting Skills

Priority setting is a skill that all nursing students must demonstrate. The difference between nursing school and the real world is that serious consequences occur if prioritizing is not done effectively. Flanagan (1995) suggests asking the following questions when prioritizing.

- Will patients be jeopardized if this task is not done?
- Is this task a priority because of time deadlines?
- What other personnel can perform this task?
- Do safety concerns make this task a priority?
- What will be the consequences if this task is postponed?
- What are the legal issues related to the priority of the task?

Many novice nurses need help in organization skills, and saying "no" is difficult (Gries, 2000). Novice nurses may derive more satisfaction from performing technical skills such as starting an intravenous (IV) drip than from cognitive skills such as developing a plan of care. Once they are comfortable with basic skills, they move on to critical thinking skills. Gries (2000) stresses that, with the loss of the graduate nurse role, novice nurses are propelled into practice, where they focus on what they do not know and are seemingly blind to their accomplishments. She presents a scenario of how this can happen to a novice nurse:

http://community.nursingspectrum.com/MagazineArticles/article.cfm?AID=800).

Gries also supports the idea of nurses using an organization sheet to facilitate prioritization and completion. How many people make "To Do" lists? Many make grocery lists, lists of bills to be paid, or lists of important dates. The same should be done for work, and tasks crossed off as they are completed. At the end of the day, consider what time was spent in unproductive ways, what caused interruptions, and what could have been done to save time. Huber (2000) also suggests determining the urgency of the problem, which allows for prioritization.

STRATEGIES TO EASE TRANSITION

When interviewing for their first positions, novice nurses should determine philosophies of the agencies and how orientation programs assist new nurses to enter the profession. There are many opinions on the best way to accomplish a smooth transition, and each nurse should evaluate orientation options available.

Novice nurses are even chatting on the Internet about their frustrations with the transition from student to professional nurse. One such novice nurse described herself as in a race, having only 5 minutes for meals, and having to stay overtime (Cybernurse, 2000). She searches the Internet for "words of encouragement for a novice" and to learn how others have dealt with the period of change.

Biculturalism

Biculturalism is the joining of two contradictory value systems, those of school values with those of the workplace (Gray and Arnell, 2000). Biculturalism is designed to enhance a positive self-image and help novice nurses set realistic goals for practice. This strategy, if accepted in the workplace, allows the new nurse to introduce ideas or values brought from nursing school and integrate them into the work environment. Kramer suggested that the novice nurse appraise both sides of an issue, determine how his or her behavior will have an effect on other members of the transdisciplinary health care team, and single out accessible objectives.

Role Models and Mentors

Mentoring and role modeling are often considered to be the same, but in fact they are very different. Mentoring is an interactive, mutual, and personal experience (Sullivan and Decker, 1997; Klein and Dickenson-Hazard, 2000); whereas role modeling is usually not an interactive process (Stone, 2000). A staff nurse can be a role model for a novice nurse but have no interaction with the novice. This can often be distressing for the novice (Meissner, 1999).

Mentors are experienced nurses who must be willing to commit to a 6-month relationship with novice nurses (Bozell, 2000). They help novice nurses to recognize both their limitations and assets and raise confidence (Klein and Dickenson-Hazard, 2000). Mentors help novice nurses set and reach realistic goals by reinforcing and recommending. They build self-confidence and help the novice nurse gain professional satisfaction. Mentors also serve in short-term arrangements such as preceptorships. The benefactor of mentoring is termed the protégé; Vance (2000, p. 25) lists the characteristics of both the mentor and protégé in Box 22-3.

Preceptorships

Another popular orientation program is the use of preceptors during the final semester of nursing school and on entering the workforce. Preceptor programs have gained popularity as a means to socialize the novice nurse into the profession and to ease the tension of transition from student to nurse. Preceptor programs often are incorporated during the senior nursing

BOX 22-3	*Characteristics of Mentor and Protégé*

Mentor	**Protégé**
Generosity	Takes initiative
Competence	Career commitment
Self-confidence	Self-identity
Openness to mutuality	Openness to mutuality

student's final practicum, but they also may be used as part of the orientation program in the first work experience. Preceptorship is often viewed as one method of orientation, which usually last about 3 weeks (Sullivan and Decker, 1997). Preceptors orient the novice nurse to the specific nursing area, aid in socialization, and teach skills that are deemed necessary. Preceptor programs reduce economic cost by reducing turnover of new graduates and assisting novice nurses in meeting the expectations of their employers and peers.

Self-Mentoring

No one is responsible for transition into the nursing profession except novice nurses themselves. Mentors and preceptors can ease the transition, but novice nurses can also help by using self-mentoring when preceptors or mentors are not available. Novice nurses must be willing to learn appropriate references, develop problem-solving skills, and ask questions. Novices must reflect back over times when they were self-reliant and believe in themselves.

SELF-CONFIDENCE AND SELF-ESTEEM

"Even though this is my dream, I can still get discouraged. I can still forget that this is what I want to do" (Klein and Dickenson-Hazard, 2000, p. 21).

A relationship woven with encouragement can inspire self-esteem and self-confidence. It is easy to become discouraged and disillusioned when reality doesn't quite match our dreams and fantasy. Self-esteem, or belief in oneself, comes as the novice nurse passes through the stages of reality shock and into a career in nursing.

Self-esteem = Self confidence + Self-respect

Individuals with high self-esteem can critically problem solve, tackle obstacles, take sensible risks, believe in themselves, and take care of themselves (Positive Way, 2000). Nurses with self-esteem are effective and respond to themselves and others in healthy ways (Fig. 22-1). They can accomplish more because they feel comfortable with themselves.

Take the following self-esteem questionnaire in Box 22-4, and then go to the "Create Positive Relationships" website. If your score is low, learn how to stop the inner critic:

http://positive-way.com/stopping%20your%20inner%20critic.htm.

We have discussed ways such as implementing biculturalism, preceptorships, mentoring, and self-mentoring that the employer and novice nurse can use to ease the transition period. However, each new nurse must begin by evaluating his or her own self-esteem. In addition, the novice nurse must realize his or her uniqueness and rely on instinct and past experiences when maturing and moving to a higher level of responsibility. The new nurse should remember to seek a role model for guidance through the transition. It is important to remember that it is difficult to be successful if personal and social life are not kept in

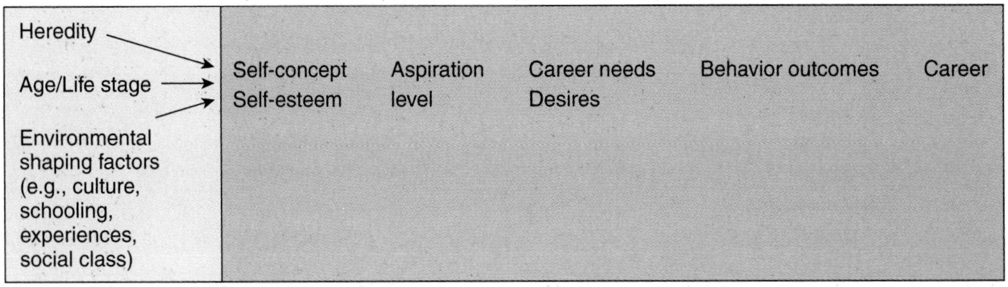

FIG. 22-1 Behavior model. (From Schutz C, Decker PJ, Sullivan EJ: *Effective management in nursing: an experiential/skill building workbook,* Menlo Park, 1992, Addison-Wesley Nursing, A Division of Benjamin Cummings Publishing Co.)

BOX 22-4	*Self-Esteem Questionnaire*

Answer Yes or No to the following questions:

                                                       Yes   No

Do you have a hard time nurturing yourself?

Have you ever turned down an invitation to a party or function because of the way you felt about yourself?

Do you get your sense of self-worth from the approval of others?

Are you supportive of others who berate you?

When things go wrong in life, do you blame yourself?

Do you react to disappointment by blaming others?

Do you begin each day with a negative attitude?

Do you feel undeserving?

Do you ever feel like an impostor and that soon your deficiencies will be exposed?

Do you have an inner critic who is disparaging or demeaning?

Do you believe that being hard on yourself is the best motivation for change?

Do your good points seem ordinary and your failings all important?

Do you feel unattractive?

Have you ever felt that your accomplishments are due to luck, but that your failures are due to incompetence or inadequacy?

Have you ever felt that, if you are not a total success, then you are a failure, and that there is no middle ground with no points for effort?

Do you feel unappreciated?

Do you feel lonely?

Do you struggle with feelings of inferiority?

Do other people's opinions count more to you than your own?

Do you criticize yourself often?

Do others criticize you often?

Do you hesitate to do things because of what others might think?

The more yes answers you have, the greater it is that opportunity exists for improving your self-esteem.

The Positive Way, 2000, PO Box 1703, Williamsville, NY 14231-1703, mailto:positive-way@positive-way.com.

balance (e.g., in high school it was great to solve all the chemistry equations on an examination, but if "personal chemistry" was neglected, a void was felt that could plague future attempts at maturing).

KEYS TO SURVIVAL DURING TRANSITION

Tingle (2000, p. 6) suggests transition strategy using the analogy NURSES (Box 22-5).
Melissa Groggin (2000) suggests 10 ways to help nurses cope and reduce stress:

1. Think before answering—take a few minutes before you answer and decide what is best for you.
2. Take vacations—what can seem like a crisis before the break may become manageable with distance.
3. Get rid of minor things that drain your energy—bring your lunch and eat in a quite space rather than spending most of your break waiting in line, only to "swallow your lunch whole" or, even worse, eat on the unit.
4. Support your co-workers—be a good listener.
5. Wear comfortable uniforms and shoes—you can't think if your feet hurt and your pants are too tight.
6. Treat yourself—do something nice every week.
7. Avoid people who irritate or hassle you—pessimistic people can bring you down.
8. Keep in touch with yourself—don't take on everyone else's responsibilities.
9. Say NO—and don't feel guilty.
10. Remember, nursing is a noble profession.

MEETING SPECIAL NEEDS OF THE NOVICE NURSE

It is important to review some common problems perceived by novice nurses and to offer suggestions to ease the transition period.

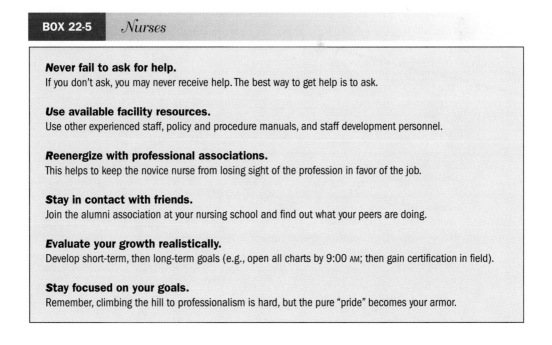

BOX 22-5   *Nurses*

Never fail to ask for help.
If you don't ask, you may never receive help. The best way to get help is to ask.

Use available facility resources.
Use other experienced staff, policy and procedure manuals, and staff development personnel.

Reenergize with professional associations.
This helps to keep the novice nurse from losing sight of the profession in favor of the job.

Stay in contact with friends.
Join the alumni association at your nursing school and find out what your peers are doing.

Evaluate your growth realistically.
Develop short-term, then long-term goals (e.g., open all charts by 9:00 AM; then gain certification in field).

Stay focused on your goals.
Remember, climbing the hill to professionalism is hard, but the pure "pride" becomes your armor.

Organizational Skills

Lack of organization is common when the novice nurse's assignment becomes much heavier than that of a student nurse. The use of a report sheet can enable the novice nurse to note important information received during the shift report and from other members of the transdisciplinary health care team as the day progresses. The report sheet can also be used to document occurrences during the shift. Another suggestion for the novice nurse is to contact a former nursing instructor. Most students have developed a special rapport with one or two instructors. Novice nurses might telephone one of their former instructors to discuss the challenges they face during transition so that the instructor can help with problem solving.

The basic report sheet (Box 22-6) also can be transformed into a unit-specific sheet. For instance, if the novice nurse is on a telemetry floor, there might be a section for "Rhythms." The orthopedic nurse could include "Traction." This form also can be used to establish and set priorities. Once the care has been prioritized, the nurse can begin those critical interventions.

BOX 22-6	*Worksheet*

Patient's name _____

Room # _____

Diagnosis _____

Diet _____

Activity status _____

Lab ordered/time _____

IV fluids _____

Intake/output

    Urine _____ Stools _____

    Other _____

    IV primary _____

    IV secondary _____

Other _____

Patient's name _____

Room # _____

Diagnosis _____

Diet _____

Activity status _____

Lab ordered/time _____

IV fluids _____

Intake/output

    Urine _____ Stools _____

    Other _____

    IV primary _____

    IV secondary _____

Other _____

Patient's name _____

Room # _____

Diagnosis _____

Diet _____

Activity status _____

Lab ordered/time _____

IV fluids _____

Intake/output

    Urine _____ Stools _____

    Other _____

    IV primary _____

    IV secondary _____

Other _____

Patient's name _____

Room # _____

Diagnosis _____

Diet _____

Activity status _____

Lab ordered/time _____

IV fluids _____

Intake/output

    Urine _____ Stools _____

    Other _____

    IV primary _____

    IV secondary _____

Other _____

However, it also may be possible to delegate tasks to ancillary staff if the tasks are within their scope of practice. This requires the novice nurse to become familiar with the job descriptions of other nursing personnel, such as licensed professional nurses, nursing assistants, or unlicensed personnel, so delegation will be within their defined roles. Remember that the RN cannot do everything.

Clinical Skills

Suggestions for developing skills needed in practice now will be addressed. Based on Benner's model, the graduate nurse must be allowed to develop clinical skills based on experiences. The novice nurse can develop competence with clinical skills during the orientation phase by asking to observe an experienced nurse perform those skills with which the novice nurse is less familiar. The novice nurse also can provide the nurse manager and mentor with a list of skills that need further practice. The unit's policy and procedure book is a valuable asset. It should describe in detail the steps to follow when performing a procedure. Spend time reviewing the manual before observing the procedure being performed and then ask questions. The novice nurse must take into consideration that there is more than one correct way to perform a skill; however, it is not acceptable to take shortcuts that jeopardize the safety of the patient.

Interpersonal Skills

Developing interpersonal skills may be achieved by attending unit meetings, volunteering for committees on the unit or within the agency, and taking an active interest in the nursing unit. These activities aid in socialization into the unit and profession. It is important for all nurses, regardless of their experience, to take part in professional organizations at the local, regional, state, or national level. Specialty organizations often provide valuable information and continuing education pertinent to the nurse's area of practice.

As the nurse becomes more confident in his or her nursing abilities and is less stressed by performing tasks, positive relationships with physicians and other members of the transdisciplinary health care team can be developed. Various methods that may be used to develop professional relationships should be emphasized during the orientation period. Nurses in staff development positions can be key players in assisting the novice nurse in developing professional communication skills. Making rounds with physicians and assisting them with procedures opens the door for communication. Asking pertinent and relevant questions ensures that the door remains open.

Delegation Skills

How to best master delegation skills will be considered now. First, nurses should consider how others have delegated to them. Body language is important when delegating. Look at the person, be pleasant, and leave room for suggestions from the delegate; however, do not allow the delegate to resist or intimidate you so that you complete the task yourself. After communicating face-to-face, give a list of tasks in writing or post it at the nurse's station. This leaves little room for misunderstanding. Be willing to change the assignment if there are changes in a patient's condition, new patients are admitted, or you realize that the time needed to perform a task was underestimated. If time allows, it is always good to help those to whom you have delegated tasks. For example, if a nurse passes by a door and the attendant is trying to turn a very large patient, enter the room and ask, "How can I best help you turn the patient?" Always take time to give sincere positive reinforcement and say "thank you."

Priority-Setting Skills

Now consider the best way to prioritize. How did you prioritize in nursing school? What worked then will probably work now with a few modifications. Remember, if it is not written down, it probably is forgotten. Keep a notepad and pen in a pocket. Jot down reminders of things to be done, and place a number indicating their importance. For example, consider the following list.

   _3_ Start the IV in room 211.
   _1_ Check the IV site in room 300.
   _2_ Call the laboratory and check on blood sugar in room 215.

Then a call is received from the licensed practical nurse that the IV line is not dripping on the patient in room 212. The dietary worker calls to say that, when she brought the patient in room 217 her food tray, he vomited. The emergency light goes off in the bathroom of an elderly confused patient. Now prioritize! First answer the emergency light; don't even take time to write down this one. Now reprioritize; pretend the following is a list of tasks to be completed. How would you prioritize the following?

   ___ Start the IV in room 211.
   ___ Check the IV site in room 300.
   ___ Call the laboratory and check the blood sugar in room 215.
   ___ Check the IV that is not dripping.
   ___ Assist the patient who is vomiting.

In the space provided, prioritize the tasks to be completed. Indicate tasks that can be delegated with a D.

   ___ Start the IV in room 211.
   ___ Check the IV site in room 300.
   _D_ Call the laboratory and check on blood sugar in room 215; delegate to unit secretary and ask him or her to report results to you.
   ___ Check IV in room 212 that is not dripping.
   _D_ Assist the patient who is vomiting; delegate to the licensed practical nurse or nursing assistant, but remember to follow up on the patient's condition.

What had to be considered when prioritizing these situations? First, you needed to consider how much time was required for the task. It usually takes longer to start a new IV line than to check an IV site. It also requires less time to determine why an IV is not dripping. However, this is insignificant if the patient needing the IV line started is critical and needs the medication to reduce his or her blood pressure. Delegation may be needed. What tasks can other members perform? A nurse knows how to prioritize. Think through the situation. Change the priority as needed or as situations change throughout the shift.

Now that you know ways to develop organization skills, refine clinical and interpersonal skills, delegate, and set priorities; take time to remember other important areas of your life. Remember the people you may have neglected during school and make it a priority to reestablish special relationships with friends, family, and loved ones.

Try the following; these activities show appreciation for yourself and your significant others for all they have endured during your education.

- Reintroduce yourself to spouse and close friends. You might even treat them to a special dinner at your favorite restaurant.
- Participate in your children's activities at school.
- Read a romance or war novel, depending on your taste or mood at the time.
- Clean your house or apartment. There really is furniture under all those papers.
- Get a cookbook and try those recipes you haven't had time to prepare.
- Call old friends whom you knew before nursing school.
- Participate in a health club, learn aerobic exercise, or just walk to improve your health.
- Enjoy the nursing profession—it really is the best.

Experienced RNs should consider the following to help ease the transition of the novice nurse to the profession of nursing. The novice nurse should not be expected to enter the work environment and be as productive as experienced staff members. It is important for experienced nurses serving on agency committees to serve as advocates for novice nurses by reminding nurse managers and hospital administrators that it is not possible for nursing students to learn everything necessary for professional practice during school. Also, remind members of the nursing unit about this fact. If a nurse develops initiative, autonomy, and a desire to become a team member, he or she will succeed.

SUMMARY

The period of transition from novice to competent practitioner is critical. New skills must be learned and refined, professional relationships established, and autonomy in nursing practice gained. Knowledge and skills must be refined over time. The transition from student to RN can be compared with that of butterflies as they emerge from the cocoon. It is unfair to judge them while still nymphs; therefore the nursing profession must withhold scrutiny until novice nurses fly with their beautiful wings spread.

Critical Thinking Activities

1. What kind of nurse do I want to become?
2. What are the roles of the professional nurse as seen by the student compared with those as seen by the experienced nurse?
3. What type of nursing environment eases transition from student to professional nurse?
4. Analyze important factors affecting transition from novice to experienced nurse?

REFERENCES

Benner P: *From novice to expert,* Menlo Park, 1984, Addison-Wesley.

Boyle DK, Taunton RL: Socialization of new graduate nurses in critical care, *Heart Lung* 25(2):141-153, 1996.

Bozell J: Career path, Nursing Library, August 2000, www.findarticles.com/cf_0/m3231/8_30/64427504/pl/article.jhtml

Brown S: Shock of the new, *Nurs Times* 96(38):27, 2000.

Charnley E: Occupational stress in the newly qualified staff nurse, *Nurs Standard* 13(29):32-37, 1999, www.nursing-standard.co.uk/archives/vol13-29/research.htm.

Cybernurse: Reality shock, 2000, http://www.cybernurse.com/wwwboard/messages/1173.html.

Domrose C: *Staying power: keeping nurses isn't about showing them the money,* July 24, 2000, http://www.nurseweek.com/news/Feature/00-07/retain.htm.

Flanagan L, editor: *What you need to know about today's workplace: a survival guide for nurses,* Washington, DC, 1995, American Nurses Publishing.

Groggin M: Managing your career, *Nurs Spectrum,* 2000, www.nsweb.nursingspectrum.com/Articles/CalmWithinStrm.htm.

Gray J, Arnell Y: February 1, 2000, www.jps.net/yvonnea/www.NewGradProgram.htm.

Gries M: Don't leave grads lost at sea, *Nurs Spectrum,* March 06, 2000: http://community.nursingspectrum.com/MagazineArticles/article.cfm?AID=800.

Huber D: *Leadership and nursing care management,* ed 2. Philadelphia, 2000, WB Saunders.

Klein E, Dickenson-Hazard N: The spirit of mentoring, *Reflect Nurs* 26(3):18-22, 2000.

Kramer M: *Reality shock: why nurses leave nursing,* St Louis, 1974, Mosby.

Larsen C: *Reality shock and preventing burnout in nursing,* 2000, http://www4.allencol.edu/~lmh0/CindyL/Burnout.html.

Meissner JE: Nurses, are we still eating our young? *Nursing* 29(2):42, 1999.

Positive Way: *Self-esteem questionnaire,* 2000, www.positive-way.com/self-est1.htm.

Stone S: Mentoring and modeling for the millennium, 2000, www.ajj.com/jpi/deannote/backissu/mar2000/mentor.htm.

Strader MK: Role transition to the workplace. In Strader MK, Decker PJ, editors: *Role transition to patient care management,* Norwalk, Conn, 1995, Appleton & Lange.

Sullivan EJ, Decker PJ: *Effective leadership and management,* ed 4, Menlo Park, 1997, Addison-Wesley.

Tingle CA: Workplace advocacy as a transition tool, June, 2000, http://www.lsna.org/newpage12.htm.

Vance C: Discovering the riches in mentor connections, *Reflect Nurs* 26(3):24-25, 2000.

Zerwekh J, Claborn JC: Reality shock. In Zerwekh J, Claborn JC, editors: *Nursing today: transition and trends,* ed 2, Philadelphia, 2000, WB Saunders.

Managing Time: AKA Managing Yourself

23

Charold L. Baer, PhD, RN, FCCM, CCRN

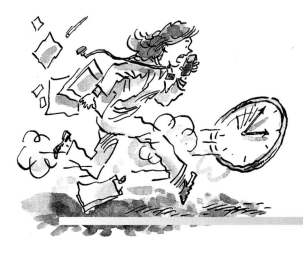

Our lives revolve around time; use it as
a self-management tool.

Vignette

The charge nurse, Karen Jordan, RN, approaches a staff nurse, Susan Williams, RN, to give her a report about a patient who is being transferred from the intensive care unit. Karen begins the report, only to be interrupted by Susan, who states, "I can't possibly take that patient now. I am so behind in my patient care." Karen responds, "Well, your assignment was such that you were first on the list to take a new admission. What can I do to help you get caught up?" Susan replies, "I couldn't begin to tell you. I don't feel like I have accomplished much today." Karen continues, "Does that mean that Mr. Smith can't go home because he hasn't been taught about the dressing change for his leg? Did you start Mrs. Jones on her subcutaneous insulin and 1800-calorie diet so we can discontinue the IV and the insulin drip? Did you give Mr. Wilson the vancomycin so we can start the peak-and-trough regimen and get him stabilized so he can go home tomorrow?" Susan replies, "No, none of it has been done. Nor has Mr. Anderson been ambulated or the dressing changed on Mr. Gregory's abdominal wound. I swear I don't know where the time has gone." Karen suggests, "Well, tell me what you have done, and I'll see if I can get someone else to help get you caught up." Susan responds somewhat defensively, "I really have been very busy all day. I guess I just haven't gotten the important things done. I started by doing some of the easy things that I was sure wouldn't take much time. You know, like helping Mrs. Johnson contact her relatives, washing Ms. Pearson's hair, and cleaning and restocking the top of the med cart that was so messy and devoid of supplies. All of those "easy" things took much more time than I expected because we had to make six calls to find Mrs. Johnson's relatives, Ms. Pearson had lots of IVs and lines, and we didn't have some of the med cart supplies in stock. It all seemed to take forever, but I got it done. Then I helped Dr. Swanson collect some data for his

517

research, which took longer than expected because we had to find three separate files for each patient. Now, here you are trying to give me a new admission, and I haven't even begun to do those things that should be done for my patients. I am so frustrated! I'm tired of never having enough time to get the really important things done for my patients."

Questions to consider while reading this chapter

1. When Susan initially received her patient care assignment, what are some time management strategies she could have implemented to be sure her patient needs were met?
2. What factors should Susan consider when deciding how to prioritize her patient care assignment?
3. What time wasters have interfered with Susan's ability to complete her patient care assignment?
4. What strategies can help Susan find "extra time" so that she could accomplish more in her workday?
5. What resources are available to help Susan learn more about managing herself and her time to accomplish goals?

Key Terms

Concentration The process of systematically controlling those things that can be controlled.

Priority Superiority in rank, a preferential rating, or the state of coming first in order or ahead of others in some process.

Procrastination The art of never doing today what can be put off until tomorrow.

Segmentation The process of separating those things over which you have control from those over which you do not.

Time management Self-management strategies to better use time.

Learning Outcomes

After studying this chapter, the reader will be able to:

1. Integrate the value of time management as a self-management process.
2. Critique 14 myths associated with time management.
3. Differentiate between external and internal time wasters.
4. Create an action plan to overcome procrastination.
5. Write an action plan that outlines 10 time management strategies designed to promote more effective self-management.

CHAPTER OVERVIEW

The previous scenario is typical of what happens daily in the lives of many busy professionals. It occurs in conjunction with work, education, community service, and their personal lives. It is simplistically referred to as not having sufficient time to accomplish all of a person's goals. In reality it is a lack of self-management that results in underuse of the time available. Thus, to accomplish the important goals in life, it is necessary to better manage ourselves to make the most of the time available. This chapter is designed to assist students and busy professionals implement self-management strategies to better use their time. The topics included are the concept of time, perspectives of time, common myths of time management, time wasters, time management strategies, and methods for continued success.

THE CONCEPT OF TIME

Time is one of the most important, most discussed, and most often misused resources available to humans. In essence time is life, and as such, our lives tend to revolve around the concept of time. For example, we plan our lives according to specific times for getting up in the morning, arriving at work, carrying out procedures, administering medications, going to lunch, leaving work, participating in evening activities, and going to bed (Baer, 1979). In addition, we frequently misuse time by intentionally or unintentionally wasting it, thus adding to its scarcity.

Time also is a unique and paradoxic resource. It is unique because it cannot be accumulated or saved. Instead people are forced to expend it at a fixed rate of 24 hours per day. It is paradoxic because few people ever have enough time, yet everyone has all that is available. Time is available to everyone, regardless of status, in equal amounts. Thus, because each person has the same amount of available time, people really cannot refer to time in terms of deficient quantities. So, if time is not the problem, what is? The answer to that question is, of course, that people are the problem. It is not about how much time a person has, but instead about how that person chooses to manage himself or herself to use the available time. From this perspective, time management more appropriately becomes self-management. Peter Drucker suggests that the old prescription for wisdom of "know thyself" may be too difficult for mortals, but everyone can "know thy time" and be well on the road to making important contributions and improving personal effectiveness (Drucker, 1967).

Historically the concept of time management dates back to the sixth century AD before the advent of even the most primitive clocks. However, the emphasis on efficiency and effectiveness in association with time did not occur until the Industrial Revolution in the eighteenth century. This emphasis soon was followed by the linkage between the proper use of personal time and success, which was postulated by Benjamin Franklin, who is considered the father of modern time management. The mid-twentieth century saw the attention regarding time management shift to the organizational skills of the person (Brunicardi and Hobson, 1996). That shift resulted not only in the realization that time management is a self-management process, but also in the development of several time management models and the delineation of specific strategies for managing yourself in relation to time. The subsequent question that resulted from this trend toward better self-management for better time management was, "Why should I bother with this whole concept of time management?" The answers that were forthcoming were persuasive for the busy health care professional. Included among the benefits were:

- Greater personal job satisfaction because more goals are met.
- Increased productivity as a result of focusing on the priorities and eliminating unnecessary tasks.
- Improved interpersonal relations because of less stress and anxiety.
- Better future direction because of continuous goal setting and achievement.
- Reduced stress because of an increased ability to meet deadlines and accomplish established goals.
- Improved personal health because of decreased anxiety and increased self-esteem from accomplishing established goals (Morano, 1984).

Thus it appears that improved self-management to better use time is beneficial and worthy of pursuit.

PERSPECTIVES ON TIME

Each person has a specific perspective of time that influences behavior. It is essential to understand your own perspective on time to understand your behavior in relation to the use of time. It is also important to remember that the perspective on time is influenced by personality type, education, culture, and socioeconomic factors. Webber devised a series of four tests to determine a person's perspective on time. Those four tests included time metaphors, adjectives describing time, the recollection of the dates of past events, and a determination of the setting of a person's watch as being fast or slow in relation to the actual time (Webber, 1972). He then related the perspective of time to a person's achievement orientation. For example, if a person selected the active metaphor of a "galloping horseman" rather than the passive metaphor of a "quiet, motionless ocean," that person was thought to have a higher achievement orientation. Likewise, if adjectives such as sharp, active, tense, and clear were selected to describe time rather than empty, soothing, sad, cold, and deep, a higher achievement orientation was indicated. In addition, people with a higher achievement orientation were more likely to underestimate the passage of time when asked to recall the dates of important events from the past and almost always wore watches that were set faster than the actual time. Thus it appears that those with a higher achievement orientation tend to have a perspective on time that reflects movement, direction, and value. In addition, it seems that most of these people also have a type A personality which is characterized by a habitual sense of urgency regarding time (Norville, 1984).

It is easy to apply the perspectives-on-time concept to nurses because most nurses tend to be high achievement–oriented and many also possess a type A personality. Because most nurses are high achievers, they are more likely to encounter stress when they mismanage themselves and do not use time appropriately. The reason for this phenomenon becomes clear when some of the common characteristics of high achievers are examined. High achievers are identified as those who gain satisfaction through the process of achieving a goal and not just in the goal itself. In addition, they gain intrinsic satisfaction through (1) performing a task well and meeting high standards, (2) trying to overcome difficult but not impossible obstacles, and (3) trying different ways or implementing novel and creative solutions to problems (Webber, 1972). Thus as high achievers nurses usually are attracted to activities that are challenging, difficult, and risky. In most cases the activities are complex and time-consuming, which forces the person to use self-management to meet the goals and gain internal satisfaction. When these people mismanage themselves in relation to time, frustration and stress are the result. To assist nurses in improving their self-management and time management, it is first necessary to explore the common myths that are associated with time management and how these myths might affect the busy clinician.

COMMON MYTHS OF TIME MANAGEMENT

Mackenzie (1972, 1974) formulated 14 myths of time management based on years of research, lecturing, and writing about the topic. These myths, which have widespread applicability and generalizability, involve the aspects highlighted in Box 23-1. Further explanation of these myths will clarify their impact on the professional nurse.

The Myth of Activity

The myth of activity implies that those who are the most active get the most done. This is definitely a myth because activity is not synonymous with results. Unfortunately the two com-

BOX 23-1	*The Myths of Time Management*

- The myth of activity
- The myth of decision level
- The myth of delayed decisions
- The myth of delegation
- The myth of omnipotence
- The myth of overworking
- The myth of efficiency

- The myth of hard work
- The myth of the open door
- The myth of problem identification
- The myth of saving time
- The myth of time shortage
- The myth that time flies
- The myth that time is against us

ponents are often confused, and clinicians believe they are accomplishing something when they really are not. For example, nurses can become involved and active in rearranging their work environment, restocking shelves, checking linen, or ordering supplies without ever accomplishing any of their patient care goals that will provide them with the internal satisfaction they need. In the opening vignette Susan was a perfect example of the myth of activity. She was so busy stocking the medicine cart and doing other tasks that she never really got to the important patient care activities. Thus the results were less than satisfactory, and she was frustrated.

The Myth of Decision Level

This myth states that the higher the level at which a decision is made, the better the decision. It suggests that the people at the top of the hierarchy will make the best decisions for everyone. This is a myth because decisions should ideally be made at the lowest level possible, consistent with good judgment and the relevant facts. In general, those who are the most affected by the decision should be involved in making the decision because they are more familiar with the circumstances and relevant data. In addition, making the decision at a lower level may be more cost-effective for the organization. This myth is operational at the clinical level. For example, staff nurses often allow charge nurses or supervisors to make the daily patient care assignments without providing adequate input. The result may be an assignment that is not congruent with the skills of the nurse or that constitutes too heavy a workload. In the vignette Karen suggests that Susan's assignment should have allowed time for her to accept a new admission. When Susan states that she cannot take the new admission, Karen realizes that perhaps the assignment may have been too heavy and offers to help. However, Susan's response clearly indicates that the assignment may not have been the problem. Instead, it appears to be a case of poor use of time resulting from personal mismanagement.

The Myth of Delayed Decisions

This myth implies that, by delaying making a decision, the quality of the decision will be improved. Experts suggest that the delay occurs because the decision maker either is afraid to commit to the decision that is being made or fears the consequences of the decision. This state has been referred to as "paralysis of analysis." The longer it takes to make a decision, the more crucial and difficult it becomes. In addition, there is less time to correct problems if the decision proves to be wrong or has dire unforeseen consequences. A clinical example that happens too frequently is the nurse who detects changes in a patient but cannot decide whether to notify the physician. For example, when a patient's level of consciousness, respiratory pattern, or urine output decreases, the nurse decides not to notify anyone, but continues to monitor the patient. The hope is that this decrease is transient and that the parameter will return to normal at the next assessment. The problem occurs when the nurse gets busy with another patient, and the next assessment is delayed or omitted. The change in the patient may continue to progress to a crisis level.

The Myth of Delegation

The myth of delegation assumes that delegation saves time, worry, and responsibility. This is a myth because it may take more time to delegate a task than it does to do it, and the responsibility always remains with the delegator. Effective delegation may save time overall, but initially it requires a significant amount of planning, selection, and communication. In addition, accountability can never be delegated. Professionals are responsible for their own actions, even when the action is the process of delegation. If a task is delegated inappropriately or without sufficient information, the delegator is still responsible for the results. For example, in the vignette Karen basically has delegated the care of certain patients to Susan. The fact that those patients have not received the appropriate care is Karen's responsibility as much as it is Susan's. Susan, however, may have a greater sense of frustration because it was not bad delegation that resulted in insufficient care, but rather poor self-management.

The Myth of Omnipotence

The myth of omnipotence implies that, by personally doing a task yourself, it will get done faster and better than if anyone else does it. This is a myth because no one is indispensable or omnipotent. However, if a person chooses to function in such a manner, the result is that the person will need to continue doing the task and accept responsibility for it. The impact could be overall decreased staff morale and an on-call status for the omnipotent nurse. An example of such an omnipotent nurse is one who attends a conference to learn how to implement a new clinical procedure, such as continuous renal replacement therapy. The nurse then hoards the information and is unwilling to teach anyone how to perform the procedure. Thus the nurse needs to be available 24 hours a day, 7 days a week to cover that procedure. As you might imagine, that schedule could become intrusive rather quickly.

The Myth of Overworking

This myth stems from a person creating an internal aura of being indispensable and thus needing to work longer and harder than anyone else to ensure the survival of the organization. Again, no one is indispensable. In addition, many people who participate in perpetuating this myth do so by dealing with detail and clutter in their attempt to be seen as indispensable. Often they are doing tasks that do not need to be done, or at least not by them. Examples of this myth abound on clinical units. Some nurses always stay on duty long after their shift has ended because there is always something more to be done that the next shift will never get done; others constantly work double shifts and avoid taking vacations because they believe that the unit could not survive without them.

The Myth of Efficiency

This myth assumes that the most efficient person also is the most effective. This is a myth because a person can be efficient doing the wrong task or doing the right task at the wrong time.

Being efficient means doing things right; being effective means doing the right things right. For example, a nurse might be efficient in administering an intramuscular antibiotic before drawing a peak-and-trough level. However, the nurse may not be effective if the antibiotic was ordered to be given intravenously. Or a nurse could be efficient at infusing intravenous (IV) fluids, but less than effective if the IV had infiltrated. A nurse may be efficient at administering pain medication, but less than effective because the etiology of the pain is never discerned.

The Myth of Hard Work

The myth of hard work implies that the harder a person works, the more work gets done. This is a myth because it requires more than hard work to ensure that a task will be completed correctly and efficiently. It takes thorough planning and refined organizational skills to meet a specified goal. It is estimated that every hour spent in effective planning saves 3 to 4 hours in execution and ensures better results. Thus the key is not to work harder, but to work smarter to get more done in less time. This myth has direct clinical application. A nurse could work hard preparing a patient psychologically and gathering equipment and supplies to perform a complex dressing change on a thigh wound. However, unless there is a plan for how the dressing is going to be done, it is likely to require more time than necessary or perhaps be omitted entirely. For example, the plan would need to consider questions such as: (1) Does the patient need pain medication before the dressing change? (2) What is the proper position for the extremity? (3) Is a second person required to hold or stabilize the extremity during the dressing change? (4) Are there sufficient, appropriate supplies to complete the dressing change? (5) Is there sufficient time to complete the dressing change before the patient's next scheduled test? (6) Is the timing appropriate for the dressing change in relation to the next scheduled change or other therapeutic interventions? Contemplating such questions and having preplanned solutions will ensure that the dressing change is completed in a timely fashion with few interruptions.

The Myth of the Open Door

This myth suggests that being open and available to others at all times will improve a person's effectiveness. This is a myth because being open and available to others often results in not being able to complete your own workload. Certainly it is appropriate to want to help others, but not at the expense of your own responsibilities. Perhaps having planned availability times for assisting or interacting with others would be more appropriate. This myth frequently is seen on clinical units. Some nurses become so involved in the activities of others or so intent on assisting another team member with patient care that their own patients' care suffers. Their care becomes negligent by virtue of acts of omission, rather than of commission. In the opening vignette Susan is a perfect example of this myth in action. She was so busy helping a physician gather data and restocking the medication cart that her patients did not receive the requisite care.

The Myth of Problem Identification

This myth abounds in everyday life. It implies that identifying the problem is the easiest part of problem solving. It is a myth because identifying the right problem is often a difficult task. Significant amounts of time, energy, and money are expended daily solving the wrong problems. A prime example is a nurse who works diligently teaching a patient how to administer subcutaneous insulin in preparation for discharge, only to be frustrated when the patient can never get the dose correct. The nurse repeats the teaching process many times with little improvement. The nurse is close to concluding that the patient cannot learn the procedure sufficiently well for self-care, when it becomes clear that the real problem is that the patient's vision is too diminished to view the units on the syringe. Thus much time and energy have been expended, and much frustration has been generated by trying to solve the wrong problem.

The Myth of Saving Time

Saving time probably is the biggest myth of all. Technically there is no time bank, and time cannot be saved. Instead it can only be better used. People often try to "save" time by taking shortcuts in their work. All too frequently such shortcuts actually end up taking more time in the long run. Such may be the case when important conversations are curtailed in a manner that results in only part of the communication occurring or when decisions are made hastily based on incomplete data. The result is that actions are taken that are inappropriate or inadequate and thus will necessitate further action at a later time. The overall effect is a loss of time rather than the intended time savings. In the vignette Susan exhibited an example of timesaving mentality. She started by doing some "easy" things first because she was certain that they would not take much time; then she would have extra time to spend on her other patient care. When the "easy" things took more time than expected, she was at a loss for a strategy to compensate for the time mismanagement.

Another clinical example that illustrates this myth involves a nurse teaching a patient about insulin administration for self-care. The nurse teaches the patient all of the steps of the procedure but neglects to instruct the patient about those instances when decision making is necessary to decide when and how much insulin to administer. The patient is left with the caveat of not missing the morning insulin dose. The patient follows the caveat even when not eating because of an episode of the flu and is admitted in a hypoglycemic coma. Thus the shortcut of including all of the decision making into one caveat resulted in an unnecessary trip to the hospital for the patient and more time involvement for both the patient and the nurse.

The Myth of Time Shortage

This myth stems from the fact that everyone complains about not having enough time. Since everyone has the same amount of time 24 hours per day, this is definitely a myth. Thus the shortage of time is merely an illusion perpetuated by personal mismanagement, resulting in a misuse of time in relation to attainment of goals. The illusion often results from inadequate preplanning, not setting priorities, confusing priorities, or an inability to say "no." Once again Susan is a perfect example. If she had approached her patient care from a prioritization aspect and chosen not to rearrange the medication cart and not to help the physician with his research, she may have had enough time to complete her patient care assignment and not been so frustrated.

The Myth That Time Flies

This myth also stems from personal mismanagement. The image of time flying also is an illusion that usually results from inadequate preplanning so that a person has too much to do in too little time. Susan also illustrates this myth. Because she chose not to attack the priorities of her patient care assignment first, she found herself well into the shift with little accomplished and an expectation that she could do even more by admitting a new patient. Her lack of preplanning was evident when she could not tell Karen how to help her get caught up with her assignment.

The Myth That Time Is Against Us

This myth is perpetuated by busy people who always are missing deadlines and dealing with crises instead of preplanning. It is definitely a myth because time is totally inanimate and cannot possibly fight us. So, if time is not the problem, what is? In the words of the comic strip character Pogo, "We has met the enemy, and they is us." People are the problem. Personal mismanagement results in the illusion of an adversarial relationship with time. After a person becomes organized, time becomes an ally. Susan certainly could benefit from some self-management strategies to assist her in accomplishing her goals. Before such strategies are presented, it is beneficial to explore how people waste time. Such an exploration may help identify specific time wasters that should be addressed with specific management strategies to help improve self-management for better time use.

TIME WASTERS

Many factors influence how time is wasted. These factors have been documented by several authors and are collectively referred to as time wasters. Time wasters are any activities that have fewer benefits and generate less internal satisfaction than another activity that you could be doing. Mackenzie (1972) was one of the first to document time wasters, and he did so for managers by categorizing them according to seven management functions: planning, organizing, staffing, directing, controlling, communicating, and decision making. Lancaster (1984) added to the documentation by categorizing time wasters as being either internal or external. Other authors (Baer, 1979; Douglass and Douglass, 1980; Fuqua, 1988; Perry and Rowe, 1993; Thompson and Huston, 1994) continued to add to the list or to explicate time wasters that had already been documented. Box 23-2 presents an eclectic list of external and internal time wasters. Numerous strategies can be used to minimize or eliminate these time wasters and assist in better managing ourselves to better use our time.

TIME-MANAGEMENT STRATEGIES

The self-management process for better time use begins with two activities: segmentation and concentration.

Segmentation

According to Webber, segmentation is the process of separating those events over which a person has control from those over which a person does not have control (Webber, 1972). For example, a nurse may not have control over which shift he or she works, but the nurse does have some control over what he or she does when at work. A nurse may not be able to control the types of therapeutic interventions that a patient requires, but he or she can control when the interventions are implemented. A nurse may not be able to control the numbers and types of patients for whom he or she cares, but he or she can control how to deliver their care.

Concentration

The second activity is concentration, or the process of systematically controlling those events that can be controlled (Webber, 1972). Concentration is the heart of self-management for better time use. It consists of planning, organizing, and implementing activities to control the use of time.

Planning. Planning is the *most* important step in time management. Unfortunately few people expend as much energy planning as they should. Some shy away from planning because

BOX 23-2	*Time Wasters*

External time wasters	**Internal time wasters**
Telephone interruptions	Procrastination
Socializing or visitors	Inadequate planning
Meetings	Ineffective delegation
Excessive paperwork to read	Failure to set goals and priorities
Excessive paperwork to write	A cluttered desk or mind
Lack of information	Personal disorganization
Ineffective communication	Inability to say "NO"
Lack of feedback	Lack of self-discipline
Travel	Responding to crises
Inadequate policies and procedures	Haste
Incompetent co-workers	Indecisiveness
Poor filing systems	An "open door" policy
Understaffing	Shifting priorities without sound rationale
Personnel or co-workers with problems	Leaving tasks unfinished
Lack of teamwork	Not setting time limits
Duplicating efforts	Daydreaming
Confusing lines of authority, responsibility, and communication	Attempting too much at once
	Overinvolvement in routine details
Bureaucratic red tape	Making numerous errors
	Surfing the Internet
	Not listening

they believe it is too time-consuming and never leads to closure. In reality, planning allows people to better use their time and can lead to closure in relation to goals that will produce the most internal satisfaction. Those who plan well tend to encounter fewer problems when Murphy's Laws become a reality. Three of Murphy's Laws that always seem to be true when working on a project are: (1) nothing is as simple as it seems; (2) everything takes longer than it should; and (3) if anything can go wrong, it will. Thus it is important to plan before beginning any task, project, or day's activities. Planning involves (1) setting priorities, (2) scheduling activities, and (3) establishing "To Do" lists.

Setting Priorities. The term priority is synonymous with a superiority in rank, a preferential rating, or the state of coming first in order or ahead of others in some process (Feldman, Monicken, and Crowley, 1983). A major component of planning is deciding what should be done first and what activities should follow sequentially. Many factors influence how to establish priorities. These factors include the urgency of a situation, demands of others, closeness of deadlines, existing time frame, degree of familiarity, ease of the task, amount of enjoyment involved, consequences involved, size of the task, and congruence with personal goals. Unfortunately, when considering the use of time, not all of these factors are of the same weight. Factors that are most likely to assist in meeting your goals need to be given more consideration. Several processes have been proposed to help people set priorities, including the ABC approach, the Pareto Principle, and the continuum approach.

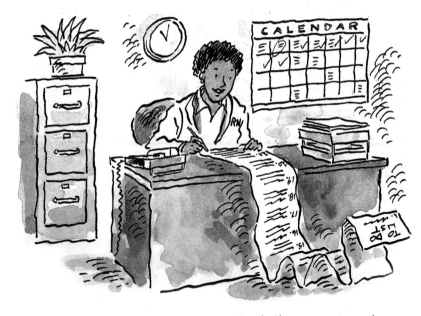

Planning is the *most* important step in time management.

The ABC approach is advocated by Lakein (Lakein, 1973). In this approach a person lists every task that needs to be done. Then an A is assigned to the high-value items, a B to the medium-value items, and a C to the low-value items. The A items should stand out from the other items because of their worth to the person. The A items also are likely to require more energy and time, but they should be completed before any of the B or C items. As the A items are completed, you actually may find that the C items were of such low value that they did not need to be done at all. It is also possible that Monday's C item could become an A item on Friday, reflecting a change in values. This is, of course, an arbitrary system that is based on the person's estimation of the value of activities within his or her life. It allows for reflection and change while maintaining focus. The Pareto Principle is another process that is suggested for setting priorities. This principle also is referred to as the 80-20 rule, and it states that 80% of the time expended produces 20% of the results, and 20% of the time expended produces 80% of the results (MacKenzie, 1972). The essence is in determining the "vital few" activities that should be done and eliminating the "trivial many." This principle emphasizes selecting the most productive activities, eliminating trivia, and learning to say "no."

The continuum approach to setting priorities encourages a person to select priorities by categorizing or ranking items according to four continuums. As you read about the four continuums, think about Susan's patient care assignment and what tasks would have been priorities based on this approach. The first continuum is intrinsic importance, and the range of categorizations include:

- Very important and must be done
- Important and should be done
- Not so important and may not be necessary, but may be useful
- Unimportant and can be eliminated entirely

The second continuum is urgency, and the range of responses is:
- Very urgent and must be done now
- Urgent and should be done soon
- Not urgent and can wait
- Time is not a factor

The third continuum is delegation, with the range of categorizations being:
- Must be done by me because I am the only one who can do it
- Can be delegated to A; and can be delegated to B

The fourth continuum is visitations and conferences, and the range of responses is:
- People I must see each day
- People to see frequently but not daily
- People to see regularly but not frequently
- People to see only infrequently

Obviously these continuums would have varying usefulness, depending on the activity being scrutinized.

Overall it does not matter which method is used to establish priorities, as long as they are established using sound rationale. If Susan had established her patient care priorities for the day, it is unlikely that washing a patient's hair, rearranging and restocking the medication cart, or helping with the research project would have taken precedence over the teaching, the antibiotic administration, or the insulin. Thus setting priorities would have allowed Susan to better use her time and would have decreased her frustration with not having completed her patient care assignment appropriately.

Scheduling Activities.   Scheduling activities is an important component of planning. It is one way to control Parkinson's Law, which states that work will expand to fill the time that is available. By scheduling activities, a person determines how much time is spent on a specific activity. Such time delineations tend to focus attention and activity so that the task gets completed more efficiently and effectively. A schedule of activities can be constructed using a variety of different methods, including hourly time schedules, Gantt Charts, or even Program Evaluation and Review Techniques (PERT) charts (Marriner, 1981). Hourly time schedules are not new to most people because they have been used continuously throughout life. Everyone has had an hourly schedule for appointments, classes, or leisure activities. In addition, nurses are adept at using them to administer medications appropriately. Unfortunately most people, including nurses, do not use time schedules frequently or consistently enough.

Gantt Charts are visualizations that depict a task and its progress in relation to a specific time frame. Such charts usually are used for long-term projects. Thus the chart would have the activities to be completed on one axis and the hours, days, months, or years on the other. PERT charts are planning models that identify key activities in a project, sequence the activities in a flow diagram, and assign the duration time for each phase of the work. These charts are constructed based on the premise that activities are executed in a well-defined sequence and that the interrelationships between steps can be depicted by arrows that carry a time estimate. They can be used to schedule large or small projects, including household activities such as a dinner party.

The process of scheduling activities is an important part of planning to use your time better. However, scheduling must be done appropriately to ensure adherence. Remember to schedule activities so that they coincide with your internal "prime" time, when you concentrate best, and your external "prime" time, when you deal best with people. Also, be sure to include some flexible time just for yourself. In addition, schedules have proven to be most useful when they are written in ink. Having a written schedule tends to motivate people, particularly high achievers, because they cannot bear to deviate from that which challenges them in black and white. Having the schedule completed in ink seems to compel people to adhere to it.

Establishing "To Do" Lists. Writing something on paper often is the first step to accomplishing it. "To Do" lists tend to keep people on track and focused on specific activities. Thus they should be reflective of your priorities and goals. "To Do" lists should be made and revised daily to be the most useful in managing your time. Sometimes they require revision more frequently, even hourly, when priorities shift for valid reasons. They also should be written in ink on something that can be kept with the person at all times during the waking hours. Individuals have elected to construct their lists on note cards, in day planner calendars, on pocket calendars, in electronic recall devices, on computers, and in a myriad of other ways. There is no right or wrong way to make a "To Do" list; it just must always be accessible to you.

Organizing. Organizing yourself and the environment is an important component of time management. Such organization mandates that you be able to deal effectively with the following:
- The stacked desk syndrome
- No detourism
- The art of wastebasketry
- Memo mania

The Stacked Desk Syndrome. This syndrome is exactly what the label implies—a cluttered desk full of stacks of papers, books, and things (Mackenzie, 1972; Minar-Baugh, 1998). The syndrome can also apply to the mind when it is cluttered with many thoughts and ideas. Both are distractors to accomplishing your goals. Both will divert your attention sufficiently so that you do not know where to begin, and, when you lose your concentration even a little after beginning, you will again become distracted by the "clutter." To deal effectively with this syndrome, you must clear both the work area and the mind. To effectively organize or clear a work area you should:
- Remove everything from the work surface that does not directly relate to the project at hand.
- Place the phone out of sight, but within reach.
- Remove all personal items, such as calendars, clocks, or photographs, that might prove to be distractors.
- If possible, close the door to the work area (Kozoll, 1982).

For the nurse, it usually means eliminating the clutter from the patient's room so that care can be more effectively and efficiently delivered.

No Detourism. To effectively organize, or clear the mind, you must practice the art of "no detourism." "No detourism" requires complete concentration on one activity or task until it is accomplished. It mandates that only one activity at a time be undertaken and that it should be completed before moving to a different task. This method also implies that the task should be completed correctly the first time so that you do not waste time redoing it. Inherent in the concept of "no detourism" is the fact that the tasks undertaken are directly related to personal goals and objectives, and thus completing them eventually will result in internal satisfaction. Susan may certainly have benefited from practicing "no detourism." Perhaps she would not have become so absorbed in restocking the medication cart or helping with the research project if she had been focused on her other priority patient care goals.

The Art of Wastebasketry. Perfecting the art of wastebasketry is mandatory to improving self-management for better use of time. The art of "physical" wastebasketry involves "circular filing" any document or other paperwork that has limited use or needs no response. This art involves being sufficiently knowledgeable and skilled to ascertain which documents and paperwork are appropriate candidates for the circular file and then daring and aiming to follow through. Practicing this art daily will also help in managing the stacked desk syndrome by reducing much of the clutter. The art of "mental" wastebasketry involves organizing your mind to deal with the established priorities. This requires using selective perception to attend only to those tasks at hand. It also assists in discarding useless information. "Mental" wastebasketry is a valuable skill to perfect to effect a better use of time.

Memo Mania. The general consensus regarding memos is that too many of them are generated for useless reasons and they constitute a major time waster. Furthermore, it seems to be irrelevant whether the time is wasted in constructing or reading the memos. Eric Webster in his classic article described several types of memos that clearly illustrate how the consensus regarding memos as being a time waster evolved (Ulrich, 1985). The six types of memos that Webster described are:

1. Postponing work memos state a person's intent to do something, but really enable the person to do nothing for a little while longer with a clear conscience.
2. Demonstrate efficiency memos usually begin with the phrase, "Following the memo of (any specific date) . . ." and translate into "I know what it says, but can you find your copy?"
3. Militant memos usually are from people who are afraid of face-to-face interactions; thus their memos say things that the person would not dare to say in person.
4. "For the record" or accusatory memos constitute the "gotcha" memos and mandate a response, which, if given, can be refuted. If a response is not given, this is clearly documented in the files, and the accusation becomes valid.
5. "See-how-hard-I'm-working" memos are sent from subordinates to the boss to demonstrate productivity; unfortunately the sender often expends more energy writing the memos than he or she spends doing the job.
6. Carbon copy memos are intended more for the people who are sent copies than for the person to whom the memo is directed.

Recently it seems that another type of memo should be added to the list. The addition would be status-making memos, or those that are "from the desk of . . ." "to the desk of . . .," signifying the importance of the two people talking to each other. Thus it is evident why people view memos with such disdain. In general, the rule regarding memos and time management is to use them as infrequently as possible. Some experts suggest never using them. They believe that, if communication is necessary, it should be done in person so that it is clear, accurate, and timely. In addition, if a response is required, it can be obtained more rapidly.

Implementing for Control. Implementing for control refers to carrying out the activities that assist people in better self-management for better time use. The implementing activities include:

- Attacking the priorities.
- Finding "extra" time.
- Handling paperwork appropriately.
- Avoiding procrastination.
- Delegating appropriately.
- Controlling interruptions such as phone calls, meetings, and visitors.
- Learning the art of saying "no."
- Rewarding yourself.
- Using technology.

Further exploration of these activities will clarify how they can be implemented fairly easily within the context of daily life.

Attacking the Priorities. It is important to attack the priorities early to gain control of your time. Delaying beginning tasks will only result in crises when deadlines or personal goals are not met. One of the most cited reasons for delaying attacking priorities is fear. Usually it is the fear of failure, although it could be a fear of something else. In either case it is important to analyze a person's fears to be able to identify the source and to determine if the fear is real or exaggerated.

Procrastination wears many disguises, and fear is just one of them (Lancaster, 1984). If the priority is a big project or large task, it can be approached successfully using Lakein's Swiss Cheese method, chunking, or the "SWAP" approach. The Swiss Cheese method involves "poking" small holes in the task until it is completed (Lakein, 1973). The method requires planning several short time periods of sufficient length to complete the creation of a small hole in the task. To use the Swiss Cheese approach, it is important to first define smaller aspects of the task that can be accomplished in a relatively short time frame. As the smaller aspects are completed and accumulate, the larger task is also accomplished. Chunking is a process similar to the Swiss Cheese approach. Chunking involves dividing a task into smaller pieces and doing a little at a time. The following are the suggested steps of the chunking process:

1. Divide the task into smaller components.
2. Start anywhere in the task with any of the smaller components.
3. Make a list of the chunks and cross them off as they are completed to add incentive.
4. Set deadlines for completing each of the chunks.
5. Involve other people or resources to assist with specific chunks.
6. Make a list of advantages and disadvantages of completing the chunks and the overall task (Time Management, 1994).

The "SWAP" approach is also similar to the previously mentioned processes. This approach requires that the task be broken down into several smaller, more manageable parts that have a logical order for completion. A person then "SWAPs," or starts with a part and logically completes parts until the project is completed (Berner, 1997). Using any of these methods help to attack the priorities and accomplish the larger goal.

Finding "Extra" Time. The concept of finding "extra" time seems paradoxic because people all have the same amount of time and it is all that is available. In reality, the concept relates to how people choose to use their time. In some cases a little different use of time may result in additional time for accomplishing goals. Examples of different uses of time that could produce "extra" time are:

1. Using commuting time and coffee breaks to relax so that designated working hours are more productive.
2. Instituting working lunches periodically, such as twice a week.
3. Posing a question to the subconscious before sleep.
4. Decreasing the usual sleeping time by 30 minutes per night to create a whole week of extra time per year.

There certainly are other ways individuals might choose to alter their use of time. The key is knowing which activities can be altered without being detrimental to overall functioning. For example, perhaps giving up 30 minutes of television watching or reading each evening would work for some, but not if that is the only relaxation time that is available daily. Sacrificing "down" time for more work may decrease overall productivity. It may be a case of working longer, but not smarter, so less actually gets accomplished.

Handling Paperwork Appropriately. The rule regarding paperwork is to handle it only once. Either decide to act on the paperwork or circular file it. Shuffling papers, filing, and retrieving are all time wasters. Plan to avoid becoming mired in paperwork. If a person needs to communicate with someone, it should be done either face-to-face or by telephone. It takes less time to convey information verbally than it does in writing, and responses are received more quickly. Perfecting the art of wastebasketry also will assist in handling paperwork appropriately. Other tips for dealing with paperwork include:

1. Setting aside a specific time each day for dealing with all paperwork, particularly related to "in" and "out" boxes.
2. Responding to paperwork immediately so it never has to be handled a second time.
3. Simplifying all paperwork by streamlining it, incorporating response boxes to be checked, and using form letters when appropriate (Volk-Tebbitt, 1978).

Avoiding Procrastination. Procrastination is a bad habit that ranks high on the list of time wasters. It has been referred to as an obstacle to success, a close relative of incompetency, a handmaiden of inefficiency (Mackenzie, 1972), and a tyranny of the trivial (Berner, 1997). It can wear many disguises, including fear, laziness, indifference, overwork, and forgetfulness. Procrastination most frequently is evident when a person is faced with an unpleasant task, a difficult task, or a difficult decision. It usually is easily recognizable because it involves doing low-priority tasks rather than high priority ones, and it always welcomes interruptions. Procrastination is the art of never doing today what can be put off until tomorrow. The result is less productivity, less internal satisfaction, and more stress.

The first step in avoiding procrastination is being able to recognize it when it is occurring. The second step is being able to admit that what is occurring is procrastination. Once these two steps are accomplished, the work of overcoming procrastination can begin. The following have been proposed as mechanisms for overcoming procrastination:

1. Identify the tasks that are being put off.
2. Ask why the task is being avoided.
3. Determine if the task could or should be done by someone else.
4. Identify consequences of the procrastination.

5. Set priorities in relation to the task.
6. Establish deadlines and adhere to them.
7. Focus on one aspect at a time.
8. Do not strive for perfection if 95% or 98% will be just as effective (Lancaster, 1982).

It also helps if a person can eliminate the tasks that comprise the procrastination. For example, if rearranging the desk, the furniture, or even the medication cart is part of how a person procrastinates, then eliminate that activity by changing the work location or environment. Most important, emphasize the benefits that are to be gained by completing the task and accomplishing the goals that will provide internal satisfaction.

Delegating Appropriately.   Most simplistically, delegation is the art of giving other people tasks to be accomplished. In reality, there is nothing simplistic about delegation. It usually requires considerable time and energy to delegate, but the rewards are greater in the overall context of accomplishing goals. Mackenzie (1972) identifies the following four important benefits of delegating. It extends the results that can be accomplished from what one person can do alone to what he or she can control through others; it frees time for more important tasks; it assists in developing the initiative, skills, knowledge, and competence of others; and it maintains the responsibility and decision level. With these possible benefits, it would seem that everyone would want to use delegation. Unfortunately this is not the case. There are many barriers, both internal and external, that can hinder the delegation process.

The internal barriers (within the person delegating) include a personal preference for how tasks get accomplished, demanding that everyone know all the details, believing that no one else can complete the task as well, lack of experience in delegating, insecurity, fear of being disliked, lack of confidence in others, perfectionism resulting in overcontrol, lack of organizational skill, failure to delegate authority commensurate with the responsibility delegated, indecision, poor communication skills, and lack of commitment to contributing to the development of others. The external barriers are inherent in either the situation or the person to whom something is being delegated. External barriers within the situation may include stringent policies that mandate who can do what, low tolerance of mistakes, the criticality of the decisions, implementation of a management-by-crisis style, confusion regarding responsibilities and authority, and understaffing. External barriers to delegation that reside within the person to whom tasks are being delegated include lack of experience, lack of competence, avoidance of responsibility, overdependence on others, disorganization, procrastination, work overload, and immersion in trivia and clutter (Mackenzie, 1972). When the barriers are identified and overcome, the delegation process can proceed.

Implementing the following steps will facilitate appropriate delegation: (1) identify exactly what is to be delegated and why; (2) select the best person for the task, meaning either the most qualified person or the person whom one chooses to develop; (3) communicate the assignment in detail, perhaps even including written instructions; (4) involve the delegatee in establishing the objectives and deadlines for the task; (5) have the delegatee repeat the details of the task; (6) give the person the authority for accomplishing the task; (7) provide adequate resources and support as needed; (8) schedule regular meetings for progress reports; (9) establish controls and monitor the results; (10) evaluate the process and progress of the delegatee; (11) let the person do the job; and (12) enjoy the results of having the delegated task completed and being able to accomplish other tasks simultaneously (Volk-Tebbitt, 1978). It is not prudent to take shortcuts when delegating tasks because the results might be different from those originally intended. Avoiding delegation shortcuts is an important consideration because the nurse who delegates retains accountability for the task.

Delegation would have been useful to Susan in the vignette. It could have helped her meet her patient care goals and decreased her frustration. Unfortunately, Susan was so disorganized that she could not even identify the things that needed to be done, let alone direct someone else to do them. In addition, she had not established any priorities, so it was difficult for Susan to plan for appropriate delegation. Chapter 18 discusses delegation in more detail.

Controlling Interruptions. To be able to focus on priorities, it is important to establish uninterrupted blocks of time. Data suggest that the most frequent causes of interruptions are telephone calls, meetings, and visitors, particularly the drop-in type. Learning how to control such interruptions will assist in accomplishing more in less time. One of the easiest ways to manage incoming calls is to not answer them during the time that was scheduled for other activities. An answering machine, voice mail, or a secretary can take the message to be responded to later. "Later" should refer to the time that was preestablished for returning telephone calls. Most people schedule call-backs for times when their productivity level is lower or during their "down" time. Telephone calls also can be controlled by the tone and verbiage that is used to begin the conversation, as well as by being prepared for the content of the call. If a person chooses to invite conversation and ensure a longer call, using a vague, open-ended greeting accomplishes that purpose. If a person chooses to focus the call specifically on its purpose, a specific, factual, informative greeting enhances the productivity of the call and shortens its length. For example, "Hi Bill, how are you and how are things going?" definitely invites the person to expound at length, whereas, "Hi Bill, I have two questions that I need for you to answer," tends to condense the telephoning session. Also, being prepared for the conversation with all of the relevant facts readily available helps to focus the conversation and shortens the call.

Meetings can become a major time waster if they are poorly managed and nonproductive. The first step in controlling this interruption is deciding whether to attend. Such a decision should be based on an evaluation of the potential productivity of the meeting. For example, is the meeting absolutely necessary, does the agenda contain items that you should be informed about; is it necessary for you to contribute to the discussion, will decisions be made that will impact you and your functioning, or are you conducting the meeting (Schwartz and Mackenzie, 1979)? Once a person is committed to attending a meeting, he or she is responsible for helping to ensure that the meeting remains focused and productive so that the goals can be accomplished. The person conducting the meeting not only shares those same responsibilities but also has a more direct role in effecting the outcome. Some of the components of conducting a productive meeting are presented in Box 23-3.

Visitors, particularly unplanned visitors, also constitute an interruption. One way to decrease the number of visitors is to be secluded during specific times by closing the door to others, physically and mentally. When unplanned visitors appear, practice the following: ask them if they want to make an appointment, do not ask them to sit down, suggest that there is only a short amount of time before the next activity, and dismiss them gracefully. Remember, you have the right to control your time. This does not mean that you must be insensitive to the needs of others; it simply means that you decide when to deal with visitors. The cost-benefit ratio of visitors must be weighed against expending the time in performing a task that will help to accomplish the overall goals.

> **BOX 23-3**   *Components of Conducting a Productive Meeting*
>
> 1. Create an agenda and circulate it in advance.
> 2. Compose a fact sheet in relation to specific agenda items if appropriate and circulate it with the agenda.
> 3. Start on time in accordance with the preestablished time and do not wait for latecomers.
> 4. Have a preestablished adjournment time and adhere to it.
> 5. Cover only important topics and adhere to the agenda.
> 6. Control interruptions and personal outbursts.
> 7. Restrict negative input to factual information.
> 8. Maintain a solution-oriented structure to the meeting.

From Nursing Times: Time management: the role of the nurse, *Nurs Times* 90:6 (Professional Development section), 1994.

Learning the Art of Saying "NO." No is such a small word, but it is sometimes more difficult to say than any 14-syllable word. The first step in learning the art of saying no is determining when to say it. The cost-benefit ratio of each opportunity must be evaluated in relation to the overall goals. If the activity will be a benefit overall, obviously it must be given careful consideration. If it will not be a significant benefit, decline gracefully but emphatically. Do not buffer the "no" with a plausible excuse, unless you are willing to say "yes" when someone finds a way to dispose of the excuse (Pagana, 1994). For example, when asked to review a clinical guideline, do not decline because you are overworked and do not have a free minute for 3 weeks. The person requesting the review is likely to agree that the later time frame will be fine. At that point you are either committed to doing something that has low benefit or creating another excuse. Instead be polite and gracious in the refusal, but do not allow leeway to be manipulated into saying "yes." Some busy individuals have signs posted above all of their telephones that say "NO." It serves as a reminder to consider the opportunity in terms of the overall goals.

Rewarding Yourself. All people function more productively when they are motivated. The sources of motivation vary from person to person. A person needs to identify his or her motivators and use them as rewards for accomplishing goals. It is important to identify long- and short-term rewards so they can be implemented appropriately. Most people are familiar with rewarding themselves in exchange for doing something, and they do it frequently. For some it is a way of life. It usually amounts to bargaining with yourself to facilitate the completion of a task. For example, "If I finish reading these two work-related articles, then I can read my novel for 30 minutes." Or, "If I complete this paper, I will treat myself to an ice cream cone." You should know which rewards work best and use them appropriately to accomplish long-term goals.

Using Technology. Many of today's technologic advances can be used to improve self-management for better use of time. However, there are advantages and disadvantages to most of the new technologic devices. Table 23-1 includes an overview of selected technologic devices, their impact on time management, and their advantages and disadvantages. Technologic devices may be very valuable adjuncts to other time management strategies. However, as Bergeron states, "Technology is of value only when it decreases time spent on labor-intensive

TABLE 23-1	*Time Management Technologies*

Technologic device	Impact on time management	Advantages	Disadvantages
Books on tape and CD-ROM	Decreases reading time and allows for multitasking	Can be used while doing other things (i.e., commuting, gardening, cooking)	May be more expensive than books; may be difficult to focus while multitasking
Cellular phone	Can return calls or check messages at any time or place	Instant communication with anyone near a telephone or any site using a phone line	Instant communication with you if it is turned on; additional costs and another number to remember
Digital voice recorder with graphic display	Easy to keep track of information quickly	Direct access to information; can be tailored to meet one's needs; can be used to create to do or to call lists	Additional expense; audio quality may not be clear; limited recording time
Digital camera	Decreases scanning waiting time for images	Less expensive and faster than traditional photography; no film to develop	Limited image capacity and decreased image quality
Educational materials on tape or CD-ROM	Decreases conference attendance and allows for individual pacing of learning	Inexpensive, self-paced and self-timed	Need the correct hardware; variable quality; limited topics
Laptop computer	Increases productivity while traveling or away from home or the office	Easy access to information and work documents	Some devices are expensive and heavy
Optical character-recognition software and hardware	Decreases the time to get documents into computer readable form	Fast processing; easy access to retrieved information	Some devices require manual input; may be inefficient
Personal digital assistant	Increases access to information for self-management	Compact, portable, accessible, affordable, easy to use	Must become familiar with the device and its options; some are expensive
Voice recognition systems	Decreases the time to get spoken thoughts into a written form	Easy to use and access	Need the appropriate hardware and software; may be inaccuracies

---

BOX 23-4 *Helpful Websites*

Crazy Lady
www.crazyladyco.com

Day Runner
www.dayrunner.com

Day Timer
www.daytimer.com

Filofax
www.filofax.com
www.TheDailyPlanner.com
MrFilofax@aol.com

Franklin Covey
www.franlinquest.com

TMI/Time Manager
www.tmius.com

---

tasks and reduces overall effort. It's not how many technologies and techniques you use that counts; it's how you apply them to your goals and personal style" (Bergeron, 1998).

All of the previously discussed time management strategies have been proven effective in self-management to better use time. Additional assistance related to specific strategies can be obtained from the Internet. Box 23-4 presents selected Internet sites (Watkins, 1999). Many of these sites also contain online catalogs, ordering, user forums, tips and retail availability information. Once the strategies have been implemented, it is important to continue to use them to achieve your overall goals and gain internal satisfaction.

CONTINUING TO SUCCEED

Improving self-management to better use time is a lifelong process. It becomes easier the longer you engage in it, but it still requires attention and energy. Obviously self-management does not just happen. Thus Lakein suggests that it is important to continue doing the following to succeed: (1) when feeling overwhelmed, always stop and plan activities; (2) keep focused on priorities and act accordingly; (3) avoid favorite forms of procrastination; (4) maintain a positive attitude about the established goals or revise them so that they coincide with your value system; (5) do something for yourself everyday; (6) continue to work on overcoming your fears; and (7) resist doing the easy but unimportant tasks (Lakein, 1973).

In addition, delete the words "if only" from your vocabulary. Regret is a luxury and a great time waster. Significant time is expended rehashing mistakes or determining how to make something perfect when it was a one-time occurrence. Such time usually is not productive unless you will encounter similar situations in the future. It is more productive to admit mistakes, accept responsibility for them, and move on. Thus the words "if only" should be replaced by "next time," and the incident should be filed in the mental circular file (Lancaster, 1982). The Douglasses (1980) also have a formula for continuing success in managing time. They propose the 20 steps to successful time management presented in Box 23-5.

BOX 23-5 *Twenty Steps to Successful Time Management*

1. Clarify objectives, put them in writing, and establish priorities.
2. Focus on objectives, not on activities.
3. Set at least one major objective for each day, and achieve it.
4. Record a time log periodically to analyze how time is used and to document bad habits.
5. Analyze everything in terms of objectives.
6. Eliminate at least one time waster from your life each week.
7. Plan your time.
8. Make a "to do" list every day that includes daily objectives and priorities and time estimates to accomplish them.
9. Schedule time every day to ensure that the most important things are accomplished first.
10. Make sure the first hour of every workday is productive.
11. Set time limits for every task undertaken.
12. Take the time to do the task right the first time so that time will not be wasted doing it over.
13. Eliminate recurring crises from your life.
14. Institute a quiet hour of uninterrupted time each day to work on the most important tasks.
15. Develop the habit of finishing whatever task is started.
16. Conquer procrastination, and learn to do tasks now.
17. Make better time management a daily habit.
18. Never spend time on less important things when it could be spent on more important things.
19. Take time for yourself—time to dream, time to relax, time to live.
20. Develop a personal philosophy of time that is consistent with your values.

From Douglass ME, Douglass DN: *Manage your time, manage your work, manage yourself,* New York, 1980, AMACOM.

SUMMARY

This chapter has focused on how to better manage yourself to control one of the most precious resources—time. Time management is important to achieving any personal or professional goals, and it helps decrease frustration and anxiety in high achievers. Without time management, most professionals could never achieve their established goals. When the concept is applied to nursing, it means that many patient care activities would never get completed, perhaps resulting in additional difficulties for the patient. Susan's experience in the opening vignette is an example of what your life could be like in nursing unless strategies for better self-management are implemented. Thus it is important in your professional career to initiate habits related to time management that will continue throughout the years. Start asking "Lakein's Question" frequently throughout the day: "what is the best use of my time right now?" (Lakein, 1973). You may be surprised that the answer does not coincide with the current activity. When this occurs, stop and implement the strategies for self-management to better control time. You will become more productive and gain internal satisfaction as a result. The TIME to begin is NOW! Otherwise the words of Robert Herrick in his poem, "To the Virgins, To Make Much of Time" will become true regarding your life and nursing career. Herrick wrote:

> "Gather ye rosebuds while ye may,
> Old Time is still a-flying;
> And this same flower that smiles today,
> Tomorrow will be dying."

Critical Thinking Activities

1. Write a one-paragraph statement regarding your philosophy of time.
2. At the end of a day, make a record of how you spent your day. Analyze the record to determine what personal objectives were attacked or accomplished and which activities could be classified as either time wasters or procrastination efforts.
3. Analyze each hour of the day that was recorded to determine if it was the best use of your time.
4. For 1 day keep a record of the number and type of interruptions that you experienced. Analyze the record and develop a plan to decrease that number by at least one half.
5. Identify your three favorite time wasters and devise a plan for decreasing them somewhat each day until they finally are eliminated.
6. Identify your three favorite forms of procrastination; then create an action plan with strategies identified to eliminate procrastination.
7. List all of the patients on your unit, their ages, diagnoses, and specific therapeutic interventions. Prioritize the patient care activities in terms of how you would plan to deliver their care.
8. Evaluate the patient care assignment that you had today and replan how you would deliver the care to be able to accomplish more within the same time frame.
9. Make a "To Do" list for tomorrow's tasks, complete with time estimates. Analyze the list in terms of your objectives and priorities. Revise it as necessary and then implement it.
10. Identify three of your favorite short- and long-term rewards and implement a short-term reward at least every day.

REFERENCES

Baer CL: Effecting time management, *Topics Clin Nurs* 1:78, 82, 1979.

Bergeron BP: Taming time with technology, *Postgrad Med* 103:33, 40, 1998.

Berner AJ: Overcoming procrastination: a practical approach, *Information Outlook* 1:23, 25, 1997.

Brunicardi FC, Hobson FL: Time management: a review for physicians, *J Natl Med Assoc* 88:581, 1996.

Douglass ME, Douglass DN: *Manage your time, manage your work, manage yourself,* New York, 1980, AMACOM.

Drucker PR: *The effective executive,* New York, 1967, Harper & Row.

Feldman ES, Monicken D, Crowley MB: A systems approach to prioritizing, *Nurs Admin Q* 7:57, 1983.

Fuqua L: Diagnosing timewasters, *Diabetes Educ* 14:46, 1988.

Kozoll CE: *Time management for educators,* Bloomington, Ind, 1982, Phi Delta Kappa Educational Foundation.

Lancaster J: Making the most of every minute: reminders for nursing leaders, *Nurs Leadership* 5(2): 6-10, 1982.

Lancaster J: Making every minute count, *Nurs Success Today* 1:14-15, 1984.

Lakein A: *How to get control of your time and your life,* New York, 1973, Signet.

Mackenzie RA: *The time trap,* New York, 1972, McGraw-Hill.

Mackenzie RA: Myths of time management, *Business Q* 1974; as excerpted in *Notes Quotes* 410:2, 1974.

Marriner A: Work smarter not harder with time management, *J Contin Educ Nurs* 12(6):10-13, 1981.

Minar-Baugh, V: Survival strategies: improving time management skills, *Ostomy/Wound Manage* 44:79, 1998.

Morano VJ: Time management: from victim to victor, *Health Care Supervisor* 3:2, 1984.

Norville JL: Improving personal effectiveness through better management of time, *Nurs Homes* 33:10, 14, 1984.

Nursing Times: Time management: the role of the nurse, *Nurs Times* 90:6 (Professional Development section), 1994.

Pagana KD: Teaching students time management strategies, *J Nurs Educ* 33:381, 1994.

Perry A, Rowe M: Beating time, *Nurs Times* 89:32-34, 1993.

Schwartz EB, Mackenzie RA: Time management strategy for women, *J Nurs Admin* 9:26, 1979.

Thompson BA, Huston JL: How to break down tasks so they don't break you: coping with overwhelming demands on your time, *Health Care Supervisor* 12:40, 1994.

Time management: the role of the nurse, *Nurs Times* 90:6 (Professional Development section), 1994.

Ulrich B: Time management for the nurse executive, *Nurs Econ* 3:320, 1985.

Volk-Tebbitt B: Time: who controls yours? *Supervisor Nurs* 9:19, 1978.

Watkins D: Are you a time management junkie? *Information Outlook* 3:35, 1999.

Webber RA: *Time and management*, New York, 1972, Van Nostrand Reinhold.

Contemporary Nursing Roles and Career Opportunities

Robert W. Koch, DNS, RN

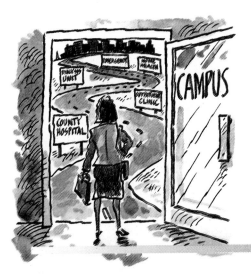

The career path for nurses
is long and wide.

Vignette

"When I graduated 15 years ago, I thought I would work in the hospital my entire career. However, with so many changes in economic forces and the resulting shift of clients outside acute care, more opportunities exist for me. I can take my skills and seek new ones to have a choice of practice roles and settings. Being a registered nurse now gives me more options for practice than I ever thought possible."

Questions to consider while reading this chapter

1. What community-based opportunities exist for graduate nurses?
2. How can a new nurse gain knowledge about the role of the parish nurse or forensic nurse?
3. What unique skills do nurses working in community settings need?

Key Terms

Nursing roles (1) Traditional duties and responsibilities of the professional nurse, regardless of practice area or setting, such as the roles of care provider, educator, counselor, client advocate, change agent, leader and manager, researcher, and coordinator of the transdisciplinary team; (2) duties and responsibilities of the professional nurse that are guided by specific professional standards of practice and usually are carried out in a distinct practice area (e.g., flight nurse, forensic nurse, and occupational nurse).

Advanced practice nursing Defined by National Council of State Boards of Nursing (1992) as "practice based on knowledge and skills acquired in a basic nursing education, through licensure as a registered nurse (RN), and in graduate education and experience, including advanced nursing theory, physical assessment, and psychosocial assessment and treatment of illness"; includes nurse practitioners (NPs), certified nurse midwives (CNMs), certified registered nurse anesthetists (CRNAs), and clinical nurse specialists (CNSs).

Learning Outcomes

After studying this chapter, the reader will be able to:

1. Evaluate the impact of the current health care environment on the future role of nurses.
2. Analyze the influence of current demographic characteristics of RNs in the United States on contemporary nursing roles.
3. Differentiate among various innovative nursing practice roles today.
4. Differentiate between the roles of advanced practice nurses and other RNs in various settings.

CHAPTER OVERVIEW

The health care system continues to undergo dramatic changes. Social and economic factors create a state of constant evolution. Professional nurses respond by creating innovative alternatives to traditional nursing practice to meet these new challenges. As nurses proactively define solutions to today's health care dilemmas, multiple career opportunities emerge.

Not long ago most nurses considered acute care hospitals to be the main practice setting available to them after graduation. Few other career choices were available. Public health nursing was one of few exceptions providing variety in the nursing job market. With health care trends moving from inpatient treatment to outpatient and home care and acute care to health promotion and disease prevention, the United States society is seeking alternative settings to meet this growing need. This shift in health care settings creates a variety of choices for nurses exploring career opportunities.

Nurses today have more liberty to explore and even create job opportunities. Nurses may continue to select the hospital or acute care setting or may venture into less traditional nursing roles. It is imperative that nurses claim ownership of nontraditional roles as they emerge in the health care job market. As a profession, nurses should exercise their influence to develop and support new nursing roles.

This chapter presents an overview of some key opportunities available for RNs today in the United States. Included are demographics of today's nurses, as well as implications for the future. This chapter examines the traditional and less traditional options available and the current and future issues for roles in professional practice.

NURSING . . . MUCH THE SAME, BUT BIGGER AND BETTER

Not so long ago describing the role of RNs was simple because there were few opportunities for variation. Today exploring job opportunities for RNs is more complicated as nurses are practicing in literally hundreds of diverse settings with a broad variety of clients. The proliferation of career opportunities for nurses is growing. Although nursing roles have expanded, the traditional functions of the nurse remain intact. Box 24-1 summarizes the roles nurses will assume in any employment role or setting.

Care Provider

The role of care provider is basic to the nursing profession. As the provider of care, the nurse assesses client resources, strengths and weaknesses, coping behaviors, and the environment to optimize the problem-solving and self-care abilities of the client and family. The nurse plans therapeutic interventions in collaboration with the client, physician, and other health care providers. In addition, the nurse takes responsibility for coordination of care that involves other health professionals or resources, providing continuity and helping the client deal effectively with the health care system. As part of the care provider role, caring will always be central to nursing interventions and an essential attribute of the expert nurse.

Educator and Counselor

Multiple factors increase the need for nurses to serve as educators. Today the new emphasis is on health promotion and health maintenance rather than on management of disease conditions. The role of nurse counselor has been elevated to new heights. More than ever before, nurses encourage clients to look at alternatives, recognize their choices, and develop a sense of control in a rapidly changing health care environment.

Client Advocate

Professional nurses find that the role of client advocate is essential in multiple situations with a multitude of client populations. Promoting what is best for the client, ensuring that the client's needs are met, and protecting the client's rights remain important responsibilities of the professional nurse.

BOX 24-1	*Professional Nursing Roles*

Care provider
Educator and counselor
Client advocate
Change agent
Leader and manager
Researcher
Coordinator of the transdisciplinary health care team

Change Agent

When nurses first adopted the role of "change agent," few individuals visualized to what extent nurses would fulfill this role. However, nurses have expanded their role as change agents in many ways. The profession continues to identify client and health care delivery problems, assess their motivation and capacity for change, determine alternatives, explore possible outcomes of the alternatives, and assess cost-effective resources in infinite health-related situations.

Leader and Manager

The leadership role of the professional nurse is paramount to the health care system. Today nursing leadership varies according to the level of application and includes:

- Improving the health status and potential of individuals or families.
- Increasing the effectiveness and level of satisfaction among professional colleagues providing care.
- Managing multiple resources in a health care facility.
- Raising citizens' and legislators' attitudes toward and expectations of the nursing profession and the health care system.

There is little doubt that the management role of the nurse has become more important. Nursing management includes planning; giving direction; and monitoring and evaluating nursing care of individuals, groups, families, and communities.

Researcher

During the past decades nursing has taken its place among other disciplines in the production and use of research specific to its profession. Although the majority of researchers in nursing are prepared at the doctoral and postdoctoral levels, an increasing number of clinicians with master's degrees are beginning to participate in research as part of their advanced practice role. Nurses prepared at the baccalaureate and associate degree levels are also participating in research. These nurses may be assisting with data collection, critiquing research findings, and using these findings in practice. More nursing interventions are based on nursing research than in the past.

Coordinator of the Transdisciplinary Health Care Team

Transdisciplinary teams consist of collaborative practice relationships among several disciplines of health care professionals. The disciplines include nursing, medicine, pharmacy, nutrition, social work, and other allied health professionals such as physical therapists, respiratory therapists, occupational therapists, and speech therapists. Chaplains or pastoral care representatives also serve a very valuable role on the transdisciplinary health care team. These teams are found in all health care delivery settings and function most effectively when their focus revolves around the needs of the client.

Transdisciplinary teams are valuable because professional members bring their in-depth and specialized knowledge and skills to the interaction process. In an age of exploding information, the roles of transdisciplinary team members complement one another. Through the formal and informal communication of ideas and opinions of team members, health care plans are determined. A plan of care developed by the transdisciplinary team is usually considered a valuable health management tool (Van Ess Coeling and Cukr, 1998).

The term *transdisciplinary health care team* may not be as familiar as the term *multidisciplinary* or *interdisciplinary team*. Multidisciplinary health care teams consist of many disciplines involved in meeting client care needs. Interdisciplinary teams refer to coordination between and among disciplines involved in providing client care. The more global and inclusive term *transdisciplinary health care teams* can be described as including multiple disciplines bonding, interacting, and uniting toward common goals of client care. The collaborative process involved in transdisciplinary health care incorporates the definitions of multidisciplinary and interdisciplinary health care and, in fact, transcends a single health profession to create comprehensive work outcomes. Studies that investigate the process of transdisciplinary health care teams in action report improved quality of care, increased client satisfaction, increased nursing satisfaction, and reduced hospital cost by decreasing hospital length of stay and increasing nursing retention (Wasserman, 1997; Baggs, 1989; Baggs et al., 1992; Knaus et al., 1986).

Successful health care team models that use concepts related to transdisciplinary health care include pain management, nutritional support, skin care, rehabilitation, mental health, and hospice. Discharge planning, which emerged as a major focus of health care delivery in the 1980s and involves developing a plan of treatment that ultimately results in the discharge of the client from the health care facility, is built on the concept of transdisciplinary care, with each discipline involved in providing care for the client included in developing the discharge plan.

Client education is another area in which collaboration and disciplines working together are absolutely essential. Health care professionals must understand one another's contributions to client education and ensure that the information clients and families receive is consistent and complete. This will lead to the best possible health outcomes for clients and families.

In Box 24-2 some of the more common roles of transdisciplinary health care team members are addressed, and the website of their associated professional organization is listed. These team members are involved in client care to varying degrees, depending on client needs for the specific talents and knowledge of each team member. Although this list contains selected professional roles contributing to the transdisciplinary health care team approach, it is not exhaustive.

The following case study provides an excellent example of the role of various members of the transdisciplinary health care team. Multiple professional caregivers provide health care within the limits of each provider's expertise. The joint efforts of all professionals provide the opportunity for a better overall outcome.

John was discussing a problem with a co-worker over his cell phone as he approached the intersection. He didn't notice the truck approaching on his left side and he didn't notice the STOP sign. After evaluation in the Emergency Department, John was diagnosed post Motor Vehicle Accident with multiple trauma, closed head injury, several rib and leg fractures, lacerations, and internal injuries. His physician ordered multiple diagnostic tests, laboratory tests, medications, and treatments. His nurse monitored his physical status and carried out the orders written by the physician. The nurse organized the tests and procedures and managed his pain and psychologic reaction. The pharmacist reviewed and supplied the medications ordered and analyzed potential interaction effects of the multiple pharmaceutic agents. A respiratory therapist was consulted to perform breathing treatments to facilitate lung expansion and prevent respiratory complications. After surgical repair of his fractured leg, physical therapy was consulted to assess John's condition and his need for physical reconditioning. A plan of care was determined to enhance his mobility. His long recuperation led to mild depression and spiritual distress. The nurse who noted these symptoms made arrangements for the chaplain to visit John. Throughout John's period of care, all practitioners involved communicated their assessments and worked together to provide collaborative interventions aimed at holistic care. In addition, all transdisciplinary team members interacted in medical rounds and discharge planning meetings collaborating and coordinating the client's care.

| BOX 24-2 | *Transdisciplinary Health Care Team Members* |

Nurse (RN): Often the coordinator of the team. RNs take licensure examinations after completing associate degree, diploma, or baccalaureate degree preparation from an accredited school of nursing. RNs are able to obtain specialty certification for advanced skills and/or advanced degrees. RNs use the nursing process in client care in any health care setting.

American Nursing Association: www.nursingworld.org/

Physician (MD or DO): Often the leader of the team, physicians diagnose and prescribe treatment interventions for clients. Medical doctors (MDs) or doctors of osteopathy (DOs) complete 4 years of medical school and board examinations. Physicians can complete postgraduate training, including internship, residency, and fellowship training in a specialty area. Doctors also complete state licensing examinations and function in all health care arenas.

American Medical Association: www.ama-assn.org

Pharmacist (RPh or PharmD): Responsible for providing drug therapy for positive client outcomes; activities include drug information services, client and health care staff education, dispensing medications and client monitoring, adverse drug reaction reporting, research, concurrent drug use evaluation, and consultative services in areas such as pain management and nutritional support. Pharmacists complete baccalaureate preparation, an internship period, and licensing board examinations. Pharmacists can complete additional specialized training, certifications, and/or advanced degrees. In some states the PharmD or doctor of pharmacy degree is now the educational requirement for entering practice.

American Pharmaceutical Association www.aphanet.org/

Physician Assistant (PA): Works under the supervision of the MD or DO and performs assessments, procedures, or protocols approved by the physician. PAs complete a baccalaureate degree with specialized PA training (usually 2 years) and state licensure.

Dietitian (RD/LD): Provides nutritional therapy and support to ensure the nutritional needs of the client are met. Activities include involving both client and family in dietary assessment and teaching, identifying resources for food purchase and preparation, and identifying areas of food-drug interactions. Dietitians complete a baccalaureate degree from an accredited nutrition or food service administration program and national board examinations and may also complete state licensure and advanced educational preparation.

American Dietetic Association www.eatrigh.org/

Physical Therapist (PT): Attends to the client's needs for movement. Activities include assessing physical strength and mobility needs and developing a plan of strengthening exercises for the client with movement dysfunction, maintaining range of motion and muscle tone, and identifying assistive devices that may be needed. A physical therapist may also be expert in the area of wound care. The basic educational requirement is a baccalaureate degree in a physical therapy program and completion of a national certifying examination. Advanced degrees are available.

American Physical Therapy Association: www.apta.org/

NURSES TODAY: WHO ARE THEY AND WHAT ARE THEY DOING?

The phrase "a typical nurse" has become a misnomer as the profession enters the twenty-first century. Nursing roles are so diverse that there literally is no typical role or practice setting. Recent surveys conducted by the Division of Nursing–Bureau of Health Professions document characteristics of the people comprising nursing today (Division of Nursing–Bureau of Health Professions, National Sample Survey, 2001).

| BOX 24-2 | *Transdisciplinary Health Care Team Members—cont'd* |

Speech Language Pathologist (SLP): Assists clients who are communicatively impaired by intervening into speech, language, and/or swallowing disorders related to receptive language, expressive language, speech intelligibility, voice disorders, alaryngeal speech, or prosody and cognitive impairments; plays an important role in evaluation and treatment of swallowing disorders. Therapists complete a master's degree from an accredited school, a 1-year fellowship, and a national certifying examination.

American Speech-Language- Hearing Association: www.asha.org/

Occupational Therapist (OT): Plans activities that assist and teach clients with physical disabilities to become independent with activities of daily living such as dressing, grooming, bathing, and eating. Once self-care goals have been met, the occupational therapist can help the client perform daily responsibilities of caring for a home and/or returning to work. Educational requirements include completion of an occupational therapy program of study at the baccalaureate, graduate certification, or master's degree level. Graduates must complete a period of supervised clinical experience and state licensure examinations.

American Occupational Therapy Association: www.aota.org/

Respiratory Therapist (RT): Responsible for assessment and maintenance of the client's airway and respiratory equipment used for diagnosis and therapy of respiratory disorders. Activities include client assessment, aerosolized medication administration, sputum sampling, arterial and mixed venous blood sampling, pulmonary function testing, cardiopulmonary stress testing, and sleep studies; may also be involved in conducting pulmonary rehabilitation programs. Respiratory therapists complete a program of study and take a national certifying examination. If the program of study is completed in an associate or bachelor's degree program, the level of credentialing examination is different.

American Association for Respiratory Care: www.aarc.org/

Social Worker: Uses skills to help clients, families, and communities address psychosocial needs. Activities include educating clients, families, and staff about community resources, discharge planning, financial counseling and identifying financial resources, crisis intervention, referring to community resources, abuse and neglect reporting, completing advanced directives, assisting with resolving ethical dilemmas, evaluating behavior and mental disorders, and conducting support groups. Social workers complete a minimum of baccalaureate preparation in the field and may pursue advanced degrees.

National Association of Social Workers: www.naswdc.org/

Chaplain or Pastoral Representative: Attends to the spiritual and emotional needs of the client and family. Activities include providing pastoral counseling and support and sacramental ministry and liturgical celebrations; not all pastoral representatives share the same religion as the client or family members but he or she is able to acknowledge the difference between religions and help to assist the person with spirituality needs. Basic education requirements vary based on the setting and religious affiliation. The Association for Clinical Pastoral Education is a multicultural, multifaith organization devoted to improving the quality of ministry and pastoral care offered by spiritual caregivers of all faiths.

www.acpe-edu.org

Registered Nurse Demographics

Preliminary findings indicate that there are an estimated 2,696,540 RNs in the United States as of March 2000. This represents a 5.4% increase from the 1996 survey, the smallest increase reported in previous surveys. Eighty-one percent of these RNs hold active licenses and are employed in nursing. Approximately 58.5% of this group are employed full time in the profession, with 23.3% of nurses working part time. In 2000 the average age of the RN population was

45.2 years, compared with 44.3 in the 1996 survey report. In 2000 31.7% are under 40 years of age, 18.3% under 35 years, and 9.1% under 30 years. Some speculate that the increase in the average age of RNs may represent the aging society or "second-career" nurses, with younger persons may be choosing other professions.

Although the profession continues to be predominantly female, the number of men working as RNs significantly increased in the past decade. The 2000 report indicates that the number of male RNs increased to 5.9%, up from 5.4% in 1996 data (Division of Nursing–Bureau of Health Professions, National Sample Survey, 2001).

Changes in racial/ethnic backgrounds were reported as well. The March 2000 survey reports that 86.6% of RNs are Caucasian/non-Hispanic, whereas 12.3% are nonwhite and ethnic minorities; 12.3% report being from one or more racial and/or ethnic backgrounds.

Changes also are occurring in the educational preparation of RNs. There has been a substantial increase in the number of nurses graduating from associate degree nursing programs during the past decade. Although not as dramatic an increase, baccalaureate-prepared nurses also are increasing in number. In 2000 graduates from basic nursing programs were 40.3% associate degree, 29.6% baccalaureate degree, and 29.3% diploma graduates. In March 2000 nurses reported their highest degree as 22.3% diploma, 34.3% associate degree, 7% baccalaureate degree, and 10.2% master's or doctoral degree (Division of Nursing–Bureau of Health Professions, National Sample Survey, 2001).

Advanced practice nurses now comprise 7.3% of the RN population, up from 6.3% in 1996. Nurse practitioners lead this group in numbers, followed by CNSs, nurse anesthetists, and nurse midwives. Nurse practitioners and CNSs make up 80% of the advance practice group. (Division of Nursing–Bureau of Health Professions, National Sample Survey, 2001).

Acute care hospitals remain the common worksite for RNs, although there has been a trend toward the outpatient settings. In 2000 59.1% of RNs reported working in hospitals. However, the area with the largest increase in employment was in community and public health settings—a total of 18.3%. About 10% work in physician-based practices, nurse-based practices, or health maintenance organizations (HMOs). Other worksites include educational settings, occupational health settings, nursing management, prisons and jails, and insurance companies (Division of Nursing–Bureau of Health Professions, National Sample Survey, 2001).

The Health Resources and Services Administration (HRSA) is part of the U.S. Department of Health and Human Services. The Bureau of Health Professions, a division of HRSA, provides national information on the health professions workforce in this country. See Box 24-3 for the website for the 2000 National Sample of Registered Nurses (NSRN), the most extensive source of statistics on the RN workforce

Hospital Opportunities

Despite enormous changes in hospital care, it seems evident that there will be jobs in the hospital environment for a long time. In the hospital the nurse in a direct-care role provides care for people who are ill and unable to provide for themselves. A function of the direct-care role also is to help the client and family in managing the illness event. Hospital positions can range from staff nurse to administrator and, in a general hospital, entail any of the clinical specialties and most of the target populations identified in Table 24-1. Determining the area of clinical interest depends mainly on personal preferences.

BOX 24-3	*Helpful Websites*

Air and Surface Transport Nurses Association: 2001, www.astna.org.

Allnurses: 2001, http://allnurses.com/.

American Academy of Nurse Practitioners: www.aanp.org.

American College of Nurse-Midwives, www.midwife.org.

American College of Nurse Practitioners: www.nurse.org/acnp.

American Forensic Nurses: 2001, www.amrn.com/aboutus.htm.

American Nurses Association Infomatics Association: http://www.ania.org/

Division of Nursing–Bureau of Health Professions, Health Resources and Service Administration: Clinical nurse specialist report executive summary, 2001, www.bhpr.hrsa.gov/dn/cnsrepex.htm.

Division of Nursing–Bureau of Health Professions, Health Resources and Service Administration: Nurse Practitioner Workforce Report Executive Summary, 2001, (on-line) Available: bhpr.hrsa.gov/dn/nprepex.htm.

Division of Nursing–Bureau of Health Professions, Health Resources and Service Administration: Preliminary findings from 2000 national sample survey of registered nurses, Washington, DC, 2001, Health Resources and Services Administration, www/hrsa.gov/newsroom/releases/2001%20Releases/nursesurvey.htm.

Forensic Nursing Services, 2001, www.forensicnursing.com/html/about.html.

Hospice concept, www.nho.org

International Association of Forensic Nurses, www.forensicnursing.com/html/about.html.

International Parish Nurse Resource Center: 2001, www.advocatehealth.com/about/faith/parishn.

National Advisory Council on Nurse Education and Practice (NACNEP), http://bhpr.hrsa.gov/dn/nirepex.htm.

National Association for Healthcare Quality: 2001, www.nahq.org.

National Association of Nurse Clinical Specialists: http://www.nacns.org.

National Committee for Quality Assurance: 2001, www.ncqa.org.

National Hospice and Palliative Care Organization: 2001, www.nho.org.

2000 National Sample of Registered Nurses (NSRN): www.bhpr.hrsa.gov (Division of Nursing)

Nelson, Valerie: Shattering the myths about forensic nursing, 1998, www.nurseweek.com/features/98-7/forensic.html.

Nursing infomatics, www.nursing.maryland.edu/~snewbold/sknfaqni.htm.

Nursing specialties, www.allnurses.com/Nursing_Specialties/.

Quality management, www.ncqa.org and www.nahq.org.

So, you wanna be a flight nurse? 2001, www.seaox.com/wannabe.html.

TABLE 24-1	*Trends in Health Care Delivery Systems*

From		To
Acute inpatient care	→	Lifespan care
Treating illness	→	Maintaining health
Focus on the individual	→	Focus on aggregates/populations
Product of care orientation	→	Value of care orientation
Number of hospital admissions	→	Number of lives covered (capitation)
Managing organizations	→	Managing networks
Managing departments	→	Managing markets
Coordinating services	→	Documenting quality and outcomes

Depending on the region of the United States in which one lives, the degree of choice a new graduate might have in the clinical setting is highly variable. However, if the desired arena for work in hospital-based acute care is not available, it may be wise to accept whatever position is offered, with an eye to seeking an internal transfer as a position becomes available in an area of clinical preference. Such an approach is perceived as a willingness to be flexible and to learn. Accepting assignments in an open, cooperative spirit provides more opportunities for the beginning nurse to learn about the organization and gain important experiences. Further, working as a staff nurse offers many learning opportunities in addition to the immediate client-centered ones.

If the choice of the clinical setting has been based on experiences as a student, the new graduate needs to be prepared to have different perceptions in a new role. At a minimum, experiences that are highly enjoyable on the limited-time basis of a student schedule may feel different when the new graduate functions in that role full time. It also is good to have a mix of experiences and learning opportunities before making a definitive decision.

Misleading perceptions about functioning in various clinical arenas are not limited to new graduates. Often a person perceives or believes that one clinical area is the ideal choice, only to find that it is not what he or she wanted. For example, Jane Patrick, RN, wanted to work with sick children and successfully landed a position on the pediatric unit after a couple of years' experience as a staff nurse on an adult surgical wing. Despite her eagerness for the position, Jane found it difficult to adjust to the unit. The distress of the children in the unit was painful to her, and she found herself depressed and unhappy. She began to dream about the children for whom she was caring and was increasingly unable to provide nursing intervention that entailed discomfort for the child. Jane was not in the right place.

It is critical that nurses stay attuned to their reactions and respond in a constructive manner to discoveries such as Jane's. Internal transfers in large hospitals and medical center complexes are common; the probability is high that Jane will find a position that is deeply satisfying in another area.

In addition to clinical emphasis, nursing within hospitals offers almost endless opportunities for diversity. Staff level positions in a hospital can be on many different units, and working different shifts on those units presents different work environments, approaches to work, and priorities of client care. Some examples follow.

Infection Control. The infection control nurse assesses the total incidence of infections within the hospital. Clients who suffer an infection while in the hospital are comprehensively reviewed to ensure prompt and accurate treatment and timely containment of the client's infection so that it is not passed to other clients or staff. The infection control nurse must also conduct a thorough analysis to determine the source of the infection and its onset. If the infection is determined to have been contracted during hospitalization, an investigation is initiated to assess the sequence of events leading up to the infection. A position such as this enables the nurse to have hospital-wide interactions and functioning. Knowledge of epidemiology and outstanding interpersonal skills foster full participation in the infection assessment process.

Quality Management. Although the parameters of a position in quality management or quality control vary from institution to institution, the basic premise is to ensure that outcomes in client care services are consistent with established standards. Benchmarking activities to establish such standards have been under way on a national level for the past few decades. Quality management nurses assess the compliance of the institution with established standards and explore variations from established standards. Chart reviews and ongoing interaction with the staff of the agency are integral components of a quality management position.

Specific Client Services. An almost endless list of specific client services can be found in hospitals, depending on the hospital's size and function within the community. Some nursing positions might be self-evident, such as the intravenous team on which the nurse provides support and interventions with the insertion and maintenance of intravenous therapies. Other services might relate to ostomy care, counseling, support groups, or health education related to a specialty area.

Coordinator Positions. Some hospitals have various coordinator positions such as trauma nurse coordinator. The nurse in this position is responsible for the coordination and integration of the clinical and administrative requirements of the trauma victim. Comprised of equal parts of program and case management, the trauma nurse coordinator role involves overseeing the care of the client from the point of injury through acute care to rehabilitation and back to society (Blansfield, 1995). Maintenance of a comprehensive database on the management of trauma victims is an important part of this position.

Another example of a coordinator position for a highly specialized area is the organ donor coordinator, who procures organs and oversees the transplantation program. Coordinators require considerable experience in the specialty in which they practice.

Variations on Traditional Roles in Nursing

As clients shift from hospital to ambulatory and home care, the role of the community nurse has evolved beyond the traditional public health nurse concept. Although they still have their basis in the framework of the traditional public health nurse concept, nurses today take their critical care skills into the home where clients recover from illness and surgery once only seen in an acute care setting. Pharmacologic and technologic advances make the care of chronic and critically ill clients in their homes a cost-effective option. For example, therapies such as dobutamine administration or chemotherapy were once considered "too risky" for home administration. Today, adequate teaching of the client and family members and careful monitoring make these therapies a daily occurrence. Clients can be monitored through home visits by RNs, expanded technology, radiographs, or telemetry at home. Uterine monitoring for high-risk obstetric clients is common as vital signs of the mother and baby are observed by telephone modem. All these changes increase the need for home care nurses who are expert clinicians and client educators.

Hospice Nurse. As more clients with terminal illness choose to stop aggressive treatment, another nursing specialty has flourished. Over 3000 hospice programs exist in the United States today. The growth of hospice is seen by the 700,000 clients receiving these services in 1999. About 29% of all Americans who died in 1999 had hospice care, an increase from 1998 (NHO, 2001). Hospice and palliative care nurses treat the symptoms of those with progressive terminal disease. These nurses work holistically with clients and families to maximize their quality of life rather than focus on the quantity of life remaining. To learn more about the hospice concept, visit the website (Box 24-3).

Informatics Nurse Specialist. As health care systems face the inevitable need for data management for decision making, another nursing role has emerged—the informatics nurse specialist. Nursing informatics (NI) is a nursing specialty whose activities center around management and processing of health care information. The Division of Nursing–Bureau of Health Professions defines the role of nurse informatics as ". . . combining nursing science, information management science, and computer science to manage and process data, information, and knowledge to deliver quality care to the public, particularly disadvantaged and underserved populations" (National Informatics Agenda, 2001). Recommendations by the National Advisory Council on Nurse Education and Practice (NACNEP) commissioned a panel of experts to advise them in setting the direction needed for NI in this country. For the executive summary of their recommendations, visit their website (see Box 24-3).

The Joint Commission on Accreditation of Healthcare Organizations (JCAHO) recognized the increased need for information management in the clinical client care settings. In 1994 JCAHO standards on information management define management information as critical to organizational success. Nurses are well positioned to assume these roles as they best understand client care processes. Certification is available through the American Nurses Association (ANA) to support this role. The ANA defines informatics as "the activities involved in identifying, naming, organizing, grouping, collecting, processing, analyzing, storing, retrieving, or managing data and information" (ANA, 1994). The ANA Infomatics Association has an information website (see Box 24-3).

Occupational Health Opportunities. Nursing within the framework of specific occupational groups has long been a career option for nurses. Within these settings the nurse designs and implements a program of health promotion and disease prevention for employees and assists with immediate health needs as necessary. In this primary care milieu the nurse assesses the need for programs about specific topics of importance to the health of the employees. Some examples of these might be breast-screening programs for female employees and information on early identification of prostate cancer for male employees. Other programs might revolve around the management of developmental events such as empty nest syndrome, menopause, caring for aging parents, or retirement.

In addition to services related to maintaining the health of employees, the occupational nurse is responsible for the assessment of the work environment to ensure the safety of the employees. Examples of work that has been significant in improving the health of U.S. workers are clean air programs, anti-smoking-on-the-job campaigns, and requirements to eliminate the use of asbestos in heating or insulation of buildings. All of these activities pose special challenges to the occupational health nurse. The nurse in these settings develops procedures to be followed in the event of illness at work, including the management of emergencies.

There also are opportunities in specific industries such as the airline industry. Within the airline industry it is the responsibility of the nurse to contribute to airline safety through maintaining the health of employees. Protection of the employee's health is a component of the role, and of equal concern is the impact of the health of the employee on the safety of the airline and its passengers (Zimmerman, 1996). The nurse must be vigilant in the assessment of employee health problems that could affect overall airline safety. An obvious function is alcohol and drug screening. Protocols for the maintenance of employee health programs in the airline industry must be strictly followed and enforced, as required by government regulation.

Nonetheless, the heart of this nursing position still lies with providing care to people, which sometimes can place the nurse in a difficult position. In the ongoing monitoring of the health of the employees, the nurse often is the first to spot the development of a deviation from health that could affect the career and livelihood of an employee. Such an example is hypertension; if an employee is developing high blood pressure, which will affect his or her employment status, that employee can apply pressure on the nurse to "hear" the blood pressure in the qualifying range.

Morris (1996), who works in an airport health center, perceives that her work is distributed in the following manner: 75% is devoted to administrative activities, 15% to education, and 10% to clinical practice. In this particular center the occupational health and employment screening activities are entwined with urgent care and travel assistance for passengers. Although occasionally an emergency situation develops with a passenger or an employee, most of the client problems are travel-related. For example, international travel to some countries requires comprehensive precautions regarding immunizations and inoculations. In addition, passengers may forget prescribed medications, or medications may be lost in baggage. Short-term problems such as fear of flying also are managed within such a clinic.

Another form of transportation provides a career opportunity: cruise ship nurse. Generally, when people think of a cruise, they do not think of getting sick or getting a job; however, some of the cruise ships in existence are like small cities. One nurse, Wrobleski (1996), describes being the chief nurse on a liner with 2000 passengers and 900 employees. The role of the nurse in this setting is similar to that of the airline nurse with respect to the health of the employees and the safety of the passengers. The unique elements of the ship relate to special sanitation requirements such as testing and culturing the water supply and managing the total health needs of the passengers. It also is the nurse's responsibility to instruct the staff on the basic elements of emergency care and transport. Primary patient care needs are similar to those found in an Emergency Department.

Quality Manager. Another role that is becoming more attractive to nurses is that of quality manager. This reflects the need for health care providers to assess opportunities for process improvement, implement changes, measure outcomes, and then start the improvement process over again. Quality management nurses research and describe findings and look for opportunities to improve care. The result of quality studies may produce critical pathways or algorithms defining care and expected client outcomes. Basic and advanced knowledge of quality management tools is essential, although practice may vary from setting to setting. For instance, in the inpatient setting the quality management nurse needs strong clinical skills as might be acquired in medical-surgical practice, intensive care units, or the operating room. Experience in home care would be an advantage for a quality management nurse in that setting. Interpersonal skills are important because to be successful this role requires building relationships and rapport. The role of quality manager is one that promotes improved care for health care recipients in a variety of settings. Visit the quality management websites for more information (see Box 24-3).

Case Manager. This role has had a rich tradition in community and public health nursing, and it recently has been gaining more prominence in acute care. Case managers coordinate resources to achieve health care outcomes based on quality, access, and cost. The complexity of case management practice is obvious in the era of chaotic systems caused by recent changes in the health care market in which providers, services, and coverage details are constantly changing. Case managers identify the best resources at the lowest cost to achieve the optimum health outcome for the client (Stanhope and Lancaster, 2000).

Flight Nurse. Flight nursing is a specialty for nurses who desire autonomous practice and the opportunity to use advanced clinical skills. Practice is as diverse since clients are all ages and from all backgrounds with different health problems. Critical care experience, with certification in advanced cardiac life support, is necessary. Most programs prefer experienced nurses in critical care and/or Emergency Department nursing. The two types of flying practice available are military, such as in the Air Force Reserves or active duty, and civilian flight nursing. Visit the website *So, You Wanna Be a Flight Nurse* (Box 24-3) to learn more. Nurses who enjoy a fast-paced diverse practice in an unstructured setting may find this role a good fit for them. For more information, call the Air and Surface Transport Nurses Association, formerly known as the National Flight Nurse Association, at 1-800-897-NFNA (6362) or visit their website (see Box 24-3).

Telephone Triage Nurse. Another emerging career is that of telephone triage nurse. In this practice nurses interact with clients on the telephone to assess needs, intervene, and evaluate. This position requires excellent communication and assessment skills, as well as problem-solving skills. Telephone triage is used in a variety of settings, including Emergency Departments and physician practices.

Forensic Nurse. Forensic nursing may well be one of the fastest-growing nursing specialties in the twenty-first century. This is likely due to the United States' epidemic increase in violence and resulting trauma. The ANA's Scope and Standards of Forensic Nursing Practice, published by American Nurses Publishing, serves as a professional guide for nurses working in or entering this evolving specialty. Forensic nursing applies nursing science to public or legal proceedings in the scientific investigation and treatment of trauma and/or death of victims of violence, abuse, criminal activity, and traumatic accidents. The nurse may provide direct services to individual clients, as well as consult with and/or be an expert witness for medical and law enforcement.

To learn more about this exciting practice, visit the International Association of Forensic Nurses (IAFN) website (see Box 24-3). The American Forensic Nurses' Organization offers distance-learning programs through the Internet (see their website in Box 24-3).

School Nurse. Most registered professional nurses employed in school health are generalists prepared at the baccalaureate level who function as consultants/coordinators. The newer role for school nurses is school health manager or coordinator and includes functions such as policy-making, case management, and program management activities; and health promotion and protection activities (Stanhope and Lancaster, 2000).

Parish Nurse. The role of parish nurse is quickly becoming a recognized specialty in growing professional practice. In 1998 the ANA, in collaboration with the Health Ministries Association, established the scope and standards of this professional practice. This role focuses on health promotion within the beliefs, values, and practices of faith communities. Health is seen as a sense of physical, psychologic, social, and spiritual well-being. Health is further viewed as being in harmony with self, others, the environment, and God. The parish nurse functions as counselor, teacher, referral agent, volunteer coordinator, and integrator of spiritual care and health. Although all communities do not have a hospital or clinic, most have a faith community, providing an exciting setting to teach disease prevention and health promotion.

The late Granger Westberg (1988), founder of this role in the mid 1980s, proposed that clergy can and already do more in the field of preventive medicine than traditional physicians. Westberg's efforts focused on getting the medical establishment to recognize faith communities as partners in keeping people well. He stated that churches, even though they may not realize it, are in the health business. In this role parish nurses participate in joint ministry with other staff members, helping to integrate faith and health for healing and wholeness. For more information on this practice, visit the website of the International Parish Nurse Association (see Box 24-3).

Other Unique Roles. Career opportunities described in this chapter should not be considered an exhaustive list of possibilities. Nurses now have multiple selections for practice areas never before considered. Nurses should be encouraged to adopt an attitude of openness, an attitude of creativity, and a willingness to take a chance to explore different possibilities. Nurses can let their imaginations take them to unknown settings or explore uncharted waters. To do this, nurses must develop confidence in their abilities and talents and be willing to venture outside the norm. One website lists over 50 categories of roles for nurses with links and discussions areas (see Nursing Specialties, Box 24-3).

There are those in the nursing profession who would limit the possibilities for the profession, claiming that alternatives are not really "nursing." However, this mindset severely limits the expansion of professional nursing in a changing health care environment. For nursing to thrive, new roles need to be defined and refined for future success of the discipline.

One way to settle this dispute within the nursing profession is to evaluate new nursing roles through the definition established by the ANA (1980). Nursing is the diagnosis and treatment of the human response to health and illness. Therefore evolving nursing roles should be evaluated based on the ability of the new role to fit this accepted definition. Does the newly created role require assessment, diagnosis, planning, implementation, or evaluation to human responses? Does the newly created role require the knowledge and expertise of a professional nurse? Through answering these questions, nurses can see that nursing is bigger, more encompassing, than what was once termed "traditional" nursing.

ADVANCED PRACTICE NURSING

There is much written in the professional and lay literature about advanced practice nursing. Although new roles in advanced nursing may be forthcoming, the term advanced practice nurse (APN) is presently a descriptor that includes nurse practitioners (NPs), CNMs, CRNAs, and CNSs. A more formal definition developed by the National Council of State Boards of

Nursing (1992) defines advanced practice nursing as ". . . practice based on knowledge and skills acquired in a basic nursing education, through licensure as a registered nurse, and in graduate education and experience, including advanced nursing theory, physical assessment, and psychosocial assessment and treatment of illness."

Each specialty of APN has unique differences, although there are key elements that the specialties share. All APNs make independent and collaborative health care decisions and engage in active practice as expert clinicians. APNs are educationally prepared through master's level education to demonstrate leadership as consultants, educators, administrators, and researchers. They are expected to provide their client populations with advanced assessment skills and to possess the ability to synthesize and analyze data beyond the level of basic nursing.

Nurse Practitioner

NPs engage in advanced practice in a variety of specialty areas such as family, adult, pediatric, geriatric, women's health, school health, occupational health, mental health, emergency, and acute care. Typically NPs assess and manage medical and nursing problems. Health promotion and maintenance, as well as disease prevention, are the emphases of their practice. Some NPs diagnose and manage acute and chronic diseases of their selected population.

Job responsibilities of NPs include taking client histories; conducting physical examinations; ordering, performing, and interpreting diagnostic tests; and prescribing pharmacologic agents, treatments, and therapies for the management of client conditions. Frequently the NP serves as a primary care provider and consultant for individuals, families, or communities.

NPs have advanced education, with specific emphasis on pathophysiology and pharmacology. Certification is achieved via written examination after the completion of a master's level program. Several professional organizations offer certification for NPs. For example, pediatric NPs are certified by the National Certification Board of Pediatric Nurse Practitioners; adult NPs or family NPs may be certified by the American Academy of Nurse Practitioners. Visit their website (see Box 24-3).

NPs achieve registration and licensure by state boards of nursing or other designated agencies. The state boards of nursing regulate NP practice and prescriptive authority.

The National Advisory Council on Nurse Education and Practice (NACNEP), established by Title VIII of the Public Health Service, provided a Nurse Practitioner Workforce report (see NACNEP, Box 24-3). The American College of Nurse Practitioners' website offers further professional information (see Box 24-3).

Clinical Nurse Specialist

CNSs are APNs who possess clinical expertise in a defined area of nursing practice for a selected client population or clinical setting. This practice specialty emphasizes the diagnosis and management of human responses to actual or potential health problems.

The CNS functions as an expert clinician, educator, consultant, researcher, and administrator. The CNS monitors the care of clients and collaborates with physicians, nurses, and other members of the transdisciplinary health care team. The emphasis of this advanced nursing practice is to provide clinical support that improves client care and client outcomes.

CNSs are educated in graduate nursing programs. Their expertise is acquired from combining graduate study with clinical experience. The educational program for CNSs features an intense study of nursing theories and knowledge from other disciplines. Programs emphasize advanced scientific concepts, research methodologies, and supervised clinical practice.

CNSs practice within a systems model paradigm, which means that in performing their role, CNSs evaluate each client in the context of his or her social environment. These APNs view clients as individuals who are part of a larger society entering a complex health care delivery system. This practice philosophy prompts the CNS to use a comprehensive approach to client care.

As consultants, CNSs are called on for expert clinical advice within and outside the clinical setting. Their consultation function frequently consists of problem solving with a client who may be a colleague, an individual, family, group, agency, or community. Problems may be related to provider competence, equipment, facilities, or health care delivery systems.

CNSs contribute to research in their area of specialization, generating and refining research questions, interpreting research findings, applying them to clinical practice, and educating other nurses about research findings. As teachers, CNSs educate clients, families, and communities. The CNS functions as a role model or preceptor for nurse generalists and students in a variety of clinical settings (ANA, 1986).

The National Advisory Council on Nurse Education and Practice (NACNEP), established by Title VIII of the Public Health Service, provided a CNS report (see NACNEP, Box 24-3).

Certified Registered Nurse Anesthetist

Established in the late 1800s, nurse anesthesia is recognized as the first clinical nursing specialty. Nurse anesthesia practice developed in response to requests from surgeons seeking a solution to the high morbidity and mortality attributed to anesthesia at that time. The most famous nurse anesthetist of the nineteenth century, Alice Magaw, "mother of anesthesia," worked at St. Mary's Hospital in Rochester, Minnesota. Magaw was instrumental in establishing a showcase of professional excellence in anesthesia and surgery. In 1909 the first formal educational programs preparing nurse anesthetists were established (Bankert, 1989).

Since World War I nurse anesthetists have been the principal anesthesia providers in combat areas of every war in which the United States has been engaged. Although nurse anesthesia educational programs existed before World War I, the war sharply increased the demand for nurse anesthetists and, consequently, the need for more educational programs.

Founded in 1931, the American Association of Nurse Anesthetists (AANA) is the professional association representing more than 27,000 nurse anesthetists nationwide. The AANA promotes education, practice standards, and guidelines and affords consultation to both private and governmental entities regarding nurse anesthetists and their practice.

The AANA developed and implemented a certification program in 1945 and instituted mandatory recertification in 1978. The association established a mechanism for accreditation of nurse anesthesia educational programs in 1952 (Thatcher, 1973). Additional information is available at the AANA website (see Box 24-3).

The educational preparation of CRNAs occurs at the graduate level or in association with traditional institutions of higher education, most commonly in schools of nursing or health sciences. The educational curriculum in the anesthesia specialty ranges from 24 to 36 months in an integrated program of academic and clinical study. The academic curriculum consists of a minimum of 30 credit hours of formalized graduate study in courses such as advanced anatomy, physiology, pathophysiology, advanced pharmacology, principles of anesthesia practice, and research methodology and statistical analysis. All programs require approximately 1000 hours of hands-on clinical experience. Students gain experience with clients of all ages who require medical, obstetric, dental, and pediatric interventions.

Admission requirements to a nurse anesthesia educational program include a Bachelor of Science degree in nursing, license as an RN, and a minimum of 1 year of acute care nursing experience. Nurse anesthetists are required to successfully complete a written examination for certification as a CRNA.

Recertification, which includes a practice and continuing education requirement, must be met every 2 years. CRNAs are qualified to make independent judgments relative to all aspects of anesthesia care based on their education, licensure, and certification. CRNAs provide anesthesia and anesthesia-related care on request, assignment, or referral by a client's physician most often to facilitate diagnostic, therapeutic, or surgical procedures. In other instances CRNAs perform consultation or assistance for management of pain associated with obstetric labor and delivery, management of acute or chronic ventilatory problems, or management of acute or chronic pain through the performance of selected diagnostic or therapeutic blocks.

The laws of every state permit CRNAs to work directly with a physician or other authorized health care professional such as a dentist without being supervised by an anesthesiologist. The JCAHO does not require anesthesiologist supervision of CRNAs nor does Medicare. In some cases a provider, payer, or medical staff bylaws may require anesthesiologist supervision. However, these decisions are not based on legal requirements (AANA, 1992).

Certified Nurse-Midwife

According to the American College of Nurse-Midwives (ACNM, 1995) nurse midwifery practice is the independent management of women's health care, focusing particularly on pregnancy, childbirth, the postpartum period, care of the newborn, and the family planning and gynecologic needs of women. This practice occurs within a health care system that provides consultation, collaborative management, or referral as indicated by the health status of the client.

A CNM is educated in the two disciplines of nursing and midwifery and possesses evidence of certification according to the requirements of the ACNM. A CNM has successfully completed prescribed studies in midwifery and has met the requisite qualifications to be certified. A CNM is legally qualified to practice in one or more of the 50 states. The ACNM supports educational programs for CNMs at the certificate and the degree level but opposes mandatory degree requirements for state licensure.

The ACNM claims that mandatory degree requirements would limit access to maternity and gynecologic services for women. Several national reports specifically recommend placing greater reliance on CNMs to increase access to prenatal care for underserved populations. These reports also recommend that state laws should be supportive of nurse-midwifery practice.

The entry-level midwife is a primary health care professional who independently provides care during pregnancy, birth, and the postpartum period for women and newborns within their communities. Therefore the CNM is an individual who has successfully completed an ACNM-accredited educational program in nurse-midwifery and passed the national certification examination administered by the ACNM Certification Council. Additional information is available at the ACNM website (see Box 24-3).

Midwifery care occurs within a variety of settings, including homes, birthing centers, clinics, and hospitals. The midwife works with each woman and her family to identify their unique physical, social, and emotional needs. Services provided by the midwife include education and health promotion.

With additional education and experience, the midwife may provide well-woman gynecologic care, including family planning services. When the care required extends beyond the midwife's abilities, the midwife should have a mechanism for consultation and referral.

CNMs are an expanding group of professionals. Each year approximately 400 nurse-midwives pass the national certification examination. Since 1991 the number of CNMs who are certified each year has increased by 25%. Currently there are 50 accredited nurse-midwifery education programs in the United States. Approximately 68% of CNMs have a master's degree. Four percent have a doctoral degree. Nurse-midwifery practice is legal in all 50 states and the District of Columbia (Division of Nursing–Bureau of Health Professionals, 2001).

Nurse Administrator/Nurse Executive

Although not formally considered an advanced practice nurse, the nurse executive has an important advanced role within nursing. It is vital that individuals be knowledgeable about the business of the health care system and the profession of nursing. Nursing administration unites the leadership perspective of professional nursing with the various aspects of business and health administration. The practice of nursing administration focuses on the administration of health care systems for the purpose of delivering services to groups of clients.

Individuals who assume a nurse executive role typically hold a master's degree. Both master's and doctoral level programs that offer degrees in nursing administration are available, although some nursing executives are educated in additional disciplines such as business.

Nursing administration research focuses on organizational factors and management practices and their impact on nurses, nursing delivery systems, and client outcomes. Nursing administration is concerned with establishing the costs of nursing care and examining relationships between nursing services and quality client care. Nurse executives are called on to view problems of nursing service delivery within a broader context of policy analysis and delivery of health care services.

Nursing administration is an integral part of any organization that provides health care. Nurse administrators lead and direct large groups of nurses and ancillary personnel. They manage large budgets and are responsible for provision of quality care at reasonable cost. They serve at all management levels in health care organizations and in the community.

WHAT ABOUT THE FUTURE?

The future of nursing is brighter than ever. Because of never-ending changes in the health care environment, many new jobs will result. Growth of the nursing profession also will be prompted by technologic advances in client care, which allow an increased number of health problems to be detected early and managed quickly. A greater number of sophisticated health-related procedures already are performed not only in hospitals but in a variety of settings such as clinics and physician's offices. Health maintenance organizations, ambulatory surgicenters, and church health centers are only a few of the places where the public will receive their health care. Nursing can be a vital component of the "alternative setting" movement that is on the forefront of health care reform.

As the focus of health care shifts to disease prevention and modification of lifestyles, the opportunities for nurses will follow. Nursing also can benefit from the increased emphasis on primary care because prevention is the only true mechanism to reduce health care expenditures. Professional nursing services should be viewed as a cost-effective way to provide disease prevention and health-promotion activities in multiple areas of the community, including industry, business, and commerce. Wellness and disease prevention, historically fundamental to the nursing profession, are now becoming more meaningful and revitalized concepts within the larger health care system.

There always will be a need for the traditional role of the hospital nurse. Although the number of acute care beds will decrease, the intensity of hospital nursing care is likely to increase. Increases in client acuity will expand the need for professional nursing within the hospital setting. However, the most rapid growth for nursing employment is expected in out-patient facilities such as same-day surgery, rehabilitation, and chemotherapy infusion centers.

Nurses also will see job opportunities continue to develop in home health care. Many factors contribute to this phenomenon. The increasing numbers of older persons with disabilities require nursing care to minimize their functional loss and optimize their quality of life. Another factor that promotes home care is the consumer's preference for care in his or her own home. Home care is a feasible option with recent technologic advances. Complex health care treatment that was once thought only possible in the hospital setting is now a reality in the home. Professional nurses who are able to perform complex procedures and comprehensive client assessments will be invaluable to the home care industry.

Financial pressures on hospitals to discharge clients as soon as possible are producing increased admissions to nursing homes, skilled nursing facilities, and long-term rehabilitation units. In addition, because many individuals are aging into their ninth and tenth decades, the number of people entering nursing homes or assisted-living facilities will increase. The opportunity for nursing is tremendous in the long-term care arena because no other discipline can offer the multiple skills nursing has to offer to the aging population.

Yet the nursing profession must heed the old cliché that "opportunity only knocks once." If nurses fail to seize their opportunity, other less qualified health care providers will attempt to move into this advantageous position. It is truly up to the individuals in the nursing profession to demonstrate their contribution to health care and publicly market their potential. The nursing profession historically has requested a chance to prove its worth in producing cost-effective, quality health care—now is the time.

SUMMARY

This chapter explores the various roles available to professional nurses today. Social and economic trends influencing the development of new nursing roles in innovative practice settings have been discussed. Encouragement for nurses who are interested in developing new roles is provided by examples of nurses who envisioned and created new roles. Traditional, nontraditional, and advanced practice nursing roles offer many exciting opportunities for professional growth and satisfaction. The diversity and challenge available to professional nurses today is unparalleled.

Critical Thinking Activities

1. Identify a setting in the community where the influences of professional nursing may be needed but do not presently exist. Develop a job description for the newly created role. What educational preparation would be required for this role? Discuss strategies to market or support the new nursing position. Evaluate the newly developed role within the context of the ANA definition of professional nursing practice.
2. Compare and contrast advanced practice roles such as clinical nurse specialist, nurse practitioner, nurse midwife, and nurse anesthetist. How would you explain the differences to a lay person?
3. Analyze the influence of current trends in health care on the development of new nursing roles.
4. Evaluate the impact of health care trends on traditional nursing roles.
5. Compare and contrast skills needed by the nurse who works in an occupational health setting and a nurse who works in a critical care unit.

REFERENCES

American Association of Nurse Anesthetists: *Qualifications and capabilities of the certified registered nurse anesthetists,* Park Ridge, Ill, 1992, AANA.

American College of Nurse Midwives: *Professional standards and practice,* Washington, DC, 1995, ACNM.

American Nurses Association: *Nursing: a social policy,* Washington, DC, 1980, ANA.

American Nurses Association: *The role of the clinical nurse specialist,* Kansas City, Mo, 1986, ANA.

American Nurses Association: *The scope and practice of nursing informatics,* Washington, DC, 1994, ANA.

Baggs J: Intensive care unity use and collaboration between nurses and physicians, *Heart Lung* 18:332-338, 1989.

Baggs J et al: The association between interdisciplinary collaboration and patient outcomes in a medical intensive care unit, *Heart Lung* 21:18-24, 1992.

Bankert M: *Watchful care: a history of America's nurse anesthetists,* New York, 1989, Continuum.

Blansfield J: Trauma nurse coordinator, *J Emerg Nurs* 22:486-488, 1995.

Division of Nursing–Bureau of Health Professions, Health Resources Service Administration: *The national sample survey of registered nurses, March 2000* preliminary findings, Washington, DC, 2001, Health Resources and Service Administration.

Knaus W et al: An evaluation of outcomes from intensive care in major medical centers, *Ann Intern Med* 104: 411-418, 1986.

Morris J: Working at an airport medical center. *J Emerg Nurs* 22:530-531, 1996.

National Council of State Boards of Nursing: *National councils of state boards of nursing position paper of the licensure of advanced nursing practice,* Chicago, 1992, NCSBN.

National Informatics Agenda for Nursing Education and Practice (NACNEP): December 1997, www.bhpr.hrsa.gov/dn/nirepex.htm.

Stanhope M, Lancaster J: *Community and Public Health Nursing,* ed 5, St Louis, 2000, Mosby

Thatcher VS: *History of anesthesia with emphasis of the nurse specialist,* Philadelphia, 1973, JB Lippincott.

Van Ess Coeling H, Cukr, P: Collaboration in practice. In Price S, Koch M, Bassett S, editors: *Health care resource management,* St Louis, 1998, Mosby.

Wasserman K: Improving the process of care: the cost-quality value of interdisciplinary collaboration, *J Nurs Care Qual* 10(2):10-16, 1997

Westberg GE: *Parishes, nurses, and health care,* Lutheran Partners, November/December, 1988.

Wrobleski D: Interview with a cruise ship nurse, *J Emerg Nurs* 22:546-549, 1996.

Zimmerman P: Airline nurse. *J Emerg Nurs* 22:549-551, 1996.

SUGGESTED READINGS

Cohjen SS, Juszczak L: Promoting the nurse practitioner role in managed care, *J Pediatr Health Care* 11(1):3-11, 1997.

Fitzgerald SM, Wood SH: Advanced practice nursing: back to the future, *J Gynecol Neonatal Nurs* 26(1):101-107, 1997.

Hester LE, White MJ: Perception of practicing CNSs about their future role, *Clin Nurse Spec* 10(4):190-193, 1996.

Hickey JV, Quimette RM, Venegoni SL: *Advanced practice nursing—changing roles and clinical application,* Philadelphia, 1996, Lippincott-Raven.

Koch RW: Intrapreneurship: bloom where you're planted, *Tenn Nurse* 59(2):15-16, 1996.

Kupina PS: Community health CNSs and health care in the year 2000, *Clin Nurse Spec* 9(4):188-198, 1995.

O'Brien C: Sexual assault nurse examiner (SANE) program coordinator, *J Emerg Nurs* 22(6):532-533, 1996.

Parker CD, Gassert C: JCAHO's management of information standards—the role of the informatics specialist, *J Nurs Admin* 26(6):13-15, 1996.

Stokes E, Whitis G, Moore-Threasher L: Characteristics of graduate adult health nursing programs, *J Nurs Educ* 36(2):54-59, 1997.

US Department of Labor, Bureau of Labor Statistics: *Occupational outlook handbook,* Washington, DC, 1996, US Department of Labor.

Watts RJ: Critical care nurse practitioner curriculum at the University of Pennsylvania: update and revision, *Am Assoc Crit Care Nurse* 8(1):116-122, 1997.

Wojner AW, Kite-Powell D: Outcomes manager: a role for the advanced practice nurse, *Crit Care Nurs Q* 19(4):16-24, 1997.

Job Search: Finding Your Match

Kathryn S. Skinner, MS, RN, CS, and Laura Day, BSN, MS, RN

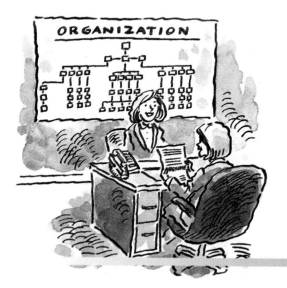

Finding the right match can
be exciting!

Vignette

"For 2 years I've struggled to meet deadlines for term papers, nursing care plans, and examinations. Now that graduation is almost here, I'm scared that I don't know enough to be a 'real nurse.' And I'm confused about where I should begin and what kind of nursing position I should seek. This first job seems so important."

Questions to consider while reading this chapter
1. How should the new graduate in the scenario decide where to apply for that first position?
2. What kinds of questions should the applicant ask about a prospective position?
3. How can the applicant demonstrate knowledge, skills, and experience to the recruiter?

Key Terms

Orientation Activities that enhance adaptation to a new environment.
Professional objective Occupational position for which one aims.
Resumé Summary of a job applicant's previous work experience and education.
Portfolio A collection of evidence acknowledging acquisition of skills, knowledge, and achievements related to a professional career.

Learning Outcomes

After studying this chapter, the reader will be able to:

1. Use the interview process to evaluate potential employment opportunities.
2. Prepare an effective resumé.
3. Compare and contrast various professional nursing employment opportunities.
4. Summarize the employment process.

CHAPTER OVERVIEW

This chapter helps student nurses prepare to successfully negotiate their first employment as professional nurses. They learn the importance of networking; researching available opportunities; and examining their personal aptitudes, interests, lifestyle priorities, and long-term goals to find the best job fit.

Readers are shown how to create and use cover letters and resumés to market themselves in written introductions and how to prepare for and actively participate in a recruitment interview. The chapter describes what can be expected from a recruiter and how to obtain the information needed to make thoughtful and rewarding job choices. Putting these recommendations into practice will ensure the new graduate of the best chance for finding a good job match as an entry-level nurse practicing in a suitable work environment.

EXPLORING OPTIONS

The job market for graduate nurses is very good. There are many opportunities in both urban and rural areas. Although health care economics ride a roller coaster from robust to lean times, with the demand and supply of nurses 1 or 2 years behind the lead, always trying to catch up, the overall need for the skills of professional registered nurses (RNs) remains constant, and the potential for finding suitable employment is excellent. Recent trends in health care dictate that today's health care providers change their orientation from disease to health and from inpatient to outpatient services. Therefore there is a growing need for professional nurses in nonacute community-based care settings such as primary care clinics; ambulatory surgery centers; and home, school, and work environments. However, although rapid changes in health care delivery systems continue to create new and varied opportunities outside the acute care settings where nurses have traditionally practiced, hospitals remain the most likely starting place for new graduates to acquire general experience helpful in opening career path doors. In fact, with the recent nursing shortage there is an increased demand for nurses to work in acute care settings.

Numerous marketing strategies have been tried in an effort to aggressively attract bright, energetic new graduates in times of demand and short supply. For some institutions cost seems irrelevant. Sign-on bonuses, expense-paid weekends to visit institutions in other parts of the United States, promises of tuition reimbursement for continued education, student loan repayment, and low interest loans for new cars, just to name a few, have been offered as enticements. However, being aware of one's own personal qualities and taking advantage of networking opportunities are keys to finding just the right match in today's job market.

Knowing Oneself

The choice of one's first nursing position deserves study. For some the opportunities seem to be a smorgasbord of possibilities, all of them attractive. The neophyte nurse should carefully explore any job under consideration and its responsibilities in light of his or her own personal qualities. Some students find it helpful to consult an instructor, job counselor, or a trusted nursing mentor for objective input and perspective. An experienced nurse can see the pros and cons that would not be visible to a new nurse. A thoughtful review of general interests, abilities, and strengths, especially those pointed out by clinical instructors, and the types of patients who have provided the greatest emotional reward is essential. Other important considerations are one's physical and emotional stamina, energy level, and responsibilities to others—spouse, children and other family members, volunteer commitments, and social activities—all of which make legitimate demands on one's schedule. Long-term goals must be factored into the first job choice as well. Is the first job a stepping stone to an advanced degree, to a narrowly specialized area of nursing, or to a management role? Selection of a position that fits the nurse's abilities, lifestyle, and career aspirations will affect job satisfaction, career advancement, and overall sense of success and happiness.

Working in an environment that does not match well with one's attributes and long-term goals could not only make the graduate nurse miserable, but it could damage future employment options. Poor job fits lead to frequent job changes, which could lead to poor references, as well as a label of "job hopper."

Ill-considered job choices not only cost the new graduate, but they also are expensive for the employer. Some estimate the cost of recruiting, placing, and orienting a new nurse to be more than $12,000. Having a new nurse join a unit, start orientation, and then become disheartened and quit lowers the morale of the staff and manager and can have negative consequences on patient care, especially if turnover is repeated.

Networking

The investigative process of researching potential employers begins with networking at school, in the community, and within student nurse organizations. One may question other nurses, employees, and former employees, especially alumni of one's own school who have worked in various settings. Faculty will have pertinent observations based on their experiences with clinical sites in the community. Perhaps most valuable is listening to neighbors, friends, and family members who have been patients.

BOX 25-1	*Helpful Websites*
www.nsna.org	www.nursingworld.org/
www.medsearch.com/	wwwnurse.com/
www.monster.com	nursingcenter.com/
www.nursingspectrum.com	www.southern-healthcare.com/
www.nursing-jobs.com/	www.springnet.com/career.htm
www.wmed.com/hospdir.html	www.nursezone.com

The Internet also offers links to actual jobs, as well as information on career planning. Most hospital and large health care systems maintain websites to post their employment needs and in many cases invite applications online. Examples of Internet sites that would be helpful in exploring job opportunities, writing resumés, and preparing for employment interviews are contained in Box 25-1.

If a new graduate is fortunate to be seeking a position in a large community with multiple job choices available, this informal research will help to narrow the best place to begin the job application process. Later in the interview, the applicant may wish to describe to the recruiter how his or her search resulted in this employer being the number one choice over others for the graduate's first job. This process of researching potential employers will continue through the interview process. Assessing the climate of the work environment is a valuable tool in "finding a match" and is discussed later in this chapter.

WRITTEN INTRODUCTIONS

Three of the most important steps in a job search are writing a cover letter, preparing a professional resumé, and assembling a professional portfolio. These tools introduce the applicant to a prospective employer. The first impression should be persuasive; there may not be a second chance. Presenting oneself on paper can make a difference, perhaps the difference between getting a desired interview and being passed over in favor of someone else. Both types of introductions should present a conscientious, mature, competent, committed professional who would be an asset to an agency that prides itself on its nursing services.

How To Write a Cover Letter

The cover letter (Box 25-2) is a chance to sell oneself and make the recruiter look forward to meeting an attractive candidate. A convincing cover letter will show how this candidate is different and will convey to the recruiter why he or she is the best fit for the position. The letter should also address why this institution is the applicant's first choice.

A cover letter should reflect the nurse's own style of writing, should never appear to have been copied from a book, and should be tailored to the particular job. Like any business document, it should be clean, direct, and letter perfect. It should be attractive and effortless to read. There must be no obvious erasures, no typing errors, no evidence of correction fluid, and no grammar or spelling mistakes. Everything should fit on a single page of 8.5 × 11-inch white, heavyweight bond paper with ample margins on the top, bottom, and sides.

The letter should be addressed to a specific person. If the person's name or title is unknown, refer to a marketing brochure or call the recruitment office to ask for correct title and spelling of the appropriate person's first and last names.

If spelling is not a strength, using spell-check on the computer is a must; using a dictionary or the assistance of a friend who will proofread the final copy is also a good idea. Poor typists would be well served to pay someone to type for them. A sloppy letter should never determine one's opportunities in the job market.

The body of the letter should be single-spaced, three or four paragraphs in length, skipping a line between paragraphs, and organized as follows:

- Paragraph one should be a statement of purpose that tells the recruiter what kind of position is being sought, the writer's expected date of graduation, state licensing status, and when the writer will be ready to begin work.
- Paragraph two should emphasize the writer's suitability. The unspoken message should be, "I'm just the person for the job!" without going into all the details that will

BOX 25-2	*Cover Letter*

April 8, 2002

Ms. Donna Henderson, RN, MS
Director of Nurse Recruitment
Charleston Memorial Hospital
1600 Beckley Avenue
Memphis, Tennessee 38104

Dear Ms. Henderson:

I would like to apply for a new graduate position on a cardiology nursing unit at Charleston Memorial Hospital. After graduating from Smith College with a BSN on June 6, I will be ready to start work immediately. I plan to take the RN licensing examination in early July.

Through reading about your hospital and my own personal experience in a recent clinical rotation at Charleston Memorial, I have learned that your institution is a modern, professional one with an emphasis on quality patient care. For this and many other reasons, I am convinced that Charleston Memorial is where I want to work as a nurse.

I will be in Memphis on April 20-25 and will call to schedule an appointment to see you then. My phone number is 555-912-3120.

I look forward to meeting you and discussing how I can contribute to Charleston Memorial Hospital.

Sincerely,

Bonnie McCray Pino

Enclosure

be included in the resumé. A sentence should describe past work or educational experiences that relate to the agency's particular needs and philosophy. The more homework the nurse has done in learning about the institution, the more convinced the recruiter will be. Finally refer to the enclosed resumé.

- Paragraph three should request an interview appointment and give a range of dates of availability. It is a good idea for the writer to promise a telephone call "next week" or "soon" to schedule a meeting time and provide a telephone number where the writer can be reached, if the number is different from the permanent telephone number listed on the resumé.
- The letter can end with a "written handshake" such as, "I look forward to meeting with you to discuss available nursing positions in your institution"—a cautious, but upbeat note.
- The letter closes with "Sincerely," and after four lines of space for a signature, the writer's name is typed. A line is skipped, and "Enclosure" is typed on the left margin to indicate that a resumé is enclosed.

- The letter should be proofread carefully, signed, and copied; and the copy filed. If the nurse has chosen to use different approaches with different institutions, it would be wise to review the cover letter before the interview.

One week later, one should follow up by telephone to be sure the letter was received. This attention to detail and follow-through will impress the recruiter or personnel office and improve chances of getting an interview soon. These telephone calls become mini-interviews, and one should be extra courteous, aware that it usually is the secretary who controls the interview schedule. By keeping a written list of all contacts made, the new graduate will be able to add the flattering personal touch of acknowledging previous telephone contacts when meeting them for the first time during the interview process.

The cover letter serves as the foundation on which all other follow-up is built: resumé, call for appointment, and interview. What is presented in the letter should prompt the person responsible for hiring to take a good look at the enclosed resumé.

How To Prepare a Resumé

A resumé is an opportunity to tell a condensed story of one's professional life (Box 25-3). It will complement the cover letter by filling in important details about educational and work experiences. An effective resumé should compress education and employment history into an attractive, easy-to-read, one-page summary. A wealth of valuable information can be communicated simply and straightforwardly by saying more with less. The key is writing concisely. For example, "BSN with High Honors" speaks for itself. Citing grade point average or Dean's list standing adds little. Succinct ways to convey a message will be found by experimenting with phrases and word choices. Avoid pompous language and passive voice. Instead use active verbs such as improved, established, trained, administered, prepared, wrote, and evaluated. Pepper the resumé with such words, and it will read easily.

A basic resumé contains three essential sections: identifying information, education, and work experience. In addition, optional information may include professional objectives, honors, achievements, and memberships in professional organizations. A well-designed resumé will mark the writer as a career-minded professional, just what recruiters are seeking. A succinct well-organized resumé indicates that the applicant is focused and organized in other areas as well.

The first section of the resumé, the identifying information, contains the name, address, and home and work telephone numbers, followed by licensure information. The states of licensure and license numbers are listed. Graduating students should indicate when and where the National Council of Licensing Examination (NCLEX) was taken or will be taken.

If the resumé writer opts to include a professional objective, it should be next. Some interviewers like to see this because it shows that the nurse has put some thought into career planning. One should beware; it is limiting to put forth a singular objective that ties the nurse to only one particular clinical area. If there is no opening available in that department, the recruiter will consider the applicant an unlikely candidate to pursue. It is better to have an objective statement that is broad and general.

The second section should include details about education, including degrees and diplomas awarded, names and locations of schools, and graduation dates, starting with the most recent graduation and degree in reverse chronologic order.

The third section will present the information apt to be the greatest help in obtaining a job: work experience and employment history. Many recruiters are nurses themselves, so a

---

BOX 25-3 *Resumé*

Bonnie McCray Pino
416 Melody Avenue
Bristol, Tennessee 37620
(555) 912-3720
Professional

Objective:	Staff nurse position (cardiology)
	Anticipated date of NCLEX: July 2002
Licensure:	Eligible to take NCLEX after June 6, 2002
	Anticipated date of NCLEX: July 2002
Education:	Smith College School of Nursing
1998-2002	Bristol, TN
	BSN, June 6, 2002
1994-1998	Oakview High School
	Nashville, TN
	Diploma, June, 1998

Experience:

May 2001–August 2001 St. Mary's Hospital, Knoxville, TN
Patient Care Assistant: assisted RNs in providing basic nursing care including feeding, bathing, ADLs, and patient teaching in a pediatric setting
June 1999–August 1999 Drs. Smith and Jones OB/GYN office, Bristol, TN
Office Assistant: accompanied patients to treatment area, weighed, and recorded vital signs
Honors: Sigma Theta Tau International, 2001
        Who's Who Among American High School Students
Professional Organizations: Tennessee Student Nurses Association, 1998–2002
References: Provided on request

---

detailed description of what a routine job entails is not needed. Instead, efforts should be directed toward illustrating any special knowledge or contributions. The new graduate's resumé might reflect student accomplishments or elaborate on jobs in which he or she has demonstrated skills also applicable to nursing responsibilities, such as organization of tasks, time management, delegation to subordinates, and ability to work well with others. Start with current or most recent position and work backward, including place of employment, job title, dates worked, and responsibilities. List accomplishments while employed, including number and type of patients cared for, any special techniques used, or any participation in the development of programs, policies, or forms pertinent to the position.

This section closes with optional information such as seminars attended, honors received, and memberships in professional organizations. It is not advisable to list community activities or activities from more than 5 years ago, unless it can be shown that they are pertinent to a nursing career. Similarly, one should exclude personal information such as marital and health status, age, number of children, and hobbies. This information is not job related and should not be used by the employer to screen applicants.

References do not need to be included in the resumé but should be ready for presentation in a neatly typed, photocopied list when the request does come from any future employer. Simply state, "References provided on request," or "References available." When someone agrees to be listed as a reference, take time to discuss what prospective employers may want to know. Former instructors or former employers may require written permission before releasing information. As the job search continues, keep references informed of the names of employers who may be inquiring.

Produce the resumé neatly and inexpensively. A good resumé will be used repeatedly with revisions, and the nurse will want to be able to produce an up-to-date version without rewriting it. Production methods should be kept as simple as possible. It is not necessary to go to the added trouble and expense of having the resumé typeset and printed; just having it neatly typed with good quality photocopying suffices. Again have someone review the final copy for typing errors and then use a photocopying service for "quick copying" onto good quality paper. It is important to remember that, when it comes to resumés, appearances do count. A well-formatted resumé that is properly organized and neatly typed makes a great first impression.

How To Prepare a Portfolio

The professional portfolio is a tool that allows the nurse to showcase his or her credentials in a manner not available on a resumé. As opposed to the resumé, the portfolio provides concrete examples of professional competence and how these events facilitated personal or professional development. Nurse recruiters appreciate the portfolio as a representation of professional accomplishments.

The graduate nurse may want to include supervisor evaluations from nonnursing positions because they may demonstrate leadership, dependability, and attention to detail, which are characteristics also relevant to the nursing work setting. In addition to supervisor evaluations, the new graduate should include clinical evaluations, papers, and other student projects that demonstrate knowledge and skills. Letters of recommendation, resumé, diplomas, transcripts, honors, awards, and professional and community activities are considered traditional documents. Items in the portfolio (Box 25-4) demonstrate professional competence and personal characteristics. Nurses who present portfolios to the recruiter often may have a competitive edge over nurses who do not have as complete a compilation of evidence reflecting their competence to practice professional nursing (Serembus, 2000).

HOW TO INTERVIEW EFFECTIVELY

No matter how qualified and self-confident a person may feel, sitting across the desk from an interviewer can be intimidating. One's conduct in the recruiter's office may determine whether a job offer is made. Being a little anxious is normal, but panic is not. When the applicant has made a good first impression in the cover letter and resumé, he or she can expect to be called for an interview. The graduate's tasks then becomes to enter the interview prepared to answer and ask questions that will help determine whether this organization with its available job opportunities is a good match.

Every agency has its own hiring and interviewing policies. Generally the smaller the organization and the more decentralized the nursing department, the more involved the lower-level manager is in the recruitment and hiring process. The same person who interviews nurse applicants also may be the manager, staff development instructor, quality assurance director,

BOX 25-4	*Documents for Professional Portfolio*

Traditional Documents	Research and Scholarly Activity
Resumé	Publications
Letters of recommendation	Abstracts
License	Book reviews
Certifications	Case studies
Specialty Practice Certifications	Picture of Poster Session
Basic Cardiac Life Support (BCLS)	Power Point outline of presentation
Advanced Cardiac Life Support (ACLS)	Student papers and projects
Diplomas	Professional activities
Transcripts	Membership cards
GRE results	Membership lists
Continuing Education certificate	Letters acknowledging committee work
Honors and Awards	Community involvement
Program from Awards Ceremony	Letters acknowledging work
Letters regarding awards	Pictures or fliers of event
Newspaper articles	

Adapted from Serembus, 2000 Nurse educator.

employee health nurse, and chair of the product standards committee. A large organization with many employees may have a separate human resources department with a nurse recruiter on staff. Within such large organizations the hiring process becomes more complicated and more formal, applicants are more tightly screened, and the hiring decisions are farther removed from the actual work position.

Not all "nurse recruiters" are nurses themselves, which may make a difference in the kind of information exchanged in the interview. A nonnurse is not likely to be able to fully discuss questions that pertain directly to a nurse's job description, patient care workload, and nursing responsibilities. The applicant does not have to answer questions that are not job related. In fact, some questions are illegal (Box 25-5). After a job offer is made, some of the out-of-bound questions may be asked, but not before. They should not be a part of deciding whether the applicant is offered a position.

How To Prepare: Planning Ahead

It is recommended that interview appointments be made as early as possible and that senior students not wait until graduation day. Job hunting takes time, and appointments are not easily scheduled near nursing school graduation dates, as these tend to be busy weeks for recruiters.

How To Prepare: Self-Talk

As the day approached, Mary obsessed about the interview, thinking to herself, "What if they ask me something I cannot answer, and I go blank like I used to do in clinicals when the instructor quizzed me about my patient's medicines. I will look like an idiot, and maybe even start to cry." The night before the appointment, she could not sleep.

BOX 25-5	*Legal and Illegal Areas of Questioning*

Some questions are inappropriate to be asked of an applicant before a job offer is made.

Legal	**Illegal**
Educational preparation	Race
Licensure status	Creed
Work experience	Color
Reasons for leaving previous jobs	Nationality
Reasons for applying to this institution	Marital status
Qualifications for this job	Sexual preference
Strengths and weaknesses	Number of children or dependents
Criminal convictions	Financial or credit status
Criminal arrests	Religious beliefs

One's thoughts dictate one's reality. Nurses, especially new nurses, should be aware of what they are saying to themselves. The applicant who thinks, "Why would anyone want to hire a graduate nurse with no practical experience like me?" will project a lack of self-trust that may be interpreted by the recruiter as lack of enthusiasm or even incompetence. If instead the graduate thinks, "I have successfully completed a difficult nursing course of study. I am now ready to take on the responsibilities of a professional. With orientation, on-the-job training, and the support of experienced nurses, I can succeed as an RN. I have everything I need to begin practice." This reality-based "self-talk" is an important internal dialog for establishing peace of mind before the job interview.

The reality is that all graduates have met the criteria for graduation from a nursing education program and have been deemed ready by that credentialing body for an entry-level position as an RN. The final test of competence to practice, the NCLEX, will provide further proof. Graduate nurses who fear failure of this final test must remind themselves of those now successfully practicing who preceded them from the same educational program with the same preparation.

How To Prepare: Rehearse

A simple visualization of how the graduate wants to appear to the recruiter can bring about the self-assurance needed to create an attractive candidate. It is helpful to mentally review and be prepared to describe pride in any past work experiences, especially the parts of any job that relate to what is required of a nurse. Even baby-sitting jobs can validate a worker as a responsible adult if that person worked consistently for the same family and showed stability and good judgment as a trusted caretaker for children. Applicants tend to discount minimum wage, part-time, teen-age, or summer employment, but would attendance records attest to the worker's dependability? Was the worker given greater responsibility over time? Was the worker allowed to open or close the business? Handle the cash receipts?

The only job Sam had before nursing school had been working the customer service desk at a large children's toy store, where he scheduled and supervised the cashiers. His title was

"Designated Key Carrier," which he listed on his resumé. The interviewer reasonably interpreted this to be a position that demonstrated the employer's trust in Sam.

It is not only the graduate's academic standing or honors and awards that measure success as a student. Perhaps the student was not in the top 10% of the class but was active in student affairs. Perhaps the student was chair of a student government committee or a contributor to the campus newspaper. The graduate should be prepared to describe other areas of student accomplishments.

Unfortunately many nurses are not accustomed to selling themselves and are uncomfortable in situations in which they need to be able to discuss their best attributes and market their qualifications. Therefore, after rehearsing in one's own mind how to present these qualifications to interviewers, it would be wise to rehearse with another person, role-playing the expected interview dialog. Role-play with another student or an experienced nurse (even better), rehearsing answers to questions the interviewer is expected to ask. Practice descriptions of the key points of past employment. A few minutes spent in rehearsing with another will contribute to composure and self-confidence in the actual situation.

Finally, it is important for the graduate to remember that the job interview is neither an examination to pass or fail nor an interrogation. It is an exchange of information: the recruiter hoping to find a potential employee to fill a staff vacancy, and the applicant hoping to find employment as a nurse in this organization. Each has responsibilities for informing the other, and each has rights to obtain information from the other (Box 25-6).

How To Prepare: the Interview Itself

Dress Appropriately. Business-like clothing such as a neat dress, suit, or pantsuit projects a professional attitude. Casual attire projects a casual attitude. Jeans are not acceptable, nor are shorts or any clothes that are too short, too tight, or too trendy. Conservative and simple always is best. "Dressing for success" not only influences the impressions others have, but also influences the wearer's own behavior. When people are dressed to look their best, attitudes improve and levels of self-confidence increase. Facial make-up should be light, and the use of

---

BOX 25-6	*Applicants' Rights*

Applicants have the right to:

- Be informed of available positions at an institution and the minimum qualifications required.
- Apply for any available position for which they are qualified.
- Be seriously and fairly considered for any available position for which they are qualified.
- An interview and to be shown a job description and be made aware of the requirements and expectations of the job.
- Have the work schedule discussed.
- Be informed of the benefits package.
- See the nursing unit and meet the manager if they are being seriously considered.
- Be made aware of the orientation program.
- Be given an expected time when a decision would be made

perfume or cologne should be avoided. Many institutions are fragrance-free because of patients' and employees' allergic reactions to perfumes. Large, distracting jewelry should be avoided.

Arrive on Time. To arrive late for a job interview creates a bad impression. Be considerate of the interviewer's time and agenda. If delayed, call to reschedule. To arrive too early can make the interviewer feel rushed or the applicant appear overanxious.

Bring a Resumé. Even if a resumé has been submitted, the applicant should bring extra copies. The recruiter may have routed the mailed copy to a manager for review. Applicants probably will be asked to complete an employment application, and the resumé is a ready reference for past employers and dates of employment. Social security card, driver's license, and the nursing license, if available, also will be requested as necessary parts of the identification process. Some agencies request that a current cardiopulmonary resuscitation card be made available to photocopy.

The Interview

The interview is the most time-consuming and subjective part of the employment process. For professionals it is appropriate for interviews to be unstructured, using open-ended questions; both recruiter and applicant will have questions. The initial interview can be expected to last 30 minutes to 1 hour. Being prepared is the key, and planning answers to the questions most likely to be asked is the best way to prepare. Eight of the most frequently asked questions follow.

What Positions Interest You? The interviewer needs to know if there are positions available in the applicant's area of interest and if the applicant has the required qualifications to fit the vacant positions. If there is no fit in interest or qualifications with jobs available, neither applicant nor recruiter need waste much more time in the interview.

Because titles and position names vary from organization to organization, it is better to answer the question with favorite clinical experiences. Applicants might share short- and long-term goals and how they visualize laying the groundwork today for tomorrow's professional roles. A good response might be, "I'm interested in a position that will help me grow as a professional and give me opportunities to develop greater competency as a nurse. Ultimately I would like to work as a critical care clinical nurse specialist." If interest, qualifications, and the available positions match, the interviewer will want to start planning secondary interviews and tours.

Tell Me About Your Work History. Even if previous jobs were not nursing related, the applicant can highlight the responsibilities carried out, the skills acquired, and how those skills can transfer to the professional nursing role. This is the point at which the interviewer will get an idea of motivation, drive, energy level, and reliability. No new graduate will be expected to have all the knowledge and skills of an experienced RN; however, when answering, the graduate may stress other aptitudes such as verbal skills or interpersonal skills. It is best to start with the current or most recent job and proceed backward. A new graduate might discuss student clinical experiences, which clinical areas were favored, and why.

How Did You Choose to Apply For a Job Here? Any previous investigative homework done on the institution is useful and helps to form honest responses. For example, an applicant might say, "This hospital has a reputation for its quality care, and I like that," or "I am interested in research and have heard you have a nursing research committee for staff nurses."

Do You Want a Full-Time or Part-Time Position, and Which Shift Do You Prefer? If there is a need or desire for a particular schedule, the nurse should be honest and ask for that schedule. If the recruiter does not have that schedule available, ask what is available, so a decision can be made. Can the nurse be flexible to accept an undesirable shift until a preferred one becomes available? Part of one's investigation of an institution should include looking at a current list of posted positions. Particularly with smaller agencies, if what the nurse desires is not posted, it may be beneficial to ask for a particular schedule but, if willing, express an interest in working a schedule that is posted. For example, "I'm willing to work the evening shift posted for the medical-surgical unit; however, I'm most interested in moving into a day position in labor and delivery."

What Are Your Strengths and Weaknesses? Sometimes this question may be asked in less direct ways such as, "What are some of the areas you know you need to improve?" or "How have your skills developed in your advanced nursing courses?" Honesty always is best. By asking this question, the interviewer may only be trying to pinpoint the special skills and preferences of the nurse. For example, with what kind of patients has the nurse been most effective, and which ones proved most difficult? The clearer the applicant can be in articulating specific talents and deficiencies, the better the recruiter will be in matching the candidate to a position suited to his or her abilities. The closer this match, the more likely the employee will flourish and be able to use special talents.

It is not advisable to avoid the issue of weaknesses. Everyone has them. It is better to admit them but to present them in a positive way. In addition, it may be helpful to tell the interviewer what is being done to correct weaknesses. For example, "Sometimes I tend to see the 'big picture' and have to remind myself to pay more attention to the details. I've started keeping lists, and they seem helpful." Another suggestion might be, "I have limited bedside nursing experience, but I am excited about building on the clinical skills I have learned in school."

What Would You Do If . . . ? The recruiter probably will ask some situational questions to find out about decision-making and critical-thinking skills. The nurse will be asked to explain how to assess a particular situation, set priorities, decide what should be implemented first for a patient, and what can be delegated. Rather than fabricate an answer about unfamiliar circumstances, one can honestly say, "I've never been in that situation, but I think I would . . . ," or "I was in a similar situation in which so and so occurred, and this is what I did in those circumstances."

Why Should We Hire You? This is an opportunity to share the special assets that the new hire brings to the institution. Without embellishment or selling oneself short, it is important to convey pride in being a nurse and conviction that one has something special to offer.

What Questions Do You Have? Usually the interview ends with the interviewer asking if there are any questions. This is an opportunity for the applicant to demonstrate initiative,

---

BOX 25-7   *What to Expect a Recruiter to Communicate*

Recruiters should inform applicants of basic human resource policies regarding job descriptions, compensation, benefits, and staff development, including:

- Conditional period
- Job descriptions
- Shift rotation
- Weekend rotation
- Salary
- Staff development
- Parking
- Security
- Health insurance and other insurance benefits
- Preemployment physical examinations

- Credit union
- Overtime
- Scheduled paydays
- Paid time off
- Leaves of absence
- Employee discounts
- Transfer and promotion policies
- Resignation policies
- Preemployment policies
- Pay increases

BOX 25-8   *Appropriate Questions for the Applicant*

1. May I see the job description for the position we are discussing?
2. How many patients are on this unit? How many will I be responsible for?
3. How many RNs, LPNs, and unlicensed assistive personnel (UAP) will be working with me?
4. What about clerical help and support services? What type of nursing is practiced here (team nursing, primary nursing, centralized, decentralized)?
5. How available are physicians? Admitting physicians and house staff?
6. How often are nursing care conferences held on this unit?
7. What type of nursing documentation is used?
8. How long is the orientation program? What does the program include? What continuing education programs are available after my initial orientation?
9. How will my performance be evaluated? How often, and by whom?
10. What exact schedule or shift will I be working in this position?
11. What will my salary be? Is there a shift differential?
12. How are pay increases decided?
13. What other benefits are there (health, life insurance, vacation time, retirement plan)?

---

and one should, although not to excess. In an effective interview with an experienced interviewer, most questions regarding salary, benefits, and human resource policies will have been addressed (Box 25-7). If not, this is the time to ask. Should a tour of the nursing unit and a meeting with the supervisor be arranged, many concerns will be answered then. Box 25-8 presents a list of suggested questions.

Mentally reviewing practiced responses to these questions will give the applicant confidence. The more information gathered, the easier it will be to make a decision, and the more likely it is that the nurse will be happy in the long term.

THE APPLICANT'S TASKS
Assess the Climate of the Work Environment

As mentioned in the previous discussion of researching potential employers, there are ways other than direct questioning to learn a lot about the institution. Every organization has its own personality and atmosphere. The first impression probably came from the secretary who answered the phone when the applicant called for an appointment with the recruiter, followed by the greeting on arrival at the recruiter's office. A tone of respect and pride in being associated with the organization may have been communicated in the first encounter. Every subsequent encounter builds on the first.

In the hallways of the agency, how do people acknowledge each other? A visit to the employee cafeteria to buy a cup of coffee or a sandwich at mealtime can be enlightening. Are nurses eating there? Does it seem that the staff members are enjoying themselves? Pick up for later reading any available in-house publications such as employee newsletters or bulletins.

Ask for a Tour

If the interviewer does not automatically offer a tour of the unit, the applicant can request to see it and will certainly want to meet with the person who will be the immediate supervisor. To get an accurate feel for the unit, the applicant should pay close attention to the pace, the tone of the staff interaction, and the morale. Is this a group the prospective employee would like to join? Are the manager's philosophy and management style similar to the applicant's own?

The astute applicant can get an accurate feel for the nursing unit's culture and personality if the manager's interactions with staff are observed. Is the manager accessible to the staff and supportive in response to them? How are telephone calls and other interruptions handled? How well do people seem to be getting along? Pay attention to the way people on the unit relate to each other—nurses to doctors, nurses to families, nurses to nurses. How are the patients responded to on the intercommunication system? Notice the efficiency with which staff work. How rushed are they? Also note bulletin boards and any public displays of staff recognition (e.g., "Employee of the Month" plaques or brag boards). Even a second visit to the unit might be requested before a final decision is made. The more information gathered, the easier it will be to make a decision.

Some managers offer opportunities for the applicant to meet with staff, and formal interviews with staff nurses may be scheduled as a routine part of the hiring process. This gives the applicant a closer view of the actual work organization and gives representative staff members a chance to have a voice in selecting new co-workers. Staff nurses provide bedside care to patients and best understand the qualities appreciated in a good team member (Allen et al., 1998). Whether the introduction to staff is a formal interview or a casual conference room encounter, the applicant can be made to feel welcome and wanted while learning about the real work and the real workers of the agency. Now that firsthand knowledge has been obtained, if the applicant confers again with these employees and former employees consulted before applying, he or she can ask more informed questions.

Follow-Up

Thank-You Letter. A follow-up letter thanking the recruiter is a courtesy and a reminder of the nurse's interest in receiving a timely response (Box 25-9). If the nurse does not hear from

BOX 25-9	*Interview Follow-up Letter*

April 24, 2002

Ms. Donna Henderson, RN, MS
Director, Nurse Recruitment
Charleston Memorial Hospital
1265 Beckley Avenue
Memphis, Tennessee 38104

Dear Ms. Henderson:
It was a pleasure meeting with you on Monday. I now have a clear picture of what I might expect as a new graduate nurse in your hospital. Everyone on the units I visited was very friendly.

I look forward to hearing from you with good news about a position at Charleston Memorial. I can be reached in the afternoons at 555-912-3720.

Thank you again for your time and interest.

Sincerely,

Bonnie McCray Pino

the employer within a reasonable length of time (1 to 2 weeks) after the interview, it is appropriate to inquire by telephone about the status of a hiring decision.

Avoid Impulse Decisions. If offered a position and time is needed to make a decision, the applicant should postpone a decision and should not feel pressured into acceptance while still unsure. An offer to telephone the recruiter with an answer within an agreed on time is appropriate.

If there are other job opportunities, certainly comparisons need to be made by weighing the pros and cons of each position and each organization. How do benefits compare? What are the possibilities for movement within the systems laterally and vertically? How available are continuing education opportunities to staff nurses? How do observations of the work culture fit with the nurse's ideas of what is needed to support professional success? Does the schedule that is offered fit the applicant's lifestyle? When a decision has been reached, a telephone call should be made promptly to the recruiter, whether the answer is "yes" or "no."

Weighing Options. What questions might be asked of oneself while weighing the merits of one position against others? Remembering that no job is perfect, the following four questions should be considered.

Does the Position Match the Nurse's Qualifications? Although it is flattering to receive a job offer for a position for which a nurse has little or no preparation, one should not be influenced by such a compliment. When there is a nursing shortage, a position that is beyond an applicant's present skills and experience may sound wonderfully challenging, when in actuality it may be overwhelming and a disastrous beginning for a new graduate. Being overzealous, overconfident, and overanxious to please can only lead to feelings of guilt and inadequacy if the job is not appropriate. It is wiser to accept a position in which adequate orientation and clinical support exists, which would allow the graduate to gain the experience and preparation necessary to accept a position requiring more skills at a later time.

What Are the Actual Responsibilities of the Job? The newly hired nurse has the right to completely understand what will be expected in the position offered, including the overall and daily responsibilities and the length and nature of on-the-job training that will be provided. What will the supervisory responsibilities be? How many and what skill level employees will be under the RN's leadership? What orientation is planned to prepare the RN for practicing independently? Are there arrangements for a preceptor to guide the graduate through the difficult transition of entering a first nursing job? Reality shock can be anticipated, and the more assistance a new graduate receives in adjusting to the new role of the nurse, the more likely is the beginner to be successful and satisfied.

Does this Position Lead the Nurse in the Direction of Projected Career Goals? Is the offered job a step toward meeting long-term career objectives? For example, a graduate who wants to be a nurse midwife someday would be better accepting a position in postpartum if labor and delivery is not available, instead of accepting a position in neurosurgery just because 10¢ more per hour in pay or a few more weekends off are promised. No position or job change should be accidental or a snap decision. Career moves should result from deliberate planning and purposeful preparation.

How Will the Work Be Compensated? Experienced nurses often advise that money, although important, is not the only reward associated with a job. But money does matter, especially to a new graduate who may have subsisted on a limited income while in school. It is common for loans to have accumulated, along with unpaid bills. Inadequate salary can be a real source of job dissatisfaction, of course, but with 24-hour responsibilities, nurses traditionally have basic salaries that include other income-contributing factors, such as shift differentials, weekend differentials, holiday pay, paid vacation days, and expected salary increases over time. Compensation comes in other packages besides paychecks. There are policies that allow for maternity leaves, medical leaves, tuition reimbursement, sick days, discounts on prescriptions and health insurance, retirement benefits, and malpractice insurance coverage, all of which affect income in indirect but important ways. As is true in other areas of consideration, the better the total compensation package fits one's needs, the greater the likelihood that one will remain satisfied with the job.

Well-prepared job applicants will have listed those benefits they consider essential, and these vary with individual circumstances. For example, the essentials for someone who is the sole family breadwinner probably include health insurance, paid time off, and an employer-provided retirement plan.

Box 25-10 further helps applicants evaluate potential employment opportunities.

BOX 25-10	*Assessment Tool for Decision Making*

When weighing options for employment, consider those measures of a professional work climate evident in written documentation and visible in the patient care areas. The following observations should guide the new graduate in making an informed decision.

- Standards of nursing practice are evident and are an integral part of patient care.
- Nurse-patient ratio is adequate and adjusted for patient acuity.
- Orientation is structured, individualized, and adequate for new graduates.
- Opportunities for horizontal transfer and advancement exist within the system.
- The salary is competitive and reasonable.
- Benefits are competitive.
- Continuing education is available, and staff members are encouraged to attend.
- A nurse administrator is responsible for delivery of nursing services.

THE EMPLOYER'S TASKS

In any agency providing nursing services, its nurses are the indispensable employees. The selection of new nurse employees is a critically important responsibility, and it is the recruiter's duty to make sure the best selection is made.

First the nurse must meet the minimum requirements for the position desired. For example, 1 year of experience might be required for a nurse to work a weekender program or in a critical care area. Operating room (OR) experience may be required for OR nursing positions, and perinatal nursing experience may be required for labor and delivery positions. A secondary consideration is the nurse's suitability for contributing to the mission of the health care delivery system. The recruiter is selling the organization to the applicant and measuring the skills and aptitudes the applicant would bring to the organization.

The bottom line for any employer who provides health care services to the public is to ensure that its nursing staff practices safely. Recruiters are looking to uncover anything that would impair a nurse applicant's ability to provide safe nursing care, such as incompetence, unprofessional conduct, unreliability in attendance, chemical dependency, or record of criminal activity. For screening, recruiters have four primary sources of information: the application, interview impressions, test results, and references.

Applications are validated. Work history and references are checked to ensure accuracy. Previous supervisors are asked about attendance, dependability, performance, attitude, ability to get along with others, integrity, and eligibility for rehire. The applicant's stated reason for termination is compared with information obtained from work references. The employer has a right to obtain reasonable information about the persons who are hired. Most employment applications ask if the applicant has ever been convicted of a crime other than a minor traffic violation. The question is about convictions, not arrests, and the response is verified by a background or criminal record check. Response to this or any other question in the application process must be honest and truthful. Each institution has its own policies regarding convictions, but most are vitally concerned about their responsibilities regarding negligent hiring. If an applicant committed a crime that, if repeated while in the employ of the institution, would cause harm to patients, families, other employees or the institution, the applicant is rejected.

A preemployment physical examination is often required. This usually is done on site and at the employer's expense. It may involve obtaining the applicant's full medical history and vital signs, routine blood tests, a urine drug screen, and sometimes a chest radiograph. The purpose of the physical examination is to ensure protection for patients and to ensure that the caregiver can carry out the necessary physical responsibilities of the job. For example, are illegal mood-altering substances evident that would impair the nurse's abilities and judgment? Are there physical limitations the institution should know about to determine if any special accommodations are necessary to allow the candidate to perform the usual duties associated with the position?

Even with a job offer made and a date for employment set, actual start dates are contingent on receipt of documentation of these final screenings, plus a reference check to verify the resumé; these items establish safety and reliability of the practitioner. Other parts of screening for safety might include paper and pencil testing such as skills tests, pharmacology tests, and in some cases, psychologic testing for specialty areas.

A preemployment pharmacology test is common. Many institutions give such a quiz to determine basic knowledge of routinely administered medications, their purposes, and side effects. Simple dosage questions and calculation methods may be asked. Some questions may be situational ones, such as, "What would you do in this case . . . ?" or "The first nursing action in this scenario should be . . . ."

A few larger institutions also may administer a clinical skills test. This might involve a laboratory where frequently used patient care equipment is set up. Usually a staff development instructor accompanies the nurse through a series of stations where the nurse would be asked to plan and perform the appropriate nursing actions. Examples might be starting cardiopulmonary resuscitation on a simulated patient, demonstrating the proper procedure for starting an intravenous line, or talking through an assessment of a patient.

It is far better to be prepared and even better to be proactive and offer to produce some of the documentation required. For instance, the nurse may be able to get a written reference from a former employer or a statement from a physician sooner than the institution can. The employment start date depends on the receipt of all the necessary information, so it would expedite the process if the hopeful employee volunteered to initiate some of the documentation gathering.

Once an applicant is selected, the agency has committed itself to costly training, orientation, and additional benefits that may cost as much as 30% to 40% of the employee's salary. A major element of control, which any organization possesses, is its ability to choose its employees. When the selection process is thorough, it is a sign to the committed professional that this is a reputable employer.

SUMMARY

If not offered a position, the new graduate should still feel good about himself or herself. There may have been several candidates for that same position. Perhaps it was not the best match for one's skills or preferences. There is victory in having had an opportunity to practice interview skills. Preparation, practice, and perseverance will reward the nurse with the job that is better suited to his or her personality, values, qualifications, and skills. New graduates have internalized standards of practice from their nursing education experience. On graduation they must decide where to begin to put those standards to work in real life terms bearing real responsibilities with real patients. The question becomes, "Can school and work values be reconciled in this nursing environment?" When adequate groundwork in pursuit of a job has been laid, the answer should come easy.

Critical Thinking Activities

1. In the interest of creating the right match for yourself with your first career choice as a graduate nurse, what personal qualities and professional strengths and weaknesses will you consider?

2. How would you evaluate the overall work environment of the agency you have selected for employment other than by asking direct questions?

3. Consider the responsibility of nurse recruiters to create an environment of safe care. How thorough should preemployment examinations be? In what positions should a new graduate be allowed to function and why? Describe what would be included in a preemployment examination.

REFERENCES

Allen SR et al: Peer interviewing: Sharing the selection process, *Nurs Management* 29(3):46, 1998.

Serembus J: Teaching the process of developing a professional portfolio, *Nurs Educator* 25(6):282-287, 2000.

SUGGESTED READINGS

Bozell J: *Anatomy of a job search,* Springhouse, Pa, 1999, Springhouse.

Fitzpatrick JJ, Montgomery KS, editors: *Internet resources for nurses,* New York, 2000, Springer Publishing.

Russo C: How to interview on your own terms. *The AJN career guide for 2001* 101:(1, Part 2):16-18, 2001.

Saver C: Make the Internet your new career partner, *Imprint* 46(3):40-42, 60, 1999.

Saver C: Nursing in the new millennium, *Imprint* 46(1):32-36, 1999.

Saver C: How to choose the right first job, *Imprint* 47(1):35-36, 2000.

SpringNet career opportunities: job interviews, 1997, www.springnet.com/career art/intview.htm.

Trossman S: The professional portfolio: documenting who you are, what you do, *Am Nurse* March/April 2, 1999.

Walden P: Tips on getting the job you want, *Imprint* 46(1):40-41, 1999.

Walton RH, Morton PG, Amig A: How to succeed in job interviewing, *Crit Care Nurse* 18 (1):68-73, 1998.

NCLEX-RN Examination

Sandra S. Swick, EdD, RN, C

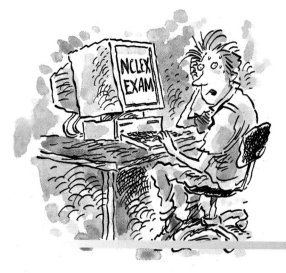

Adequate preparation for the NCLEX
can reduce panic and ensure success.

Vignette

Have you ever considered how nursing and licensure examinations have changed as society has changed? Nursing is a reflection of society's values, knowledge, and needs. Test items or questions found on the NCLEX examination today have little resemblance to questions asked on state board examinations during the early part of the century. Questions of that era dealt with practical issues and had little to do with assessment, application, evaluation, or need and consisted mainly of knowledge-based questions. Consider the following questions taken from the 1919 State Board Questions and Answers for Nurses (Foote, 1919):

- What are the advantages of fireplaces?
- How would you sterilize silkworm-gut and silk sutures?
- What care regarding nourishment would you give a gynaecological [sic] patient to prevent a common discomfort?
- Give some general rules for preparing meats.
- Give three common complaints that the public makes about graduate nurses.

Questions to consider while reading this chapter

1. What is the purpose of the NCLEX-RN examination?
2. What type of questions can I expect on today's NCLEX-RN examination?
3. What is the best way to prepare for the examination?

Key Terms

NCLEX-RN (NCLEX) Examination An examination taken by qualified graduates of approved schools of nursing. Graduates successfully taking the NCLEX are granted a license to practice as registered nurses (RNs).

Compulsory licensure Individuals working as RNs must have a license to legally practice or work as an RN. Licensure is a prerequisite to practice in each state and U.S. territory.

Computer adaptive testing (CAT) A type of computer testing in which a person is given a test question to answer and the next question is based on the answer given in the first question. CAT adapts or changes according to the answers a person gives. For example, a person missing a question dealing with assessment might be given another assessment question to determine the person's competency with assessment.

Learning Outcomes

After studying this chapter, the reader will be able to:

1. Explain the purpose of the NCLEX examination.
2. Evaluate various methods of preparation for the NCLEX examination.
3. Create a personal plan for preparing for the NCLEX examination.
4. Analyze the relationship between the nursing process and client needs as they relate to NCLEX test items.
5. Compare and contrast various review courses designed to aid in review for the NCLEX examination.

CHAPTER OVERVIEW

Graduates from approved schools of nursing cannot begin their careers and practice as RNs until they have successfully passed the National Council Licensure Examination for Registered Nurses (NCLEX-RN) examination. Success on the NCLEX-RN examination depends on many factors, such as a candidate's knowledge of the examination, the knowledge brought from his or her school of nursing, formal review before the examination, test-taking skills, and confidence level. This chapter discusses the purpose and characteristics of the NCLEX-RN examination, examples of test items based on the nursing process and client needs, how to prepare for the examination, and factors to think about when considering a review course.

THE NCLEX EXAMINATION

The NCLEX examination and licensure to practice nursing go hand in hand. To receive a license to practice as an RN in the United States and its territories, candidates must furnish evidence of competency to provide effective nursing care by successfully completing the NCLEX examination (National Council, 2000).

There currently are three types of registered nursing programs: 2-year associate degree programs usually found in community or junior colleges, hospital-based diploma programs, and baccalaureate degree programs found in 4-year colleges and universities or academic health centers. Graduates from all three programs take the same NCLEX examination. The examination tests content common to all three programs, is job related, and reflects current entry level nursing practice (National Council, 2000). Individuals taking the examination must have graduated from approved schools of nursing.

Purpose of the NCLEX Examination

All states and U.S. territories have compulsory licensure and use the NCLEX for licensure determination. The purpose of the NCLEX examination is twofold:

1. It safeguards the public from unsafe practitioners.
2. It assists state boards of nursing in determining candidates' capabilities for performing entry-level RN positions.

The National Council of State Boards of Nursing periodically ascertains entry-level capabilities by investigating the jobs that entry-level nurses are performing in various health care settings in the United States (National Council, 2000).

Characteristics of the NCLEX Examination

The NCLEX is a pass–fail examination and has been computerized since 1994. Before that time the NCLEX was a paper-and-pencil examination requiring 2 days to complete. The examination was offered twice a year in selected cities in each state. Today the NCLEX is offered at selected Sylvan Learning Centers throughout the country, can be taken at the candidate's convenience, and can be completed in 5 or fewer hours. The results of the examination are sent to candidates a few weeks after taking the examination.

Computerized Adaptive Testing. The NCLEX uses CAT, which is a technique for administering tests that uses current computer technology and measurement theory (Computerized Adaptive Testing, 2000). As a candidate answers questions on the examination the CAT adapts to the level of the candidate's knowledge, skills, and ability. All examinations are consistent with the NCLEX-RN Test Plan, which controls inclusion of current nursing content. Candidates have ample opportunity to demonstrate their competence since the examination does not end until stability of the pass/fail result is certain or time runs out (Computerized Adaptive Testing, 2000).

Candidates taking the NCLEX do not need to be computer literate. Only two keys on the keyboard are used during the examination—the space bar and the enter or return key. The remainder of the keyboard is locked during the examination and becomes unusable. A tutorial is administered before the examination actually begins, providing candidates with experience in using the computer in CAT situations (How CAT works, 2000). Questions on the NCLEX examination use a multiple-choice format with four possible answers. Candidates should carefully read an entire question and all possible answer options before selecting an answer. A multiple-choice question may have only one correct option; or all options may be correct, but one is more correct than the others. In the example mentioned previously, the candidate must determine which action has priority and should be implemented before the others.

Skipping Questions/Changing Answers. Candidates taking the NCLEX are not allowed to skip questions and return to them at a later time or to change answers to questions once an answer has been selected and entered into the computer. These actions would defeat the purpose of adaptive testing because CAT is based on the knowledge, skills, and abilities of the examination taker and selects questions based on these three measures. Candidates are not disadvantaged using this method of testing because CAT has a built-in, self-correcting mechanism (Why aren't skipping questions, 2000).

Question Format. All of the information needed to answer a particular question appears on the one computer screen so candidates do not need to see the previous or next screen for answer determination. Questions appearing on the computer screen will take one of two formats, depending on the type of question. The first question format is simply a question with four possible answers (Fig. 26-1). The question appears on the left side of the computer screen, and the four possible answers appear on the right side of the screen. In determining an answer, completely read the left side of the screen and then read all of the possible answers.

The second question format has three components (Fig. 26-2). The left side of the computer screen contains information needed to answer the question. This information may be background or short case study in nature. The right side of the computer screen contains the two additional components. The right top of the computer screen contains the actual question. The right bottom of the computer screen contains four possible answers. In reading a question, read all of the information needed to answer the question, then read the question, and lastly, read the four possible answers.

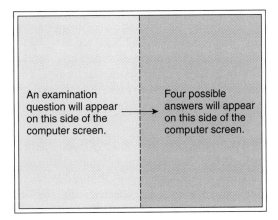

FIG. 26-1 Question format with two components (arrows do not appear on actual test screens).

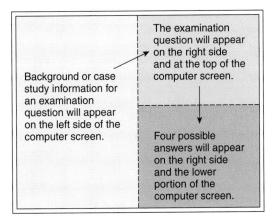

FIG. 26-2 Question format with three components (arrows do not appear on actually test screens).

NCLEX examination questions use Bloom's cognitive levels of knowledge, comprehension, application, and analysis (National Council, 2000). These levels may be viewed as four consecutive steps, with knowledge being the lowest, most fundamental step and analysis being the highest, most highly evolved of the steps.

Knowledge Questions. As the lowest and simplest level of learning within the cognitive domain, knowledge is remembering or recalling information. Included in this level is knowing specific facts, common terms, methods and procedures, basic concepts, and principles (Gronlund, 1985).

Comprehension Questions. Comprehension, the second level of Bloom's cognitive domain, is the ability to grasp or understand information or material. Included in this level are the understanding of facts and principles; explaining verbal material, graphs, and charts; translating material into mathematical formulas; estimating outcomes implied in an information base; and justifying methods and procedures (Gronlund, 1985).

Application Questions. The third cognitive level, application, refers to the ability to use learned information in new situations. This level involves applying theories and principles in new or practical situations, solving mathematical problems, constructing charts and graphs, and showing accurate usage of a procedure (Gronlund, 1985).

Analysis Questions. The final and highest cognitive level, analysis, is the ability to reduce material into its elemental parts so that its design and structure may be understood. Included in this level are questions recognizing undeclared assumptions and logical inconsistencies in reasoning, discriminating between facts and deductions, and evaluating the applicability of information (Gronlund, 1985).

The NCLEX test item pool is composed of 3000 questions of varying levels of difficulty (National Council, 2000). Candidates taking the examination answer from a minimum of 75 questions to a maximum of 265 questions. Past candidates of the NCLEX examination have asked if some candidates are randomly selected to receive longer versions of the examination. The National Council of State Boards of Nursing writes:

> It is not true that some candidates randomly receive a maximum length examination. The length of an NCLEX examination is based on the performance of the candidate on the examination. After you have answered the minimum number of questions, the computer compares your competence level to the passing standard and makes one of three decisions:
> 1. If you are clearly above the passing standard, you pass and the examination ends.
> 2. If you are clearly below the passing standard, you fail and the examination ends.
> 3. If your competence level is close enough to the passing standard that it's still not clear whether you should pass or not, the computer continues to ask you questions until a clear pass or fail decision can be made, the maximum number of questions is reached, or time runs out (More untrue rumors, 2000).

COMPONENTS OF THE NCLEX TEST PLAN

The test plan for the NCLEX is based on the current nursing practice of entry-level RNs. According to the National Council of State Boards of Nursing (2000, p. 3):

> Provision is made for an examination reflecting entry-level content and behaviors to be tested. . . . Based on the NCLEX-RN Test Plan, each unique NCLEX-RN® examination reflects the knowledge, skills and abilities essential for the nurse to meet the needs of clients requiring the promotion, maintenance and restoration of health.

The NCLEX test plan is composed of two components or parts: the nursing process and client needs. The nursing process is a five-step process composed of assessment, analysis, planning, implementation, and evaluation. The client needs section addresses psychosocial integrity; physiologic integrity; health promotion and maintenance; and safe, effective care environment.

Each question in the NCLEX test item pool relates directly to one step of the nursing process and one client need category. For example, a question may be an assessment question that has to do with health promotion and maintenance or an implementation question that concerns psychosocial integrity. All questions relate to some activity in which an entry-level nurse may engage when caring for or managing a patient.

The Nursing Process

Success on the NCLEX examination relies on a sound working knowledge of the nursing process. The nursing process provides the foundation for nursing practice and is the tool that nurses use to assess, plan, implement, and evaluate the care given to their patients. The nursing process is applicable to all situations in which the nurse and patient interact and may be used with any theoretic framework. Cox and others (1997, p. 2) write:

> Basically, the nursing process provides each nurse with a framework to use in working with a patient. The process begins at the time the patient needs assistance with health care through the time the patient no longer needs assistance to meet health care maintenance. The nursing process represents the cognitive (thinking and reasoning), psychomotor (physical), and affective (emotions and values) skills and abilities used by the nurse to plan care for a patient.

Assessment. Assessment is the first step of the nursing process and establishes a database for the client. Just as the nursing process provides a foundation for nursing practice, assessment provides the foundation for the nursing process. Assessment includes gathering information or data about an identified client. Depending on the nurse's focus, the client may be a person, a family, a group of people, or a community.

Information about a client will come from a variety of sources, including the client, the family and significant others, laboratory or radiographic reports, physician records, hospital or clinic records, and other caregivers. Client data are typically classified as subjective and objective. Simply put, subjective data are the client's perception or understanding of a specific event or phenomenon. It is his or her opinion, such as the degree of pain experienced during an episode of angina. Objective data are observable and measurable by the nurse and come from various patient records. Blood pressure, heart rate, and the presence of absence of edema are examples of objective data.

Cox and others (1997) suggest two additional classifications of client data—historical and current. Historical data relate to health events occurring before the current health problem or admission to the health care system. Current data include information specific to the current health problem or admission. Historical and current data may occur as subjective or objective information.

Assessment also includes verification and communication of data. Seeking additional patient-related information such as laboratory work or talking with the family may confirm data. Communication of data may be accomplished by verbal report to other health care workers or by written or computerized record.

Twenty percent of NCLEX questions address assessment. The following is an example of an assessment question.

A 33-year-old man comes to the emergency room. Subjective assessment reveals polyphagia, polyuria, polydypsia, and visual disturbances. Objective assessment reveals dehydration and lethargy. Diabetes mellitus is suspected, and blood chemistries are drawn to aid in confirmation of a diagnosis. Chemistries supporting a diagnosis of diabetes mellitus would show which of the following?

   A.   Increased glucose, potassium, chloride, ketones, cholesterol, and triglycerides.

   B.   Decreased glucose, potassium, chloride, ketones, cholesterol, and triglycerides.

   C.   Increased glucose, potassium, chloride, with decreased ketones, cholesterol, and triglycerides.

   D.   Decreased glucose, potassium, chloride, with increased ketones, cholesterol, and triglycerides.

Option A is the correct answer. Glucose, potassium, chloride, ketones, cholesterol, and triglyceride levels are increased in patients with poorly controlled diabetes mellitus.

Option B is incorrect. Glucose, potassium, chloride, ketone, cholesterol, and triglyceride levels are increased, not decreased, in patients with poorly controlled diabetes mellitus.

Option C is incorrect. Ketones, cholesterol, and triglyceride levels are increased in patients with diabetes mellitus, not decreased.

Option D is incorrect. Glucose, potassium, and chloride levels are increased in patients with diabetes mellitus, not decreased.

Analysis. Analysis is the second step or phase of the nursing process. Client-related data gathered during assessment provide the basis for analysis. During this phase the nurse classifies or groups assessment data and identifies actual or potential client problems. During classification data also are validated and interpreted, and additional data may be required. Numerous frameworks exist for categorizing data. Included in the frameworks are Gordon's Functional Health Patterns, Maslow's Hierarchy of Needs, and the North American Nursing Diagnosis Association's (NANDA) Human Response Patterns (Cox and others, 1997).

Nursing diagnoses are determined based on classification of data. A working definition of nursing diagnosis is provided by NANDA.

> A nursing diagnosis is a clinical judgment about individual, family, or community responses to actual or potential health problems/life processes. Nursing diagnoses provide the basis for selection of nursing interventions to achieve outcomes for which the nurse is accountable (Carroll-Johnson, 1991, p. 65).

As with assessment, nursing diagnoses must be communicated in a reliable format. It is important to remember that there must be congruency between the client's needs or problems and the nurse's ability to realistically meet those needs.

Twenty percent of the questions on the NCLEX examination relate to analysis. An example of an analysis question follows.

A 68-year-old female is admitted to the rehabilitation unit after discharge from the orthopedic floor 6 days after having a total knee replacement. In analyzing the rehabilitation unit admission data, the nurse should:

   A.   Determine the impact of rehabilitation unit nursing care on the patient.

   B.   Observe for toxic effects of ibuprofen.

   C.   Assist the patient in performing all activities of daily living.

   D.   Communicate the results of analysis to other transdisciplinary team members who will be working with the patient.

Option D is the correct answer. Analysis has to do with identification of actual or potential problems. For health care professionals to meet the needs of patients, the results of analysis must be communicated to other health care professionals caring for the patient. Most rehabilitation units have a transdisciplinary focus that includes nurses; occupational, physical, and speech therapists; nutritionists; social workers; and physicians.

Option A is incorrect. The effect of nursing care cannot be evaluated because the patient has just been admitted to the rehabilitation unit and because only minimal nursing care has been given. Determining the effect of nursing care on the patient is evaluation, not analysis.

Option B is incorrect. There is no information to suggest that the patient is taking ibuprofen. Observing for toxic effects of medication is implementation, not analysis.

Option C is incorrect. There is no information to suggest the amount of assistance the patient needs. Assisting a patient is implementation, not analysis.

Planning. Planning is the third phase of the nursing process and includes setting realistic and measurable mutual goals, designing strategies to meet or resolve identified patient needs or problems, and modifying goals as necessary. Included in planning of care are ranking nursing diagnoses, documenting expected outcomes for each goal, and setting realistic target dates for the accomplishment of each goal. Goal setting should include the collaboration of members of the transdisciplinary health care team, the client, his or her family, and significant others as indicated.

As with the previous phases of the nursing process, the plan must be communicated to other members of the health care team to ensure continuity of care. Again communication is in a verbal or written format.

Twenty percent of the NCLEX examination addresses planning. An example of a planning question follows.

A 50-year-old unconscious female with a known history of type I diabetes mellitus is brought to the Emergency Department by ambulance. Family members tell the nurse that the woman has had the flu for the past 4 days. Assessment reveals a fruity breath odor. After appropriate laboratory studies are done, a diagnosis of ketoacidosis is made. The emergency department nurse should expect to do which of the following?

A. Administer Humulin 70/30, intramuscularly
B. Administer Humulin R by intravenous infusion
C. Administer one-half cup of apple or orange juice by mouth
D. Administer three glucose tablets by mouth

Option B is the correct answer. Humulin R is appropriate to give by intravenous infusion. Regular insulins are short acting and start to work quicker than other types of insulin.

Option A is incorrect. Humulin 70/30 is inappropriate insulin to give to a patient in a ketoacidotic state. Insulin is not given intramuscularly.

Options C and D are incorrect. Fruit juices and glucose tablets are indicated for patients with episodes of low blood sugar, not extremely high blood sugar. Unconscious patients should never be given food, fluids, or medications by mouth.

Implementation. The fourth phase of the nursing process is implementation. This stage includes initiating and carrying out nursing interventions or nursing actions to achieve the goals set in the planning phase of the nursing process. In discussing nursing actions, Cox and others (1997) write:

> Nursing action is defined as nursing behavior that serves to help the patient achieve the expected outcome. Nursing actions include both independent and collaborative activities. Independent

actions are those activities the nurse performs using his or her own discretionary judgment and that require no validation or guidelines from any other health care practitioner; for example, deciding which noninvasive technique to use for pain control or deciding when to teach the patient self-care measures. Collaborative actions are those activities that involve mutual decision making between two or more health care practitioners (e.g., a physician and nurse deciding which narcotic to use when meperidine is ineffective in controlling the patient's pain).

Each nursing action should be geared toward achieving a particular goal of care. Included in the implementation phase are: (1) organizing and managing care; (2) actually performing patient care; (3) overseeing and coordinating the delivery of care; (4) delegating nursing actions to other health care workers; (5) teaching or counseling the client, his or her family, significant others, and other caregivers; and (6) communicating and exchanging patient-related information with other health care workers (Cox and others, 1997).

As with the other phases of the nursing process, 20% of the NCLEX examination is devoted to questions pertaining to implementation. An implementation question follows.

A patient admitted to the hospital with pneumonia develops a temperature of 103.4° F. The nurse administers Tylenol 500 mg by mouth. By the end of the shift the patient's temperature is 100.2° F. In giving the end-of-shift report on this patient to the oncoming nurse, the most appropriate information to be conveyed is:

A. "The patient had a temperature earlier today, but it is down now."
B. "The patient had a temperature of 103.4° F earlier in the day. I gave him Tylenol 500 mg by mouth. His temperature has gradually come down during the shift. His last temperature, taken 30 minutes ago, was 100.2° F."
C. "The patient had a temperature earlier today. I gave him some medicine, and the temperature came down. He's now doing fine. You know, my cousin had this same type of pneumonia, and his temperature did the same thing—it would always come up in the morning."
D. It is not necessary to tell the oncoming nurse about the elevated temperature. The oncoming nurse will see this information when the chart is reviewed in preparing to care for the patient during the shift.

Option B is the correct answer. The nurse is giving accurate information to another member of the health care team (i.e., the oncoming nurse). The report given to the nurse provides information regarding the patient's previous and current status, the patient's response to the Tylenol, and nursing actions taken to reduce the elevated temperature.

Option A is incorrect. The nurse is giving vague and unusable information to the oncoming nurse. Temperature may be interpreted as the hotness or coldness of an object, but it does not indicate how hot or how cold the object is. Temperature also may indicate an elevation in normal body temperature, but it does not indicate the amount of elevation.

Option C is incorrect. The nurse is giving vague, unusable, irrelevant information to the oncoming nurse. The use of the word temperature tells little about the patient's condition. The medication the nurse administered could have been any medication given for any number of conditions the patient might have. The report does not demonstrate that the administered medication was specifically for the elevated temperature. Sharing information about a relative who had a similar pneumonia is irrelevant to the implementation of patient care.

Option D is incorrect. The purpose of the end-of-shift report is to communicate accurate, relevant information regarding the patient's status and responses to any changes that may have occurred; nursing actions taken; and any other information relevant to the implementation of patient care. There is nothing to suggest that the oncoming nurse will review the patient's chart before implementing care.

Evaluation. Evaluation is the fifth and final phase of the nursing process. Evaluation includes comparing what actually happened (the actual outcomes) with what the nurse hoped would happen (the anticipated outcomes or goals). This phase measures the progression the patient has made toward a specific goal.

To evaluate, data must be collected to document the progress the patient has made, or not made, in relation to the stated goal. Once data have been collected and analyzed, the nurse must decide what action to take or what modification to make regarding the goal. In all instances the nurse will make one of three choices:
1. Resolve the plan because the patient has achieved the goal
2. Continue the plan because the patient is still making satisfactory progress toward the goal but did not achieve the goal during the original time frame
3. Revise the plan because the patient is not making satisfactory progress toward the goal (Cox and others, 1997).

As with the other phases of the nursing process, evaluation involves documenting and illustrating the patient's responses to the care provided. In accordance with the percentage given to the other phases of the nursing process, 20% of NCLEX examination questions pertain to evaluation. The following is an example of an evaluation question.

A home health nurse visits a patient recently diagnosed with diabetes mellitus. The patient complains of having episodes of shakiness, dizziness, and diaphoresis. In reviewing the patient's home record of blood glucose levels, the nurse notices that each blood glucose level made by the home health nurse is within physician-set limits but that each blood glucose level made by the patient is outside of the physician limits and requires insulin according to the sliding scale. What is the most appropriate action for the nurse to take?
A. Ask the patient why he thinks his blood glucose levels are always different from those of the home health nurses
B. Ask the patient to describe to the nurse how he obtains his blood glucose levels
C. Ask the patient to always do his blood glucose levels twice to validate that a correct reading is obtained
D. Ask the patient to demonstrate for the nurse how he obtains his blood glucose levels

Option D is the correct answer. Having the patient demonstrate how he obtains his blood glucose levels is an excellent method to determine if the patient is correctly performing the measurement. Actual demonstration validates or invalidates the procedure that the patient is using to obtain his blood glucose levels.

Option A is incorrect. In many instances the patient is the best source of information regarding his or her health status and maintenance patterns. In this case, however, the patient is not the best source unless he acknowledges problems in obtaining blood glucose levels.

Option B is incorrect. Asking the patient to tell the nurse how he obtains his blood glucose levels is a poor method to use to verify that the patient is performing the measurement correctly. The patient may be able to correctly state how he obtains his blood glucose levels but may not be able to correctly perform the measurement.

Option C is incorrect. Asking the patient to perform blood glucose levels twice is not an effective method to determine if blood glucose levels are accurate. Both determinations could be wrong, both could be right, or one could be right and the other wrong.

Client Needs

The second component of the NCLEX examination is client needs. This is a broad component that addresses the health care needs of clients (National Council, 2000).

Safe and Effective Care Environment. The first section relating to client needs is safe and effective care environment. Within this section the nurse should have the knowledge, skills, and ability to meet the client's needs for a safe and effective environment. Included in this section are management of patient care, patient safety, and infection control (National Council, 2000).

Twelve to thirty-four percent of questions on the NCLEX examination deal with a safe and effective environment (National Council, 2000). The following is an example.

A 75-year-old woman is admitted to the hospital for open reduction, internal fixation of her left radius and ulna. She fell at home and sustained the injury. Assessment reveals that the woman has fallen at home on numerous occasions. Each fall has been associated with an episode of dizziness. Physician's orders allow the patient to be up ad lib. In planning, the nurse would:

A. Ask the physician to change the activity order to strict bed rest.

B. Ask the patient to call for assistance when she wants to get out of the bed to go to the bathroom, sit up in a chair, or ambulate.

C. Place the patient in a vest restraint and tell her that she cannot get out of bed because she may have an episode of dizziness and fall and hurt herself again.

D. Keep the patient's room free of clutter and obstacles on the floor that may cause a fall.

Option B is the correct answer. Having someone with the patient when she is out of bed will reduce her risk of injury if she has an episode of dizziness. Assistance with mobility will not prevent an episode of dizziness, but the presence of another person may keep her from falling.

Option A is incorrect. There is no indication that the patient needs to have her activity level changed to strict bed rest. Keeping the older adult up and active is paramount in maintaining optimal health. Strict bed rest would place the patient at risk of developing respiratory, gastrointestinal, and skin problems.

Option C is incorrect. Restraints are not indicated in this situation and should never be used unless no other course of action is available. There is nothing to indicate that the patient is unable or unwilling to call for assistance when she wants to get out of bed. Telling this patient that she must stay in bed because she might have an episode of dizziness and fall is unwarranted.

Option D is incorrect. Keeping the patient's room free of clutter and obstacles will not prevent her from falling during an episode of dizziness. Part of the routine care afforded every patient should include keeping the room free of clutter and obstacles. This is not only for the patient's safety but also for the safety of any other person entering the room.

Included in safe, effective care environment is the management of care. Although nurses typically view themselves as caregivers, nurses also may function in a managerial role when coordinating, supervising, or collaborating with other members of the health care team (Job Analysis, 1996). A question dealing with management of care follows.

As the nurse manager for a medical-surgical unit, you are called on by two of the staff nurses working on the unit to assist in resolving a scheduling conflict. Both nurses should have off for an upcoming holiday, but short staffing requires that one work the holiday. After gathering pertinent data from each staff nurse, you realize that the type of conflict occurring between the two nurses is:

- A. Intrapersonal conflict.
- B. Interpersonal conflict.
- C. Organizational conflict.
- D. There is no conflict because staff nurses do not determine their work schedules.

Option B is the correct answer. Interpersonal conflict occurs among two or more people. Interpersonal conflict is common because each person perceives the world in a fashion that is unique to himself or herself.

Option A is incorrect. Intrapersonal conflict occurs within the person.

Option C is incorrect. Organizational conflict occurs when dealing with policies and procedures that relate to patient care or employee behavior.

Option D is incorrect. Conflict exists because the two staff nurses are unable to resolve an issue. Whether the staff nurses determine their work schedules has nothing to do with the issue presented in the question.

Psychosocial Integrity.   The second section of dealing with client needs is psychosocial integrity. As with the previous section, the nurse needs to possess the knowledge, skill, and ability to assist the client in meeting this need. Included in this section are coping, adaptation, and psychosocial adaptation (Job Analysis, 1996).

Ten to twenty-two percent of NCLEX examination questions address psychosocial integrity (National Council, 2000). The following is an example of a psychosocial integrity question.

A 23-year-old woman underwent a radical mastectomy for breast cancer. Three weeks after surgery during a postoperative visit to the surgeon, the nurse discovers that the woman refuses to look at her surgical scar, is reluctant to leave her home and socialize with her friends, and feels she is not a "real woman" anymore. In assisting the woman, the nurse would:

- A. Counsel the woman regarding her knowledge and treatment of breast cancer.
- B. Encourage the woman to increase her level of mobility and socialization.
- C. Teach the woman the importance of follow-up care.
- D. Collaborate with the physician for a mental health referral for alterations of self-concept and body image.

Option D is the correct answer. The woman is involved in a situational crisis and is having difficulty with coping and adapting to her postoperative status. To successfully cope, adapt, and get on with her life, mental health counseling is indicated.

Option A is incorrect. Increasing the woman's knowledge and treatment of breast cancer will not help her strengthen her self-concept or body image. Increasing knowledge and treatment of breast cancer has to do with a safe, effective care environment, not psychosocial integrity.

Option B is incorrect. There is nothing to suggest that the woman's level of mobility needs to be increased. A reluctance to leave her home and socialize with others does not suggest that she is immobile. Mobility has to do with physiologic integrity, not psychosocial integrity.

Option C is incorrect. Although follow-up care always is important and should be encouraged, follow-up care for a surgical patient usually has to do directly with the surgical procedure and its aftercare and does not routinely address mental health problems. Follow-up care is related to health promotion and maintenance, not psychosocial integrity.

Physiologic Integrity. The third section included in client needs is physiologic integrity. As with the previous two sections, the nurse needs to possess the knowledge, skills, and abilities to assist the patient in this area. Aspects included in physiologic integrity are basic patient care and comfort, pharmacologic and parenteral therapies, reduction of risk potential, and physiologic adaptation (National Council, 2000).

Thirty-six to sixty percent of questions on the NCLEX examination address physiologic integrity (National Council of State Boards of Nursing, Inc., 2000). An example follows.

A 75-year-old man is hospitalized and diagnosed with congestive heart failure. When he is discharged, his physician prescribes a low-sodium diet and furosemide 20 mg orally twice daily. He asks the nurse caring for the patient to make sure the patient understands the need to include high-potassium foods in his diet each day. In teaching the patient, the nurse should encourage the patient to include which of the following in his diet?

A. Whole grain breads, dried dates, cantaloupe, and sweet potatoes
B. Hominy, noodles, spaghetti, and rice
C. Canned meats, corned beef, sauerkraut, and bouillon drinks
D. Raw lettuce, turnips, green beans, and beets

Option A is the correct answer. All items are high in potassium and low in sodium.

Options B and D are both incorrect. All items are low in potassium and would be found on a potassium-restricted diet.

Option C is incorrect. All items are high in sodium.

Health Promotion and Maintenance. The final section relating to client needs is health promotion and maintenance. As with previous sections of client needs, the nurse needs to possess the knowledge, skill, and ability to assist the client to meet these needs. In this section 12% to 34% of NCLEX examination questions address health promotion and maintenance (National Council, 2000). The following is an example of a health promotion and maintenance question.

An RN works at a hospital that is actively involved in the community with health promotion and maintenance programs for older adults. Which of the following is an appropriate project activity for the nurse to institute at the county fair?

A. Screening for blood pressure and blood glucose abnormalities
B. Determining a patient's ability to perform self-care activities.
C. Identifying the coping abilities of children of recently divorced couples
D. Distributing acquired immune deficiency syndrome (AIDS)/human immunodeficiency syndrome information to health care workers

Option A is the correct answer. Health promotion and maintenance includes the prevention and early detection of disease. Blood pressure and blood glucose screening at a county fair would provide screening for adults of the community who may not seek medical care unless serious illness occurs.

Option B is incorrect. People attending a county fair would not be considered patients just because they sought blood pressure and blood glucose screening. In most instances, determining the ability of a patient to perform self-care activities would be accomplished in a health care setting such as a hospital, clinic, or home where a nurse intervenes and would include psychosocial integrity.

Option C is incorrect. In most instances, identifying the coping abilities of children of recently divorced couples would occur in a formal health care setting such as a hospital or clinic. Identification of coping abilities relates to psychosocial integrity, not health maintenance and promotion.

Option D is incorrect. It would be illogical to provide AIDS information for health care workers attending a county fair. Such a program relates to providing a safe and effective environment in the management of patient care and has nothing to do with health promotion and maintenance.

PREPARING FOR THE NCLEX EXAMINATION

There is no one best method for preparing to take the NCLEX examination. Success depends on a candidate's nursing knowledge and ability to use that knowledge, test-taking skills, and confidence level. The best preparation any candidate can have is what the candidate brings from his or her nursing program.

Some measure of preparation for the NCLEX examination after graduation from nursing school is a must for all candidates seeking success on the examination. Candidates should not convince themselves that they do not need to review because average or above-average grades were made in their academic and nursing course work, nor should they decide that review will serve no purpose because average or below-average grades were made in their course work.

In preparing for the NCLEX examination it is important to remember that review is a personal undertaking. What works for one candidate may not work for another and vice versa. Use study and review methods that have proven successful in the past.

Consider the following when preparing for the NCLEX examination:

- *Perform a needs assessment.* Determine content areas of strengths and weaknesses. Look at previous academic and nursing course work, class notes and handouts, examination grades, and grades made on nursing care plans or process papers. Talk with faculty in courses in which weakness or difficulty existed. Determine where the greatest amount of review is needed. Candidates should be honest in performing the needs assessment. The foundation for success or failure on the NCLEX examination may be determined here.
- *Determine the number of days or weeks necessary for review.* Candidates with a strong nursing knowledge base may need less time than candidates with weaknesses. As with the needs assessment, candidates should be realistic in planning the amount of review time needed.
- *Decide what method of review will be used.* Personal and group study has strong and weak points.
  Strong points of individual study include having total control over content and time spent in review.
  Weak points include having no immediate resources to explain or assist with understanding difficult concepts. Candidates with weakness in disciplining themselves may have problems sticking to review schedules and focusing on specific content with individual study.
  Strong points of group study include the support that members can give each other and learning from others in the group. Also, many minds working together are stronger than one working alone.
  Weak points of group study include a lack of preparation of some group members, weaker members of the group holding the rest back, and a tendency of the group

to focus on topics that have more to do with socialization than review. Candidates using study groups should insist on members coming to sessions prepared to work and discuss.

■ *Decide what materials or resources will be used during review.* Textbooks and class notes from nursing or nursing-related courses, such as anatomy and physiology, psychology, or nutrition, will prove helpful. Computer-assisted instructions used during the nursing program may be available. Numerous NCLEX review books are available. Their prices range from around $20 to $50. Many review books include a computer disk or CD-ROM to be used with review. Make sure that these computer aids are compatible with the computer being used.

■ *Talk with nursing faculty* about using any NCLEX preparation aids the school of nursing may have available for candidates.

■ *Structure review time.* Schedule review during times of peak performance. Learning is enhanced when reviewing for short blocks of time, around 50 minutes, instead of reviewing for several unbroken hours at a time. Candidates should remember that they are reviewing for an examination, not cramming for one.

■ *Control the review environment.* Keep noise and distraction at a minimum. Have adequate space and lighting for review. Control the room temperature when possible; if not possible, dress for the environment. Have all materials, including soft drinks and snacks, needed for review close at hand so time is not wasted gathering these items during review time. Make sure that friends and family know not to interrupt during review time.

■ *Have a game plan for each review session.* Develop a review schedule complete with subject matter to be considered and specific tasks to be completed during each session. Stick to the schedule.

■ *Learn concepts and principles, not isolated facts.* The NCLEX examination tests a candidate's ability to apply, analyze, and evaluate nursing knowledge and does not focus on isolated events. Candidates whose past test-taking success has been based on memorization rather than actual learning will increase their risk of failure on the NCLEX examination.

■ *Use learning techniques that have proven successful in the past,* such as flash cards or note cards, underscoring of key points, taking notes or outlining material, or capturing pertinent information on a tape recorder for later playback. One should either quiz himself or herself or ask others to pose questions.

■ *Seek qualified help when reviewing information that is particularly difficult.* Faculty are an excellent resource. Be cautious when asking peers for assistance because they may not understand materials as well as they think they do.

■ *Practice taking "NCLEX-type" examinations,* paying particular attention to the rationales or reasons provided for correct and incorrect answers. Successful test takers know why a specific option is correct or incorrect. Even though candidates may spend as much time as they want on a question when actually taking the examination, they should get into the habit of taking about 1 minute for each question. Poor time management may cause a candidate to not have enough time to complete the test and therefore be unsuccessful on the NCLEX examination. Practice also will help reduce test anxiety. NCLEX-type examinations are commonly found in NCLEX review books.

BOX 26-1	*Helpful Websites*

NCLEX-RN® examination
http://www.ncsbn.org

Study strategies and test preparation
http://www.sas.calpoly.edu
http://www.iss.stthomas.edu/studyguides/

Nursing site
http://www.nursing.about.com/health/nursing

- *Use the Internet.* It provides numerous sources that may aid in preparation for the NCLEX examination. Box 26-1 provides a partial listing of available sites that might be helpful.
- *Avoid excessive stimulants* (e.g., caffeine) to increase review time. The best learning takes place when heads are clear.
- *Maintain a healthy, positive attitude* toward reviewing and taking the NCLEX examination. Have confidence in your abilities to be successful on the examination. Plan to do the best that you can. Remember that even practicing nurses with years of experience don't know everything there is to know about every aspect of nursing and that the goal on the NCLEX examination is to demonstrate competency for an entry-level RN position, not competency for an advanced RN position.

FOOD FOR THOUGHT WHEN SELECTING AN NCLEX REVIEW COURSE

Just as there is no one best method for preparing to take the NCLEX examination, there is no one best review course for a candidate to take in preparation for the NCLEX examination. The most important thing to remember when considering a review course is that a review course is exactly what it says it is—a review course. Such courses are designed to reconsider or reexamine content common to the three types of nursing programs.

The purpose of a review course is to enhance or polish what candidates already know from their nursing programs. Review courses are not intended to teach totally new concepts. If candidates have an extreme weakness in one or more content areas, the review course may not provide enough content to bring the candidate up to speed on the topic.

Numerous companies and people offer review courses. Each review offering has strong and weak points, and what appeals to one candidate may not appeal to another. Some offer financial discounts or other incentives if more than one candidate from a school of nursing registers for their course.

Review courses usually are expensive and last from 1 or 2 days to a complete work week. Some courses provide books or other written materials. Others may offer additional materials for a fee. Some courses will refund a part or all of the cost of the review if a candidate takes their review course and is unsuccessful in taking the NCLEX examination.

Review courses may or may not be taught by competent people. Nurse educators who are teaching faculty at schools of nursing teach many courses. People who teach the material without any substantial background in nursing teach other courses. A review course is no better than the person or people teaching it.

The decision to take a review course in preparation for taking the NCLEX examination is a personal one. Some candidates find the structure and schedule of a review course helpful in preparation. Other candidates may find the structure and schedule restrictive and overly time consuming.

Candidates seriously interested in taking an NCLEX review course should look to the faculty at their school of nursing for guidance. Many faculty have had experience with review courses or may teach review courses. Serious candidates also should obtain written information from several different review course offerings and compare and contrast among the offerings. Selection of a review course should be based on more than the cost of the review program—it should meet the candidate's unique needs.

SUMMARY

Success on the NCLEX examination is needed to obtain a license and practice as an RN. Most candidates taking the NCLEX examination are successful. Of the approximate 72,000 first-time, United States–educated candidates taking the examination during the first three quarters of 2000, around 81% were successful (Number of Candidates, 2000). The key to success on the NCLEX examination is sound preparation from the nursing program, adequate preparation for the examination, and confidence in oneself.

Critical Thinking Activities

1. Develop a realistic plan for reviewing for the NCLEX examination. Include what you think is important in developing your plan and include the following:
    a. Areas of strengths and weaknesses
    b. Time frame for review
    c. Methods of review
    d. Specific plans for each review session
    e. Resources
    f. Barriers to effective review
    g. Realistic solutions to barriers
2. Investigate at least three different NCLEX review courses and determine the strengths and weaknesses of each.

REFERENCES

Carroll-Johnson RM: *Classification of nursing diagnoses: proceedings of the ninth conference,* Philadelphia, 1991, JB Lippincott.

Computerized adaptive testing (CAT) overview, 2000, www.ncsbn.org/files/nclex/cattop.asp.

Cox HC et al: *Clinical applications of nursing diagnosis: adult, child, women's, psychiatric, gerontic, and home health considerations,* Philadelphia, 1997, FA Davis.

Foote J: *State board questions and answers for nurses,* Philadelphia, 1919, JB Lippincott.

Gronlund NE: *Measurement and evaluation in teaching,* New York, 1985, Macmillan Publishing.

How CAT works: A candidate primer. 2000, National Council of State Boards of Nursing Web Site, www.ncsbn.org/files/nclex/overview.asp.

Job analysis of newly licensed registered nurses, Chicago, 1996, National Council of State Boards of Nursing.

More untrue rumors regarding the NCLEX examination, National Council of State Boards of Nursing Web Site, 2000, www.ncsbn.org/files/nclex/news.asp.

National Council of State Boards of Nursing: NCLEX-RN examination test plan for the National Council Licensure Examination for Register Nurses, Chicago, 2000, Author.

Number of candidates taking NCLEX-RN examination and percent passing, 2000, by type of Candidate, 2000, www.ncsbn.org/research/nclexstats/nclex.asp.

Why aren't skipping questions and changing answers allowed? 2000, www.ncsbn.org/files/nclex/overview.asp.

Appendixes A to D

APPENDIX A: NURSING ORGANIZATIONS

Academy of Medical-Surgical Nurses
http://www.medsurgnurse.org/
East Holly Ave., Box 56
Pitman, NJ 08071
Phone: 609-256-2323
Fax: 609-589-7463

Aerospace Nursing Association
North Carolina Central University
Dept. of Nursing, PO Box 19798
Durham, NC 27707
Phone: 919-560-6431

American Academy of Nurse Practitioners
http://www.aanp.org/
Capital Station, PO Box 12846
Austin, TX 78711
Phone: 512-442-4262
Fax: 512-442-6469

American Academy of Nursing
http://www.nursingworld.org/aan/index.htm
600 Maryland Ave., SW, Suite 100 West
Washington, DC 20024-2571
Phone: 202/651-7238
Fax: 202/554-2641

American Assembly for Men in Nursing
http://aamn.freeyellow.com/
AAMN % NYSNA
11 Cornell Rd.
Latham, NY 12110-1499
Phone: 518-782-9400 Ext. 346

American Association for the History of Nursing
www.aahn.org
PO Box 175
Lanoka Harbor, NJ 08734
Phone: 609-693-7250
Fax: 609-693-1037

American Academy of Ambulatory Care Nursing
http://aaacn.inurse.com
AAACN National Office, East Holly Ave., Box 56
Pitman, NJ 08071-0056
Phone: Main number 856-256-2350; Toll Free:
   800-AMB-NURS
Fax: 856-589-7463

American Association of Colleges of Nursing
http://www.aacn.nche.edu
One Dupont Circle
Suite 530
Washington, DC 20036-1120
Phone: 202-463-6903
Fax: 202-785-8320

American Association of Critical Care Nurses
www.aacn.org
101 Columbia
Aliso Viejo, CA 92656
Phone: 949-362-2000
Fax: 949-362-2020

American Association of Legal Nurse Consultants
http://www.aalnc.org/
4700 West Lake Ave.
Glenview, IL 60025
Phone: 877-402-2562
Fax: 877-734-8668

American Association of Neuroscience Nurses
http://www.aann.org
4700 W. Lake Ave.
Glenview, IL 60025
Phone: 847-375-4733
Fax: 847-375-4777

American Association of Nurse Anesthetists
www.aana.com
222 South Prospect Ave.
Park Ridge, IL 60068-4001
Phone: 847-692-7050

American Association of Nurse Attorneys
http://www.taana.org
7794 Grow Dr.
Pensacola, Fl 32514
Phone: 877-538-2262
Fax: 850-484-8762

American Association of Occupational Health Nurses
http://www.aaohn.org
Suite 100 Brandywine Rd.
Atlanta, GA 30341
Phone: 770-455-7757
Fax: 770-455-7271

American Association of Spinal Cord Injury Nurses
www.aascin.org
75-20 Astoria Blvd.
Jackson Heights, NY 11370-1177
Phone: 718-803-3782
Fax: 718-803-0414

American College of Nurse Practitioners
http://www.nurse.org/acnp/
1111 19th St. NW
Suite 404
Washington DC 20036
Phone: 202-659-2196
Fax: 202-659-2191

American College of Nurse-Midwives
http://www.acnm.org
818 Connecticut Ave. NW, Suite 900
Washington, DC 20006
Phone: 202-728-9860
Fax: 202-728-9897

American Forensic Nurses
www.amrn.com
255 N. El Cielo, Suite 195
Palm Springs, CA 92262
Phone: 760-322-9925
Fax: 760-322-9914

American Holistic Nurses Association
http://ahna.org
PO Box 2130
Flagstaff, AZ 86003-2130
Phone: 1-800-278-2462

American Nephrology Nurses Association
http://www.anna.inurse.com
East Holly Ave.
Box 56
Pitman, NJ 08071-0056
Phone: 609-256-2320
Fax: 856-589-7463

American Nurses Association
http://www.ana.org
600 Maryland Ave. SW, Suite 100 West
Washington, DC 20024-2571
Phone: 800-274-4ANA

American Nurses Credentialing Center
600 Maryland Ave. SW, 100 West
Washington, DC 20024-2571
http://www.ANCC@ana.org

American Organization of Nurse Executives
http://www.aone.org
325 Seventh Street NW, Suite 700
Washington, DC 20004
Phone: 202-626-2240
Fax: 202-638-5499

American Psychiatric Nurse Association
www.apna.org
Colonial Place Three
2107 Wilson Blvd, Suite 300-A
Arlington, VA 22201
Phone: 703-243-2443
Fax: 703-243-3390

American Radiological Nurses Association
www.rsna.org/about/orgs/arna
820 Jorie Blvd
Old Brook, IL 60523
Phone: 630-571-9072
Fax: 630-571-7837

American Society of Ophthalmic Registered Nurses
http://webeye.opth.uiowa.edu/asorn/
PO Box 193030
San Francisco, CA 94119
Phone: 415-561-8513
Fax: 415-561-8575

American Society of Pain Management Nurses
www.aspmn.org
7794 Grow Dr.
Pensacola, FL 32514
Phone: 888-342-7766
Fax: 850-484-8762

American Society of PeriAnesthesia Nurses
http://www.aspan.org
10 Melrose Ave, Suite 110
Cherry Hill, NJ 08003-3696
Phone: 877-737-9696
Fax: 856-616-9601

Association of Black Nursing Faculty, Inc.
www.abnfinc.org

Association of Nurses in AIDS Care
http://www.anacnet.org/
80 S. Summit St.
500 Courtyard Square
Akron, Ohio 44308
Phone: 330-762-5739
Fax: 330-762-5813

Association of Operating Room Nurses
http://www.aorn.org
2170 South Parker Rd.
Suite 300
Denver, CO 80231-5711
Phone: 303-755-6304
Fax: 303-750-2927

Association of Pediatric Oncology Nurses
www.apon.org
4700 West Lake Ave.
Glenview, IL 60025-1485
Phone: 847-375-4724
Fax: 847-375-6324

Association of Rehabilitation Nurses
http://www.rehabnurse.org
4700 West Lake Rd.
Glenview, IL 60025-1485
Phone: 800-229-7530
Fax: 877-734-9384

Association of Women's Health, Obstetric and Neonatal Nursing
http://www.awhonn.org
2000 L Street, N.W. Suite 740
Washington, DC 20036
Phone: 800-673-8499

Commission on Graduates of Foreign Nursing Schools
www.cgfns.org
3600 Market St.
Suite 400
Philadelphia, PA 19104

Dermatology Nurses Association
http://dna.inurse.com
Box 56
East Holly Ave.
Pitman, NJ 08071
Fax: 609-582-1915

Developmental Disabilities Nurses Association
www.ddna.org
1733 H St.,
Suite 330, PMB 1214
Blaine, WA 98230
Phone: 800-888-6733
Fax: 360-332-2280

Emergency Nurses Association
http://www.ena.org
915 Lee St.
Des Plaines, IL 60016-6569
Phone: 800-900-9659
Fax: 847-460-4001

Federation of Nurses and Health Professionals
http://www.aft.org/fnhp/
555 New Jersey Ave.
Washington, DC 20001
Phone: 202-879-4491
Fax: 202-879-4597

Haitian Nurses Association
113-63 Hook Creek Blvd.
Valley Stream, NY 11580

Hospice and Palliative Nurses Association
www.hpna.org
Penn Center West One
Suite 229
Pittsburgh, PA 15276
Phone: 412-787-9301
Fax: 412-787-9305

International Council of Nurses
http://www.nursingworld.org/icn/
3 Place Jean-Marteau
Geneva, Switzerland 1201
Phone: 41-22-908-01-00
Fax: 41-22-908-01-01

International Society of Nurses in Genetics, Inc.
Foundation for Blood Research
http://www.nursing.creighton.edu/isong/
Phone: 603-643-5706

Intravenous Nurses Society (Therapy)
http://www.ins1.org
220 Norwood Park South
Norwood, MA 02062
Phone: 781-440-9408
Fax: 781-440-9409

National Association Directors of Nursing Administration in Long Term Care
www.nadona.org
10999 Reed Hartman Highway
Suite 233
Cincinnati, OH 45242
Phone: 1-800-222-0539

National Association of Hispanic Nurses
www.thehispanicnurses.org
1501 16th Street NW
Washington, DC 20036
Phone: 202-387-2477
Fax: 202-483-7183

National Association of Neonatal Nurses
http://www.nann.org
4700 W. Lake Ave.
Glenview, IL 60025-1485
Phone: 800-451-3795
Fax: 888-477-6266

National Association of Nurse Practitioners in Women's Health
www.npwh.org
503 Capitol Court, N.E.
Suite 300
Washington, DC 20002
Phone: 202-543-9693
Fax: 202-543-9858

National Association of Orthopedic Nurses
http://www.naon.inurse.org
Box 56
East Holly Ave.
Pitman, NJ 08071-0056
Phone: 856-256-2310
Fax: 856-589-7463

National Association of Pediatric Nurses and Practitioners
http://www.napnap.org
1101 Kings Highway North
Cherry Hill, NJ 08034
Phone: 856-667-1773
Fax: 856-667-7187

National Association of School Nurses
www.nasn.org
PO Box 1300
Scarborough, ME 04070-1300
Phone: 207-883-2117
Fax: 207-883-2683

National Black Nurses Association, Inc.
www.nbna.org
8630 Fenton St
Suite 330
Silver Spring, MD 20910-3803
Phone: 202-589-3200

National Consortium of Chemical Dependency Nurses
167 Cleveland St.
PO Box 2749
Eugene, OR 97402
Phone: 800-876-2236
Fax: 541-485-7372

National Council of State Boards of Nursing, Inc.
http://www.ncsbn.org
676 North St. Clair
Suite 550
Chicago, IL 60611-2921
Phone: 312-787-6555
Fax: 312-787-6898

National Federation of Specialty Nursing Organizations
http://www.nfsno.org
East Holly Ave.
Box 56
Pitman, NJ 08071
Phone: 609-256-2333
Fax: 609-589-7463

Air and Surface Transport Nurses Association aka National Flight Nurses Association
www.astna.org
9101 E. Kenyon Ave.
Suite 3000
Denver, CO 80237

National Gerontological Nursing Association
www.ngna.org
7794 Grow Dr
Pensacola, FL 32514
Phone: 800-723-0560
Fax: 850-484-8762

National Institute of Nursing Research
http://www.nih.gov/ninr/index.html
NIH Building 31
Bethesda, MD 20892-2178
Phone: 301-496-0207
Fax: 301-480-4969

National League for Nursing
http://www.nln.org
61 Broadway, 33rd Floor
New York, NY 10006
Phone: 1-800-669-1656

National Nursing Staff Development Organization
7794 Grow Dr.
Pensacola, FL 32514
Phone: 1-800-489-1995
Fax: 850-484-8762

National Organization for Associate Degree Nursing
http://www.noadn.org/adnursing
11250 Roger Bacon Drive
Suite 8
Reston, VA20190-5202
Phone: 703-437-4377

National Student Nurses Association
http://www.nsna.org
555 W 57th St.
Suite 1327
New York, NY 10019
Phone: 212-581-2211
Fax: 212-581-2368

Navy Nurses Corps
www.nnca.org
2300 East Street NW
Washington, DC0372-5300
Phone: 202-762-3040
Fax: 202-762-3727

North American Nursing Diagnosis Association
www.nanda.org
1211 Locust St.
Philadelphia, PA 19107
Phone: 215-545-8105
Fax: 215-545-8107

Nurses Christian Fellowship
www.ncf-jcn.org
POBox 7895
Madison, WI 53707-7895
Phone: 608-274-4823 ext. 401

Nurses in Transition (Holistic Medicine)
PO Box 104
Glencoe, CA 95232

Nurses Organization of Veterans Affairs
www.vanurse.org
1726 M St. NW
Suite 1101
Washington, DC 20036
Phone: 202-296-0888
Fax: 202-833-1577

Oncology Nursing Society
http://www.ons.org
501 Holiday Drive
Pittsburgh, PA 15220-2749
Phone: 412-921-7373
Fax: 412-921-6565

Philippine Nurses Association of America
www.pna-america.org
151 Linda Vista Dr
Daly City, CA 94014
Phone: 415-468-7995
Fax: 415-468-7995

Respiratory Nursing Society
www.respiratorynursingsociety.org
RNS c/o NYSNA
11 Cornell Rd
Latham, NY 12110
Phone: 518-782-9400 ext 286

Sigma Theta Tau International
www.nursingsociety.org
550 West North Street
Indianapolis, IN 46202
Phone: 317-634-8171
Fax: 317-634-8188

Society for Vascular Nursing
www.svnnet.org
7794 Grow Dr.
Pensacola, FL 32514
Phone: 1-888-536-4786
Fax: 850-484-8762

Society of Gastroenterology Nurses and Associates
www.sgna.org
401 North Michigan Ave.
Chicago, IL 60611
Phone: 800-245-7462
Fax: 312-527-6635

Society of Gynecologic Nurse Oncologists
www.sgno.org
6024 Welch Ave
Fort Worth, TX 76133
Phone: 1-800-446-3180

Society of Trauma Nurses
www.traumanursesoc.org
2743 S. Veterans Parkway
Springfield, IL 62704
Phone: 217-787-3281
Fax: 217-787-3285

Transcultural Nursing Society
www.tcns.org
36600 Schoolcraft Rd.
Livonia, MI 48150
Phone: 1-88-432-5470
Fax: 734-432-5463

Wound, Ostomy, and Continence Nurses Society
www.wocn.org
1550 South Coast Highway
Suite 201
Laguna Beach, CA 92651
Phone: 1-888-224-WOCN
Fax: 949-376-3456

APPENDIX B: STATE BOARDS OF NURSING (INCLUDING U.S. TERRITORIES)

Alabama State Board of Nursing
www.abn.state.al.us/
770 Washington Ave.
RSA Plaza, Ste. 250
Montgomery, AL 36130-3900
Phone: 334-242-4060
Fax: 334-242 4360

Alaska Board of Nursing
Department of Commerce and Economic Development
Division of Occupational Licensing
www.dced.state.ak.us/occ/pnur
P.O. Box 110806
Juneau, AK 99811-0806
Phone: 907-269-8161

Arizona State Board of Nursing
www.azboardofnursing.org
1651 East Morten Ave.
Suite 210
Phoenix, AZ 85020
Phone: 602-331-8111

Arkansas State Board of Nursing
www.state.ar.us/nurse
University Tower Building
Suite 800
1123 South University Ave.
Little Rock, AR 77204
Phone: 501-686-2700
Fax: 501-686-2714

California Board of Registered Nursing
www.rn.ca.gov
400 R St., Ste. 4030
Sacramento, CA 95814-6239
Phone: 916-322-3350
Fax: 916-327-4402

Colorado State Board of Nursing
www.dora.state.co.us/nursing
1560 Broadway, Suite 880
Denver, CO 80202
Phone: 303-894-2430
Fax: 303-894-2821

Connecticut Board of Examiners for Nursing
Dept. of Public Health
410 Capitol Ave., MS# 13PHO
Hartford, CT 06134-0328
Phone: 860-509-7624
Fax: 860-509-7553

Delaware Board of Nursing
Cannon Building, Suite 203
861 Silver Lake Blvd
Dover, DE 19904
Phone: 302-739-4522
Fax: 860-739-2711

District of Columbia Board of Nursing
Dept. of Public Health
825 N. Capitol St., NE, 2nd Floor
Room 2224
Washington, DC 20001
202-442-4778
Fax: 202-442-9431

Florida Board of Nursing
www.doh.state.fl.us/mqa
4080 Woodcock Dr., Suite 202
Jacksonville, FL 32207
904-858-6940
Fax: 904-858-6964

Georgia Board of Nursing
www.sos.state.ga.us/ebd-rn
237 Coliseum Drive
Macon, GA 31217-3858
912-207-1640
Fax: 912-207-1660

Hawaii Board of Nursing
Professional and Vocational Licensing Division
www.state.hi.us/dcca/pvloffline/
Box 3469
Honolulu, HI 96801
808-586-3000
Fax: 808-586-2689

Idaho State Board of Nursing
www.state.id.us/ibn/ibnhome
280 N. 8th Street, Suite 210
P.O. Box 83720
Boise, ID 83720
208-334-3110
Fax: 208-334-3262

Illinois Department of Professional Regulation
www.dpr.state.il.us/
James R. Thompson Center
100 West Randolph, Suite 9-300
Chicago, IL 60601
312-814-2715
Fax: 312-814-3145

Indiana State Board of Nursing
Health Professions Bureau
www.state.in.us/hpb/noards/isbn/
402 West Washington Street, Suite W041
Indianapolis, IN 46204
317-232-2960
Fax: 317-233-4236

Iowa Board of Nursing
www.state.ia.us/government/nursing/
400 S.W. 8th Street Suite B
Des Moines, IA 50309-4685
515-281-3255
Fax: 515-281-4825

Kansas State Board of Nursing
www.ksbn.org
Landon State Office Building
900 SW Jackson Street
Suite 551-S
Topeka, KS 66612
785-296-4929
Fax: 785-296-3929

Kentucky Board of Nursing
www.kbn.state.ky.us
312 Whittington Parkway, Suite 300
Louisville, KY 40222
502-329-7000
Fax: 502-329-7011

Louisiana Board of Nursing
www.lsbn.state.us
3510 N. Causeway Blvd., Suite 501
Metairie, LA 70002
504-838-5791
Fax: 504-838-5279

Maine State Board of Nursing
www.state.me.us/nursingbd/
158 State House Station
Augusta, ME 04333
207-287-1133
207-287-1149

Maryland Board of Nursing
www.mbon.org
4140 Patterson Ave.
Baltimore, MD 21215
410-585-1900
Fax: 410-358-3530

Massachusetts Board of Registration in Nursing
www.state.ma.us/reg/boards/rn
239 Causeway Street
Boston, MA 02114
617-727-9961
Fax: 617-727-1630

Michigan Board of Nursing
CIS/Office of Health Services
www.cis.state.mi.us/bhser/genover
Ottawa Towers North
611 West Ottawa
4th Floor
Lansing, MI 48933
517-373-9102
Fax: 517-373-2179

Minnesota Board of Nursing
www.nursingboard.state.mn.us
2829 University Ave. SE
Suite 500
Minneapolis, MN 55414
612-617-2270
Fax: 612-617-2190

Mississippi Board of Nursing
www.msbn.state.ms.us
1935 Lakeland Dr, Suite B
Jackson, MS 39216-5014
601-987-4188
Fax: 601-364-2352

Missouri State Board of Nursing
www.ecodev.state.mo.us/pr/nursing/
PO Box 656
Jefferson City, MO 65102-0656
573-751-0681
Fax: 573-751-0075

Montana State Board of Nursing
www.com.state.mt.us/license/pol/index
301 South Park
Helena, MT 59620-0513
406-444-2071
Fax: 406-841-2343

Nebraska Board of Nursing
Department of Health and Human Services
Regulation and Licensure
Nursing Section
www.hhs.state.ne.us/crl/nns
301 Centennial Mall South
Lincoln, NE 68509-4986
402-471-4376
Fax: 402-471-3577

Nevada State Board of Nursing
www.nursingboard.state.nv.us
1755 East Plumb Lane
Suite 260
Reno, NV 89502
702-786-2778
Fax: 775-688-2628

New Hampshire Board of Nursing
www.nursingboard.state.nv.us
PO Box 45010
78 Regional Drive Bldg B
Concord, NH 03301
603-271-2323
Fax: 973-648-3481

New Jersey Board of Nursing
www.state.nj.us/lps/ca/medical
PO Box 45010
124 Halsey St, 6th Floor
Newark, NJ 07101
973-504-6586
Fax: 973-648-3481

New Mexico Board of Nursing
www.state.nm.us/clients/nursing
4206 Louisiana Blvd., NE
Suite A
Albuquerque, NM 87109
505-841-8340
Fax: 505-841-8347

New York State Education Department
www.nysed.gov/prof/nurse
89 Washington Ave
2nd Floor, West Wing
Albany, NY 12234
518-474-3817 Ext. 120
Fax: 518-474-3706

North Carolina Board of Nursing
www.ncbon.com
3724 National Drive
Raleigh, NC 27612
919-782-3211
Fax: 919-781-9461

North Dakota Board of Nursing
www.ndbon.org
919 South 7th Street
Suite 504
Bismarck, ND 58504
701-328-9777
Fax: 701-328-9785

Ohio Board of Nursing
www.stae.oh.us/nur
17 South High St, Suite 400
Columbus, OH 43215-3413
614-466-3947
Fax: 614-466-0388

Oklahoma Board of Nursing
2915 N. Classen Blvd., Suite 524
Oklahoma City, OK 73106
405-962-1800
Fax: 405-962-1821

Oregon State Board of Nursing
www.osbn.state.or.us
800 NE Oregon Street, Box 25, Suite 465
Portland, OR 97232
503-731-4745
Fax: 503-731-4755

Pennsylvania State Board of Nursing
www.dos.state.pa.us/bpoa/nurbd/mainpage
124 Pine Street
Harrisburg, PA 17101
717-783-7142
Fax: 787-725-7903

Rhode Island Board of Nurse Registration and Nursing Education
www.health.state.ri.us/
105 Cannon Building
Three Capitol Hill
Providence, RI 02908
401-222-5700
Fax: 401-222-3352

South Carolina State Board of Nursing
www.llr.state.sc.us/pol/nursing
110 Centerview Drive, Suite 202
Columbia, SC 29210
803-896-4550
Fax: 803-896-4525

South Dakota Board of Nursing
www.state.sd.us/dcr/nursing
4300 South Louise Ave., Suite C-1
Sioux Falls, SD 57106-3124
605-367-2760
Fax: 605-362-2768

Tennessee State Board of Nursing
http://170.142.76.180/bmf-bin/bmfproflist.pl
426 Fifth Ave. North
1st Floor–Cordell Hull Building
Nashville, TN 37247
615-532-5166
Fax: 615-741-7899

Texas Board of Nurse Examiners
www.bne.state.tx.us
333 Guadalupe, Suite 3-460
Austin, TX 78701
512-305-7400
Fax: 512-305-7401

Utah State Board of Nursing
www.Commerce.state.ut.us/
160 East 300 South
Salt Lake City, UT 84111
801-530-6628
Fax: 801-530-6511

Vermont State Board of Nursing
http://vtprofessionals/org/nurses/
109 State St.
Montpelier, VT 05609-1106
802-828-2396
Fax: 802-828-2484

Virginia Board of Nursing
www.dhp.state.va.us/
6606 West Broad Street, 4th Floor
Richmond, VA 23230
804-662-9909
Fax: 804-662-9512

Washington State Nursing Quality Assurance Commission
Department of Health
www.doh.was.gov/nursing
1300 Quince St. SE
Olympia, WA 98504-7864
360-236-4740
Fax: 360-236-4738

West Virginia Board of Examiners for Registered Nurses
www.state.wv.us/nurses/rn
101 Dee Dr.
Charleston, WV 25311
304-558-3596
Fax: 304-558-3666

Wisconsin Department of Regulation and Licensing
www.drl.state.wi.us/
1400 E. Washington Ave.
Madison, WI 53708
608-266-0145
Fax: 608-261-7083

Wyoming State Board of Nursing
http://nursing.state.wy.us/
2020 Carey Ave., Suite 110
Cheyenne, WY 82002
307-777-7601
Fax: 307-777-3519

United States Territories

American Samoa Health Services Regulatory Board
LBJ Tropical Medical Center
Pago Pago, American Samoa 96799
684-633-1222
Fax: 684-633-1869

Guam Board of Nurse Examiners
PO Box 2816
Barrada, GU 96913
671-475-0251
Fax: 671-477-4733

Northern Mariana Islands Commonwealth Board of Nurse Examiners
Public Health Center
PO Box 1458
Saipan, Northern Mariana Islands 96950
011 670-234-8950
Fax: 011 670-234-8930

Commonwealth of Puerto Rico Board of Nurse Examiners
Call Box 10200
Santurce, PR 00908
787-725-8161

Virgin Islands Board of Nurse Licensure
Veterans Drive Station
St. Thomas, VI 00803
340-776-7397
Fax: 340-777-4003

APPENDIX C: STATE NURSING ASSOCIATIONS

Alabama State Nurses Association
www.nursingworld.org/snas/al/
360 North Hull Street
Montgomery, AL 36104-3658
334-262-8321
Fax: 334-262-8578

Alaska Nurses Association
www.aknurse.org
237 East Third Ave.
Anchorage, AK 99501
907-274-0827
Fax: 907-272-0292

Arizona Nurses Association
www.nursingworld.org/snas/az/
1850 E. Southern Ave.
Suite 1
Tempe, AZ 85282
480-831-0404
Fax: 480-839-4780

Arkansas Nurses Association
www.arna.org
804 N. University
Little Rock, AR 72205
501-664-5853
Fax: 501-664-5859

American Nurses Association/California
www.anacalifornia.org
Sacramento, CA 95814
916-447-0225
Fax: 916-447-5568

Colorado Nurses Association
www.nurses-co.org
950 South Cherry St
Suite 508
Denver, CO 80246
303-757-7483
Fax: 303-758-0190

Connecticut Nurses Association
www.nursingworld.org/snas/ct
377 Research Parkway
Suite 2D
Meriden, CT 06450-7160
203-238-1207
Fax: 203-238-3437

Delaware Nurses Association
www.nursingworld.org/snas/de
2644 Capitol Trail
Suite 330
Newark, DE 19711
302-368-2333
Fax: 302-366-1775

District of Columbia Nurses Association, Inc.
www.dcnaonline.com
5100 Wisconsin Ave., NW
Washington, DC 20016
202-244-2705
Fax: 202-362-8285

Florida Nurses Association
www.floridanurse.org
PO Box 536985
Orlando, FL 32853-6985
407-896-3261
Fax: 407-896-9042

Georgia Nurses Association
www.nursingworld.org/snas/ga
1362 West Peachtree Street, NW
Atlanta, GA 30309-2904
404-876-4624
Fax: 404-876-4621

Guam Nurses Association
PO Box CG
Haganta, Guam 96932
011 671-477-6877

Hawaii Nurses Association
www.hawaiinurses.org
677 Ala Moana Blvd., Suite 301
Honolulu, HI 96813
808-521-8361
Fax: 808-524-2760

Idaho Nurses Association
www.nursingworld.org/snas/id
200 North 4th Street, Suite 200
Boise, ID 83702-6001
208-345-0500
Fax: 208-385-0166

Illinois Nurses Association
www.illinoisnurses.com
105 West Adams St
Suite 2101
Chicago, IL 60603
312-419-2900 ext. 231
Fax: 312-419-2920

Indiana State Nurses Association
2915 North High School Rd.
Indianapolis, IN 46224
317-299-4575
Fax: 317-297-3525

Iowa Nurses Association
www.iowanurses.org
1501 42nd Street, Suite 471
West Des Moines, IA 50266
515-225-0495
Fax: 515-225-2201

Kansas State Nurses Association
www.nursingworld.org/snas/ks
1208 S.W. Tyler
Topeka, KS 66612-1735
785-233-8638
Fax: 785-233-5222

Kentucky Nurses Association
www.kentucky-nurses.org
1400 South First Street
PO Box 2616
Louisville, KY 40201
502-637-2546
Fax: 502-637-8236

Louisiana State Nurses Association
www.lsna.org
5700 Florida Blvd.
Suite 720
Baton Rouge, LA 70806-4820
225-201-0993
Fax: 225-201-0971

Maine State Nurses Association
PO Box 254
Auburn, ME 04212-0254
207-667-0260

Maryland Nurses Association
www.nursingworld.org/snas/md
849 International Dr.
Suite 255
Linthicum, MD 21090
410-859-3000
Fax: 410-859-3001

Massachusetts Nurses Association
www.nursingworld.org/snas/ma/home.htm
340 Turnpike Street
Canton, MA 02021
Phone: 617-821-4625
Fax: 617-821-4445

Michigan Nurses Association
www.minurses.org
2310 Jolly Oak Rd.
Okemos, MI 48864-4599
1-800-832-2051
Fax: 517-349-5818

Minnesota Nurses Association
www.mnnurses.org
1625 Energy Park Drive
St. Paul, MN 55108
1-800-536-4662
Fax: 651-647-5301

Mississippi Nurses Association
www.msnurses.org
31 Woodgreen Place
Madison, MS 39110
601-898-0670
Fax: 601-898-0190

Missouri Nurses Association
www.missourinurses.org
1904 Bubba Lane, Box 105228
Jefferson City, MO 65110
573-696-4623
Fax: 573-636-9576

Montana Nurses Association
www.nursingworld.org/snas/mt
104 Broadway
Suite G-2
PO Box 5718
Helena, MT 59601
406-442-6710
Fax: 406-442-1841

Nebraska Nurses Association
www.nursingworld.org/snas/ne/index
715 South 14th St.
Lincoln, NE 68508
402-475-3859
Fax: 402-475-3961

Nevada Nurses Association
PO Box 530399
Henderson, NV 89053-0399
702-260-7886
Fax: 702-260-7052

New Hampshire Nurses Association
http://nhnurses.myassociation.com/home.jsp
48 West Street
Concord, NH 03301-3595
603-225-3783
Fax: 603-228-6672

New Jersey Nurses Association
1479 Pennington Rd.
Trenton, NJ 08618
609-883-5335 Ext. 10
609-883-5343

New Mexico Nurses Association
PO Box 80300
Albuquerque, NM 87198-0300
505-268-7744
Fax: 505-268-7711

New York State Nurses Association
www.nysna.org
11 Cornell Rd.
Latham, NY 12110
518-782-9400
Fax: 518-782-9530

North Carolina Nurses Association
www.ncnurses.org
103 Enterprise St.
PO Box 12025
Raleigh, NC 27605-2025
919-821-4250
Fax: 919-829-5807

North Dakota Nurses Association
www.ndna.org
549 Airport Rd.
Bismarck, ND 58504-6107
701-223-1385

Ohio Nurses Association
www.ohnurses.org
4000 East Main St.
Columbus, OH 43213-2983
614-237-5414
Fax: 614-237-6074

Oklahoma Nurses Association
www.oknurses.com
6414 North Santa Fe, Suite A
Oklahoma City, OK 73116
405-840-3476
Fax: 405-840-3013

Oregon Nurses Association
www.oregonrn.org
9600 SW Oak, Suite 550
Portland, OR 97223-6599
503-293-0011
Fax: 503-293-0013

Pennsylvania Nurses Association
www.psna.org
PO Box 68525
Harrisburg, PA 17106-8525
717-657-1222
Fax: 717-657-3796

Rhode Island State Nurses Association
www.risnarn.org
550 S. Water St.–Corliss Landing
Providence, RI 02903-4344
401-421-9703
Fax: 401-421-6793

South Carolina Nurses Association
www.scnurses.org
1821 Gadsden Street
Columbia, SC 29201
803-252-4781
Fax: 803-779-3870

South Dakota Nurses Association
www.nursingworld.org/snas/sd/index
818 East 41st St.
Sioux Falls, SD 57105
605-338-1401
Fax: 605-338-0516

Tennessee Nurses Association
www.tnaonline.org
545 Mainstream Dr., Suite 405
Nashville, TN 37228-1296
615-254-0350
Fax: 615-254-0303

Texas Nurses Association
www.texasnurses.org
7600 Burnet Rd.
Suite 440
Austin, TX 78757-1292
512-452-0645
Fax: 512-452-0648

Utah Nurses Association
www.utahnurses.org
3761 S. 700 East, #201
Salt Lake City, UT 84106
801-293-8351
Fax: 801-293-8458

Vermont State Nurses Association
www.nesna.org/html/vtnurses/vt.htm
One Main St #26, Fifth Floor Champlain Mill
1 Main Street
Winooski, VT 05401-2230
802-655-7123
Fax: 802-655-7187

Virgin Islands State Nurses Association
PO Box 583
Christiansted, St. Croix
U.S. Virgin Islands 00821-0583
809-773-1261

Virginia Nurses Association
www.virginianurses.com
7113 Three Chopt Rd., Suite 204
Richmond, VA 23226
804-282-1808
Fax: 804-282-4916

Washington State Nurses Association
www.wsna.org
575 Andover Park West, #101
Seattle, WA 98188
206-575-7979
Fax: 206-575-1908

West Virginia Nurses Association
www.wvnurses.org
POBox 1946
Charleston, WV 25327
304-342-1169
Fax: 304-342-6973

Wisconsin Nurses Association
www.wisconsinnurses.com
6117 Monona Dr.
Madison, WI 53716
608-221-0383
Fax: 608-221-2788

Wyoming Nurses Association
Majestic Building
Room 305
1603 Capitol Ave.
Cheyenne, WY 82001
307-635-3955
Fax: 307-635-2173

APPENDIX D: CANADIAN NURSING ASSOCIATIONS

Aboriginal Nurses Association of Canada
www.anac.on.ca
ODAWA Native Friendship Centre
12 Stirling Ave, 3rd Floor
Ottawa, ON K1Y1P8
1-613-724-4677
Fax: 1-613-724-4718

Alberta Association of Registered Nurses
www.nurses.ab.ca
11620 168 St
Edmonton, AL T5M 4A6
780-451-0043
Fax: 780-452-3276

Association of Registered Nurses in Newfoundland
www.arnn.nf.ca
55 Millitary Rd., PO Box 6116
St. John's, Newfoundland AIC5X8
709-753-6040
Fax: 709-753-4940

Canadian Association of Critical Care Nurses
www.caccn.ca
PO Box 25322
London, ON N6C 6B1
519-652-1989
Fax: 519-652-5545

Canadian Association of University Schools of Nursing
http://www.causn.org/new/causn/causn.htm
Suite 325
Ottawa, ON K1R 1B1
613-235-3150
Fax: 613-563-7739

Canadian Intravenous Nurses Association
http://web.idirect.com/~csotcina/cina.html
18 Wynford Dr.
Suite 516
North York, ONT, Canada M3C 3S2
416-445-4516
Fax: 416-445-4513

Canadian Nurses Association
http://www.cna-nurses.ca/default.htm
50 Driveway
Ottawa, ONK2P 1E2
613-237-2133
Fax: 613-237-3520

Canadian Nurses Foundation
http://www.cna-nurses.ca/cnf/
50 Driveway
Ottawa ONK2P 1E2
613-237-2133
Fax: 613-237-3520

The Canadian Nursing Students' Association
http://www.cnsa.ca/
325-350 Albert St.
Ottawa, ONK1R 1B1
613-563-1236
Fax: 613-563-7739

National Federation of Nurses' Unions
2841 prom Riverside Dr.
Ottawa ON K1V 8X7
613-526-4661
Fax: 613-526-1023

Registered Nurses Association of British Columbia
http://www.rnabc.bc.ca/
2855 Arbutus St.
Vancouver, BCV6J 3Y8
604-736-7331
Fax: 604-738-2272

Index

A

AANA. *See* American Association of Nurse Anesthetists (AANA).

ABC approach to time management, 527

Academic programs for nursing informatics, 308

Access
  to electronic health data, 187-188
  to health care, 117-118, 236

Accountability, 278
  challenge of, 215

Accreditation Council of Development Disabilities, 460

Accuracy in written communication, 399

Acland, Henry Wentworth, 98

ACNM. *See* American College of Nurse-Midwives (ASCNM).

ACS. *See* American Cancer Society (ACS).

Activity myth of time management, 520-521

Acupuncture, 336

Acute care, 139
  in continuum of care, 139
  nursing care delivery models for, 451

Acure care facilities,
  nurse-patient ratio in
    legislation affecting, 156
  registered nurses employed in, 548

Ad hominem abusive, 391

Adaptation model, 61, 62f

Adequacy of Nurse Staffing in Hospitals and Nursing Homes, 277

Administrators, strategies promoting research, 489-490

Adolescents, developing moral values, 205

Advanced nurse practitioners (ANPs), 555-559
  development of, 21
  number of, 548

Advanced practive nursing
  certification of, 107
  definition of, 100

Advocacy, patient, 280-283

Advocates, nurses as, 543

Aetna US. Health Care Plan, enrollment of, 143

AFCE. *See* Aid to Families with Dependent Children (AFDC).

AFL-CIO. *See* American Federation of Labor-Congress of Industrial Organization (AFL-CIO).

African-American nurses during Civil War, 12

African-Americans
  biological variation in, 251
  communication with, 251-252
  health education of, 253
  health indicators of, 240
  poverty rates of, 241
  recruitment of 244
  syphilis research in, 495
  time-orientation among, 254t
  view of nature, 250

Against Medical Advice (AMA) form, 192

Agency for Health Care Research and Quality (AHRQ)
  funding research, 480-481
    website for, 480
  practice guidelines of, 450
  website for, 327

Aggressive communication, 406

Aging population, 127
  growth of, 240

Aging workforce and retention, 271

AHRQ. *See* Agency for Health Care Research and Quality (AHRQ).

Aid to Families with Dependent Children (AFDC), 124

AIDS epidemic, 22

Air Surface Transport Nurses Association, 554

Airline industry, occupational health nurses in, 553

Alcott, Louisa May, 12

Alexander technique, 344b

Algorithms, 466, 467f

All one team for quality management, 458-459

Almshouses, 9

Altair 8800, 319

Alternative healing, 332-350
  categories of, 335
  overview of, 336-346
  popularity of, 334
  principles underlying, 334-335
  terminology of, 333
  use of, 333-334
  websites for, 338b-339b

Alto, 319

AMA. *See* American Medical Association (AMA).

Ambulatory care facilities, registered nurses employed in, 548

Ambulatory care services
  nursing care delivery models for, 451
  shift towards, 137

Ambulatory care surgery, development of, 20-21

American Accreditation Healthcare Commission/Utilization Review Accreditation Commission, 147-148

American Association of Managed Care Nurses, 126

American Association of Nurse Anesthetists (AANA), 557

American Board of Nursing Specialties, organization of, 106-107

American Cancer Society (ACS), website for, 327

American College of Nurse-Midwives (ACNM), 558

American Federation of Labor-Congress of Industrial Organization (AFL-CIO), 293-294

American Medical Association (AMA), union activities of, 300-301

American Medical Informatics Association (AMIA), 311

American Nurses Association (ANA)
  affirmative action resolution of, 19-20
  and collective bargaining, 303-304
  and policy making, 235
  clinical nursing practice standards of, 419
  Code of Ethics, 200b
  funding research studies, 481
  informatics workgroups of, 311
  licensure by, 98
  model nursing practice acts, 98-99
  Nursing's Agenda for Health Care Reform, 125
  precursor off, 14
  professional practice advocacy definition of, 265
  Scope and Standards of Forensic Nursing Practice, 554

American Nurses Credentialing Center (ANCC), 271, 308, 311
  and case manager certification, 446-448
  formation of, 106
  programs of, 107b

American Nurses Foundation
  and minority recruiting, *247*
  funding research studies, 481